# The Ophthalmic Office Procedures Handbook

# The Ophthalmic Office Procedures Handbook

**Leonid Skorin, Jr, DO, OD, MS, FAAO, FAOCO**

Consultant, Department of Surgery
Community Division of Ophthalmology
Mayo Clinic Health System in Albert Lea and Austin
Albert Lea, Minnesota
Assistant Professor of Ophthalmology
Mayo Clinic College of Medicine and Science
Rochester, Minnesota

**Selina R. McGee, OD, FAAO**

CEO and Visionary Founder
BeSpoke Vision
Edmond, Oklahoma
Adjunct Faculty
Northeastern State University Oklahoma College of Optometry
Tahlequah, Oklahoma

**Karl Stonecipher, MD**

Clinical Professor of Ophthalmology
University of North Carolina
Chapel Hill, North Carolina
Clinical Adjunct Professor of Ophthalmology
Tulane University
New Orleans, Louisiana
Medical Director, Laser Defined Vision
Physicians Protocol
Physicians Protocol Cosmetics
Greensboro, North Carolina

**Nate Lighthizer, OD, FAAO**

Professor of Optometry
Associate Dean
Director of Continuing Education
Chief of Specialty Care Clinics
Northeastern State University Oklahoma College of Optometry
Tahlequah, Oklahoma

**Richard E. Castillo, OD, DO, FASOS**

Senior Director of Clinical Examination Development and Administration
National Board of Examiners in Optometry
Charlotte, North Carolina
Co-Chair
Contemporary Practice Task Force
American Optometric Association
St. Louis, Missouri
President
American Society of Optometric Surgeons
Tahlequah, Oklahoma

Wolters Kluwer

Philadelphia • Baltimore • New York • London
Buenos Aires • Hong Kong • Sydney • Tokyo

*Acquisitions Editor:* Chris Teja
*Product Development Editor:* Eric McDermott
*Editorial Assistant:* Vinodhini Varadharajalu
*Marketing Manager:* Kirsten Watrud
*Senior Production Project Manager:* Alicia Jackson
*Manager, Graphic Arts & Design:* Stephen Druding
*Manufacturing Coordinator:* Lisa Bowling
*Prepress Vendor:* S4Carlisle Publishing Services



9 8 7 6 5 4 3 2 1

Printed in Mexico

---

**Library of Congress Cataloging-in-Publication Data**

ISBN-13: 978-1-975222-04-8
ISBN-10: 1-975222-04-0

Cataloging in Publication data available on request from publisher.

---



QUADM1123

*This book is dedicated to our trainers and trainees. Without them, this book would not exist.*

*It is also dedicated to our families. Thank you very much for your support throughout the years.*

# CONTRIBUTORS


**Audrey E. Ahuero, MD, FACS**
Ophthalmic Plastic and Reconstructive Surgeon
Ophthalmic Plastic Surgeons of Texas
Houston, Texas

**John Berdahl, MD**
Ophthalmologist
Vance Thompson Vision
Sioux Falls, South Dakota

**Matthew Bills, OD**
Optometrist
Barnet Dulaney Perkins Eye Center
Flagstaff, AZ

**Richard E. Castillo, OD, DO, FASOS**
Senior Director of Clinical Examination Development and Administration
National Board of Examiners in Optometry
Charlotte, North Carolina
Co-Chair
Contemporary Practice Task Force
American Optometric Association
St. Louis, Missouri
President
American Society of Optometric Surgeons
Tahlequah, Oklahoma

**Bibin Cherian, OD**
Optometrist
BeSpoke Vision
Edmond, Oklahoma

**Griffin Christenson, OD**
Optometrist
Christenson Vision Care
Hudson, Wisconsin

**Thai Do, MD**
Clinical Assistant Professor
Ophthalmology
Dean McGee Eye Institute
Oklahoma City, Oklahoma

**Jason Ellen, OD**
President/Cofounder
Oklahoma Medical Eye Group
Tulsa, Oklahoma

**Michael D. Greenwood, MD**
Clinical Associate Professor of Surgery
University of North Dakota
Grand Forks, North Dakota
Ophthalmologist
Vance Thompson Vision
West Fargo, North Dakota

**Aaishwariya A. Gulani, MD**
Ophthalmology Resident
Department of Ophthalmology
University of Tennessee Memphis
Memphis, Tennessee

**Arun C. Gulani, MD, MS**
Founding Director and Chief Surgeon
Gulani Vision Institute
Jacksonville, Florida

**Nicole Harris, OD**
Comprehensive Optometrist
Associated Eye Care
Stillwater, Minnesota

**Jessica Haynes, OD**
Consultative Optometrist
Charles Retina Institute
Germantown, Tennessee

**Edward H. Jaccoma, MD**
Director
Dry Eye and Aesthetic Services
Excellent Vision
Stoneham, Massachusetts and Portsmouth, New Hampshire
Clinical Associate Professor of Surgery
University of New England College of Osteopathic Medicine
Biddeford, Maine

**Brianna Johnson, OD**
Associate Optometrist
Lifetime Vision Source
Jamestown, North Dakota

**Andrew W. Krein, OD**
Optometrist
Devon Eye Clinic
Devon, Alberta, Canada

**Jacob Lang, OD, FAAO**
Medical Director, Dry Eye Services
Associated Eye Care
Stillwater, Minnesota

**Sophia Leung, OD, FAAO, Dipl ABO, Dipl Ant Seg**
Principal Optometrist
Seema Eye Care Centre
Calgary, Alberta, Canada

**Nate Lighthizer, OD, FAAO**
Professor of Optometry
Associate Dean
Director of Continuing Education
Chief of Specialty Care Clinics
Northeastern State University Oklahoma College of Optometry
Tahlequah, Oklahoma

**Bryan E. Lusk, MD**
Cornea and Cataract Surgeon
Lusk Eye Specialists
Shreveport, Louisiana

**Carolyn Majcher, OD, FAAO, FORS**
Residency Program Director
Associate Professor
Northeastern State University Oklahoma College of Optometry
Tahlequah, Oklahoma

**Steven L. Maskin, MD**
Director
Dry Eye and Cornea Treatment Center
Tampa, Florida

**Vlad M. Matei, MD**
Vitreoretinal Surgeon
Rocky Mountain Retina Associates
Colorado Retina Associates
Denver, Colorado

**Selina R. McGee, OD, FAAO**
CEO and Visionary Founder
BeSpoke Vision
Edmond, Oklahoma
Adjunct Faculty
Northeastern State University Oklahoma College of Optometry
Tahlequah, Oklahoma

**Jeff M. Miller, OD**
Professor of Optometry
Northeastern State University Oklahoma College of Optometry
Tahlequah, Oklahoma

**Kristin Mohr, OD**
Ocular Disease Optometrist
Cataract, Cornea, Glaucoma, and Refractive Surgery Specialist
Vance Thompson Vision
Sioux Falls, South Dakota

**Rachna Murthy, BSc (Hons), MBBS, FRCOphth**
Oculofacial Plastic Surgeon
FaceRestoration
London, United Kingdom

**Komal Patel, OD, FAAO**
Assistant Professor of Optometry
Northeastern State University Oklahoma College of Optometry
Tahlequah, Oklahoma

**Douglas K. Penisten, OD, PHD**
Dean
Professor of Optometry
Northeastern State University Oklahoma College of Optometry
Tahlequah, Oklahoma

**Karina Richani, MD**
Ophthalmic Plastic and Reconstructive Surgeon
Ophthalmic Plastic Surgeons of Texas
Houston, Texas

**Nicholas C. Risbrudt, OD**
Optometrist
Vance Thompson Vision
West Fargo, North Dakota

**Jonathan Roos, BA (Hons), MB BChir, MA (Cantab), PhD (Cantab), FRCOphth, FEBO**
Oculofacial Plastic Surgeon
FaceRestoration
London, United Kingdom

**Brandon Runyon, OD, FAAO**
Optometrist
Virginia Eye Consultants
Norfolk, Virginia

**Justin Schweitzer, OD, FAAO**
Director, Optometric Externship Programs
Adjunct Professor
Illinois College of Optometry
Chicago, Illinois
Vance Thompson Vision
Sioux Falls, South Dakota

**Joseph L. Shetler, OD**
Associate Professor
Chief NSUOCO Clinics
Northeastern State University Oklahoma College of Optometry
Tahlequah, Oklahoma

**Scott C. Sigler, MD**
Oculoplastics Specialist
Member
American Society of Ophthalmic Plastic and Reconstructive Surgeons
Edmond Eye Associates
Edmond, Oklahoma

**Inder Paul Singh, MD**
President
The Eye Centers of Racine and Kenosha
Racine, WI

**Leonid Skorin, Jr, DO, OD, MS, FAAO, FAOCO**
Consultant, Department of Surgery
Community Division of Ophthalmology
Mayo Clinic Health System in Albert Lea and Austin
Albert Lea, Minnesota
Assistant Professor of Ophthalmology
Mayo Clinic College of Medicine and Science
Rochester, Minnesota

**Seth J. Stofferahn, OD**
Optometrist
Vance Thompson Vision
West Fargo, North Dakota

**Karl Stonecipher, MD**
Clinical Professor of Ophthalmology
University of North Carolina
Chapel Hill, North Carolina
Clinical Adjunct Professor of Ophthalmology
Tulane University
New Orleans, Louisiana
Medical Director, Laser Defined Vision
Physicians Protocol
Physicians Protocol Cosmetics
Greensboro, North Carolina

**Cole Sutherland, OD**
Assistant Professor of Optometry
Northeastern State University Oklahoma College of Optometry
Tahlequah, Oklahoma

**Zurriat Syed, MS**
Osteopathic Medical Student
DeBusk College of Osteopathic Medicine
Lincoln Memorial University
Knoxville, Tennessee

**Pamela Theriot, OD, FAAO**
Clinical Director
Dry Eye Relief Centre
Lusk Eye Specialists
Shreveport, Louisiana

**Claire Toland, MS**
Education and Research Coordinator
Dry Eye and Cornea Treatment Center
Tampa, Florida

**Natalia A. Warren, MBA, MHA**
Chair and Cofounder
Not A Dry Eye Foundation
Daytona Beach, Florida

**Neal Whittle, OD**
Associate Professor
Northeastern State University Oklahoma College of Optometry
Tahlequah, Oklahoma

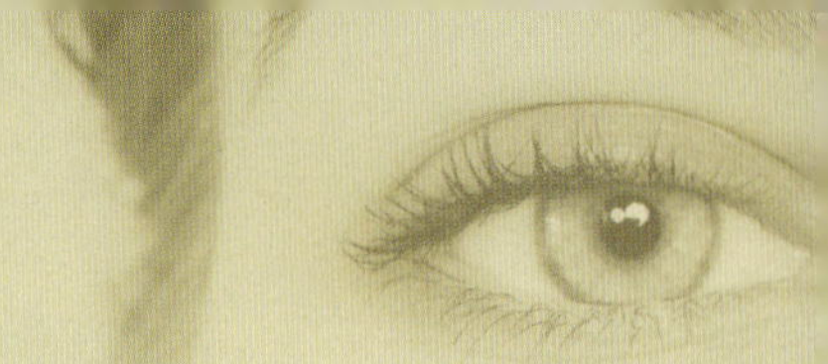

# ACKNOWLEDGMENTS

A special acknowledgment and thank you to all of the contributors for this book. Your knowledge, expertise, and experience are truly appreciated.

We would also like to thank the staff at Wolters Kluwer, especially Eric McDermott and Chris Teja, for their support and work on this project.

# PREFACE

The eye is the second most complex organ in the body. There are a myriad of procedures available to the eye care professional today. Many of these ophthalmic procedures can be performed in an office setting. Keen knowledge and skill are required to fully address patients' needs. Utilizing this handbook can complement and elevate all eye care providers, no matter their current skill level.

The core principles of all surgery are structure and function. Structure is the anatomy. Every clinician who performs any simple procedure or intricate surgery must have an intimate knowledge of the structure they plan to manipulate. Function involves the structure's physiology. Not only does one need to know the structure's actions, but one needs to appreciate the downstream effects of any potential dysfunction that manipulation of the structure may cause. To be a truly adept, efficient, and overall competent surgeon, one needs to connect this knowledge of anatomy and physiology of any body part one wants to command in the operative arena. Most surgeons who consistently achieve this higher stratum of proficiency routinely admit to being able to visualize the surgical procedure before they even step into the operative suite. Since human beings are not widgets, these same surgeons are readily cognizant of both the human anatomic differences and the various physiologic exceptions. It is quite simple to encounter a surgical obstacle or, worse yet, a complication during any procedure one performs. This may occur even in those cases considered to be routine. It brings all the skill that the surgeon possesses to mitigate the untoward event and, if possible, rectify any complication to minimize its overall effect.

How does one attain and build these procedural and surgical skills? Traditionally, formal training programs and continuing education skills-transfer lectures and hands-on workshops have been utilized. We propose an additional mode to use, at your convenience, which covers office-based surgical procedures available in written, pictorial, and video presentations. It will be especially beneficial to those in training yet equally valuable to the seasoned practitioner. We have compiled such a resource for you: *The Ophthalmic Office Procedures Handbook.*

*The Ophthalmic Office Procedures Handbook* has been devised to equip the reader with detailed and relevant surgical information constructed in a consistent and easy-to-use format. Most of the chapters contain specific key indications, contraindications, preoperative considerations, and procedural points. Postoperative considerations are also thoroughly addressed. This part of the chapter should be of considerable value to those who are comanaging surgical patients. One of the most unique aspects of this surgical procedural handbook is its contributors. All have significant procedural and surgical experience in either performing the surgery or comanaging postoperative patients. This handbook's contributors readily share their expertise with you, the reader. This is accomplished by having *The Ophthalmic Office Procedures Handbook* as both a soft cover text and eBook. The eBook contains all the material found in the soft cover text with an extensive collection of procedural and surgical videos. As a bonus, we have included several chapters covering the fundamentals of performing any procedure or surgery. These include periorbital and ocular anatomy, essential instrumentation, anesthesia requirements, and surgical pathology.

In addition, *The Ophthalmic Office Procedures Handbook* is a welcome complementary companion text to *The Ophthalmic Laser Handbook* (ISBN: 978-19-75170-17-2) and its Spanish-language edition (ISBN: 978-84-18892-20-2). These handbooks cover the complete and essential surgical and laser spectrum that every eye care practitioner needs to know.

Leonid Skorin, Jr
Nate Lighthizer
Selina R. McGee
Richard E. Castillo
Karl Stonecipher

# CONTENTS

SECTION 1

# History and Medicolegal Matters

# 1 History of Ophthalmic Office-Based Procedures

**Douglas K. Penisten**

In the past century, health care practitioners have witnessed and experienced revolutionary changes in how they diagnose and treat patients. These changes have manifested in various ways including new diagnoses, new treatment modalities, technological advances in instrumentation, and new pharmacologic creations. Propelling these changes forward has been the product of basic and applied research in all facets of science: physics, biochemistry, materials science, pathophysiology, pharmacology, and clinical trials. Where patients receive their treatment has also been changing. This brief essay will highlight the changes in ophthalmic office-based procedures in recent decades.

An eye examination includes evaluating visual abilities including the ocular refractive status and examining the health of the eyes and adnexa. These procedures have always been conducted in the doctor's office or clinic setting. In contrast, the treatment of ocular conditions runs the full spectrum from simple to highly complicated, and many of the more advanced procedures have historically been conducted in hospital operating rooms. Much has changed in the past 40 years. Many of the more invasive ophthalmic procedures have shifted and are now commonly performed in the practitioner's office.

This shift in ophthalmic care to office-based procedures has been possible due to advances in technology and new treatment modalities. Examples include ophthalmic lasers, specialized surgical instrumentation, imaging devices, and radiofrequency technology. With many ophthalmic procedures shifting from inpatient hospital settings to the practitioner's office, much of ophthalmic care has gone from tertiary care settings into primary care settings.

There have been numerous benefits of performing more ophthalmic office-based procedures.[1] These include patient convenience and cost reductions by the elimination of operating room time.[2] Patients have responded favorably to having ophthalmic office-based procedures because they feel less anxiety in a familiar setting where they can interact with office personnel they know.[3] Patients' access to care has increased due to the simplicity of a single site for delivering eye care.

Decreasing the cost of health care, increasing access to care, and providing patient preference, the shift to office-based ophthalmic procedures has been found to be a safe and efficacious means of delivering quality eye care.[3,4] The sum total is a significant positive for improved public health care.

In the United States, the shift from inpatient hospital surgery to ambulatory surgery in general began over 50 years ago and has taken decades to evolve. There have been many obstacles to this transition, including the government, hospital administrators, and insurance companies.[5] In eye care, the shift to ambulatory cataract surgery in the United States began in the mid-1980s.[2] In 1980, the Omnibus Reconciliation Act authorized reimbursement for outpatient surgery.[6] The move from inpatient hospital ophthalmic surgery to ambulatory surgical centers (ASCs) and, now, to office-based surgical suites is gradually growing in the United States. Some ophthalmologic practices are now performing retinal surgeries in their office surgical suites.[3] A large study conducted by Kaiser has shown that cataract surgery can be successfully performed in an in-office surgical suite.[7] Although office-based cataract surgery in the United States is not currently the standard, a robust analysis of the processes is presently underway.[8]

This volume is a snapshot of many of the ophthalmic office-based procedures currently being performed by eye doctors in the United States. With the continuing advances in technology, clinical trials, and the inevitable resultant new treatment modalities, the list of ophthalmic office-based procedures will increase in the future. This book stands as a testament to the benefits for public health when eye care clinicians move their work to a more patient-friendly environment.

## REFERENCES

1. Stephenson M. Office-based surgery: the pros and cons. *Rev Ophthalmol.* Published December 10, 2021. Accessed March 19, 2023. https://www.reviewofophthalmology.com/article/officebased-surgery-the-pros-and-cons
2. Durrie DS, McCabe C, Whitman J. Office-based surgery vs. ASC surgery. *Ophthalmol Manage.* 2020; 24(11):34,36,38,40,42,44.
3. Kent C. Office-based surgery: tales from the front. *Rev Ophthalmol.* Published October 10, 2022. Accessed March 19, 2023. https://www.reviewofophthalmology.com/article/officebased-surgery-tales-from-the-front
4. Aquavella JV. The ambulatory ophthalmic surgery unit: concepts, regulation, and guidelines. *Surv Ophthalmol.* 1985:29(5):366-370.
5. Hedley-Whyte J, Milamed DR. The evolution of sites of surgery. *Ulster Med J.* 2006;75(1):46-53.
6. Aquavella JV. Ambulatory surgery in the 1990's. *J Ambul Care Manage.* 1990;13(1):21-24.
7. Ianchulev T, Litoff D, Ellinger D, et al. Office-based cataract surgery: population health outcomes study of more than 21,000 cases in the United States. *Ophthalmology.* 2016;123(4):723-728.
8. Hillman L. The pros and cons of office-based cataract surgery. *ASCRS Eyeworld.* Published March 2021. Accessed March 23, 2023. https://www.eyeworld.org/2021/office-based-cataract-surgery/

# 2 Procedures, Liability, and the Doctrine of Informed Consent

**Richard E. Castillo**

The issue of liability over patient injury at the hands of the health care practitioner predates the profession's formal establishment. Health care practitioners have been dealing with the risk of litigation over the unintended or unexpected consequences of their actions or lack thereof for centuries. As early as the year 1164, in the case of *Everad v. Hopkins*, a servant and his master collected damages against a physician for the practice of "unwholesome medicine." The 1374 case, *Stratton v. Swanlond*, is frequently cited as the "fourteenth-century ancestor" of modern medical malpractice law. Then, Chief Justice John Cavendish presided over the case, in which one Agnes of Stratton sued surgeon John Swanlond for breach of contract after he failed to treat and cure her severely mangled hand.[1,2]

Moving ahead into the 21st century, the number of both medical and optometric malpractice cases has seen a dramatic increase.[2-4] Several arguments have been suggested to account for this:

1. The nature of both medical and optometric practice has changed and continues to evolve. Health care today is more dependent than at any time in the past on continuously evolving technology for complicated drug therapies, surgery, and even diagnostics to address more and more illnesses with a broader range of therapies. As more invasive treatments are devised, more patients are injured as a consequence.
2. Malpractice litigation itself has become simpler to initiate and more accessible to the average citizen.
3. Juries today are less sympathetic toward physicians, and more physicians are willing to testify against other physicians in courtrooms.
4. Malpractice law itself continues to evolve, with new causes of action and new concepts of damages being introduced, such as mental distress and manufacturer or product liability.

## THE DOCTRINE OF INFORMED CONSENT

The doctrine of informed consent evolved out of recognition and respect for the individual's inherent right to autonomy with regard to all aspects of their being, establishing that the individual has a right to be free from nonconsensual interference with their person or to be forced to act knowingly or unknowingly in a manner against their will.[5] In the present day, the doctrine of informed consent, therefore, guides medical decision-making by establishing limits to the doctor–patient relationship. Therefore, the patient's informed consent to treatment is essential to the practitioner for reducing liability risk insofar as claims of battery or negligent nondisclosure are concerned. A properly executed informed consent serves to underscore the patient's inherent right to autonomy in medical or optometric decision-making, which is the underlying principle in all consent cases, be they medical negligence (specifically negligent nondisclosure) or battery, the two circumstances upon which the majority of medical liability actions are based.[1,5,6]

## MEDICAL BATTERY

*Battery, at common law, is defined as an intentional unpermitted act causing harmful or offensive contact with the "person" of another.*[3]

The legal doctrine of battery protects a patient's physical integrity and dignity from harmful contacts or unwanted physical contacts. Note that physical injury is not required for a battery to have occurred. The doctrine only requires that the patient show they were not informed of the very nature of the touching or contact, as might occur, for example, during a laser or surgical procedure. If a practitioner operates on a structure other than that which they and the patient discussed, a battery has occurred. If the patient is not made aware that the practitioner will perform a specific procedure and has not consented, a claim for battery may be brought forth.

Health care practitioners have legal liability exposure to claims for battery, negligent nondisclosure, and the failure to obtain informed consent. Battery is an intentional tort that does not require proof of negligence or of the intent to harm. Generally, a person commits battery by intentionally touching another individual without consent. The individual may be permitted to recover monetary damages absent bodily injury, although the damages awarded in such circumstances may be nominal. Battery is also a crime punishable by fines and imprisonment, although charges of criminal battery are usually only attached if there has been a significant injury to the recipient of the offense.[4]

## CONSENT: EXPRESS OR IMPLIED

In eye care practice, consent may be expressed (permission that is explicitly given, either verbally or in writing) or implied (an assumption of permission that is inferred from actions) by the patient seeking treatment or their legal guardian. In cases of an emergency, mainly when the patient is unable or incapable of giving express consent, consent may be implied by law. Whether consent is given or implied, some boundaries limit the practitioner's actions. A practitioner exposes themselves to liability for battery if the treatment furnished exceeds the limits of the consent either given or implied.[4]

## ELEMENTS OF PROPER DISCLOSURE

Although a properly executed informed consent may be enough for the practitioner to defend a battery claim successfully, several elements must be addressed to deliver a proper and complete disclosure.[1,7,8] These elements include:

- Diagnosis
- Nature and purpose of treatment

- Risks and outcomes
- Disclosure of skill or status of risks
- Alternatives to treatment
- Prognosis if treatment is delayed
- Prognosis with treatment
- Disclosure of conflicts of interest

With regard to a discussion of the anticipated benefits and risks of a procedure, if the consent, or the patient's refusal, was not preceded by disclosure of the known material benefits, risks, and alternatives, the practitioner may be open to liability, even if the procedure itself was performed competently without technical error, or if the procedure was declined in the case of patient refusal.[1,9]

## PATIENT REFUSAL

In the case of patient refusal, for there to be liability for lack of informed consent, the patient generally must show that the physician was negligent, that there was an injury with sustained damages, and that the negligent nondisclosure was a proximate cause of the injury and damages. A claim brought forth for lack of informed consent is based on professional negligence (medical malpractice). Unlike a claim of battery, which requires proof of an intentional touch without consent, a negligent nondisclosure claim requires proof that the health care practitioner failed to furnish care in conformity with the applicable standard of care, alongside proof of injury, damages, and causation. The determination of whether the standard of care has been met or breached is generally established through the testimony of expert witnesses.[1,2]

## MEASURING THE STANDARD OF CARE: THE REASONABLE PHYSICIAN VERSUS THE REASONABLE PERSON STANDARD

The standard of care is generally measured and evaluated in either one of two ways when a charge of negligent nondisclosure or lack of informed consent is made. The first way is from the physician's perspective, known as the reasonable physician standard. Under the reasonable physician standard, current information must be disclosed to the patient regarding accepted standards of practice among physicians with similar training and experience in the community or nationally for care furnished by a subspecialist. This reasonable physician standard is followed by slightly more than one-half of the jurisdictions in the United States. The alternate perspective, followed by slightly less than one-half of the jurisdictions in the United States, is from the patient's perspective, known as the reasonable person standard. Under the reasonable person standard, the patient must be informed of the risks and alternatives that a reasonable person in their position would consider significant and material in deciding whether to undergo the proposed treatment or procedure.[1,10]

Both the reasonable physician standard and the reasonable person standard are evaluated and measured in the objective sense, rather than by the opposing parties' subjective intent to a malpractice suit. Risks that are rare or remote, not deemed severe, or which the average patient would typically know, are generally not considered to be material within the context of the charges alleged.[3]

## THE INCOMPETENT PATIENT

Patients not competent to make decisions about their health may not give or withhold consent. Cognitive impairment and decision-making capacity should be documented in the medical record. Likewise, minors may not consent to medical treatment, although some states have enacted exceptions by statute. For these individuals, consent must be obtained from a legal guardian or parent. In emergencies, it is usually permissible to perform procedures or furnish treatment necessary to save the patient's life or a vital organ (such as the eye) without express consent when it cannot be obtained in a timely fashion. In this case, like the ubiquitous "Good Samaritan laws," the legal theory of emergency implied consent applies.[7,9]

## WITHHOLDING INFORMATION

In atypical cases where the information to be disclosed might have a detrimental effect on the patient's physical or psychological well-being (i.e., a depressed or suicidal patient), some jurisdictions may excuse obtaining informed consent. The scope of this so-called therapeutic privilege varies from state to state, and the practitioner should use great caution and consult with their liability carrier's risk management adviser or legal counsel before exercising this option.[2,3,6]

In these exceptional cases, the practitioner needs to consider the ethical issues raised by postponing the disclosure of information to the patient. Ethically, it may be appropriate in these circumstances to postpone or delay the disclosure of certain information if early communication could exacerbate the patient's mental status or pose a significant threat to their well-being.[6] However, withholding medical information from patients is generally not an acceptable practice or ethically permissible. Although all information need not be communicated to the at-risk patient immediately or all at once, the practitioner should carefully assess the amount of information a patient can and should receive at any given time.[6]

## THE LIMITS OF LICENSURE AND SCOPE OF PRACTICE

Health care practitioners should be aware of the limits of their licensure and scope of practice (statutes and licensing board regulations) as well as the laws in their respective states. Practitioners often have many resources available on consent issues, such as national and state medical and optometric associations. Additionally, professional liability carriers will often guide their insured practitioner on consent issues and may have readily available templates or model consent forms for their client's use.

## THE INFORMED CONSENT FORM

In general, an informed consent form identifies the patient, the procedure, the indications, the benefits, and the risks. A generic space on the form can be used to document the physician's disclosures and discussion with the patient and their consent. Some jurisdictions require a witness to sign the consent form. Practitioners in office settings may ask technicians or other office staff to witness. Due to potential conflict of interest issues that may be raised in litigation, the practitioner should consider having a family member or friend of the patient also witness the consent process when possible, in addition to the office staff. Furthermore, there is a requirement of certified translators for patients who do not speak English and a requirement for documents written in the language used by the patient.[3]

In recent years, courts have been criticized for setting standards that do not reflect contemporary medical or optometric practice, interfering with the traditional doctor–patient relationship. Usually, the fault lies with the implementation, not in the actual concept. The concept of informed consent includes the legal concept of consent, but it goes further in that it requires that the patient be a partner in the decision-making process.[3,8,10]

## THE DECISION-MAKING PROCESS

Similar to how laws have evolved to clarify and refine informed consent, there has been a transition toward involving the patient more and more in the decision-making process. Conceptually, there are essentially four descriptive models of decision-making:

1. Conventional medical model: The health care practitioner decides which procedure(s) to perform; the patient's trust and confidence in the doctor replace the need for consent.
2. Conventional informed consent model: The health care practitioner decides which procedure(s) to perform with the patient's express or implied informed consent.
3. Collaboration: The health care practitioner and the patient work together to make a joint decision about the procedure.
4. Patient choice: The patient decides with the health care practitioner's advice.

In today's health care environment, few patients choose the traditional model, and few choose the fourth model. Most patients and health care practitioners alike are more comfortable with either conventional informed consent or collaboration. Health care practitioners should learn how to use both of these two models of decision-making and determine which model to use for a specific patient.[4]

Regardless of the model of decision-making utilized, the practitioner will be held to the standard of informed consent adopted by the state or jurisdiction in which they practice. The health care practitioner must take care to perform all due diligence in assuring that all the necessary disclosures have been made and are adequately documented in the medical record and that a written and signed consent form is utilized at every opportunity.

## VERBAL CONSENT

Except in the case of a life- or vital organ-threatening emergency, there is seldom an exception to the rule that all procedures, whether office or facility based, require a written and signed informed consent. The consent process should include a discussion and disclosure of the material risks and benefits and an opportunity to allow the patient to ask questions and participate in the ultimate decision as to whether they have or reject the procedure or alternative treatment.[7] In some instances (i.e., an illiterate patient), it may be permissible to obtain the patient's verbal consent. Verbal consents should be carefully documented by the health care practitioner in the medical record addressing all the essential points (diagnosis, procedure, material risks, benefits, known complications, and treatment alternatives). Whenever possible, written consent is always advised.[3]

## ADDITIONAL ELEMENTS OF THE INFORMED CONSENT PROCESS

The act of discussing the diagnosis and proposed procedure with the patient (parent or guardian), reviewing the possible complications, and the required aftercare is considered part of the consent process.[8] The consent form also serves as a patient education tool, and a copy (with the patient's signature) should be given to the patient or their caregiver as a reference. Patients should be educated during the consent process that the results of medical and surgical procedures are not guaranteed. Furthermore, the procedure's consent form should include postprocedure instructions and instructions for contacting the practitioner or an on-call associate if complications occur outside of regular office hours.[11]

Many offices, professional societies, and even liability insurance carriers recommend or even provide patient videos discussing the proposed procedure. Standardized recordings ensure that each patient receives consistent and complete information and can consider all the pertinent information. Standardized video instruction also serves as a record for the defense of a lawsuit. However, a video does not replace and should not be substituted for the patient and the practitioner's discussion.[3,11]

## INFORMED CONSENT IS A PROCESS, NOT JUST A FORM

Surgical complications (including those caused by ophthalmic procedures) are the foundation of many malpractice suits. The health care practitioner should not rely exclusively on a signed consent form to defend a malpractice suit. Instead, a better strategy would be to strengthen and highlight the entire process that resulted in the patient's consent. This includes all facets of the patient's participation in that process. Understand that during litigation, a practitioner who brings out a convoluted and highly technical consent form, which was signed by the patient at the last minute, with little opportunity for questions or discussion, is not likely to be viewed favorably from the perspective of a jury.[2,8]

The fact is that no printed form, regardless of signature, may necessarily be viewed as prima facie evidence that the patient's consent was informed. A consent form is only one piece in the totality of the evidence accrued, and in current lawsuits, other pieces of evidence, such as the patient's testimony, will be introduced and considered as well. The consent form itself is not a substitute for a candid discussion with the patient about the procedure and the patient's inclusion in the decision-making process. Neither is a preprinted consent form a substitute for documentation in the medical record of the discussion and opportunity to ask and have questions answered before the patient signs the form. This aspect of the process should be explicitly stated in the patient's chart.[9,10]

It is counterproductive from the standpoint of defending a lawsuit to utilize a consent form that uses language that is too technical and too long to read and interpret during an office visit. Consent forms are often handed to patients during registration by nonprofessional office staff, and many are unable to comprehend the procedure even after the written explanation. The consent form should be meaningful to the patient if it is to be of value to the defendant during litigation. Also, as stated earlier, the practitioner should include a narrative of the discussion between doctor and patient during the decision-making process in the medical record.

The health care practitioner should be careful not to overpromise or oversell a procedure. Furthermore, one should never offer a "guarantee" of what a procedure can do. "Never say never and never say always." Medicine, optometry included, is not a science of precision, like physics, for example, where problems typically have exact solutions and answers are calculated to the *n*th decimal place. The practice of both medicine and optometry is as much an art as a science, and there are simply too many intangibles when it comes to performing procedures on patients to ever offer a guarantee of results.

## CONCLUSION

It is essential to understand that no consent form will protect a health care practitioner from an actual malpractice lawsuit. Competence, experience, and staying current with the ever-evolving science, advances in technology, and the art of clinical care are essential. Recognizing one's professional limits and knowing when to seek advice from a colleague or refer for definitive care is equally essential to avoid litigation.

## REFERENCES


1. Beauchamp TL, Childress JF. *Principles of Biomedical Ethics*. 6th ed. Oxford University Press; 2009.
2. Emanuel EJ. Bioethics in the practice of medicine. In: Goldman L, Schafer AI, eds. *Goldman-Cecil Medicine*. 26th ed. Elsevier; 2020:4-10 e2.
3. Berg JW, Appelbaum P, Lidz C, et al. The legal requirements for disclosure and consent: history and current status. In: Berg JW, Appelbaum PS, Lidz CW, Parker LS, eds. *Informed Consent: Legal Theory and Clinical Practice*. 2nd ed. Oxford University Press; 2001:41-74.
4. U.S. Department of Health and Human Services. Informed consent. Accessed December 5, 2019. www.hhs.gov/ohrp/regulations-and-policy/guidance/informed-consent/index.html
5. Faden RR, Beauchamp TL. *A History and Theory of Informed Consent*. Oxford University Press; 1986.
6. Grisso T, Appelbaum PS. *Assessing Competence to Consent to Treatment: A Guide for Physicians and Other Health Professionals*. Oxford University Press; 1998.
7. Barry MJ. Involving patients in medical decisions: how can physicians do better? *JAMA*. 1999;282:2356-2357.
8. Robinson G, Merav A. Informed consent: recall by patients tested postoperatively. *Ann Thorac Surg*. 1976;22:209-212.
9. Solomon J, Schwegman-Melton K. Structured teaching and patient understanding of informed consent. *Crit Care Nurse*. 1987;7:74-79.
10. Lloyd A, Hayes P, Bell P, Naylor AR. The role of risk and benefit perception in informed consent for surgery. *Med Decis Making*. 2001;21:141-149.
11. Dawes PJ, O'Keefe L, Adcock S. Informed consent: using a structured interview changes patients' attitudes towards informed consent. *J Laryngol Otol*. 1993;107:775-779.


## SUPPLEMENTAL READINGS


1. Brennan K. Malpractice: minimizing your exposure. *Rev Ophthalmol*. Published October 14, 2018. https://www.reviewofophthalmology.com/article/malpractice-minimizing-your-exposure

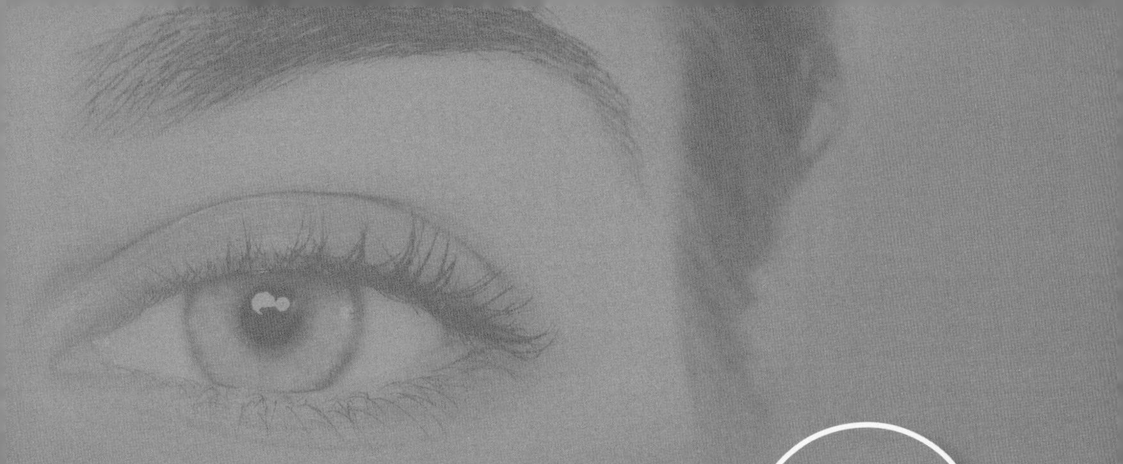

# SECTION 2

# Office Procedures Fundamentals

# 3 Surgical Anatomy of the Eyelids and Periorbita

**Richard E. Castillo**

The eyelids serve several critical physiologic functions. Primarily, they protect the eye. The inner surface of the eyelids, the conjunctiva, contributes to the tear film, and mechanically, the eyelids help distribute the tear film evenly across the eye's surface.[1] During a blink, the edges of the eyelids move tears toward the puncta, where they enter the lacrimal drainage system. The eyelashes also help to move any airborne particles away from the front of the eye, and blinking movements help to protect the cornea from injury and regulate glare. The vertical height of the palpebral fissure is typically 10 to 11 mm in a young adult, 8 to 10 mm in middle age, and 6 to 8 mm or less in old age. The horizontal length of the palpebral fissure remains constant throughout life at 30 to 31 mm[2,3] (Figure 3-1).

In adults, the upper and lower eyelids form an angle of 60° at the canthi (corners of the eye). In the primary position, the upper eyelid sits 1.5 to 2.0 mm below the superior limbus (the border between the cornea and the sclera), with this distance decreasing with age.[1-3] The lower eyelid sits at or slightly above the inferior limbus. The eyelid margin is approximately 2 mm thick. The gray line, also known as the muscle of Riolan, represents

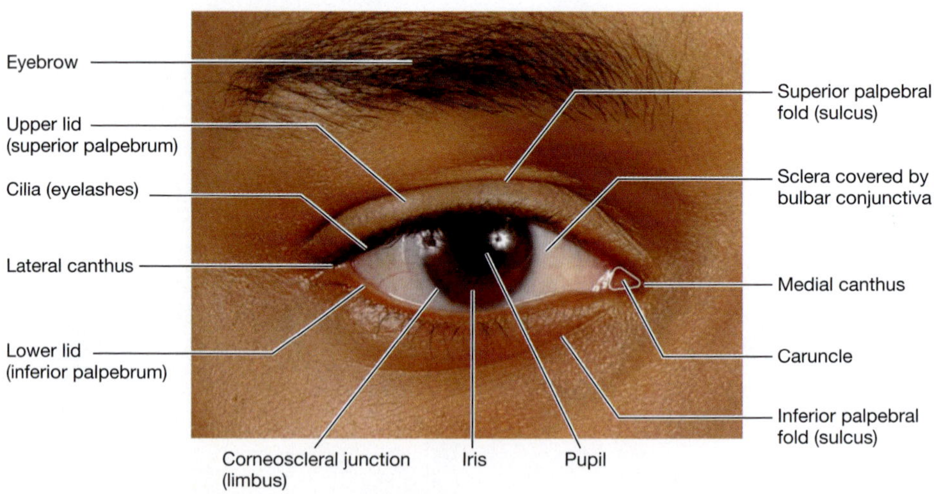


**FIGURE 3-1** Principal anatomical landmarks of the eyelids and visible portion of the eye. (From Freddo TF, Chaum E. *Anatomy of the Eye and Orbit: The Clinical Essentials*. Wolters Kluwer; 2018.)

the superficial extension of the pretarsal orbicularis muscle onto the surface of the eyelid margin.[4] The gray line is an external landmark that separates the eyelid into the anterior and posterior lamellae. Clinically, the anterior lamella of the eyelid consists of the skin and orbicularis muscle. The anterior lamella (anterior to the gray line) of the eyelid margin is covered with keratinized epidermis and contains the eyelashes. The posterior lamella (posterior to the gray line) of the eyelid margin is covered with the nonkeratinized epithelium of the palpebral conjunctiva and contains the orifices of the meibomian glands.[3-5]

The meibomian glands are located vertically within the tarsal plate, with their orifices opening onto the margin of the eyelid posterior to the gray line. The lacrimal puncta are located adjacent to the medial canthus (inner corner of the eye) on all four eyelids. The puncta admit the tears into the lacrimal drainage system.[1-3,6]

## PERIORBITAL SKIN

The integument or skin is the body's outermost covering. The skin protects against external trauma, extremes in temperature, actinic damage, and dehydration. It further serves as the sensory interface with the external environment.[7] The eyelid skin, owing to only a scant dermis and subcutaneous fat, is the thinnest in the body. The epidermis consists of epithelial cells of ectodermal origin. The epidermis of the eyelids, considered the body's thinnest skin, is approximately 0.05 mm thick. The epidermis is avascular, contains no blood vessels, and depends upon the underlying dermis for nourishment.[8] The epidermis of the periorbita and eyelids is composed of four layers consisting of keratinocytes (keratin-producing cells) stratified from the innermost stratum basale to the outermost stratum corneum in progressive stages of differentiation. The keratinocytes undergo mitosis, divide, and push more mature cells upward toward the superficial layers. Keratinocytes produce a protein called keratin, hence the term keratinocytes[8,9] (Figure 3-2).

The histologic layers of the epidermis are from innermost to outermost:

- Stratum basale
- Stratum spinosum
- Stratum granulosum
- Stratum corneum

At the base of the epidermis is the stratum basale consisting of columnar cells arranged in a single row containing large nuclei (Figure 3-2). The basal layer serves as the stem cells for keratinocyte proliferation. The stratum spinosum is the layer immediately above the stratum basale and is composed of polygonal cells that are attached to their neighbors via attachments (spines) visible following histologic preparation.[8] This is an artifact due to the presence of desmosomes between adjacent cells. The next layer, the stratum granulosum, lies on top of the stratum spinosum. The stratum granulosum is 2 to 3 cells thick, and these cells contain keratohyalin granules rich in histidine, a protein called loricrin, and precursors of the protein filaggrin, promoting keratin aggregation.[8,9] Within this layer, the cells undergo apoptosis, lose their nuclei, and become flattened. The outermost layer of the epidermis is the stratum corneum. The stratum corneum is composed of dead, flattened keratinocytes that shed about every 14 days via a process known as desquamation. This layer provides a waterproof barrier and resists minor trauma.[7-9]

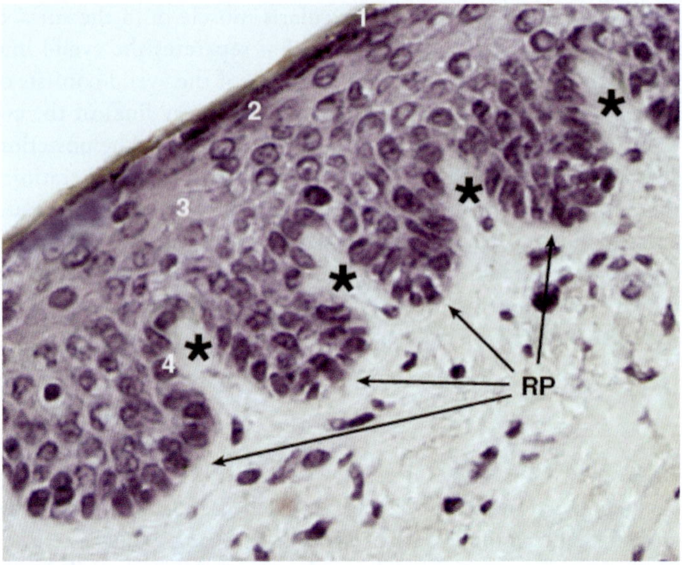


**FIGURE 3-2** Photomicrograph of eyelid skin showing stratum corneum (1), stratum granulosum (2), stratum spinosum (3), and stratum germinativum (4). Rete pegs (RPs) are evident. The underlying dermis is divided into papillary dermis between adjacent rete pegs (*) and reticular dermis below the RP. (From Freddo TF, Chaum E. *Anatomy of the Eye and Orbit: The Clinical Essentials*. Wolters Kluwer; 2018.)

The epidermis also has several specialized types of cells. Melanocytes are nonepithelial cells of neural crest origin found interspersed among the cells of the stratum basale and occasionally the deeper layers of the stratum spinosum. Melanocytes are pale cells that produce dendrites that extend between the keratinocytes of the stratum spinosum and produce melanin stored in granules called melanosomes. These are ingested by the keratinocytes, which accumulate on the apical side of the nucleus to protect it from external ultraviolet (UV) radiation. Langerhans cells are macrophages that migrate into the epidermis, primarily the stratum spinosum. Langerhans cells serve an immune function as antigen-presenting cells.[8,9]

Merkel cells are neuroendocrine cells that also exist within the epidermis, primarily the basal cell layer. Their function is not entirely understood. They are cells of neural crest origin and are attached to keratinocytes by desmosomes. Merkel cells are always associated with nonmyelinated nerve endings. It is thought that they may function as mechanosensory receptors for light touch.[8,9]

Beneath the epidermis is the basement membrane, secreted by the basal cells of the stratum basale. The basal cells are anchored to the basement membrane via hemidesmosomes. Below the basement membrane is the dermis. While the epidermis is ectodermal, the dermis derives from the embryonic mesenchyme. The dermis is anchored to the overlying basement membrane of the epidermis by collagen fibers.[10,11] The basement membrane is irregular, and downward epidermal extensions project into the dermis to form the rete ridges of the epidermis. These are more numerous in areas where the skin is under shearing stress. Between the epidermal rete ridges lie the dermal papillae. Within the dermal papillae lie a rich network of capillaries and lymphatics, which nourish and remove waste products from the overlying avascular epidermis.[10-12]

The dermis of the eyelids and periorbital skin is about 0.3 to 0.5 mm in thickness compared to other body parts, which may be up to 3 mm thick. The dermis includes three types of tissues: collagen, elastic tissue, and reticular fibers.[11] The uppermost papillary dermal layer contains an arrangement of fine collagen fibers. The lower reticular dermis is thicker and contains coarse collagen fibers oriented parallel to the surface. The reticular dermis contains fibroblasts, mast cells, nerve endings, lymphatics, and the epidermal appendages embedded in a ground substance comprised of mucopolysaccharides, chondroitin sulfates, and glycoproteins.[12] The fibroblast is the resident cell of the dermis. These cells are responsible for maintaining the dermis and secrete elastin and a procollagen cleaved by proteolytic enzymes into collagen, which becomes cross-linked. Collagen makes up 70% of the dermis by weight.[11]

The epidermal appendages, comprised of epithelium, lie within the dermis. These include hair follicles and the apocrine sweat glands (Glands of Moll), holocrine glands (sebaceous glands), and eccrine (sweat) glands. Apocrine glands are coiled structures in the reticular dermis that shed the apical portion of the secretory cell via a long ductule into the uppermost portion of the hair follicle. They are concentrated along the eyelid margins.[12-14]

Sebaceous (holocrine) glands are composed of epithelium. They shed the entire secretory cell as a unit comprised of oils, fatty acids, and cholesterol-based esters, termed sebum. Sebaceous glands are located adjacent to hair follicles and empty directly into the follicle. The hair follicle/sebaceous gland combination is termed the pilosebaceous unit.[12]

Sebaceous glands (Glands of Zeis) are found between follicles and empty their contents directly onto the skin's surface. Eccrine sweat glands are also in the dermis but are not associated with a hair follicle. They open directly onto the skin's surface via a long straight ductule. Eccrine glands produce a clear fluid composed of water, salts, glycogen, and mucin, which we recognize as sweat.[13,14]

Blood vessels and nerves can be found coursing through the dermis, deriving from similar structures in the hypodermis and the deep fascia. Specialized sensory structures called Meissner's and Pacinian (Lamellar) corpuscles within the dermis transmit sensation for touch and pressure.[14]

Below the dermis, one typically encounters a hypodermis consisting of subcutaneous fat and connective tissue. Subcutaneous fat is scant beneath the preseptal portion of the eyelid skin and absent altogether from the pretarsal portion. On the internal aspect of the eyelid, the accessory lacrimal glands of Krause and Wolfring are located beneath the conjunctiva, concentrated primarily on the medial and lateral aspects of the eyelid. The holocrine meibomian glands are located within the tarsal plates.[14-16]

## ORBICULARIS OCULI

The orbicularis oculi is a broad, striated muscle that lies below the skin. Anatomically, it consists of three contiguous parts: the orbital, preseptal, and pretarsal orbicularis. The orbital portion of the muscle originates from the nasal aspect of the frontal bone, the frontal process of the maxilla, and the medial palpebral ligament. Muscle fibers pass along the orbital rim, forming a continuous ellipse around the eye and blending with other muscles of the face[17] (Figure 3-3).

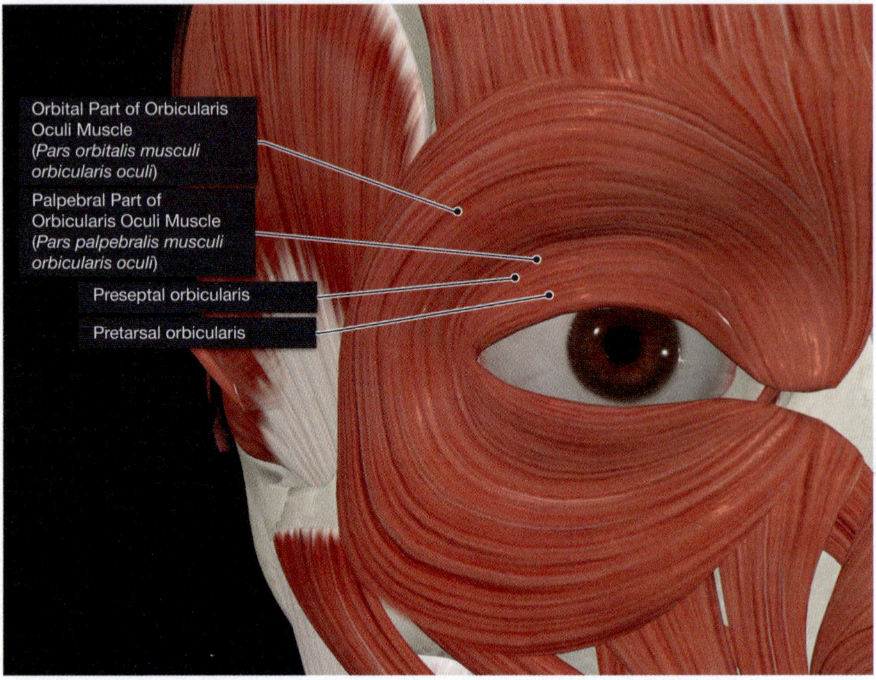


**FIGURE 3-3** The orbicularis oculi muscle. (Graphic created using Complete Anatomy by 3D4Medical/Elsevier, with permission from Elsevier.)

The palpebral portion of the orbicularis muscle originates from the medial palpebral ligament, overlying the eyelid from the orbital rim to the eyelid margin. The muscle fibers arc around each lid as a half ellipse, inserting medially and laterally at the canthal tendons. The palpebral orbicularis is further divided topographically into two parts, the preseptal and pretarsal orbicularis.[17]

The preseptal portion of the orbicularis muscle is located over the orbital septum in both the upper and lower eyelids. This muscle has fibers with origins perpendicular to the upper and lower margins of the medial canthal tendon. These fibers encircle the eyelids and insert along the lateral horizontal raphe, which is adjacent to the lateral canthus.[17,18]

The pretarsal orbicularis muscle lies directly anterior to the tarsal plates. It originates from the superficial and deep heads of the medial canthal tendon, arching around the eyelids and inserting into the lateral canthal tendon along the horizontal raphé. The contraction of these fibers contributes to the lacrimal pump mechanism. The medial heads of these pretarsal fibers fuse to form Horner's muscle, which lies behind the posterior limb of the medial canthal tendon. Horner's muscle inserts onto the posterior lacrimal crest, which helps maintain the medial canthal angle's posterior position, tightening the eyelids against the globe during eyelid closure and aiding in the lacrimal pump mechanism.[17,18]

## ORBITAL SEPTUM

The orbital septum is a multilayered fibrous membrane that originates at the arcus marginalis along the orbital rim (Figure 3-4). Distal fibers of the orbital septum fuse with the anterior surface of the levator aponeurosis. Its fibers insert 3 to 5 mm above the tarsal plate in the upper eyelid, but it may be as much as 10 to 15 mm in certain demographic groups. The septum of the lower eyelid fuses with the capsulopalpebral fascia several millimeters below the inferior tarsus, and the capsulopalpebral fascia then inserts onto the inferior tarsal border. Posterior to the orbital septum are two fat pockets that lie anterior to the levator aponeurosis in the upper lid, whereas in the lower eyelid, three fat pockets lie superficial to the capsulopalpebral fascia. It is essential to understand the regional anatomy, including the identification of the levator aponeurosis or capsulopalpebral fascia, as it is critical to many lower eyelid procedures.[17]

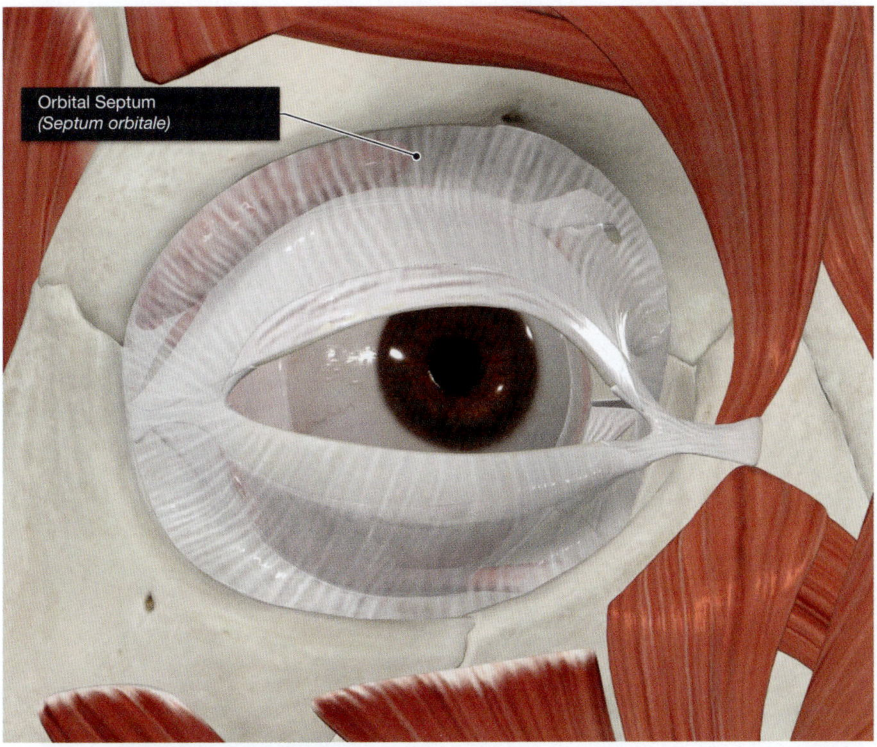


**FIGURE 3-4** The orbital septum. (Graphic created using Complete Anatomy by 3D4Medical/Elsevier, with permission from Elsevier.)

## PREAPONEUROTIC AND PRECAPSULOPALPEBRAL FAT POCKETS

The two preaponeurotic (preseptal) and three precapsulopalpebral fat pockets in the eyelids are anterior extensions of retrobulbar (extraconal) adipose tissue. These fat pockets are essential landmarks and help identify the surgical plane immediately anterior to the primary eyelid retractors of the upper lid (the levator aponeurosis) and the lower lid (the capsulopalpebral fascia). The upper eyelid typically has central and medial fat pockets. Laterally, care must be taken not to confuse the lacrimal gland for a third fat pocket. The lower eyelid has three pockets, medial, central, and lateral[10,18] (Figure 3-5).

## RETRACTORS OF THE EYELIDS

The retractors of the upper eyelid include the levator palpebrae superioris and Müller's muscle. The levator muscle originates from the lesser sphenoid wing just above the annulus of Zinn and runs anteriorly in the orbit just above the superior rectus muscle. Near the superior orbital rim, a

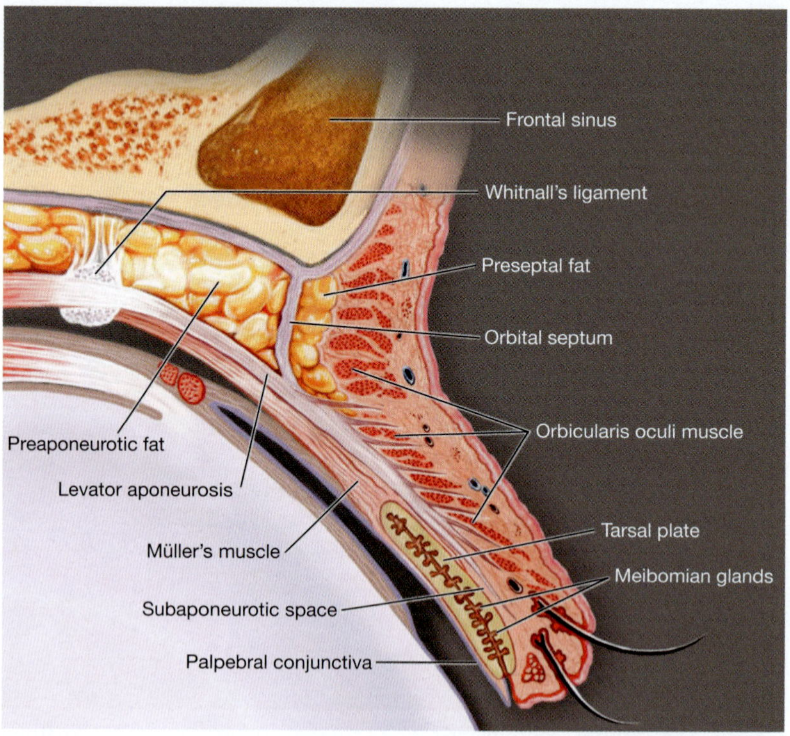


**FIGURE 3-5** Cross section of the upper lid, identifying layers. (From Freddo TF, Chaum E. *Anatomy of the Eye and Orbit: The Clinical Essentials*. Wolters Kluwer; 2018.)

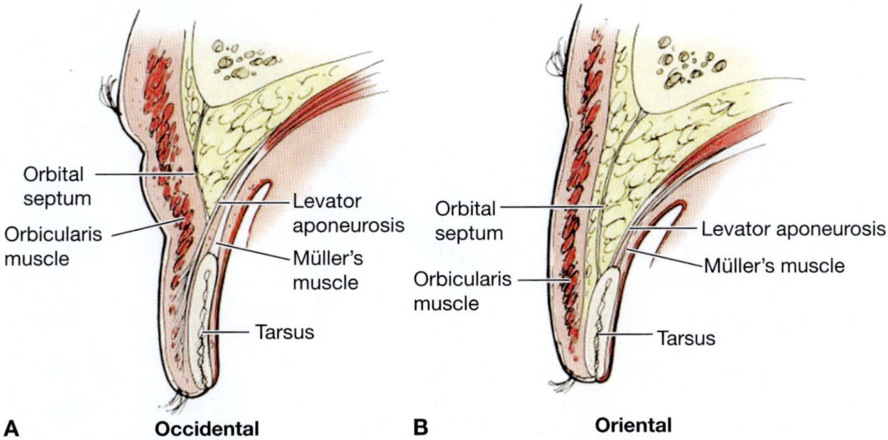


**FIGURE 3-6** Sketches of cross sections of occidental (**A**) and oriental (**B**) eyelids. Note that in the occidental lid, the orbital septum connects to the levator aponeurosis at a point above the tarsus. In the oriental lid, the orbital septum extends much further into the lid, connecting directly to the tarsus. This allows the fat of the extraconal compartment of the orbit to extend into the space between the orbital septum and levator aponeurosis, all the way to the superior margin of the tarsus. (Modified from Tse DT, ed. *Color Atlas of Oculoplastic Surgery*. 2nd ed. Wolters Kluwer; 2011.)

fibrous condensation, Whitnall's ligament, is seen along the muscle sheath and attaches medially and laterally to the orbital walls. Whitnall's ligament supports the fascial system that serves to keep proper spatial relationships between the various tissue planes and anatomic structures in the orbit[17,19] (Figure 3-6).

Inferior to Whitnall's ligament, the levator muscle continues anteriorly as the levator aponeurosis. It continues downward from 14 to 20 mm to insert near the superior tarsal border. The aponeurosis is most adherent to the tarsus at 3 to 4 mm above the superior eyelid margin. Near the superior border of the upper tarsus, the aponeurosis sends interconnecting slips anterior and inferior to insert into the interfascicular septa of the pretarsal orbicularis muscle and subcutaneous tissue. These connective tissue fibers form the lid crease (in western eyes) and maintain the close apposition of the skin, orbicularis, aponeurosis, and tarsus, combining the distal layers of the eyelid into a single functional unit.[18,19]

The levator aponeurosis is a fibrous structure that extends from Whitnall's ligament into the eyelid. As it extends, it becomes more expansive and forms the medial and lateral horns. The lateral horn forms a distinct fibrous sheet that divides the lacrimal gland into orbital and palpebral lobes. It inserts onto the lateral orbital tubercle of the zygomatic bone at the lateral retinaculum. The medial horn is the less prominent of the two. It joins with fibers from the orbital septum and then inserts onto the posterior crus of the medial canthal tendon at the posterior lacrimal crest. The two horns work together, distributing the levator's action across the aponeurosis and the superior tarsus.[20]

The capsulopalpebral fascia originates from Lockwood's ligament and the sheaths surrounding the inferior rectus and inferior oblique muscles. It extends upward and fuses with the orbital

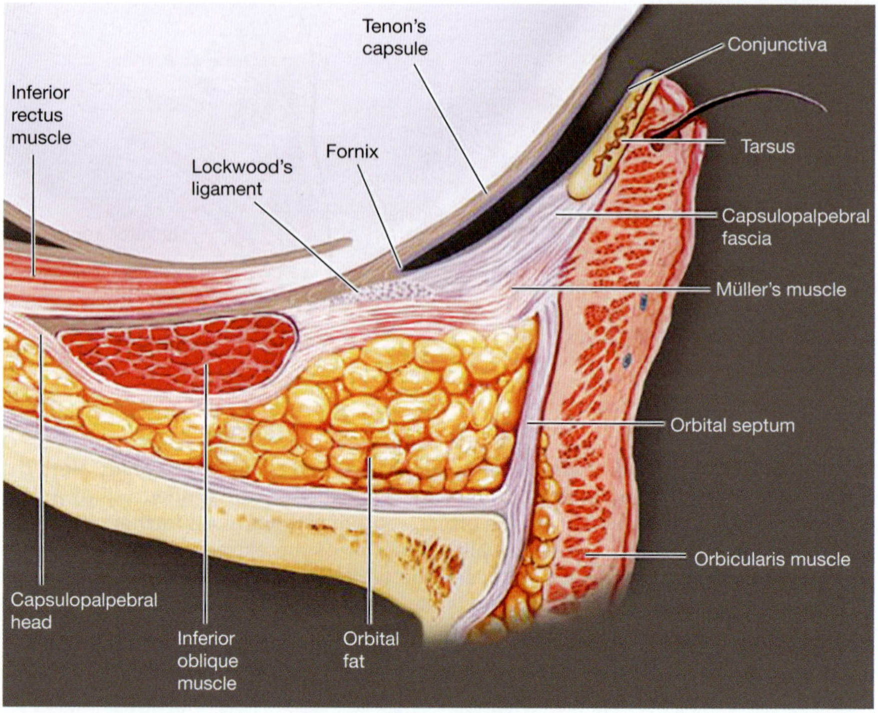


**FIGURE 3-7** Sketch showing the sagittal cross section through the lower lid. (From Rootman J. *Orbital Surgery*. 2nd ed. Wolters Kluwer; 2013.)

septum 4 to 5 mm beneath the inferior tarsus, continuing upward and inserting onto the lower border of the inferior tarsus. Fine fibrous slips extend from this common sheet into the overlying orbicularis intermuscular septae and subcutaneous tissue plane. This results in forming the lower eyelid crease and unifying the anterior and posterior lamellae into a single functional unit[19,20] (Figure 3-7).

The sympathetic nervous system innervates smooth muscles in the upper and lower eyelids that serve as accessory retractors. In the upper eyelid, Müller's muscle originates abruptly from the underside of the levator muscle just in front of Whitnall's ligament.[18] It extends downward and backward from the levator aponeurosis, to which it is attached, and inserts onto the front edge of the superior tarsal border. In the lower eyelid, the sympathetic retractor is more rudimentary. Its fibers run behind the capsulopalpebral fascia to insert onto the lower border of the tarsus, though they may end 2 to 5 mm below the tarsus.[20]

Interruption of sympathetic innervation to these muscles results in Horner's syndrome, characterized by the classic triad of ptosis, miosis, and ipsilateral anhidrosis. The specific clinical findings will vary depending on the location of the lesion(s) along the synaptic path. The degree of ptosis of the upper lid and reverse ptosis (elevation) of the lower eyelid results from the loss of sympathetic smooth muscle tone and accessory lid retraction[21] (Figure 3-8).

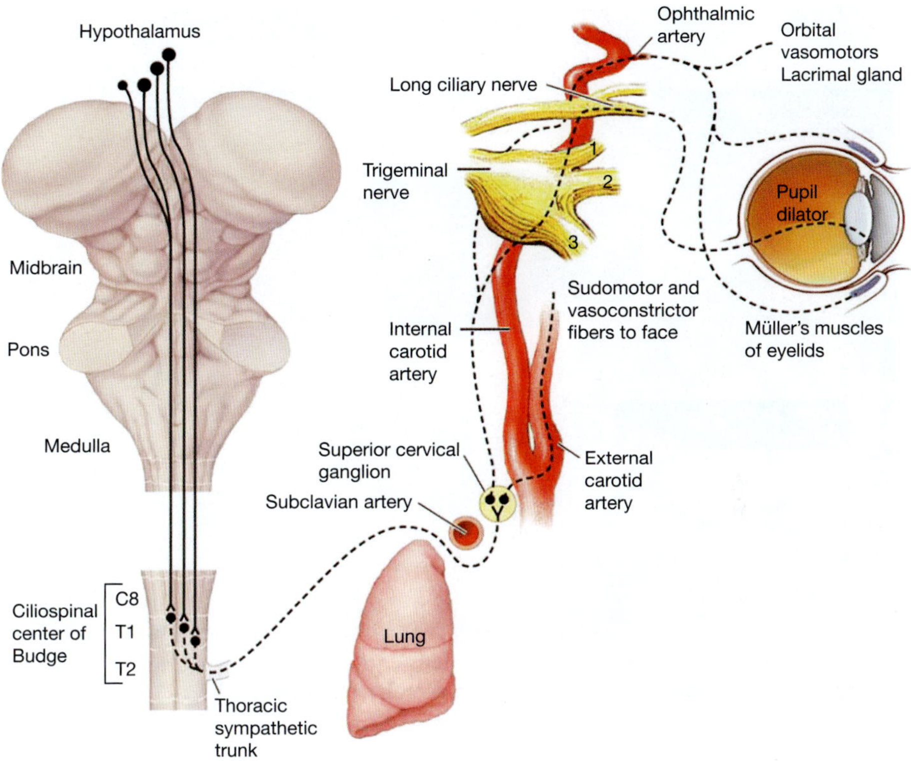


**FIGURE 3-8** Ocular sympathetic pathways. Sympathetic stimuli begin with "first-order neurons" in the hypothalamus, descending through the brainstem to reach the intermediolateral column of the spinal cord at levels C8–T2. This region is termed the ciliospinal center of Budge. The second-order neuron follows the sympathetic chain to the superior cervical ganglion where these "preganglionic" sympathetic fibers synapse. Third-order neurons (postganglionic fibers) leave the ganglion as a plexus surrounding the internal carotid artery and are distributed to the orbit via the ophthalmic artery and ophthalmic division of the trigeminal nerve. Numbers 1 to 3 indicate the following: 1, ophthalmic division; 2, maxillary division; 3, mandibular division. (Modified from Tasman W. *Duane's Ophthalmology*. 2012 ed. Wolters Kluwer; 2012.)

## TARSAL PLATES

The tarsal plates, made of dense fibrous tissue, some 1 to 1.5 mm thick, provide structural support to the eyelids. Each tarsus is approximately 25 mm in horizontal length and is curved to conform to the shape of the front of the eye. The central vertical height of the superior tarsus is 8 to 12 mm, whereas the inferior tarsus is 3.5 to 4.0 mm in vertical height.[6,19] The tarsi taper to 2 mm in height medially and laterally as they fuse with the medial and lateral canthal tendons. As the tarsi approach the canthal tendons, they broaden slightly toward the margin and narrow toward the proximal surface, thus taking on a more triangular cross section. The meibomian glands are embedded within each tarsus.[6,19] Approximately 25 glands are in the superior tarsus,

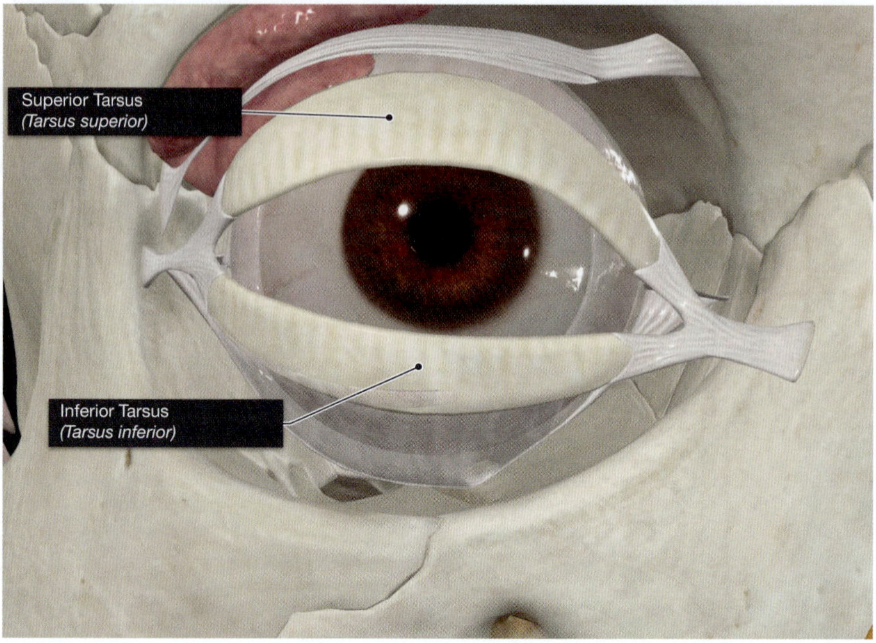


FIGURE 3-9 The upper and lower tarsal plates. (Graphic created using Complete Anatomy by 3D4Medical/Elsevier, with permission from Elsevier.)

and 20 are in the inferior tarsus. Meibomian glands are holocrine-secreting sebaceous glands. Each gland is multilobulated and empties into a central ductule that opens onto the posterior margin of the eyelid behind the gray line (muscle of Riolan). They secrete the lipid layer of the tear film[19] (Figure 3-9).

## MEDIAL AND LATERAL CANTHAL TENDONS

Medially, the tarsal plates transition into fibrous bands that continue as the crura of the medial canthal tendon. These bands are located between the orbicularis muscle and the conjunctiva. The superior and inferior crura of the medial canthal tendon fuse to form a common tendon that inserts through three limbs. The first (anterior) limb inserts onto the orbital process of the maxilla, anterior–superior to the anterior lacrimal crest, providing the principal means of support for the medial canthus. The second (posterior) limb arises near the junction of the superior and inferior crura, passing between the canaliculi and inserting onto the posterior lacrimal crest anterior to Horner's muscle.[17] This limb holds the canthal angle back to maintain a close approximation with the globe. The third (superior) limb of the medial canthal tendon arises from both of the other two limbs, traveling upward and inserting into the orbital process of the frontal bone. The posterior head of the preseptal orbicularis inserts onto this limb, forming the soft-tissue roof of the lacrimal sac fossa. This tendinous extension provides vertical support to the canthal angle and supports the lacrimal pump function.[17,20]

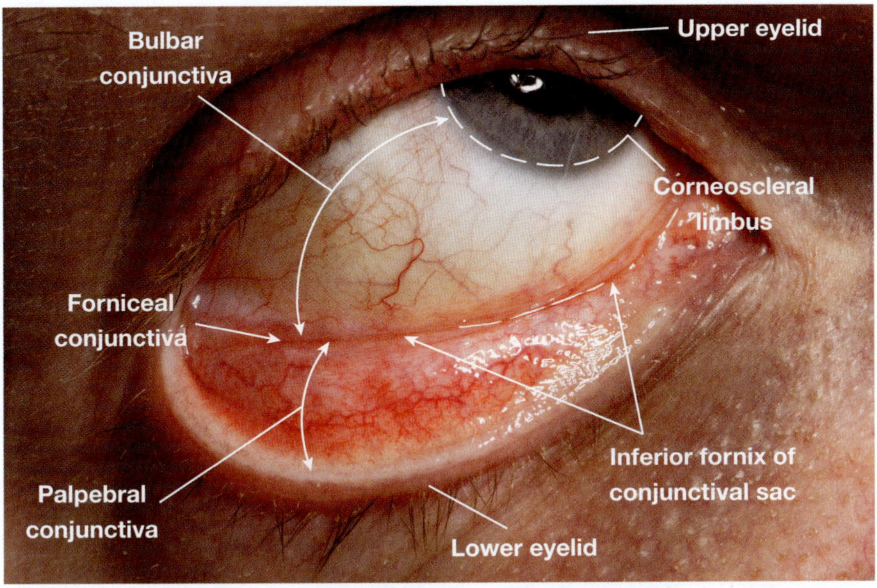


**FIGURE 3-10** Conjunctiva and conjunctival sac. This photograph of the lower part of the eyeball with a reflected lower eyelid shows different regions of the conjunctiva that line the conjunctival sac. The area shown is located between the inner surface of the eyelid and the anterior surface of the eye. The bulbar conjunctiva extends from the corneoscleral limbus covering the sclera of the eye (it does not cover the cornea) to its reflections onto the internal surface of the eyelid, at which point it is called the palpebral conjunctiva. This photograph shows the inferior point of reflection onto the lower eyelid (called the inferior fornix of the conjunctival sac). The conjunctiva in these regions is recognized as the forniceal conjunctiva. (Reprinted with permission from Pawlina W. *Histology: A Text and Atlas*. 9th ed. Wolters Kluwer; 2024:1005; Figure 24.18.)

The tarsal plates continue laterally as the crura of the lateral canthal tendon. The tendon is approximately 1 mm thick, 3 mm wide, and 5 to 7 mm long. Tendinous fibers continue posteriorly along the lateral wall of the orbit, where they fuse with fibers from the check ligament of the sheath of the lateral rectus muscle[20] (Figure 3-10).

## CONJUNCTIVA

The nonkeratinized conjunctiva is an epithelial (mucous) membrane that is subdivided into the palpebral (posterior eyelid) and the bulbar (anterior surface of the globe, excluding the cornea) conjunctiva. The palpebral conjunctiva is adjacent to the posterior surface of the tarsal plate and the sympathetically innervated Müller's muscle. It extends to the fornices and reflects onto the globe's face as the bulbar conjunctiva. Accessory lacrimal glands are located within the conjunctiva's epithelial layers[3,4,17] (Figure 3-11).

The caruncle (caruncula lacrimalis) is a small fleshy nodule found at the medial canthus. The caruncle contains modified hair-bearing skin, sebaceous glands, and sweat glands. Lateral to the caruncle lies a vertical fold of conjunctiva termed the plica semilunaris. The submucosa of plica semilunaris contains adipose cells and smooth muscle fibers. The plica represents a vestigial structure modified to permit enough horizontal slack at the shallow medial fornix for the globe's unimpeded rotation.[2,3,17]

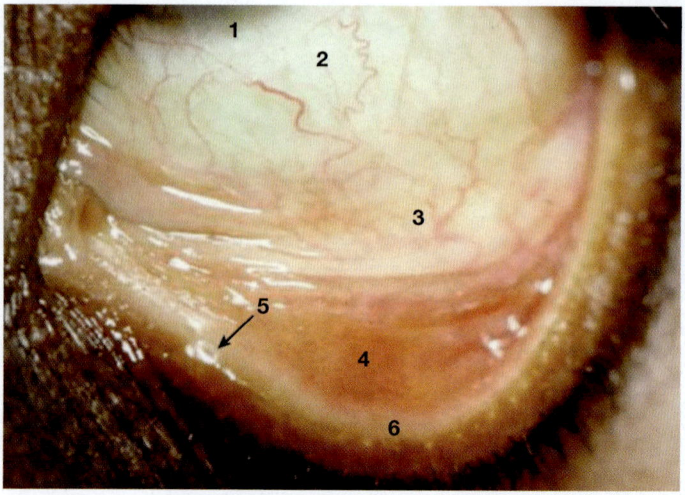


**FIGURE 3-11** Clinical photograph of conjunctiva with lower eyelid pulled inferiorly. (1) Limbus; (2) bulbar conjunctiva; (3) fornix; (4) palpebral conjunctiva; (5) lacrimal punctum; (6) mucocutaneous junction of lid margin. (Courtesy of Mission for Vision and Dr. Ben Glasgow [www.missionforvision.org].)

## INNERVATION

The facial nerve (CN VII) is a motor nerve that innervates the orbicularis oculi via temporal and zygomatic branches. The facial nerve divides into upper temporofacial and lower cervicofacial divisions. The upper division is further subdivided into temporal and zygomatic branches, which innervate the frontalis and orbicularis muscles. The lower cervicofacial division innervates the muscles of the lower face and neck.[21]

Sensory innervation to the eyelid derives from the ophthalmic ($V_1$) and maxillary ($V_2$) divisions of the trigeminal nerve (CN V). Sensory innervation from the upper lid passes along the ophthalmic division ($V_1$) via its terminal branches, the supraorbital, supratrochlear, and lacrimal nerves.[22] The infratrochlear nerve transmits sensory information from the medial aspect of both the upper and lower eyelids. The lacrimal nerve's zygomaticotemporal branch innervates the lateral aspect of the upper eyelid and adjacent brow and forehead portions.[22,23] Sensory innervation to the medial two-thirds of the lower eyelid is via the maxillary division of the infraorbital nerve. The lacrimal nerve's zygomaticofacial branch innervates the lower lid's lateral third[16,24] (Figure 3-12).

## BLOOD VESSELS AND LYMPHATICS

The eyelids possess an extensive vascular supply. The posterior lamella of each eyelid receives blood via the palpebral arcade. The anterior lamella of the upper eyelid receives blood via two vascular arcades, a marginal arcade that runs about 2 mm from the eyelid margin and a

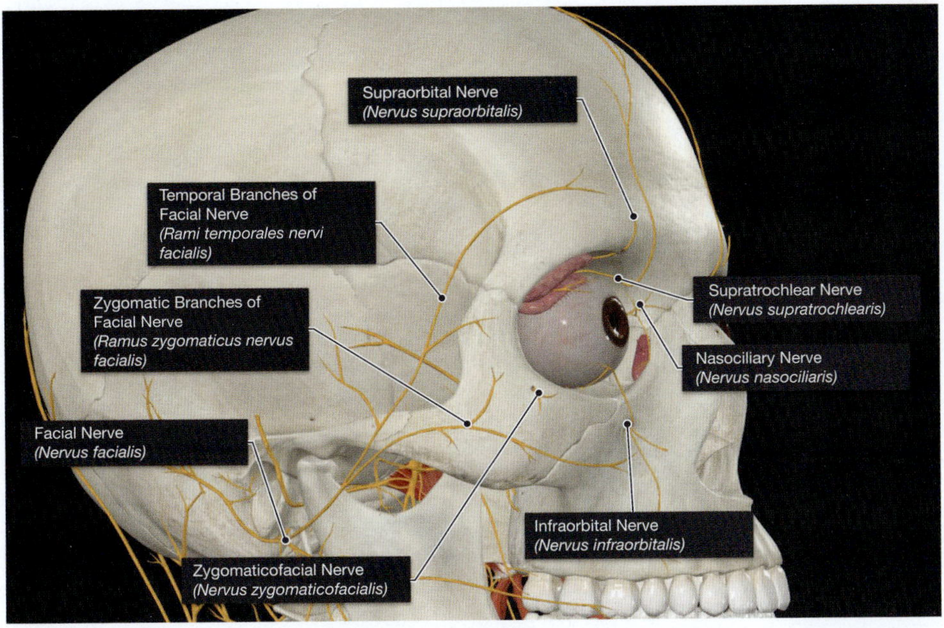


**FIGURE 3-12** Innervation of the periorbita. (Graphic created using Complete Anatomy by 3D4Medical/Elsevier, with permission from Elsevier.)

peripheral arcade that runs along the upper border of the tarsus, posterior to the levator aponeurosis.[10] These vascular arcades are supplied by the superior-medial palpebral vessels from the terminal ophthalmic artery medially and by the superior latero-palpebral vessel from the lacrimal artery laterally. Vessels of the lower eyelid are supplied by the medial and lateral inferior palpebral vessels[17,21] (Figure 3-13).

The venous system of the eyelids is not as well defined as the arterial system. Venous drainage from the eyelids is primarily into several large vessels of the facial system. Lymphatic drainage is limited to the area in front of the orbital septum. The lateral two-thirds of the upper eyelid, along with the lateral one-third of the lower eyelid, drain inferiorly and laterally into the deep and superficial parotid and submandibular nodes. Eyelid lymphatics from the upper medial one-third and the lower medial two-thirds drain medially and inferiorly into the submandibular and anterior cervical nodes[17,21] (Figure 3-14).

## EYEBROWS AND FOREHEAD

The eyebrows are histologically a part of the forehead. They lie at the junction between the upper eyelid and the forehead. The eyebrows are comprised of thickened skin overlying the supraorbital rim and present with course hairs that emerge at an oblique angle. The movements of the brows are provided by the joint actions of the frontalis, procerus, depressor supercilii, corrugator, and orbicularis muscles, which insert partially along the brow. The facial nerve (CN VII) innervates these five muscles.[25]

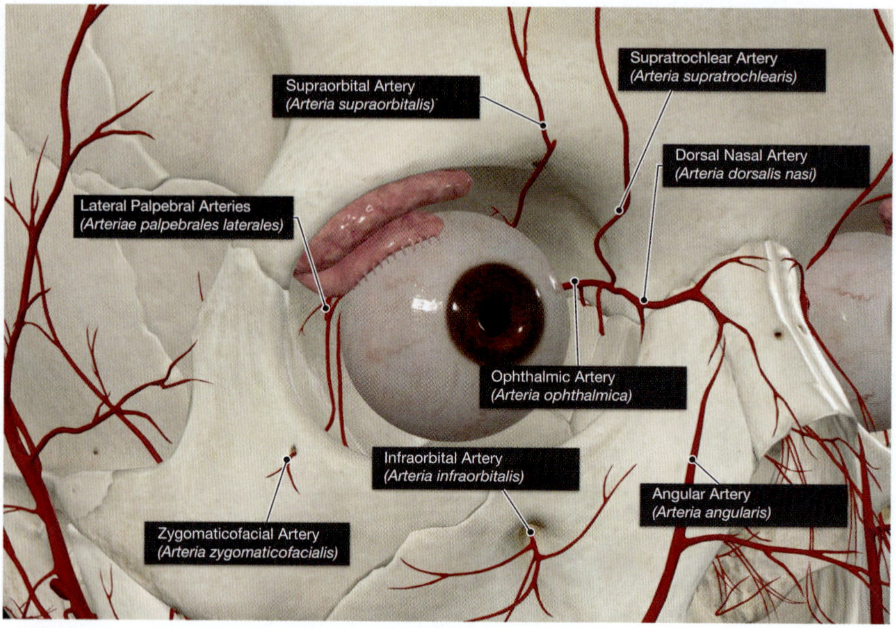


**FIGURE 3-13** Arterial supply of the periorbita. (Graphic created using Complete Anatomy by 3D4Medical/Elsevier, with permission from Elsevier.)

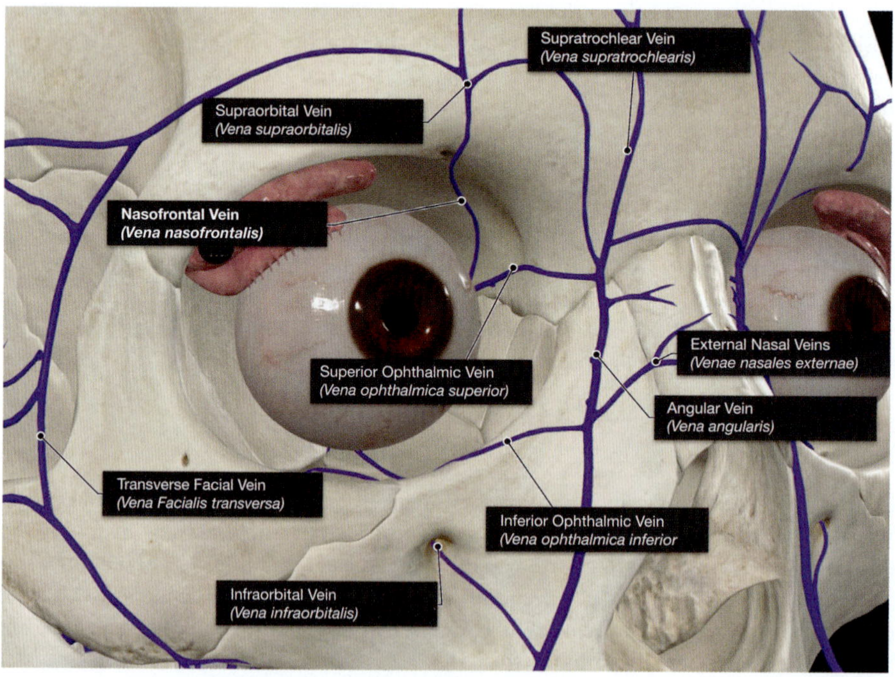


**FIGURE 3-14** Venous drainage of the periorbita. (Graphic created using Complete Anatomy by 3D4Medical/Elsevier, with permission from Elsevier.)

The fibers of the frontalis muscle run vertically on the forehead. They start at the level of the coronal suture line at the top of the head and extend downward toward the superior rim of the orbit. The galea aponeurotica splits into a thin superficial portion above the frontalis muscle and a deeper, thicker layer that extends beneath the frontalis to insert onto the superior rim of the orbit at the arcus marginalis. A deep layer of adipose tissue underneath the muscle divides the frontalis muscle from the underlying deep fascia along the orbital rim. This sub-brow fat pad may extend into the upper eyelid, which can be mistaken for the preaponeurotic fat pockets. It may contribute to a thicker, fuller upper lid appearance in certain individuals.[17,19,25]

The procerus muscle is a rectangular muscle that arises from tendinous fibers of the periosteum covering the lower portion of the nasal bone. The muscle fibers pass vertically between the brows to insert on the skin over the lower forehead. Contraction of this muscle draws the medial angle of the brows inferiorly and produces transverse wrinkles over the glabellar region. The depressor supercilii muscle lies lateral to the procerus that depresses the medial (head) of the eyebrows. The corrugator muscle forms a pyramidal band of fibers beneath the central portion of the frontalis muscle complex, lateral to the depressor supercilii. Corrugator fibers arise from the superomedial orbital rim at the medial end of the frontal bone and pass obliquely, superiorly, and laterally, inserting into the deep frontalis fascia along the medial one-third of the brow through two heads, the oblique and the transverse heads[17,25] (Figure 3-15).

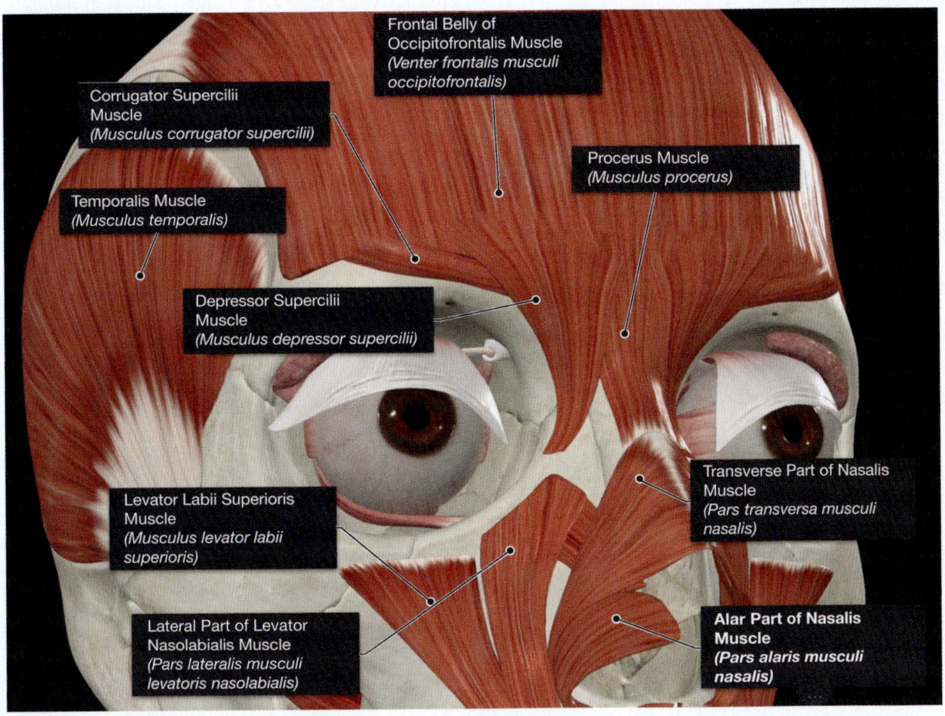


**FIGURE 3-15** Muscles of the forehead and periorbital region. (Graphic created using Complete Anatomy by 3D4Medical/Elsevier, with permission from Elsevier.)

## REFERENCES


1. Dortzbach RK, Ying Y. Anatomy of the eyelids and periorbita. *Curr Opin Ophthalmol.* 2006;17(2):78-86.
2. Jones DT. Anatomy of the eyelids. *Clin Exp Optom.* 2005;88(4):184-196.
3. Neumann A, Marx S. Anatomy of the eyelids and periorbital region. *Oper Tech Otolaryngol Head Neck Surg.* 2012;23(3):283-290.
4. Patel PV, De Paiva CS. Anatomy of the eyelids, lacrimal system, and periorbital region. *Surv Ophthalmol.* 2017;62(2):223-229.
5. Peredo AM, Malhotra R. *Ophthalmic Plastic and Reconstructive Surgery.* Springer International Publishing; 2015.
6. Trobe JD. The anatomy and physiology of the eyelids. *Surv Ophthalmol.* 2005;50(3):199-213.
7. Draelos ZD, Goldman L. Periorbital wrinkles and rejuvenation. *Dermatol Clin.* 2017;35(3):493-505.
8. Hwang SY, Kim JH, Kim KH. The anatomy and histology of the periorbital region. *Ann Plast Surg.* 2018;80(5):519-524.
9. El-Domyati M. Histological and histochemical study of the periorbital skin in Egyptians. *J Cutan Pathol.* 2013;40(9):751-758.
10. Sclafani AP, Fagien S. Periorbital rejuvenation: a review of anatomy and current treatment options. *Aesthet Plast Surg.* 2012;36(5):961-971.
11. Freddo TF, Chaum E. Chapter 2: Anatomy of the eye and orbit. In: *The Eyelids and Adnexa.* Wolters Kluwer, Wolters Kluwer Health; 2017:44.
12. Freddo TF, Chaum E. Chapter 2: Anatomy of the eye and orbit. In: *The Eyelids and Adnexa.* Wolters Kluwer, Wolters Kluwer Health; 2017:46-47.
13. Elder DE. Chapter 3: Histology of the skin. In: *Lever's Histopathology of the Skin.* Wolters Kluwer Health; 2015: 35-36 (Kindle 11th ed.).
14. Elder DE. Chapter 3: Histology of the skin. In: *Lever's Histopathology of the Skin.* Wolters Kluwer Health; 2015: 59-60 (Kindle 11th ed).
15. Bobonich MA, Nolen ME, Honaker J, DiRuggiero D. Section 1: Fundamentals of the skin. In: *Dermatology for Advanced Practice Clinicians.* 2nd ed. Wolters Kluwer: 2021: 2-3.
16. Shams PN, Ortiz-Pérez S, Joshi N. Clinical anatomy of the periocular region. *Facial Plast Surg.* 2013 Aug;29(4):255-263.
17. Miller PJ, McCord CD. Anatomy and biomechanics of the eyelid and periorbital region. *Ophthalmic Plast Reconstr Surg.* 2015;31(2):75-80.
18. Kikkawa DO. The anatomy and function of the orbicularis oculi muscle. *Plast Reconstr Surg.* 2015;135(5):965-972.
19. Hu Y, Lin Z, Chen J. Anatomy and surgical strategies of the eyelid retractors. *Curr Opin Ophthalmol.* 2016;27(2):130-136.
20. Léonard G, Barrau C. The retractors of the upper eyelid: a review of the literature. *J Plast Reconstr Aesthet Surg.* 2018;71(7):989-995.
21. Kim JH, Hwang SY, Kim KH. The anatomy of the orbicularis oculi muscle. *Ann Plast Surg.* 2018;80(5):525-529.
22. Eustachon DE. Innervation of the face. *J Am Acad Dermatol.* 2013;69(3):459-466.
23. Kuwabara T, Cogan DG, Johnson CC. Structure of the muscles of the upper eyelid. *Arch Ophthalmol.* 1975 Nov;93(11):1189-1197.
24. Sand JP, Zhu BZ, Desai SC. Surgical anatomy of the eyelids. *Facial Plast Surg Clin North Am.* 2016 May;24(2):89-95.
25. Kim JH, Hwang SY, Kim KH. The muscles of the forehead. *Ann Plast Surg.* 2018;80(5):535-539.

# 4 Equipment, Instrument Selection, and Setup

**Richard E. Castillo**

The minimum requirements for safe office surgery in terms of instruments and equipment are discussed in this chapter. Microsurgical instruments, including ophthalmic instruments, are designed ergonomically with efficiency and safety in mind.[1] Likewise, office equipment and instrumentation must be available to promote safety and good outcomes with regard to the diversity of office procedures performed. All invasive procedures must be performed in an environment set up for that purpose, with proper attention to space, lighting, equipment, instruments, and sterile technique. Resuscitation equipment and drugs must be readily available in case of an emergency in anticipation of potential complications. Periodic certification and recertification in basic and advanced life support should be prerequisites, as training and confidence will ensure patient safety and good outcomes.

## INSTRUMENTS AND SETUP

### Key Points

- Ophthalmic microsurgical instruments are ergonomically designed for efficiency and safety.
- Proper regard for sterile technique is essential to any operative setup.
- Resuscitation equipment must be regularly inspected, maintained, and easily accessible.
- The ideal assistant should be calm, reassuring, and vigilant.
- Written protocols should exist in case of spillage of caustic or biohazardous materials.
- Dirty and infected materials and sharps must be inaccessible to patients and staff.
- Reusable instruments must be sterilized in an autoclave.
- Chemical disinfection may not render instruments sterile.
- Skin markers are used before anesthetic administration to ensure accurate incisions.
- The choice of suture material affects the final appearance of the wound.

## PROCEDURE ROOM

The shape and size of the procedure room are usually dictated by available space. However, space around the procedure table or chair must be sufficient for easy access to an instrument stand, and there should be access at the head for airway protection should the patient faint. A sink for handwashing should be available nearby, although not necessarily in the same room. A dedicated dirty area for collecting contaminated instruments and a biohazard waste container must also be provided. However, biohazardous material waiting to be discarded should be kept outside the clean procedure area. A biohazard disposal service must be retained to remove biohazardous waste properly. The procedure space should also have adequate work surfaces and storage facilities.[2]

## RESUSCITATION EQUIPMENT

Office-based surgery inevitably involves some blood loss and the use of local anesthetic. Although the patient is unlikely to become hemodynamically compromised, some individuals may faint from the psychological effect of seeing their blood or the discomfort of needle sticks and manipulation around the eyes. Administration of local anesthesia also carries a small risk of syncope, allergy, or, much less frequently, anaphylaxis, so that the patient may need cardiac and respiratory support. Resuscitation equipment and supplies should always be available in the same room in case of a vasovagal or anaphylactic attack. Resuscitation equipment, including an automated external defibrillator (AED), a crash kit with emergency pharmaceuticals such as epinephrine, various sized airways, a manual resuscitator bag, a mask (Figure 4-1), and oxygen must all be easily accessible in the same room.

Table 4-1 lists the minimum requirements and some optional extras for resuscitation equipment. The practitioner and all assistants should be fully trained to use the equipment, which must be regularly inspected and maintained. It is helpful to keep a laminated sheet showing appropriate drug doses printed in a large typeface with the equipment; one thing less to worry about in an emergency. Such sheets are commercially available and typically included in a crash kit purchase.

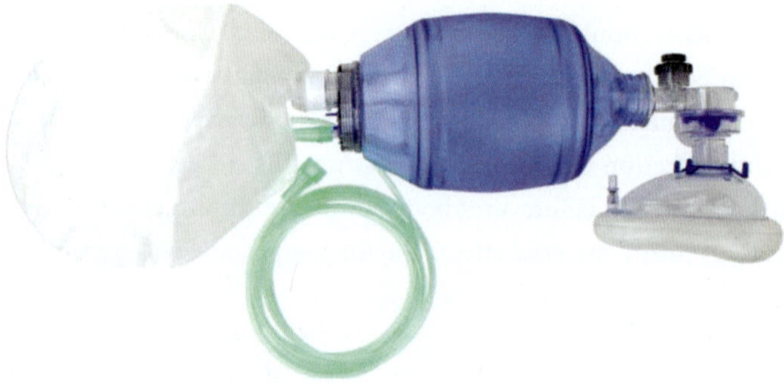

**FIGURE 4-1** Manual resuscitator bag and mask.

**TABLE 4-1 RESUSCITATIVE EQUIPMENT AND SUPPLIES**

| ESSENTIAL ITEMS | OPTIONAL ITEMS |
| --- | --- |
| • Defibrillator (auto) | • Intravenous fluids (D5W) |
| • Ambu bag (for ventilation) | • Intubation equipment |
| • Oxygen masks<br>• Various sizes<br>• Tubing | • Hemodynamic monitoring equipment<br>• Automatic blood pressure cuff<br>• Pulse oximeter |
| • Airways (multiple sizes) | • IV steroid (e.g., hydrocortisone 100 mg) |
| • Oxygen (full tank with regulator valve) | |
| • Intravenous cannulas | |
| • Epinephrine 1:1,000 | |
| • Diazepam 5 mg IV | |
| • Chlorpheniramine 10 mg IV | |
| • Needles and syringes (variable sizes) | |
| • Albuterol inhaler | |

## PROCEDURAL LIGHTING

The procedure room should have bright background lighting to ensure practitioner and assistant safety. If the operating field is well lit, but the remainder of the room is dim, used instruments or sharps on the instrument stand may be overlooked, resulting in needlestick injury. A well-lit room is also safer for a patient requiring resuscitation in an emergency.

Procedure lighting should be mounted on a flexible arm to allow variation in position and focus. Depending on the room layout, this may be achieved conveniently with a ceiling or wall-mounted lamp. Floor-based lamps (Figure 4-2) are popular and convenient, but care must be taken with power cords across floors that can be dangerous. Also, the lamp should not emit too much heat as this may cause patient or practitioner discomfort during lengthy procedures and can lead to the drying of surgically exposed tissues. Many cool LED lights with adjustable rheostats and varying color temperatures are available.

## PROCEDURE TABLE OR CHAIR

The type of table or chair required for the procedure room will depend on the practitioner's preference and the procedures performed. If long, complex procedures are routinely scheduled, a good-quality table, with articulations for height and tilt adjustments (Figure 4-3), is advisable in the event it is necessary to position the patient in Trendelenburg or reverse Trendelenburg position or accommodate issues with the patient's neck, upper or lower spine. Furthermore, an articulating backrest and headrest are essential. A simpler design may be adequate if the table or chair is used primarily for minor procedures.

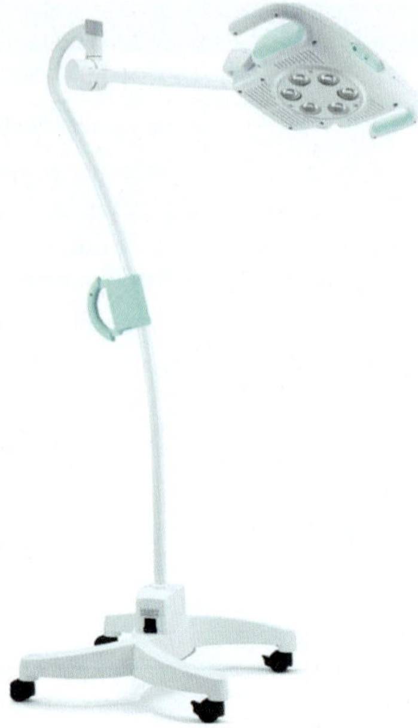

FIGURE 4-2 Floor-based procedure light.

## HEMOSTASIS

Disposable ophthalmic cautery units (Figure 4-4) are inexpensive and are sufficient for all but the most complex ophthalmic skin surgery. If more complex surgery is undertaken or the practitioner performs many procedures, an electrocautery or radiosurgical device may be a viable

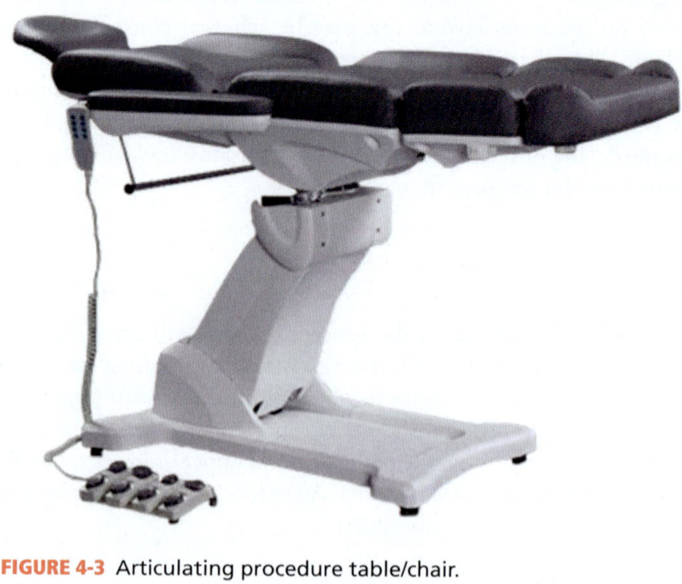

FIGURE 4-3 Articulating procedure table/chair.

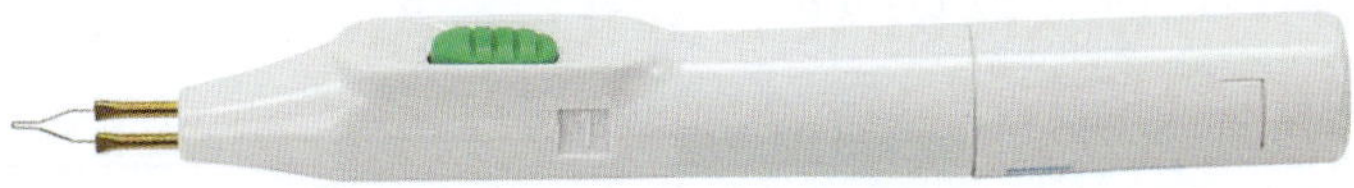

FIGURE 4-4 Disposable ophthalmic cautery unit.

alternative. A radiosurgical device (see Chapter 8) in the coagulation mode can be used on the tissues of the eyelid and periorbita, achieving hemostasis with less eyelid and collateral tissue damage than thermal or electrocautery. However, these units are expensive and unnecessary for superficial eyelid surgery or minor excisions in which bleeding can be controlled by direct pressure.

Chemical agents for hemostasis include aluminum hydrochloride, trichloroacetic acid, phenol, and silver nitrate (Table 4-2). These agents act either by precipitating proteins, thus triggering coagulation pathways, or by simple tissue destruction. Chemical cautery is used primarily for superficial wounds following shave excision or curettage. Care must be taken when applying these substances to the eyelids so that the substance does not contact the eyelid margin, the palpebral conjunctiva, or the globe's surface.[3]

**TABLE 4-2 CHEMICAL AGENTS USED FOR HEMOSTASIS**

| AGENT | ADVANTAGES | DISADVANTAGES |
|---|---|---|
| • Aluminum hydrochloride (20%–50%) | • Lack of tissue necrosis<br>• No tattooing | • Irritating to the eyes |
| • Trichloroacetic acid (30%–50%) | • Strongly hemostatic | • May damage surrounding epithelial tissues |
| • Phenol (50%–100%) | • Strongly hemostatic | • May damage surrounding epithelial tissues |
| • Silver nitrate (20%–50%) | • Germicidal | • Slow acting<br>• Variable success<br>• Potential to tattoo |

## ASSISTANTS AND STAFF

It is advisable to train and collaborate with assistants who are familiar and comfortable working with the following:

- Resuscitation equipment and techniques
- Sterile technique
- The steps involved in the procedure
- The range of instruments required for the procedure
- Stock items, such as drugs, sutures, and dressings

An assistant may not need to scrub for some minor procedures but should know how to do so if more complex procedures are undertaken or if circumstances call for assistance. For example, an extra pair of hands may be required if a patient bleeds excessively. The ideal assistant should be calm, able to reassure the patient, and capable of always observing them for signs of distress or adverse reaction.[4]

## HAZARDOUS MATERIALS, SPILLS, AND CONTAMINATION[5,6]

- Each office should have a designated safety officer, and written protocols should exist in case of caustic or biologically hazardous materials spillage.
- Caustic materials should be stored in a locked cabinet.
- Safety Data Sheets (SDS), formally known as Material Safety Data Sheets (MSDS), should be maintained for all chemicals in the office.
- Flameproof enclosures may be required for flammable liquids.

## SHARPS AND BIOLOGICAL HAZARDS[7]

- Sharps should be placed directly into sharps containers (Figure 4-5) designed for this purpose; these items should not be accessible to patients or staff.
- Contaminated disposables such as gauze sponges, towels, and swabs should be disposed of in a marked biohazard waste bin in an area not accessible to patients or staff.
- Used nondisposable instruments should be scrubbed clean of biological debris and stored in a safe area away from the clean environment pending sterilization.
- Blood or body fluids spilled onto the floor should be cleaned with disinfectant immediately after the procedure before reusing the space.
- The operating table or chair and all counters and surfaces should be wiped down with an appropriate disinfectant between procedures.
- The procedure room should be professionally cleaned regularly, the frequency of which will depend on the range and number of procedures performed and the potential for contamination.

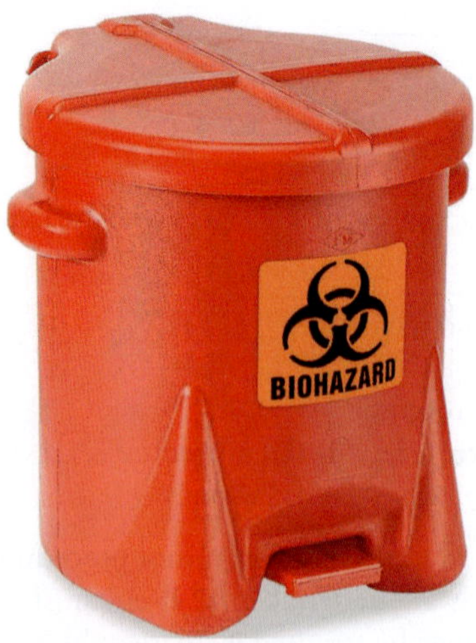


**FIGURE 4-5** Sharps disposal container.

## PREVENTION OF INFECTION

The procedure room for ophthalmic office surgery needs to be clinically clean but not necessarily sterile. Supplies for cleaning and disinfecting will need to be kept on hand. If electrosurgical or radiosurgical devices are employed, an approved HEPA-filtration electrosurgical unit smoke evacuator (see Chapter 8) must be available and utilized during procedures where these devices are used. Minimizing risk from potential sources of infection should be a matter of routine and vigilance (Table 4-3).[8,9]

## STERILE FIELD

To minimize the risk of surgical site infection, it is essential to establish and maintain a sterile operating field. The sterile field includes:

- The entire area being operated on
- The surrounding sterile drapes
- The practitioners and assistants' gloved hands
- The top of the instrument stand (which is covered with a sterile drape)
- Any gauze sponges, towels, or cotton swabs used
- All instruments and sutures on the instrument stand (Figure 4-6)

**TABLE 4-3** PREVENTION OF SURGICAL SITE INFECTION (SSI)

| POTENTIAL SOURCE OF SSI | PREVENTIVE MEASURES |
|---|---|
| • Practitioner and assistant | • Ensure handwashing and proper "gowning and gloving" technique.<br>• All attending personnel must be free from skin infection or nasal contamination.<br>• Adhere to proper sterile technique.<br>• Avoid glove tears or punctures. |
| • Patient | • Prep skin with an appropriate antiseptic agent (e.g., povidone–iodine).<br>• Use sterile drapes.<br>• Administer peri- or postoperative antibiotics if warranted.<br>• Utilize proper postoperative wound dressings.<br>• Communicate postoperative care instructions. |
| • Environment | • Meticulously clean and disinfect the procedure room and all surfaces.<br>• Dispose of biohazard waste in a container designed for contaminated waste and store it outside the clean procedure environment.<br>• Maintain proper ventilation throughout the procedure space.<br>• Assure that all surfaces, including floors, walls, ceilings, and countertops, are in good repair. |
| • Equipment | • Clean and rinse all instruments of tissue debris prior to sterilization.<br>• Sterilize nondisposable cautery devices between patients.<br>• Utilize sterile dressings and swabs.<br>• Utilize sterile packs for instrument storage. |

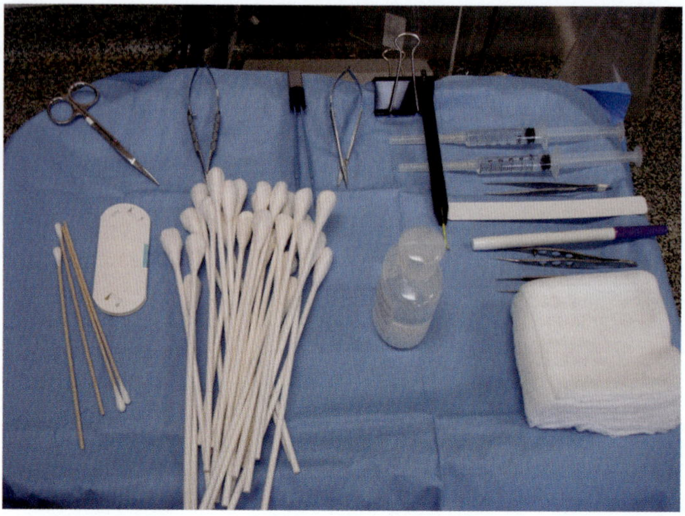

**FIGURE 4-6** Instruments for ophthalmic office surgery on a sterile stand.

A sterile pack containing swabs, gauze 4 × 4s, and towels should be opened using sterile technique. If the individual instruments are not included in the sterile pack, properly sterilized instruments should be placed on the stand again without contaminating the other items already on the field.[10-12]

After the practitioner washes their hands and dons sterile gloves, they may use the sterile field on the top of the instrument stand. An appropriate skin prep, such as povidone–iodine, is used to clean the operative area and surrounding skin on the patient. Because of the fire risk, alcohol-based solutions should not be used when thermal cautery, radiofrequency coagulation, or electrocautery (diathermy) devices are employed. A fire extinguisher should be available in a conspicuous space in the procedure room in the event of an emergency.

Following the skin prep, the operative area should be draped with sterilized linen, sterile plastic, or water-resistant paper towels. Sterile towel clips may be used to hold the drapes in place, or convenient sterile single-piece fenestrated ophthalmic drapes with adhesive backing are also available. The practitioner should not touch anything outside the prepared regions, and the assistant (unless scrubbed and sterile) should not handle areas inside the sterile field.

Sutures, extra swabs, and instruments should be placed onto the sterile field using a "no-touch" technique. The sterile field must be reestablished to the highest possible standard if it is accidentally contaminated or otherwise compromised.

## ADDITIONAL PRECAUTIONS

Establishing a sterile field and constant vigilance minimize potential surgical site infections. However, the risk of cross-contamination from the patient to the practitioner or assistant should also be considered.

Blood-borne viral infections, such as hepatitis B and HIV, are the primary concerns, but superficial cutaneous infections may be transmitted if the practitioner or assistant's skin is compromised. Active immunization against hepatitis B should be mandatory for the practitioner and all assistants, and office protocols to prevent needlestick injury should be in place. A written protocol of action should be available in case of needlestick injury. The protocol will depend on local guidelines and may be available from a local Occupational Safety and Health Administration (OSHA) office.[13,14]

It is also advisable for the practitioner and assistant to wear protective goggles or face shields to prevent blood or other biological hazards from coming into contact with their eyes during the operation.

## STERILIZATION OF INSTRUMENTS

All instruments that are to be reused must be cleaned and then sterilized. This can be achieved on the premises using a countertop autoclave or by arrangement with a local sterile supply service. It is important to realize that chemical disinfection alone may not render the instrument completely sterile. Sterilization utilizing an autoclave combines high temperatures and pressure and destroys all pathogens, including viruses, fungi, bacteria, and bacterial spores.

Prior to sterilization in the autoclave, instruments must be physically cleaned with soap and water to remove tissue debris; otherwise, the sterilization process may be hindered. The instruments must then be rinsed with distilled water, dried, and placed in the sterilization pouch, ready to be placed in the autoclave unit. Countertop autoclaves must be operated per the manufacturer's instructions and should be serviced and tested regularly. A logbook of their service history and test results should be kept. At a minimum, sterilization procedures and standards should adhere to institutional and Occupational Safety and Health Administration (OSHA) and Centers for Disease Control and Prevention (CDC) regulations and recommendations.[15]

## OPHTHALMIC SURGICAL INSTRUMENTS FOR OFFICE PROCEDURES[16,17]

Microsurgical and ophthalmic instruments are designed ergonomically for efficiency and safety. The choice of instruments for ophthalmic office procedures depends on personal preference; however, sufficient instruments must be available to perform the planned procedure and deal with any complications. For example, small hemostats (mosquito hemostats, Figure 4-7) are essential in case of excessive bleeding. Most ophthalmic instruments are no more than 6 inches long and designed to be manipulated with the fingertips to minimize extraneous arm movements above the wrist. They are available in various styles, for example, rounded handles versus flat handles, straight tips versus curved tips, and titanium and stainless steel.

- Scalpel handle (No. 3) and blades No. 15 and 15C are ideal for most skin surgery and ophthalmic office procedures (Figure 4-8). The No. 15C has a slightly longer cutting edge than the No. 15. Relative to other commercially available blades, each has a small, easily controlled cutting surface shaped to facilitate incisions that start and finish at 90° to the skin surface. Larger blades are more clumsy and are not advisable for delicate periocular work. Scalpel handle No. 3 will accommodate blade sizes from No. 6 through 16. Disposable scalpels with plastic handles are also available as an alternative.

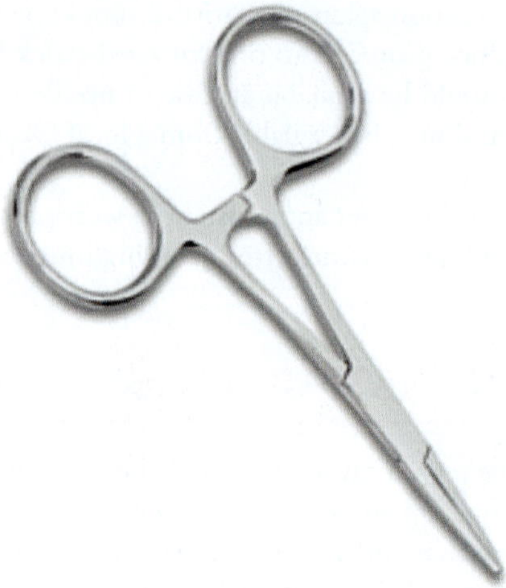

FIGURE 4-7 Small (mosquito) hemostats.

- Toothed tissue forceps, 0.12 or 0.3 mm (Figure 4-9) for ophthalmic procedures, grip the tissue specimen and offer up the wound's edge for suture insertion. They are available in various styles, with and without suture-tying platforms, and in stainless steel and titanium.
- Using nontoothed (dressing or atraumatic) forceps to grasp tissue is not good practice, as the pressure applied may crush the wound edges. It is preferable to potentially micropuncture (with toothed forceps) rather than crush skin, as crushing will impede healing.
- Chalazion forceps are a self-retaining type of thumb forceps that have discoid ends. One arm has a flattened plate at its end, which is oval and solid. The other arm has a matching

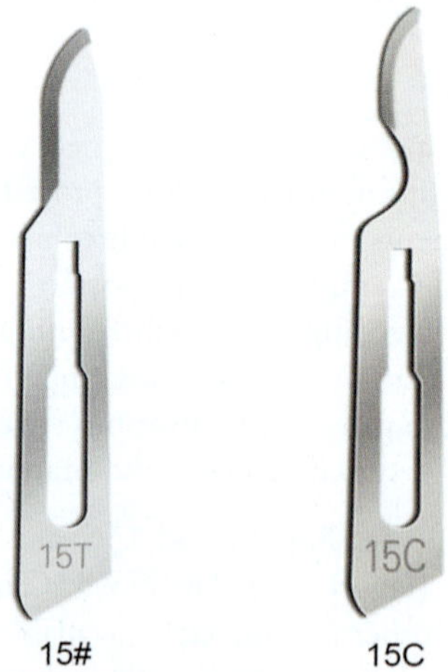


FIGURE 4-8 Scalpel blades: No. 15 versus No. 15C. The 15C has a slightly longer cutting reach.

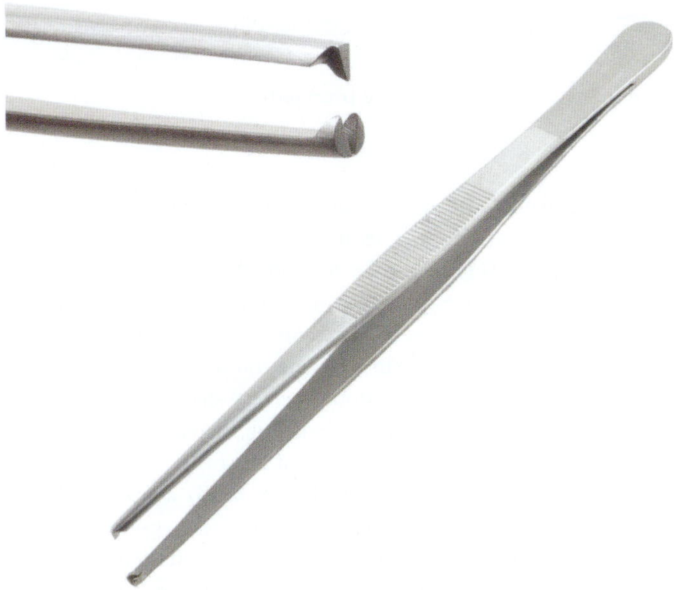

FIGURE 4-9 Toothed tissue forceps (0.3 mm).

ring that fits into the opposite arm's solid plate. An adjustable screw in the middle of the handles can be tightened until a firm tissue purchase is made (Figure 4-10).

- Skin hooks (Figure 4-11) may be preferred to tissue forceps for work on wound edges. If manipulated with care and skill, a skin hook will cause less tissue damage and prevent crushing the tissue, especially the wound margins.

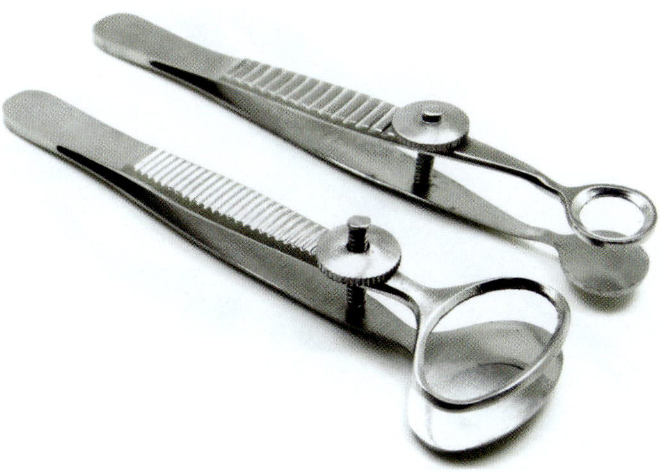

FIGURE 4-10 Chalazion forceps.

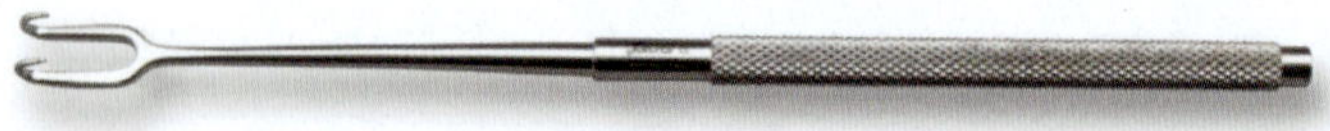

**FIGURE 4-11** Skin hook (double pronged).

- Scissors perform several tasks in skin surgery, including cutting tissue, undermining, and cutting sutures following placement. The blades may be straight or curved and are available with sharp or rounded tips (Figure 4-12). Straight sharp-tipped Iris scissors are useful for cutting tissue. Most practitioners prefer to use rounded-tipped curved scissors for tissue dissection and undermining, as there is more control over the positioning of the blade and less chance of puncturing overlying skin with the rounded ends. The choice of scissors depends on personal preference, but they should be very sharp, and the blades should oppose smoothly to enable tissue cutting without crushing. Separate scissors should be used for cutting sutures, as this may quickly blunt surgical scissors.
- Needle holders for ophthalmic procedures (Figure 4-13) are available in many different styles, but the jaws must be short and very finely serrated or nonserrated. Coarse serrations can damage fine suture material, and the small jaws avoid flattening the curve in fine ophthalmic needles. Available in both stainless steel and titanium.
- Hemostats clamp veins and arterioles that may be cut during surgery. They should be available during all incisional procedures without other hemostatic thermal, radiosurgical, or electrocautery equipment. Hemostats are available with straight or curved blades and have serrated surfaces; the Halsted mosquito is commonly used for ophthalmic procedures (Figure 4-7).

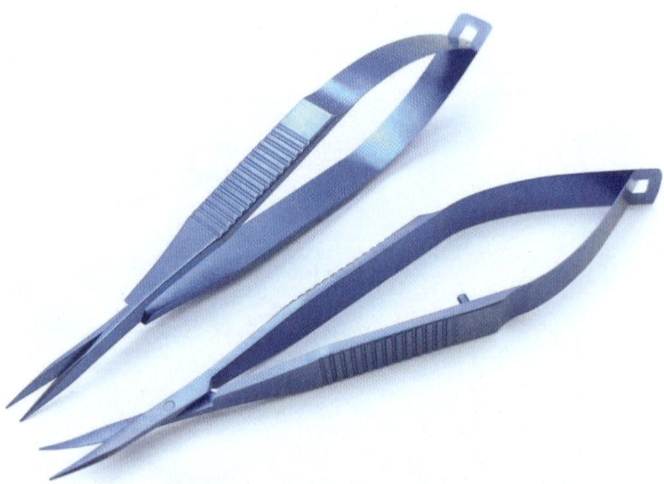

**FIGURE 4-12** Westcott-style spring-loaded scissors (Titanium).

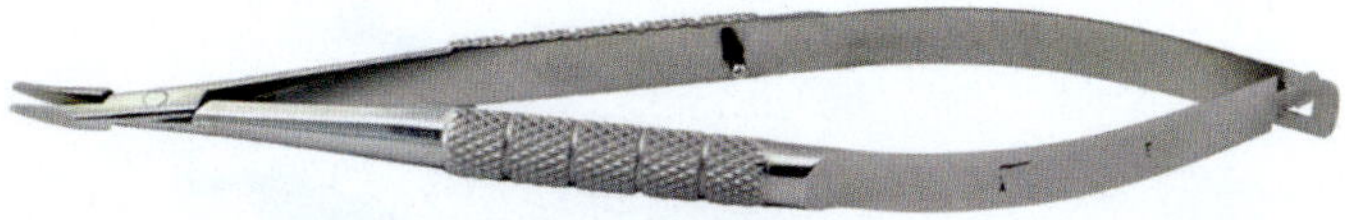

FIGURE 4-13 Micro-needle holder (Barraquer style 10 mm curved jaws).

- Curettes are invaluable instruments for a variety of skin procedures. Meyerhoefer or Mueller chalazion curettes provide a precise, sharp scoop, effective for curettage of chalazia (Figure 4-14). Disposable dermal curettes are useful for softer, more friable superficial cutaneous lesions. The sharp disposable curette has a circular loop, one edge of which is a surgical blade, while the opposite edge may be used for "blunt" curettage (Figure 4-15). Both types are available in several sizes.
- Skin punches are disposable cylindrical surgical blades (Figure 4-16). Punches allow for a full-thickness skin biopsy to be quickly taken, leaving a small circular deficit. Various diameters are available. A 3-mm punch is usually sufficient for pathologic examination of a skin tumor such as basal cell carcinoma, squamous cell carcinoma, or Bowen's disease.
- Sterile skin marking pens used before administration of anesthetic are essential and advisable. Lesions and their margins may become indistinct if the anesthetic swells the skin or epinephrine blanches the skin surface. Marking also ensures the removal of adequate margins of surrounding normal skin when excising skin malignancies.

The orientation of skin incisions should be preplanned, considering skin tension lines. Anatomic structures such as periocular wrinkles can be marked to ensure the scar is oriented in the most cosmetically desirable direction. Marking the incision allows accurate, straight, and sure manipulation of the scalpel. Also, in areas of oblique skin tension, the first incision will cause the wound to gape obliquely, so the second incision to complete the ellipse may be inaccurate if not previously marked, leading to the formation of a dog ear.

Commercially available presterilized pens should be used. Ordinary ballpoint or felt-tip pens should never be used, as there is a small risk of tattooing with the ink left behind after wound closure.

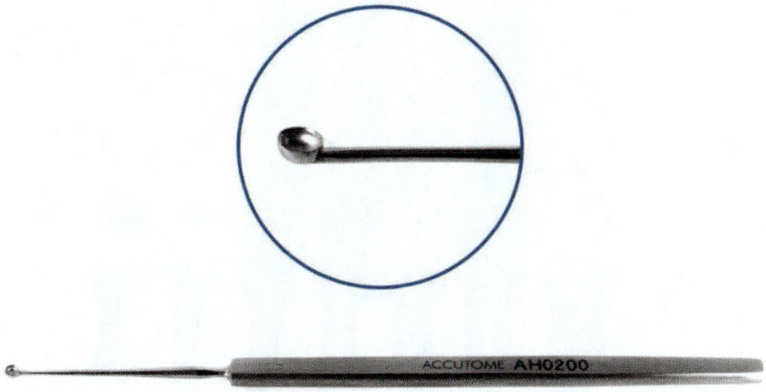


FIGURE 4-14 Meyerhoefer chalazion curette.

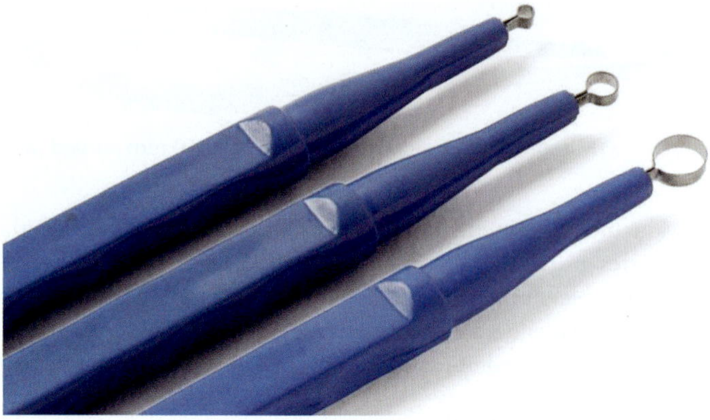

FIGURE 4-15 Disposable dermal curettes (varying diameters).

## SUTURES[18-21]

The choice of suture material affects the final appearance of the wound. Sutures are classified as either "absorbable" if the body breaks down and absorbs the material or "nonabsorbable" if it is not. Absorbable sutures are used in the subcutaneous tissue plane to reduce surface skin

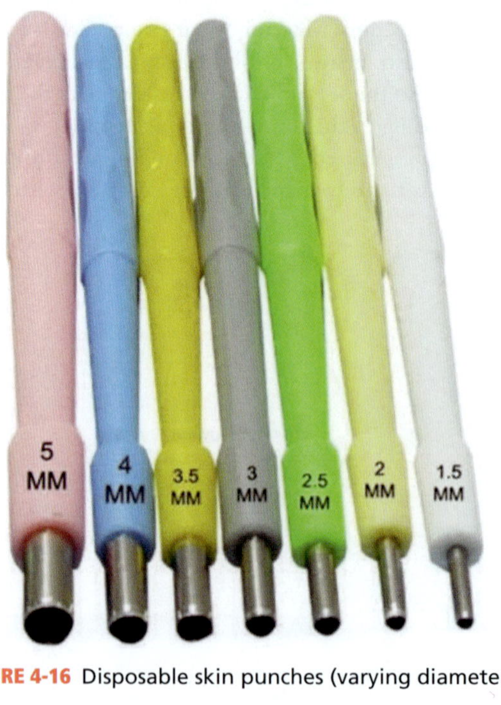


FIGURE 4-16 Disposable skin punches (varying diameters).

tension and strengthen the wound while the scar matures. Nonabsorbable sutures are usually used to approximate the skin surface and, on the eyelids, are usually removed within 5 to 7 days. Many different types of sutures are commercially available, and the practitioner's preference will determine the type used (Tables 4-4 and 4-5).

In skin surgery, sutures are usually mounted on a reverse-cutting curved needle. The needle is triangular in outline. The apex of the triangle (the cutting edge) points away from the skin's surface, helping to minimize any tendency of the suture to cut or cheese wire back out through the skin's surface. Sutures are sized according to the approximate cross section of the material. The higher the number in front of the "O," the thinner the material; for example, 4-0 is thicker than 6-0; 6-0 suture is a common size used on the face and eyelids.

Some suture materials may attempt to revert to their original configuration after they are placed in the tissue and tied. If this occurs, the suture is said to have memory. This is not a desirable characteristic, as knots may untie. Synthetic monofilament sutures, although preferred because they are inert and do not stimulate significant inflammatory reactions within the tissue, are a particular problem with regard to memory.

Absorbable sutures vary in composition, and this variation defines their respective properties. Polymerized materials that are dissolved by the body with a much-reduced inflammatory response, such as polyglycolic acid (Dexon), polyglactin (Vicryl), and polydioxanone (PDS), have superseded the older catgut and are now commonly used.

**TABLE 4-4 NONABSORBABLE SUTURE**

| SUTURE | ADVANTAGES | DISADVANTAGES | USES |
|---|---|---|---|
| • Silk | • Easy to tie<br>• Handles well with no memory<br>• Soft | • Bioactive<br>• May be colonized by microorganisms | • In areas where cosmetic appearance may be less important |
| • Ethilon | • Monofilament<br>• Relatively inert<br>• Has the least memory of the synthetic monofilament sutures | • Black color may be difficult to identify in hair.<br>• Blue-dyed is available. | • All superficial cutaneous suturing |
| • Prolene | • Monofilament<br>• Relatively inert<br>• Bright blue<br>• Easily identified in hair | • Memory is the greatest of all monofilament sutures. | • All superficial cutaneous suturing<br>• Useful in hair |
| • Novafil | • Monofilament<br>• Relatively inert<br>• High degree of elasticity<br>• Expands and contracts slightly with the wound tissues | • Intermediate memory | • All superficial cutaneous suturing |

**TABLE 4-5 ABSORBABLE SUTURES**

| SUTURE | ADVANTAGES | DISADVANTAGES | USES |
|---|---|---|---|
| • Dexon | • Less inflammatory response than with catgut<br>• Excellent knot security | • Intermediate longevity within the wound | • Buried sutures in all areas |
| • Vicryl | • Less inflammatory response than with catgut<br>• Excellent knot security<br>• More pliable and retains tensile strength longer than Dexon | | • Buried sutures in all areas |
| • PDS | • Less inflammatory response than catgut<br>• Retains tensile strength longer than Vicryl | • Has less pliability and more memory<br>• Knots may be less secure. | • Excellent for wounds under greatest tension or in areas where movement occurs |

## REFERENCES


1. Shen KT, Chang HC, Chen WL, et al. Design of microsurgical instruments for ophthalmology. *Proc Inst Mech Eng Part H: J Engineer Med.* 2005;219(4): 223-229.
2. Kosins TR. Designing an efficient and safe office-based surgery suite. *Clin Plast Surg.* 2012;39(3):405-411.
3. Kheirabadi GT, Crissey JL. Topical hemostatic agents for the management of bleeding in patients undergoing surgery. *J Blood Med.* 2015;6:245-256.
4. Tsung JW. Judkins SS. Roles and responsibilities of the surgical assistant in office-based surgery. *Clin Plast Surg.* 2013;40(4):521-530.
5. Rainchuso DL. Hazardous materials management in the dental office. *Dent Clin N Am.* 2019;63(4):553-567.
6. Mehta DK, Selvaraj BR. Handling and disposal of hazardous materials in the physician office. *Am Fam Physician.* 2019;99(12):759-766.
7. Petrilli JM. Sharps safety in the physician office setting. *J Am Board Fam Med.* 2015;28(5):655-661.
8. Bono AL, Cash JC. Infection control in office-based surgery. *J Am Acad Orthop Surg.* 2014;22(12):771-777.
9. DeLong KR, Siegel EL. Infection control in office-based dermatologic surgery. *Dermatol Clin.* 2018;36(3):239-247.
10. Clayton JL, Hoehn RA. Establishing a sterile field for office-based surgery. *Am Fam Physician.* 2014;89(5):342-348.
11. Glaser ME, Hsu KG. Establishing and maintaining a sterile field in the outpatient setting. *Aesthet Surg J.* 2017;37(2):237-243.
12. Linberg JA, Friedman AS. Sterile technique for office-based procedures. *Am Fam Physician.* 2015;92(6):516-522.
13. Tackett EJ, Kremer T, Rich JD, Alfandre D. Risk of blood-borne infection transmission in office-based surgical facilities. *J Gen Intern Med.* 2017;32(9):1016-1021.
14. Gershon KM, Karkashian CD, Vlahov D, et al. Transmission of blood-borne pathogens in US outpatient settings: a systematic review. *BMC Infect Dis.* 2009;9(1):1-23.
15. Centers for Disease Control and Prevention. Guideline for disinfection and sterilization in healthcare facilities. 2008. https://www.cdc.gov/infectioncontrol/guidelines/disinfection/index.html
16. Dozier JW, Culbertson JM. Surgical instrumentation for office-based ophthalmic surgery. *Surv Ophthalmol.* 2005;50(3):265-272.
17. Widder RP, Dietlein KA. Surgical instruments for office-based ophthalmic surgery. *Ophthalmologe.* 2016;113(10):828-834.
18. Hwang SM, Goldberg RA. Suture selection in oculoplastic surgery. *Curr Opin Ophthalmol.* 2014;25(5):441-447.
19. Yoon D, Kim JH. Surgical sutures in ophthalmic plastic surgery: a review. *Arch Plast Surg.* 2020;47(5):419-425.
20. Park SB, Lee JY, Kim SG. Surgical sutures in ophthalmic plastic surgery: a practical review. *J Korean Ophthalmol Soc.* 2017;58(11):1162-1168.
21. Yen JT. Suture materials and techniques in oculofacial plastic surgery. *Asia Pac J Ophthalmol.* 2016;5(4):274-281.

# 5 Local Anesthesia of the Eyelids and Periorbita

Richard E. Castillo

## INTRODUCTION TO PERIOCULAR LOCAL (INFILTRATIVE) ANESTHESIA AND REGIONAL BLOCKS

Periocular wound evaluation, creation, and management often necessitate using anesthetic agents for anesthesia, analgesia, or akinesia. Local infiltration of anesthetic agents directly into a wound site is an effective method of anesthesia administration for many distinct types of wounds. The standard technique of local infiltrative injection has several benefits, including ease of administration, reliability, and safety when proper procedures are employed and toxicity levels are not exceeded. Additionally, the infiltration of anesthetic agents containing epinephrine facilitates local hemostasis.[1-3]

Infiltrative local anesthesia also presents some disadvantages when dealing with the thin skin of the eyelids and periorbita. The infiltration of anesthetic agents in and around wounds can alter the anatomy and make the subsequent repair more challenging. Infiltrative anesthesia also frequently requires multiple injections.[4] Table 5-1 provides an overview of the

**TABLE 5-1** ADVANTAGES AND DISADVANTAGES OF TYPES OF CUTANEOUS ANESTHESIA

| TYPE OF ANESTHESIA | ADVANTAGES | DISADVANTAGES |
|---|---|---|
| Local | Ease of administration<br>Reliability | May require large volume of anesthetic<br>May be painful in certain locations<br>Distorts anatomy, impeding optimal wound edge approximation |
| Topical | Painless<br>Does not distort anatomy | Not always dependable (works best on face)<br>Danger of absorption if used on mucus membranes<br>Cannot be used on areas with end-arteriolar circulation |
| Regional | Does not distort anatomy<br>Requires lower volume of anesthetic<br>Fewer injections | Only useful in certain locations<br>Not as dependable as local anesthesia |

advantages and disadvantages of local anesthetic agents, topical anesthetic agents, and nerve blocks. This chapter will focus on direct infiltrative anesthesia and the two common methods of regional anesthesia administered around the eyelids and periorbita, the supraorbital and infraorbital block. Unless otherwise stated, the local anesthetic agent being referenced will be lidocaine.

Lidocaine is the most common local anesthetic employed for infiltrative and regional anesthesia.[5] It is available in several concentrations, 0.5%, 1%, 2%, and 4%, although the latter is not used for infiltrative anesthesia or regional block. Lidocaine is also frequently available as a solution containing epinephrine at concentrations of 1:100,000 or 1:200,000. For vasoconstriction and hemostasis of superficial skin procedures, epinephrine at a concentration of 1:100,000 offers little advantage over half the concentration at 1:200,000. The maximum adult dose of lidocaine is 4.5 mg/kg, not to exceed 300 mg total. The maximum adult dose of lidocaine with epinephrine is 7 mg/kg, not to exceed 500 mg total.[6]

## INFILTRATIVE ANESTHESIA: MINIMIZING THE PAIN OF INJECTION

Local infiltration of anesthetic agents directly into the area requiring anesthesia is highly effective and dependable; however, it is also associated with appreciable pain and anxiety.[7] Several strategies can be implemented to reduce the discomfort associated with an anesthetic injection, particularly in the office setting, without the need for conscious sedation.[8,9] Numerous studies have identified five principal factors that have been shown to impact the pain of anesthetic infiltration into the tissue; these include the following:

- Type of anesthetic
- Needle size (gauge)
- pH
- The temperature of the solution
- Speed and depth of injection

The following strategies and techniques may be employed to minimize the pain of local anesthetic injection:

- Buffering the anesthetic solution[10]
    - Raising the pH (alkalinization) with sodium bicarbonate 8.4% (one part sodium bicarbonate 8.4% to nine parts lidocaine solution) increases the bioavailability of lidocaine entering the nerve axon speeding up the onset of the anesthetic effect.
    - Buffered lidocaine can be utilized up to 1 week postpreparation without observing a notable change in its efficacy.
- Warming the anesthetic solution[3,10]
    - Warming the anesthetic solution to just slightly above body temperature (98°F–100°F) also raises the pH of the solution, hastening the onset of the anesthetic effect and minimizing discomfort.
- Injecting deeper into the tissue[2,3,11]
    - For example, administering a subcutaneous injection instead of an intradermal injection

- Note that a conventional subcutaneous injection is not possible in the eyelid itself due to the absence of a defined subcutaneous tissue plane. Administration of infiltrative anesthesia into the eyelid should always be delivered via an intradermal approach.
- Exceptions to the "intradermal rule in the eyelid" above would include an intralesional injection (e.g., injection of a chalazion with steroid) or chemical denervation with botulinum toxin, where an intramuscular injection technique is utilized.

- Slowing down the injection rate[2,3,11]
  - Allows for the nociceptors (pain receptors) in the skin to accommodate for the distortion caused by the dissection and separation of the respective tissue plane by the anesthetic bolus.
- Injecting from inside an open wound[11]
  - Injecting below the level of the dermis bypasses most cutaneous nociceptors, which are located primarily in the epidermis and upper dermis (epidermal–dermal junction).
- Using no larger than a 27-gauge or 30-gauge needle to administer injections to the sensitive skin of the eyelids and periorbita[8,11]
- Pretreating wounds with topical tetracaine has been shown to reduce the pain of anesthetic injection by close to 50% compared to a placebo.[10,11]
  - The topical application of a compounded solution of lidocaine, epinephrine, and tetracaine (LET) has been shown to reduce the pain of an injection.[12]
  - Note: LET is safe on intact skin but should *never* be used in the eye or on mucous membranes such as the conjunctiva or the cornea.
- The topical application of a eutectic mixture of lidocaine 2.5% and prilocaine 2.5% (EMLA Cream) is more expensive than LET but has also been shown to reduce the pain of anesthetic injection. EMLA cannot be used in the eye, the conjunctiva, or the cornea.[12]

Buffering the anesthetic solution with sodium bicarbonate before infiltrating the tissue is the most effective technique to reduce the pain associated with the injection. Local anesthetic agents are weak bases prepared in moderately acidic solutions to extend their shelf life. Numerous studies have confirmed that buffering the solution to near physiologic pH can reduce the pain of infiltration.[10] This may be due to increasing the ratio of uncharged to charged molecules as the pH of the solution approaches the anesthetic's pKa (the point at which you have equal concentrations of charged and uncharged species). Because only uncharged molecules are readily diffusible across cell membranes, the onset of anesthesia is more rapid, leading to potentially less painful infiltration. Anesthetic agents can be buffered by adding a small amount of sodium bicarbonate (1 mEq/mL) in a 9:1 or 10:1 dilution to the anesthetic solution. For example, this can be achieved by adding 2 mL of sodium bicarbonate to a 20-mL vial of anesthetic agent.[10,11]

## PERIOCULAR INFILTRATIVE ANESTHESIA: SAFETY

Several techniques should be utilized to maintain safety when administering injections into the eyelid or around the eye. Knowledge of the regional anatomy (Chapter 3), particularly the distribution of nerves and vasculature, is essential for the safe administration of anesthetic agents around the eye.[12-15]

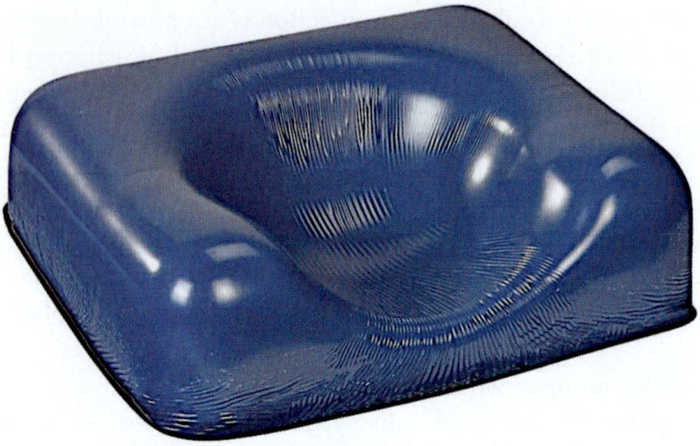

FIGURE 5-1 Gel headrest.

The following strategies should be employed whenever possible to maximize safety during eyelid or periocular anesthetic injection:

- Utilize a corneal shield to protect the globe (Video 5-1).
- Never point the tip of the needle in the direction of the globe.
- When injecting the eyelids, use an intradermal technique.
- After inserting and advancing the needle, aspirate and check for a flash of blood at the needle's hub. If a flash is observed, withdraw the needle, reposition the needle, and check again.
- To minimize the risk of intravascular injection, never inject the anesthetic solution, especially epinephrine-containing solutions, while advancing the needle. Insert and position the needle at the far point of its travel first, then aspirate and check for a flash, and only inject as you withdraw the needle.
- Adequately support the patient's head and neck when performing eyelid and periocular injections. Ideally, the patient should be supine and immobilized in a headrest. Various options are available today, including convenient gel-filled headrests, which are economical, easy to care for, and provide a safe level of immobilization (Figure 5-1).

## INFILTRATIVE ANESTHESIA

Local or infiltrative anesthesia refers to injecting an anesthetic agent such as lidocaine directly into the tissue. Local anesthesia is commonly used for superficial excisions, curettage procedures, skin biopsies, and other minor surgical procedures involving the eyelids and the periocular skin. Local anesthesia is typically administered via intradermal or subcutaneous injection.[1-4]

- Indications[1-4]
  - Analgesia
  - Anesthesia
  - Akinesia

- Primary wound closure
- Adjunct to general anesthesia
- Contraindications[16,17]
  - Allergy or sensitivity to the anesthetic agent or a component of the anesthetic solution
  - Distortion of anatomical tissue planes and landmarks
  - Preexisting infection at the proposed injection site
  - An uncooperative patient
- Preoperative preparation
  - Anesthetic agent
    - Lidocaine 0.5%, 1%, or 2% with or without epinephrine 1:100,000 or 1:200,000
    - Bupivacaine 0.25% with or without epinephrine 1:100,000 or 1:200,000
    - Hypodermic needles
      - 27 gauge to 30 gauge to inject the eyelids and face, varying lengths
      - 18 gauge to withdraw/prepare the syringe, 1.5 inch
    - Syringes (Luer-Lok), for example, 1 mL, 3 mL, and 5 mL
    - Nonsterile and sterile gloves
    - Isopropyl alcohol pads
    - Povidone–iodine solution
    - Sterile gauze 4 × 4
    - Sterile cotton balls
- Procedure[1-4,11,15]
  - An informed consent must be obtained.
  - The patient should be supine with the head immobilized in a headrest or comfortably reclined in a procedure chair with the head immobilized.
  - Clean the injection site with a povidone–iodine solution or isopropyl alcohol.
  - Use a 27-gauge to 30-gauge sterile needle and syringe to administer injections into the eyelids or face.
  - For injections into the eyelid, insert and advance the needle within the intradermal plane. A deeper, subcutaneous approach may be employed for injections outside the orbital rim.
  - Advance the needle, positioning it where required in the tissue, adjacent to a lesion, or surrounding it as in a field block.
  - Lacerations may be injected from inside the open wound.
  - Using the proper injection technique (aspirate before injection), raise a small skin wheal over or adjacent to the area of regard (~0.5–1 mL).
  - Eliciting paresthesia before injecting signifies that the needle tip is close to the nerve, and the needle must be withdrawn 1 to 2 mm to avoid intraneural injection.
  - Following injection, provide mechanical deturgescence of the anesthetic bolus with gentle tissue massage utilizing a gauze 4 × 4 or a cotton ball.
  - If the needle tip is in the proper position, slow injection of the anesthetic should be minimally painful and meet minor to no resistance.
  - Lidocaine exerts its full anesthetic effect in less than 2 minutes. Epinephrine in the solution requires 5 to 10 minutes to exert its full vasoconstrictive effect.
  - Check for the appropriate level of anesthesia by pinching the skin with forceps before commencing the procedure.

- Postoperative care/comanagement (follow-up schedule)
  - As local anesthesia is a component of the procedure, scheduled postoperative care is dictated by the nature and extent of the procedure.
- Potential complications and their treatment[15-17]: Known complications and their management include:
  - Bleeding and hematoma formation
    - Direct pressure with a gauze pad over the bleed or developing hematoma is usually sufficient to limit progression.
  - An allergic or systemic reaction to the anesthetic agent or components of the anesthetic solution
    - All providers should be current and certified in Basic Life Support and have a rehearsed plan of action to manage emergencies in their office should they occur.
    - Resuscitative equipment, including oxygen availability, airways, automatic defibrillators, epinephrine for intramuscular administration, and equipment to monitor vital signs, must always be available.
  - Infection
    - Anesthetic injections should never be administered through an area believed to be infected.
  - Inadvertent intravascular injection
    - Proper injection technique, familiarity with the regional anatomy (Chapter 3), and aspirating before injecting are essential for safe administration.
    - Injecting as one withdraws the needle from the tissue also helps minimize the risk of intravascular injection. As mentioned earlier, anesthetic compounds should never be injected as the needle is advanced through the tissues before aspirating.
  - Failure to achieve the desired level of anesthesia, analgesia, or akinesia
    - Adequate mechanical deturgescence to distribute the anesthetic and waiting at least 2 minutes if lidocaine was used (between 5 and 10 minutes if epinephrine was included in the solution) should allow for maximum anesthetic effect.
  - Nerve damage
    - Paresthesia (tingling, stinging, electric shock sensation) after needle advancement and before commencing the anesthetic injection implies the needle tip is too close to a nerve and should be slightly withdrawn to avoid intraneural injection.
  - Swelling of the eyelid
    - Gentle tissue massage with a gauze 4 × 4 or cotton ball (mechanical deturgescence) may help distribute the fluid bolus and reduce localized tissue edema.
- Video of procedure (Video 5-2 infiltrative anesthesia)
- Efficacy[3,5,7]
  - The efficacy of local infiltrative anesthesia depends on several factors, including the type and dose of the anesthetic agent used, the technique of administration, the location of the injection site, and the individual patient's response to the medication.
- Coding/billing and modifiers
  - Procedural anesthesia is bundled with the procedure code; no separate charges can be generated.

## REGIONAL ANESTHESIA: NERVE BLOCKS

Nerve blocks are used to provide anesthesia to several body regions. The upper eyelid and forehead are amenable to a supraorbital block, whereas the lower eyelid and upper maxilla are amenable to an infraorbital block. These blocks typically require a lower anesthetic volume than local infiltration and do not distort the regional anatomy. Nerve blocks can often be accomplished with a single injection; however, proper knowledge of anatomy is essential for a successful outcome. During the injection, patients may experience paresthesia (a burning or tingling sensation). It is important to carefully identify landmarks such as the supraorbital fissure and the infraorbital foramen to ensure the proper needle placement and anesthetic placement.[18]

Paresthesias indicate that the needle is too close to the target nerve. If paresthesias are experienced, the needle should be slightly withdrawn and the agent reinjected. Aspiring before administering the anesthetic is essential to avoid accidentally injecting into a blood vessel. Once the anesthetic has been injected, mechanical deturgescence (gentle massage) can help distribute it along the blocked nerve. It should be noted that it may take several minutes for a nerve block to take effect. If it is unsuccessful, the practitioner may choose to repeat the block or opt for local anesthesia, keeping in mind that the maximum dose should not be exceeded.[19,20]

## REGIONAL NERVE BLOCKS IN OPHTHALMIC EYELID AND PERIOCULAR PROCEDURES

Optimum cosmetic outcomes of facial lacerations require careful attention to matching wound layers precisely. Regional nerve blocks are advantageous in these instances due to their ability to preserve local anatomical relationships and because of their ease of administration. Two standard regional blocks that involve the eyelids and periorbita are the supraorbital and infraorbital blocks. These nerves, the supraorbital ($V_1$) and infraorbital ($V_2$), exit from foramina that lie along a plane passing through the pupil's medial aspect to the mouth's corner (Figures 5-2 and 5-3).[18,20]

The sensory innervation of the face is depicted in Figure 5-2. Recall that the supraorbital nerve provides sensation to most of the forehead and the upper eyelid. The most medial aspect of the forehead is supplied by the supratrochlear nerve. The infraorbital nerve is responsible for sensation to the skin of the medial two-thirds of the lower eyelid and the upper lip, including the cheek. The lateral third of the lower eyelid is enervated by the zygomaticofacial nerve and is best anesthetized via a direct infiltrative block to this region.[18-21]

The supraorbital nerve can be blocked at the supraorbital foramen or notch, where it exits, and the supratrochlear nerve can be blocked 5 to 10 mm medial to the supraorbital foramen or notch. The needle is directed immediately above or adjacent to the supraorbital foramen or notch via an intradermal or subcutaneous approach after which the anesthetic agent is injected. The supratrochlear branch can be blocked by extending the supraorbital block medially, raising a subcutaneous wheal of anesthetic directly above and parallel to the medial head of the eyebrow.[22,23]

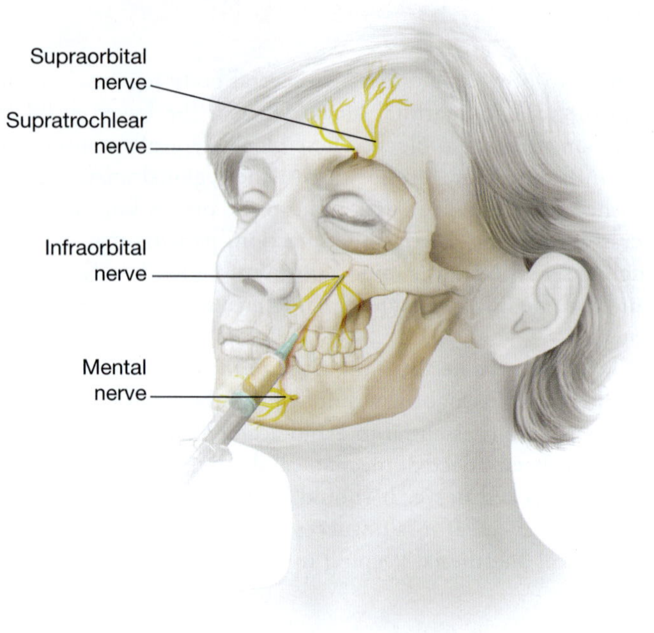


**FIGURE 5-2** Sensory distribution of the trigeminal nerve (CN V) on the face. Shown is the ophthalmic division (V1) of the trigeminal nerve also referred to as the supraorbital nerve, and the infraorbital foramen and maxillary division (V2) of the trigeminal nerve, also known as the infraorbital nerve. The mandibular division (V3) of the trigeminal nerve, also known as the mental nerve, is also included. The supratrochlear nerve is also shown medial to the supraorbital nerve. (Reprinted with permission from Chung KC. *Grabb and Smith's Plastic Surgery*. 8th ed. Wolters Kluwer; 2020:107; Figure 12.1.)

The infraorbital nerve can be blocked through either intact skin or the buccal mucosa. The infraorbital foramen, which is easily palpable, can be located along the previously described line just below the inferior border of the orbit.[24] The infraorbital nerve can be blocked by inserting a needle through the skin along a horizontal plane lateral to the infraorbital foramen, and advancing toward the infraorbital foramen, as illustrated in Figure 5-3.

Alternatively, the infraorbital nerve can be blocked through the buccal mucosa by inserting a 0.5-inch 30-gauge needle to the hub into the buccal–mucosal sulcus opposite the upper canine and palpating the foramen as the anesthetic agent is introduced. Care must be taken to introduce the needle along the surface of the maxilla to avoid the globe and not perforate through the skin of the face.[24-26]

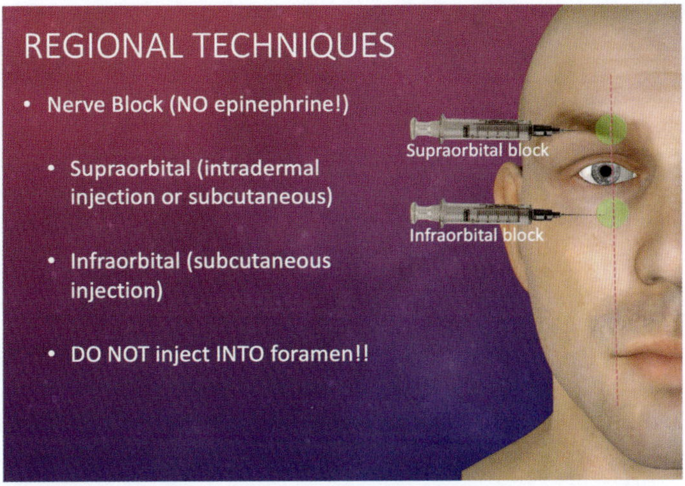


**FIGURE 5-3** Position of supraorbital foramen or notch and infraorbital foramen, depicting the lateral approach. Note the supraorbital foramen or notch and infraorbital foramen generally lie along a plane that intersects the medial aspect of the pupil and the corner of the mouth.

## LOCAL ANESTHETIC AGENTS: DOSE, TOXICITY, EPINEPHRINE AND HYALURONIDASE

Regarding the use of local anesthetic agents, it is essential to be mindful of dose-related toxicities.[17] Although dosing by weight is useful for pediatric patients, maximum safe doses for adults are typically expressed as absolute amounts because weight does not always correlate well with peak anesthetic drug levels in adults.[27] For example, the maximum safe amount of plain lidocaine in an adult patient is 300 mg, equivalent to 30 mL of a 1% solution. This dose refers to subcutaneous or intradermal injections. However, toxicity may occur at a much lower dose if the anesthetic is accidentally injected into a blood vessel. Table 5-2 provides commonly accepted maximum doses for various local anesthetics.[27,28]

Adding epinephrine to local anesthetic agents for infiltrative blocks at a concentration of around 1:100,000 or 1:200,000 can help increase the safety of injecting larger amounts of the agent.[17,27-29] Epinephrine's vasoconstrictive properties reduce systemic absorption while providing hemostasis and a less bloody surgical field. Despite these benefits, using epinephrine has some disadvantages, contraindications, and complications such as local ischemia and precipitating a hypertensive crisis must be considered.[4] Although epinephrine is commonly believed to increase the risk of wound infections, clinical trials have not proven this.[30] Additionally, injecting anesthetic agents that contain epinephrine can be more painful. Epinephrine is never used in the anesthetic solution for regional nerve blocks.

Hyaluronidase 7.5 IU/mL added to the local anesthetic has been shown to improve peribulbar block. The addition of hyaluronidase in intradermal or subcutaneous injections for

**TABLE 5-2 MAXIMUM SAFE DOSES OF COMMONLY USED LOCAL ANESTHETICS**

| DRUG | ADULT MAX DOSE (MG) | PEDS MAX DOSE (MG/KG) |
|---|---|---|
| **Lidocaine** | 300 | 4 |
| **Lidocaine with epi** | 500 | 7 |
| **Bupivacaine** | 175 | 1.5 |
| **Bupivacaine with epi** | 225 | 3 |

superficial eyelid or periocular cutaneous procedures needs to be considered by the practitioner in terms of the minimal benefit to comfort and efficacy versus the additional cost involved.[26]

## Supraorbital Block

The supraorbital nerve supplies sensory innervation to the upper eyelid, forehead, and scalp (Figure 5-2). Because the supraorbital nerve provides a large area of sensory innervation, it is a prime candidate for a regional nerve block (see Chapter 3).

- Indications[1-4]
  - Analgesia
  - Anesthesia
  - Akinesia
  - Primary wound closure
  - Adjunct to general anesthesia
- Contraindications[16,17]
  - Allergy or sensitivity to the anesthetic agent or component of the anesthetic solution
  - Distortion of anatomical tissue planes and landmarks
  - Preexisting infection at the proposed injection site
  - Uncooperative patient
- Preoperative preparation
  - Anesthetic agent
    - Lidocaine 0.5%, 1%, or 2% **without** epinephrine
    - Bupivacaine 0.25% **without** epinephrine
    - Hypodermic needles
      - 27 gauge to 30 gauge to inject the eyelids and face, varying lengths
      - 18 gauge to withdraw/prepare the syringe, 1.5 inch
    - Syringes (Luer-Lok), for example, 1 mL, 3 mL, and 5 mL
    - Nonsterile and sterile gloves
    - Isopropyl alcohol pads
    - Povidone–iodine solution
    - Sterile gauze 4 × 4
    - Sterile cotton balls

- Procedure
  - An informed consent must be obtained.
  - The patient should be supine with the head immobilized in a headrest or comfortably reclined in a procedure chair with the head immobilized.
  - The supraorbital nerve exits via the supraorbital foramen or notch, 2 cm to 3 cm lateral to the facial midline, along the inferior edge of the supraorbital ridge.
  - Clean the injection site with povidone–iodine solution or isopropyl alcohol.
  - Palpate the superior orbital ridge and locate the supraorbital foramen or notch.
  - Use a 27-gauge to 30-gauge sterile needle and syringe.
  - Insert and advance the needle within the intradermal plane, positioning it directly above the supraorbital foramen or notch along the supraorbital ridge (Figure 5-3).
  - Injecting above the supraorbital ridge rather than below and utilizing an intradermal instead of a subcutaneous approach minimizes the amount of anesthetic that infuses into the upper lid causing unwanted distortion of the tissues.
  - Using proper injection technique (aspirate before injection), raise a small skin wheal over the area (~0.5–1 mL).
  - Placing either a finger or a small gauze roll (dental roll) under the superior orbital rim below the supraorbital foramen or notch may prevent infiltration of the anesthetic into the upper lid.
  - Gently compressing/collapsing the supraorbital artery with a finger as it emerges from the supraorbital foramen or notch may further reduce the risk of inadvertent intravascular injection.
  - Eliciting paresthesia after positioning the needle and before injecting confirms that the needle tip is close to the nerve. To avoid intraneural injection, the needle must be withdrawn 1 to 2 mm before the anesthetic is injected.
  - Do not inject directly into the foramen or notch.
  - If the needle tip is in the proper position, slow injection of the anesthetic should be minimally painful and meet little to no resistance.
  - Lidocaine exerts its full anesthetic effect in less than 2 minutes.
  - Check for the appropriate level of anesthesia by pinching the skin with forceps prior to commencing the procedure.
- Postoperative care/comanagement (follow-up schedule)
  - As local anesthesia is a component of the procedure of regard being performed, scheduled postoperative care is dictated by the nature and extent of the procedure performed.
- Potential complications and their treatment[15-17]: Known complications and their management include:
  - Bleeding and hematoma formation
    - Direct pressure with a gauze pad over the bleed or developing hematoma is usually sufficient to limit progression.
  - An allergic or systemic reaction to the anesthetic agent or components of the anesthetic solution
    - All providers should be current and certified in Basic Life Support and have a rehearsed plan of action to manage emergencies in their office should they occur.
    - Resuscitative equipment, including oxygen availability, airways, automatic defibrillators, epinephrine for intramuscular administration, and equipment to monitor vital signs, must always be available.

- Infection
  - Anesthetic injections should never be administered through an area believed to be infected.
- Inadvertent intravascular injection
  - Proper injection techniques should always be followed, including being familiar with the regional anatomy (Chapter 3) and aspirating and checking for a flash of blood at the needle hub before injecting.
  - Injecting as one withdraws the needle from the tissue also helps minimize the risk of intravascular injection. As mentioned earlier, anesthetic compounds should never be injected as the needle is advanced through the tissues before aspirating.
- Failure to achieve the desired level of anesthesia, analgesia, or akinesia
  - Adequate mechanical deturgescence to distribute the anesthetic and waiting at least 2 minutes if lidocaine was used (between 5 and 10 minutes if epinephrine was included in the solution) should allow for maximum anesthetic effect.
- Nerve damage
  - Paresthesia (tingling, stinging, electric shock sensation) after needle advancement and prior to commencing the anesthetic injection implies the needle tip is too close to a nerve and should be slightly withdrawn to avoid intraneural injection.
- Swelling of the eyelid
  - Gentle tissue massage with a gauze 4 × 4 or cotton ball (mechanical deturgescence) may help distribute the fluid bolus and reduce localized tissue edema.

- Video of procedure (Video 5-3 supraorbital block)
- Efficacy[3,5,7]
  - The efficacy of local infiltrative anesthesia depends on several factors, including the type and dose of the anesthetic agent used, the technique of administration, the location of the injection site, and the individual patient's response to the medication.
- Coding/billing and modifiers
  - Procedural anesthesia is bundled with the procedure code; no separate charges can be generated.

## Infraorbital Block

The infraorbital nerve innervates the medial two-thirds of the lower eyelid, the skin of the cheek, the upper lip, the lateral aspect of the nose, and the ipsilateral upper teeth. This nerve is located along the medial pupillary line approximately 0.7 to 1.0 cm below the infraorbital rim (Figure 5-3).

- Indications[1-4]
  - Analgesia
  - Anesthesia
  - Akinesia
  - Primary wound closure
  - Adjunct to general anesthesia
- Contraindications[16,17]
  - Allergy or sensitivity to the anesthetic agent or component of the anesthetic solution

- Distortion of anatomical tissue planes and landmarks
- Preexisting infection at the proposed injection site
- Uncooperative patient

- Preoperative preparation
  - Anesthetic agent
    - Lidocaine 0.5%, 1%, or 2% **without** epinephrine
    - Bupivacaine 0.25% **without** epinephrine
    - Hypodermic needles
      - 27 gauge to 30 gauge to inject the eyelids and face, varying lengths
      - 18 gauge to withdraw/prepare the syringe, 1.5 inch
    - Syringes (Luer-Lok), for example, 1 mL, 3 mL, and 5 mL
    - Nonsterile and sterile gloves
    - Isopropyl alcohol pads
    - Povidone–iodine solution
    - Sterile gauze 4 × 4
    - Sterile cotton balls
    - Procedure
  - An informed consent must be obtained.
  - The patient should be supine with the head immobilized in a headrest or comfortably reclined in a procedure chair with the head immobilized.
  - The infraorbital nerve exits via the infraorbital foramen, approximately 3 cm lateral to the facial midline and 0.7 to 1 cm below the inferior orbital rim in line with a perpendicular plane passing through the supraorbital foramen and medial pupillary border (Figure 5-3).
  - Clean the injection site utilizing a povidone–iodine solution or isopropyl alcohol.
  - Palpate the inferior orbital ridge and locate the infraorbital foramen.
  - Use a 27-gauge to 30-gauge, 1-inch sterile needle and syringe.
  - Insert and advance the needle from the lateral aspect along the horizontal plane, positioning the needle tip approximately 2 mm lateral to the infraorbital foramen.
  - Using proper injection technique (aspirate prior to injection), raise a small skin wheal over the area (~0.5–1 mL).
  - Eliciting paresthesia before injecting confirms that the needle tip is too close to the nerve. To avoid intraneural injection, the needle must be withdrawn 1 to 2 mm before the anesthetic is injected.
  - Do not inject directly into the foramen.
  - If the needle tip is in the proper position, slow injection of the anesthetic should be minimally painful and meet little to no resistance.
  - Provide mechanical deturgescence by gently massaging the area with gauze 4 × 4 or a cotton ball.
  - Lidocaine exerts its full anesthetic effect in less than 2 minutes.
  - Check for the appropriate level of anesthesia by pinching the skin with forceps prior to commencing the procedure.

- Postoperative care/comanagement (follow-up schedule)
  - As local anesthesia is a component of the procedure of regard being performed, scheduled postoperative care is dictated by the nature and extent of the procedure performed.

- Potential complications and their treatment[15-17]: Known complications and their management include:
  - Bleeding and hematoma formation
    - Direct pressure with a gauze pad over the bleed or developing hematoma is usually sufficient to limit progression.
  - An allergic or systemic reaction to the anesthetic agent or components of the anesthetic solution
    - All providers should be current and certified in Basic Life Support and have a rehearsed plan of action to manage emergencies in their office should they occur.
    - Resuscitative equipment, including oxygen availability, airways, automatic defibrillators, epinephrine for intramuscular administration, and equipment to monitor vital signs, must always be available.
  - Infection
    - Anesthetic injections should never be administered through an area believed to be infected.
  - Inadvertent intravascular injection
    - Proper injection techniques should always be followed, including being familiar with the regional anatomy (Chapter 3) and aspirating and checking for a flash of blood at the needle hub before injecting.
    - Injecting as one withdraws the needle from the tissue also helps minimize the risk of intravascular injection. As mentioned earlier, anesthetic compounds should never be injected as the needle is advanced through the tissues before aspirating.
  - Failure to achieve the desired level of anesthesia, analgesia, or akinesia.
    - Adequate mechanical deturgescence to distribute the anesthetic and waiting at least 2 minutes if lidocaine was used (between 5 and 10 minutes if epinephrine was included in the solution) should allow for maximum anesthetic effect.
  - Nerve damage
    - Paresthesia (tingling, stinging, electric shock sensation) after needle advancement and prior to commencing the anesthetic injection implies the needle tip is too close to a nerve and should be slightly withdrawn to avoid intraneural injection.
  - Swelling of the eyelid
    - Gentle tissue massage with a gauze 4 × 4 or cotton ball (mechanical deturgescence) may help distribute the fluid bolus and reduce localized tissue edema.
- Video of procedure (Video 5-4 infraorbital block)
- Efficacy[3,5,7]
  - The efficacy of local infiltrative anesthesia depends on several factors, including the type and dose of the anesthetic agent used, the technique of administration, the location of the injection site, and the individual patient's response to the medication.
- Coding/billing and modifiers
  - Procedural anesthesia is bundled with the procedure code; no separate charges can be generated.

## Allergies to Local Anesthetics

Patients often report allergies to local anesthetics, but true anaphylaxis, particularly to amides, is rare. Testing patients with reported lidocaine allergies has shown that few reactions are true allergies. However, anaphylaxis is a dangerous complication to avoid. It is important to differentiate between a true reaction and a vasovagal reaction to evaluate a patient claiming an allergy. An anesthetic from a different class can be used if the specific allergen is known. A "true" allergy to lidocaine is often to methylparaben, the preservative in multidose vials, not the lidocaine itself. The ester anesthetics, like procaine and tetracaine, can cause a similar reaction due to para-aminobenzoic acid (PABA), a chemical related to methylparaben. If a patient is confirmed allergic to methylparaben, single-dose lidocaine without preservatives can be used. However, it is challenging to make this distinction, so alternatives to traditional anesthetics are constantly being sought.[31,32]

# ALTERNATIVES TO TRADITIONAL ANESTHETIC AGENTS

Patients who report an allergy to local anesthetic agents can consider alternative options. Two of these alternatives are 1% diphenhydramine and 0.9% benzyl alcohol.

Diphenhydramine (Benadryl) is an antihistamine that can be used instead of lidocaine. The chemical structure is similar to local anesthetics, but cross-reactivity is not a concern. Although 1% diphenhydramine provides anesthesia comparable to 1% lidocaine, it is more painful to administer and may cause side effects such as sedation, local irritation, erythema, vesicle formation, tissue necrosis, and prolonged anesthesia. As a result, another alternative to "caine" anesthetics is desirable for patients allergic to lidocaine.[33,34]

Benzyl alcohol (found in multidose normal saline as a preservative) provides good anesthesia with minimal pain of infiltration. It is low in toxicity, even when used parenterally. Compared with five other anesthetic agents, benzyl alcohol was found to be the least painful. However, its duration of action is limited and only lasts a few minutes. The duration can be extended by adding epinephrine at 1:100,000. Compared with 1% diphenhydramine and 0.9% buffered lidocaine, benzyl alcohol with epinephrine was found to be the least painful. Although it caused slightly less pain than lidocaine with epinephrine, practitioners should know that its duration may be short in the clinical setting. A solution containing benzyl alcohol with epinephrine can be made by adding 0.2 mL of epinephrine 1:1,000 to a 20 mL vial of multidose normal saline containing 0.9% benzyl alcohol.[35]

## VIDEOS OF PROCEDURES

**Video 5-1**—Inserting a corneal shield.

**Video 5-2**—Infiltrative anesthesia of lesions (seborrheic keratoses) of the lower eyelid and upper cheek.

**Video 5-3**—Supraorbital nerve block.

**Video 5-4**—Infraorbital nerve block.

# REFERENCES


1. Boyce MJ, Boulton ME. Local anaesthesia for ophthalmic surgery. *Eye (Lond)*. 2003;17(8):907-914.
2. Vagefi MR, Lin CC, McCann JD, Anderson RL. Techniques of local anesthesia for eyelid surgery: a survey of the American Society of Ophthalmic Plastic and Reconstructive Surgery. *Ophthal Plast Reconstr Surg*. 2007;23(3):194-198.
3. Dutton JJ. Local anesthesia for ophthalmic surgery. *Ophthalmol Clin North Am*. 2006;19(2):217-224.
4. Hunter-Smith DJ, Srinivasan K, Hill AG. Local anaesthesia in plastic surgery and the potential dangers of adrenaline. *ANZ J Surg*. 2004;74(10):859-863.
5. Langford AJ, Katzung JM, McKell JG. Lidocaine as a local anaesthetic: early studies and current indications. *Br J Anaesth*. 2017;118(3):333-337.
6. Lidocaine Hydrochloride—Drug Summary. Lexicomp® Online, Adult Drug Information. Wolters Kluwer Clinical Drug Information, Inc. Accessed February 28, 2023.
7. Shrestha BR, Maharjan SK, Singh R. Pain perception and management with local anesthesia. *J Inst Med*. 2019;41(2):77-80.
8. Moore PA, Boynes SG. A review of 20 years' experience with injection pain—does the needle size matter? *J Am Dent Assoc*. 1997;128(suppl):33S-40S.
9. Haas DA, Lennon D. A 21 year retrospective study of reports of paresthesia following local anesthetic administration. *J Can Dent Assoc*. 1995;61(4):319-320, 323-326, 329-330.
10. Yagiela JA, Messer HH. pH changes in dental local anesthetic solutions. *J Am Dent Assoc*. 1984;109(4):626-629.
11. Wong M, Coppola J. Techniques to reduce pain from local anesthetic injection. *J Can Dent Assoc*. 2002;68(8):497-501.
12. Moore PA, Boynes SG. The use of lidocaine-prilocaine cream for topical anesthesia prior to oral surgery in adults. *J Am Dent Assoc*. 1994;125(4):429-434. doi:10.14219/jada.archive.1994.0198
13. Bhalla M, Thami GP. Safety of local anesthesia in dermatosurgery. *J Cutan Aesthet Surg*. 2015;8(4):192-197. doi:10.4103/0974-2077.172191
14. Alam M, Posten W, Martini MC, Wrone DA. Ipsilateral hemifacial anaesthesia after injection of local anaesthesia for dermatological procedures. *Br J Dermatol*. 2006;155(6):1247-1252. doi:10.1111/j.1365-2133.2006.07514.x
15. Most SP, Antunes MB. A prospective study of the safety of local anesthesia for rhinoplasty. *Arch Facial Plast Surg*. 2008;10(3):170-174.
16. Yilmazlar A, Bilginer B, Korfali E. Intravascular injection of local anesthetics in regional anesthesia: evaluation of the complication in Turkey. *Minerva Anestesiol*. 2011;77(6):565-569.
17. Neal JM, Bernards CM, Butterworth JF, et al. ASRA practice advisory on local anesthetic systemic toxicity. *Reg Anesth Pain Med*. 2010;35(2):152-161.
18. Manku K, McCluskey P. Regional anesthesia in ophthalmology. *Curr Opin Ophthalmol*. 2007;18(1):17-21.
19. Kothari M, Modi L, Choudhary R, et al. Efficacy of peribulbar anesthesia versus retrobulbar anesthesia in ophthalmic surgery. *J Clin Diagn Res*. 2016;10(2):NC01-NC04.
20. Çelebi AR, Can E, Yüksel K, et al. The use of regional anesthesia techniques in ophthalmic surgery. *Anadolu Kardiyol Derg*. 2012;12(7):613-616.
21. Rudkin AK, Farooq N, Nessim M, Cheung N. Regional anesthesia in ophthalmic surgery. *Middle East Afr J Ophthalmol*. 2010;17(3):215-222.
22. van der Jagt M, Atebara NH. Supraorbital nerve block for post-operative pain control after trabeculectomy with topical anesthesia. *Ophthalmic Surg*. 1995;26(2):151-153.
23. Na KS, Kim YC, Song KH. Comparison of peribulbar and supraorbital nerve blocks for vitreoretinal surgery under topical anesthesia. *Korean J Ophthalmol*. 2009;23(2):88-92.
24. Czyz CN, Burns JA, Petrie TP. Anesthesia for ophthalmic plastic surgery. *Ophthalmic Plast Reconstr Surg*. 2010;26(6):441-447.
25. Chhabra N, Rao N, Radhakrishnan S. Infraorbital nerve block with or without hyaluronidase in oculoplastic surgery: a randomized, double-masked, placebo-controlled clinical trial. *Ophthalmic Plast Reconstr Surg*. 2017;33(5):333-338.
26. Wu SY, Ma L, Wu Y. Infraorbital nerve block with or without hyaluronidase in eyelid surgery: a meta-analysis of randomized controlled trials. *BMC Ophthalmol*. 2018;18(1):290.

27. Brown DL, Ransom DM, Hall JA, Leicht CH, Schroeder DR, Offord KP. Regional anesthesia and local anesthetic-induced systemic toxicity: seizure frequency and accompanying cardiovascular changes. *Anesth Analg.* 1995;81(2):321-328.
28. Weinberg G. Lipid infusion therapy: translation to clinical practice. *Anesth Analg.* 208;106(5): 1340-1342.
29. Weiner AL, Weiner SM. The systemic toxicity of local anesthetics. *JAMA.* 1983;250(14):1928-1932.
30. Pippi R, Di Franco S, Landi F, et al. The addition of epinephrine to lidocaine does not increase the incidence of wound infection after skin biopsy: a double-blind randomized controlled trial. *J Am Acad Dermatol.* 2018;79(2):379-385.
31. Fisher MM. Clinical observations on the pathophysiology and treatment of anaphylactic cardiovascular collapse. *Anesthesiology.* 1979;50(6):507-509.
32. Bhole MV, Manson AL, Seneviratne SL, Misbah SA. IgE-mediated allergy to local anaesthetics: separating fact from perception: a UK perspective. *Br J Anaesth.* 2012:108(6):903-911.
33. Johnson PN, Thomason ME. Use of diphenhydramine in local anesthesia. *J Am Dent Assoc.* 1976;92(6):1255-1257.
34. Winter CA, Flataker L. Studies on the local anesthetic action of diphenhydramine. *J Pharmacol Exp Ther.* 1949;97(2):113-117.
35. Blake KV, Gurrin L, Evans RE. Use of benzyl alcohol as an additive to local anesthetic agents. *Anesth Prog.* 1987;34(1):24-26.

# 6 Surgical Pathology: A Visual Guide

**Richard E. Castillo**

As this text primarily deals with eyelids and periorbital skin procedures, a review of relevant histopathologic terminology is merited. The practitioner must be firmly grounded in the dermatologist's and the pathologist's language and terminology to correctly interpret the biopsy result and develop an appropriate plan for the patient. A biopsy is a medical procedure in which a small tissue sample is removed and examined under a microscope. It is a standard diagnostic tool to identify and diagnose various eyelid and skin conditions. The clinician needs to understand a skin biopsy report because it is an integral part of the diagnostic process. The biopsy report provides direct information about the condition of the involved skin and any abnormalities that may be present.

The process of obtaining a skin biopsy, as detailed in Chapter 7 of this text, typically involves the use of a local anesthetic to numb the area, followed by the removal of a small sample of involved skin (lesion) using a scalpel, scissors, biopsy punch, or other instruments. The tissue sample is then placed in a fixative solution, typically 10% neutral buffered formalin, and sent to a laboratory where it is examined by a pathologist, who analyzes the tissue and prepares a report with the results of the histopathologic examination.[1]

The skin biopsy report includes information about the appearance of the tissue, the presence of any abnormal cells, changes in tissue architecture or morphology, and a diagnosis based on these findings. Rarely, a report may be returned without a specific diagnosis. In these instances, the practitioner must be conversant in the language of the pathologist if relevant information is to be extracted from the information returned and an appropriate plan developed for the patient. The report may include further testing or treatment recommendations depending on the diagnosis.[1-3]

Therefore, understanding how to analyze and interpret the biopsy report is critical for several reasons. First, it helps the practitioner determine the appropriate course of treatment for the patient. For example, a diagnosis of actinic keratosis may require different treatment options than a diagnosis of eczema. Second, the report can provide valuable information about the progression of a condition, which can help consider timely referrals or monitor the effectiveness of treatment and make any necessary adjustments. However, it is essential to remember that biopsy results are just one aspect of the diagnostic process. Other factors, such as the patient's medical history and physical examination, must also be considered when making a diagnosis and considering a treatment plan.[4-6]

Finally, being conversant in the terminology of the biopsy report can help practitioners communicate effectively with one another about the patient's condition and treatment.

Within the context of primary eye care, one typically samples lesions involving the periocular skin or other eyelid structures. The remainder of this chapter will limit itself to the histopathology and common terminology encountered when dealing with biopsies of the periocular skin and common lesions of the eyelids and periocular tissues.

- **ABSCESS**—a closed pocket containing pus (Figure 6-1).[6]
- **ACANTHOLYSIS**—loss of coherence between epidermal cells (cell separation) due to the breakdown of intercellular bridges (desmosomes) (Figure 6-2).[6]
- **ACANTHOSIS**—an increase in the thickness of the squamous cell layer (stratum spinosum) of the epidermis. Acanthosis often results in elongated projections of the epidermis into the dermis (Figures 6-3 and 6-74).[6,7]
- **ACROCHORDON**—a benign nonepithelial tumor (fibroepithelial polyp) arising from mesodermal tissue. Common on the eyelids and areas of skin folds. They are often associated with trauma, diabetes mellitus, pregnancy, and obesity (Figure 6-4).[7,8]
- **ACTINIC ELASTOSIS (aka solar elastosis)**—characterized by lightly basophilic blue-gray), irregular, thickened elastic fibers in the dermis. Individual fibers are sometimes not evident, and there may be only an amorphous mass of lightly basophilic material in the dermis. Externally, it presents as a yellowish thickened appearance to the skin, which is bumpy and covered with furrows (Figures 6-5 and 6-73).[6,9]
- **ACTINIC KERATOSIS**—an intraepidermal keratinocytic lesion secondary to solar (ultraviolet [UV]) damage. Actinic keratoses exhibit partial thickness epidermal dysplasia, parakeratosis, dermal solar elastosis, and a mild dermal lymphocytic infiltrate. Actinic keratosis

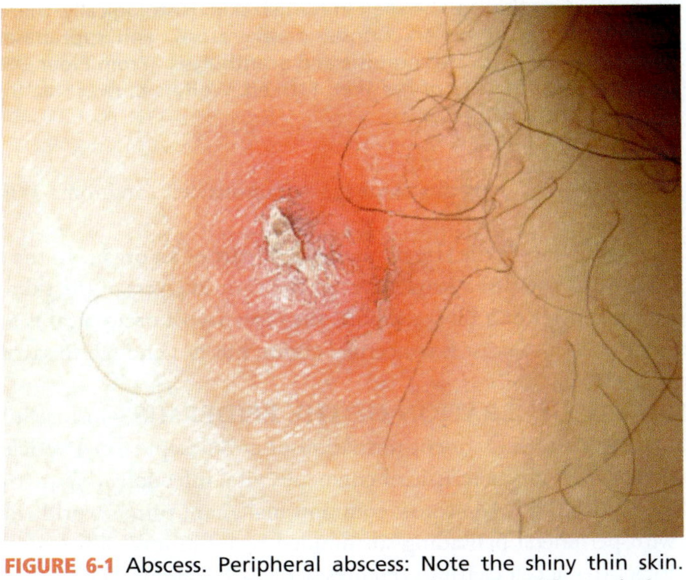

**FIGURE 6-1** Abscess. Peripheral abscess: Note the shiny thin skin. This abscess was treated by incision and drainage with resolution. (From Bobonich M, Nolen M, Honaker J, DiRuggiero D. *Dermatology for Advanced Practice Clinicians*. 2nd ed. Wolters Kluwer Health; 2021:206. Kindle Edition.)

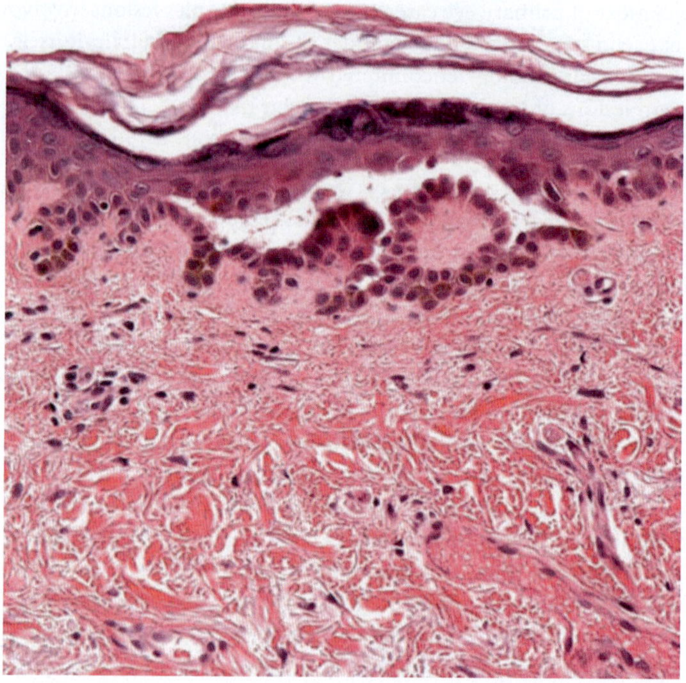

FIGURE 6-2 Focal acantholytic dyskeratosis represents another incidental finding that can be seen in normal skin. Histologically, there is a focal area of hyperkeratosis, parakeratosis, and suprabasal cleft formation with dyskeratosis and acantholysis. (From Elder DE. *Lever's Histopathology of the Skin*. 11th ed. Wolters Kluwer Health; 2019:65. Kindle Edition.)

is the most common precursor of cutaneous squamous cell carcinoma (Figures 6-6, 6-7, and 6-23).[6,10]

- **ATROPHY**—a reduction in the size of an organ or part of an organ. In the skin, it may be a reduction in the thickness of a single layer or the various layers of the skin (Figure 6-8).[12]
- **ATYPIA**—in the context of a biopsy report, the term atypia or atypical is a caution to the practitioner that the pathologist is concerned about, but not enough to say that the patient has cancer (Figure 6-9).[6,11]
- **BALLOONING DEGENERATION OF THE EPIDERMIS**—intracellular edema that leads to acantholysis and subsequent formation of an intraepidermal vesicle or bulla. Ballooning degeneration is characteristic of cutaneous viral infections (Figure 6-10).[12]
- **BASAL CELL CARCINOMA**—most common malignant tumor worldwide. Nests of basaloid cells with peripheral palisading surrounded by a fibromyxoid stroma may exhibit a retraction artifact (basal cell clefting) (Figures 6-11, 6-12, and 6-77).[6,10-13]
- **BULLA**—a bulla is a fluid-filled blister greater than 0.5 or 1 cm in diameter (depending on the author). Bullae may be subcorneal (stratum corneum), intraepidermal, or subepidermal (Figures 6-13 and 6-14).[10-13]

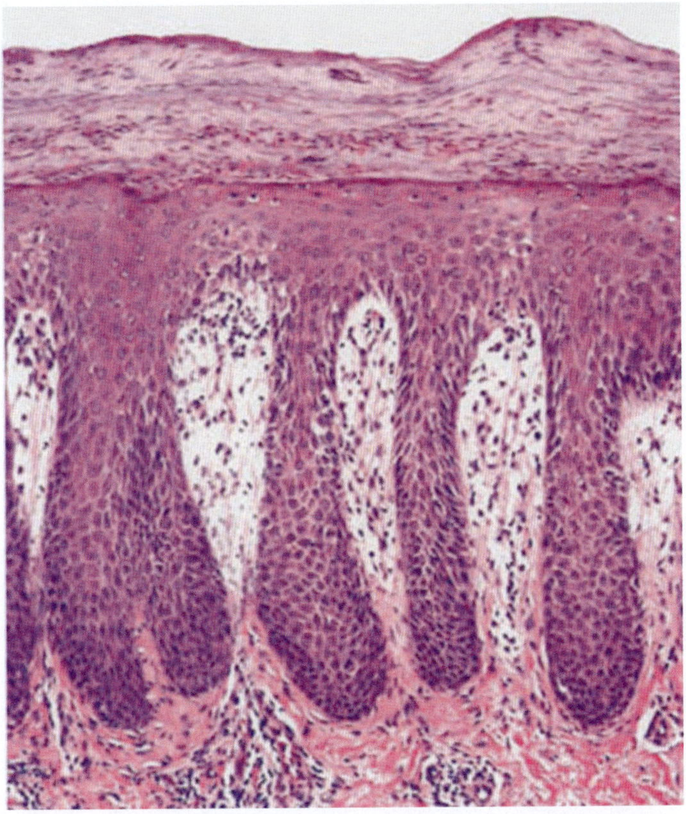

**FIGURE 6-3** Acanthosis with club-shaped rete ridges of even length, suprabasal mitoses, thin suprapapillary epidermal plates, absent granular layer, pallor of the upper epidermis, and confluent parakeratosis with collections of neutrophils. (From Elder DE. *Lever's Histopathology of the Skin*. 11th ed. Wolters Kluwer Health; 2019:202. Kindle Edition.)

- **CARCINOMA**—a malignant neoplasm of epithelial (ectodermal) origin. Carcinomas often exhibit lymphogenous dissemination (spread) (Figure 6-15).[12]
- **CHALAZION**—a common, inflammatory eyelid lesion involving the meibomian glands, characterized by granulomatous inflammation with lipogranulomas (Figure 6-16).[6]
- **CELLULITIS**—an acute inflammatory process of the dermis and subcutis caused by an infection (Figure 6-17).[10-13]
- **COLLOID BODIES**—(aka cytoid bodies, Civatte bodies, hyalin bodies, and apoptotic bodies). Colloid bodies are apoptotic epidermal cells (keratinocytes) lacking nuclei appearing as homogeneous, eosinophilic, and round structures. Colloid bodies are not specific for any disease, but they are commonly seen in lupus erythematosus, lichen planus, and graft-versus-host disease (Figure 6-18).[10-13]

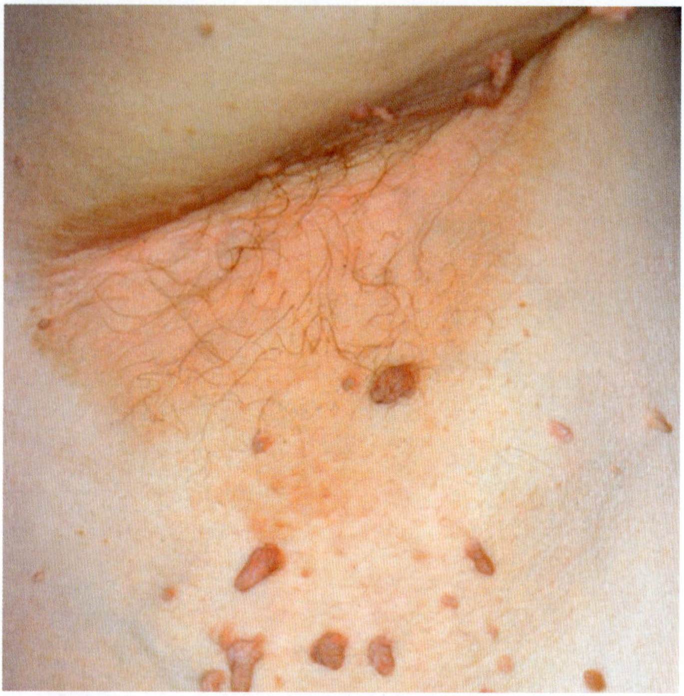

FIGURE 6-4 Skin tags or acrochordons are commonly found in areas of friction. (From Bobonich M, Nolen M, Honaker J, DiRuggiero D. *Dermatology for Advanced Practice Clinicians*. 2nd ed. Wolters Kluwer Health; 2021:81. Kindle Edition.)

- **CRUST**—a term used to describe a scab caused by leaking blood or plasma through a lesion (Figures 6-19, 6-75, and 6-77).[13]
- **CYST**—an enclosed sac in the skin that contains either fluid or a solid material (e.g., sebaceous cyst, epidermal cyst, chalazion cyst) (Figure 6-20).[13]
- **DERMATITIS**—nonspecific term for inflammation of the skin. Further classified based on etiology, for example, atopic, allergic, contact, or seborrheic (Figure 6-21).[6,11,12]
- **DESMOPLASIA**—desmoplastic change (aka, desmoplastic reaction) refers to the deposition of fibrous tissue around a pathologic process. In dermatopathology, desmoplasia may be seen with benign, as well as malignant, conditions (Figure 6-22).[12]
- **DYSPLASIA**—a term used to describe the presence of abnormal cells within a tissue or organ. Dysplasia is not cancer, but it may sometimes become cancer. Dysplasia can be mild, moderate, or severe, depending on how abnormal the cells look under a microscope and how much of the tissue or organ is affected (Figure 6-23).[11-13]
- **ECCHYMOSIS**—a bruise or visible accumulation of blood within the skin larger than 0.5 cm in diameter.
- **EPHELIDES**—a term for common freckles resulting from UV exposure (Figure 6-24).[13]

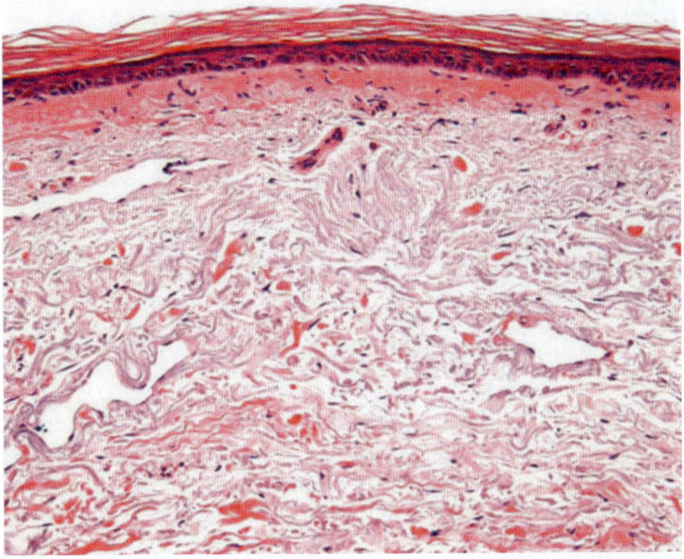

**FIGURE 6-5** Actinic (solar) elastosis. Changes associated with skin aging include a thinner epidermis with a flattened dermal–epidermal junction and telangiectatic dermal vessels associated with marked solar elastosis in the form of bluish-gray fibers, the latter related to chronic sun damage. (From Elder DE. *Lever's Histopathology of the Skin*. 11th ed. Wolters Kluwer Health; 2019:61. Kindle Edition.)

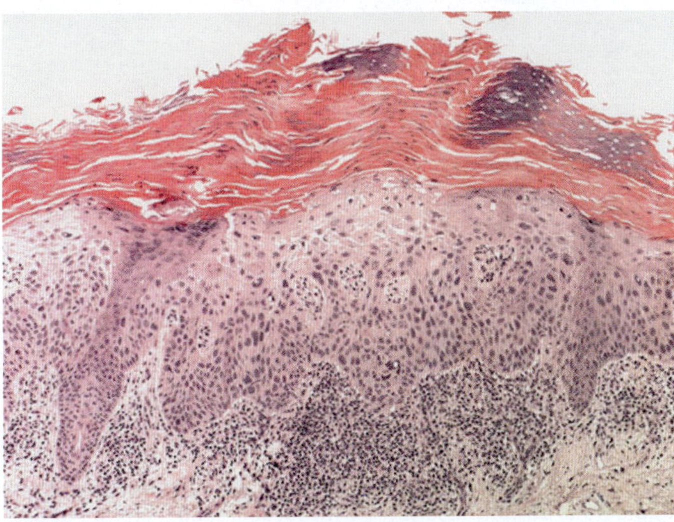

**FIGURE 6-6** Actinic keratosis. Tall columns of parakeratotic keratin alternate with bands of orthokeratotic keratin, with moderate atypia of the underlying keratinocytes. (From Elder DE. *Lever's Histopathology of the Skin*. 11th ed. Wolters Kluwer Health; 2019:988. Kindle Edition.)

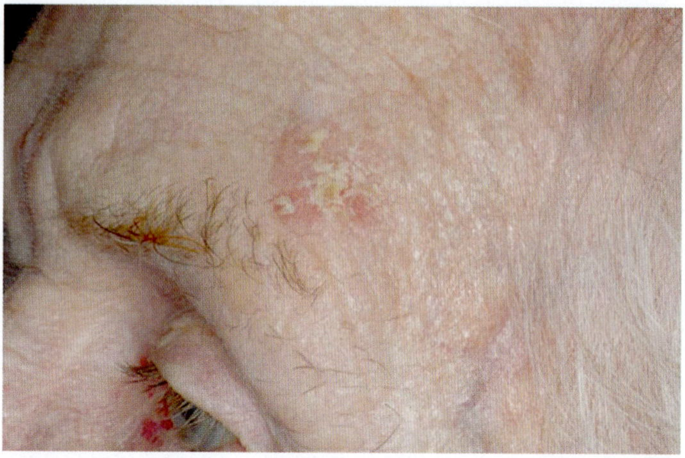

**FIGURE 6-7** Actinic keratosis. The lesion on the forehead is crusted and erythematous. (From Elder DE. *Lever's Histopathology of the Skin*. 11th ed. Wolters Kluwer Health; 2019:987. Kindle Edition.)

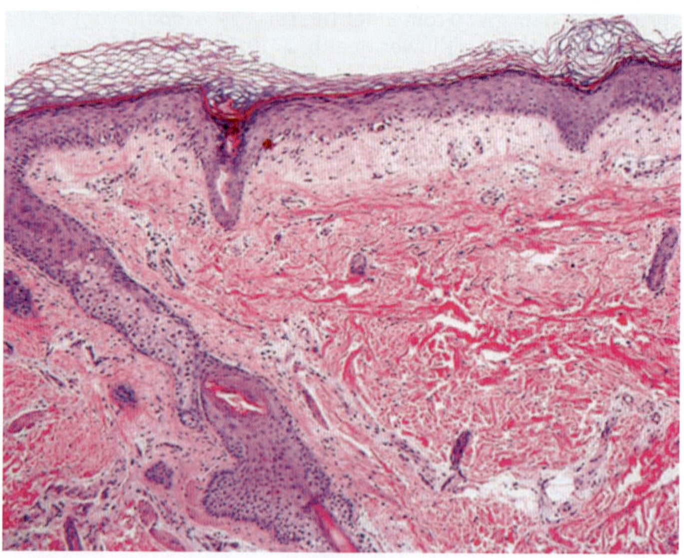

**FIGURE 6-8** Atrophy seen in poikiloderma with neutropenia. There is epidermal atrophy associated with vacuolar degeneration of basilar keratinocytes and rare dyskeratotic keratinocytes. Telangiectasias are present in the papillary and upper dermis. (From Elder DE. *Lever's Histopathology of the Skin*. 11th ed. Wolters Kluwer Health; 2019:174. Kindle Edition.)

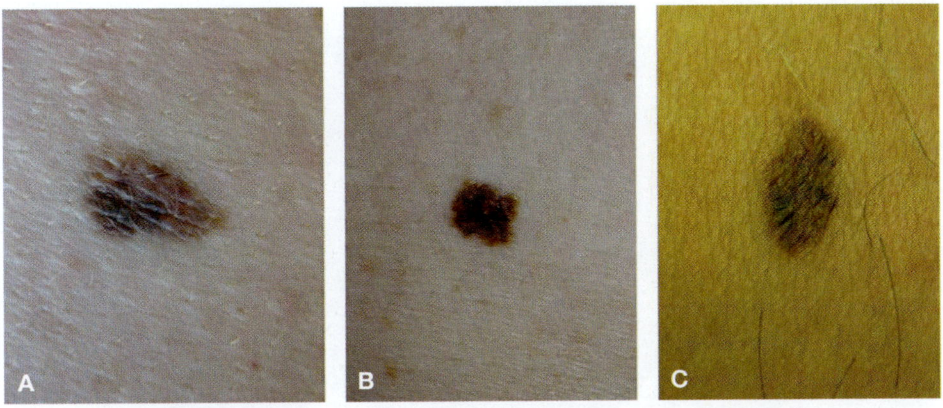


**FIGURE 6-9 A–C,** Dysplastic nevi. Note color variation, border irregularity, and asymmetry in these lesions. These lesions have a high suspicion of atypia. (From Bobonich M, Nolen M, Honaker J, DiRuggiero D. *Dermatology for Advanced Practice Clinicians*. 2nd ed. Wolters Kluwer Health; 2021:48. Kindle Edition.)

- **EPIDERMOTROPISM**—the presence of atypical lymphocytes in the epidermis without spongiosis. Characteristic of mycosis fungoides. Atypical lymphocytes in the epidermis may occur singly surrounded by a clear halo or form small clusters referred to as Pautrier microabscesses (Figures 6-25 and 6-65).[11-13]

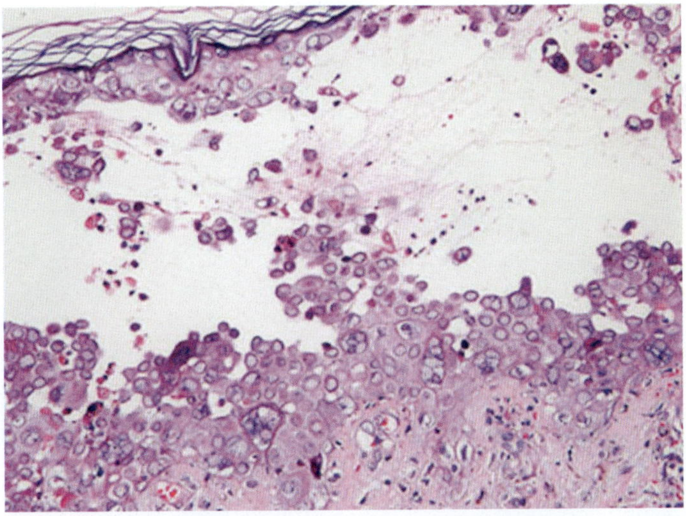

**FIGURE 6-10** Ballooning degeneration in *Herpes simplex*. On high magnification, balloon cells at the floor of a vesicle are shown; these cells exhibit characteristic ballooning degeneration with steel gray nuclei with homogeneous pale chromatin and nuclei molding. (From Elder DE. *Lever's Histopathology of the Skin*. 11th ed. Wolters Kluwer Health; 2019:785. Kindle Edition.)

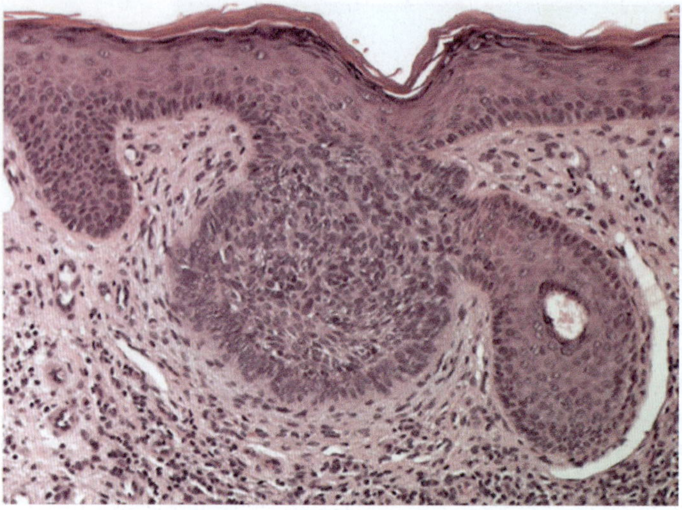

FIGURE 6-11 Superficial basal cell carcinoma. High magnification. The tumor shows a bud of cells in the bulge zone of a hair follicle similar to the primary epithelial germ buds in embryonal skin. Peripheral palisading and a cleft (retraction artifact) are also present at the interface with the dermis. (From Elder DE. *Lever's Histopathology of the Skin.* 11th ed. Wolters Kluwer Health; 2015:1009. Kindle Edition.)

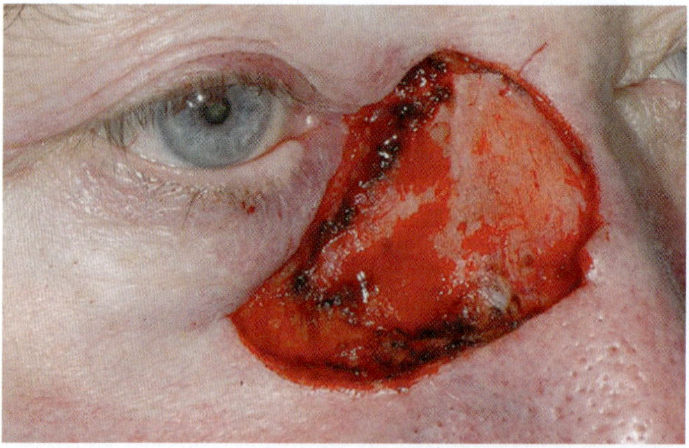

FIGURE 6-12 Micronodular basal cell carcinoma. An extensive resection was required. Mohs micrographic surgery was used to achieve clear surgical margins. (From Elder DE. *Lever's Histopathology of the Skin.* 11th ed. Wolters Kluwer Health; 2019:1008. Kindle Edition.)

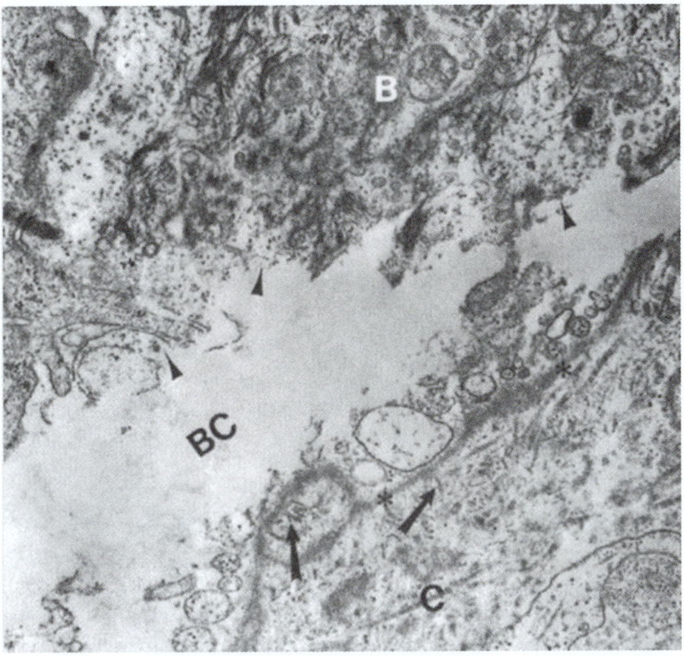


**FIGURE 6-13** Bulla observed in epidermolysis bullosa simplex. The blister formed due to degenerative, cytolytic changes in the basal cells (B). The bulla cavity (BC) is situated above the basement membrane (asterisk). The basal cells are severely damaged, lacking a plasma membrane (pointers). (From Elder DE. *Lever's Histopathology of the Skin*. 11th ed. Wolters Kluwer Health; 2019:1433. Kindle Edition.)

- **EPIDERMAL INCLUSION CYST**—a cystic structure featuring a benign keratinizing squamous epithelium lining (Figure 6-20).[6,10,11]
- **EPITHELIOID CELLS**—activated macrophages that have an epithelial-like appearance. They are large cells with oval to elongated nuclei, eosinophilic cytoplasm, and indistinct cell borders. They occur singly or may form groups termed granulomas (Figure 6-26).[6,10-13]
- **EROSION**—a focal loss of the top layer of skin (Figure 6-27).[11-13]
- **EXCORIATION**—an erosion or ulcer caused by scratching (Figure 6-28).[7,11-13]
- **FIBRINOID DEGENERATION**—(aka, fibrinoid necrosis) deposition of fibrin within vessel walls or dermal collagen. In the skin, fibrinoid necrosis of vessel walls is seen in leukocytoclastic vasculitis, whereas fibrin deposition in dermal collagen is seen in rheumatoid nodules and sometimes in lupus erythematosus (Figure 6-29).[12,13]
- **FOREIGN-BODY GIANT CELL**—a multinucleated giant cell derived from the fusion of epithelioid cells (activated macrophages). Foreign-body giant cells are characterized by their large size and haphazardly arrayed nuclei. Typically found on or around implanted biomaterials such as a suture (Figure 6-30).[11-14]
- **GRANULATION TISSUE**—the hallmark of wound healing. The term comes from the soft, pink, granular appearance when viewed from the surface of a wound. Histologically,

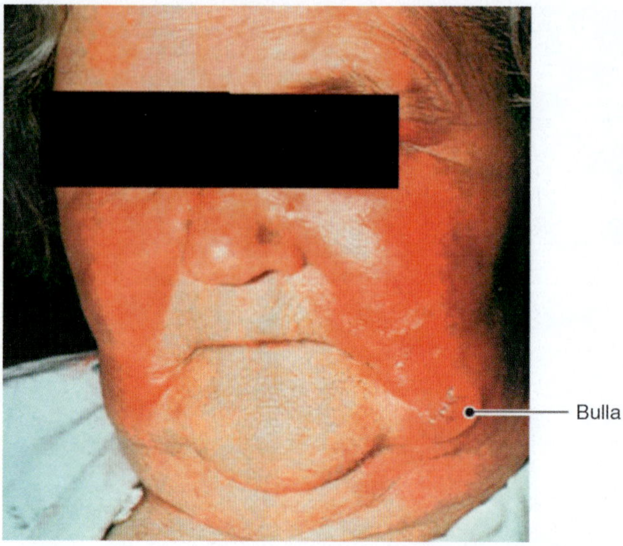


**FIGURE 6-14** Erysipelas. This patient has large, confluent erythematous plaques. A bulla is present near the angle of her jaw. (From McConnell TH. *The Nature of Disease Pathology for the Health Professions*. Wolters Kluwer Health | Lippincott Williams & Wilkins; 2007. Kindle Edition.)

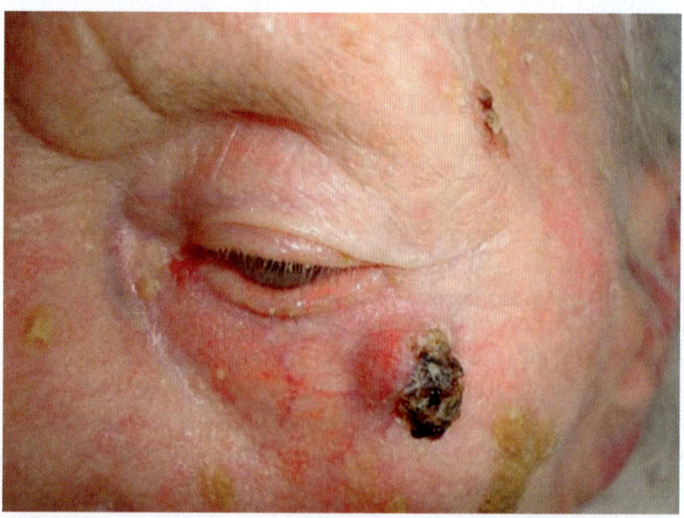

**FIGURE 6-15** Squamous cell carcinoma. There is a hyperkeratotic horn on the surface of the tumor, which has a fleshy appearance around its base. (From Elder DE. *Lever's Histopathology of the Skin*. 11th ed. Wolters Kluwer Health; 2019:999. Kindle Edition.)

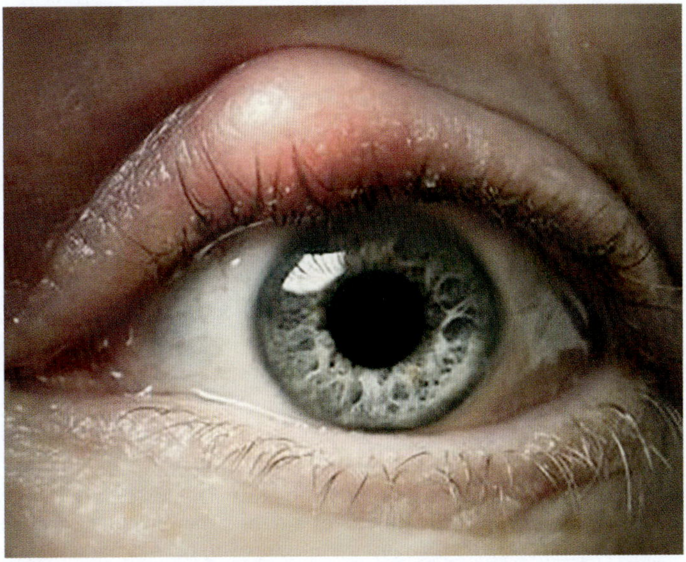

**FIGURE 6-16** Chalazion, upper lid—a common, inflammatory eyelid lesion involving the meibomian glands, characterized by granulomatous inflammation with lipogranulomas (From NSU-OCO Archives.)

granulation tissue consists of a proliferation of small blood vessels and fibroblasts, often accompanied by edema (Figure 6-31).[11-13]

- **GRANULOMA**—a microscopic aggregate containing varying proportions of activated macrophages (epithelioid cells), multinucleated giant cells resulting from the fusion of epithelioid cells, and other mononuclear leukocytes (lymphocytes, plasma cells, monocytes, and macrophages) (Figures 6-32 and 6-33).[6,12,13]

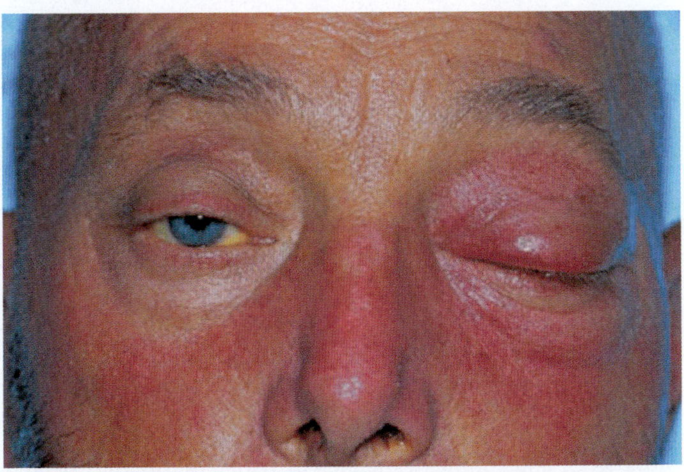

**FIGURE 6-17** Orbital cellulitis. Left orbital cellulitis with marked periorbital edema, erythema, and proptosis. (From Bobonich M, Nolen M, Honaker J, DiRuggiero D. *Dermatology for Advanced Practice Clinicians*. 2nd ed. Wolters Kluwer Health; 2021:205. Kindle Edition.)

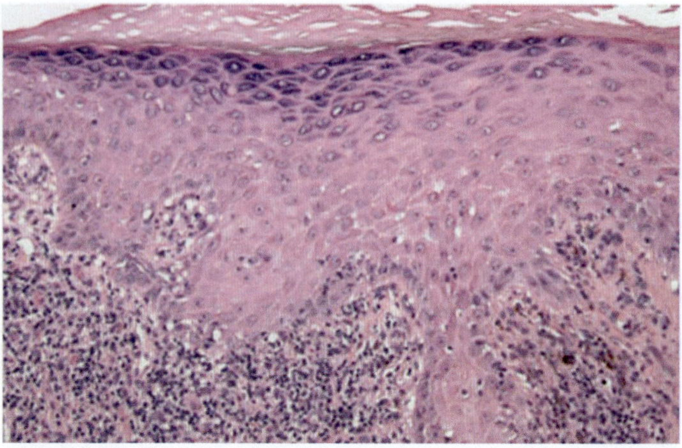

**FIGURE 6-18** A patient with hepatitis C developed an eruption that was clinically compatible with lichen planus. The histomorphology confirmed the diagnosis by virtue of a dense, bandlike lymphocytic infiltrate in apposition to an epidermis showing colloid body formation. (From Elder DE. *Lever's Histopathology of the Skin.* 2nd ed. Wolters Kluwer Health; 2019:493. Kindle Edition.)

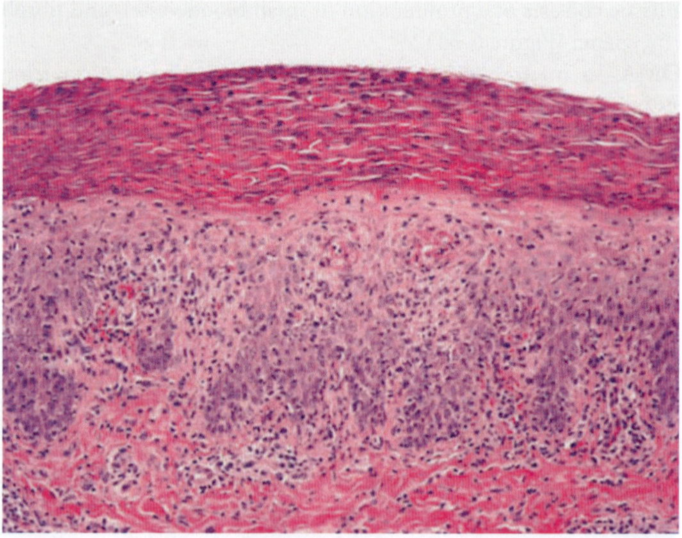

**FIGURE 6-19** Pityriasis lichenoides et varioliformis acuta. A closer view reveals a lichenoid inflammatory pattern with an infiltrate of lymphocytes, extravasated erythrocytes, irregular acanthosis, pallor of the upper layers of the epidermis, spongiosis, necrotic keratinocytes, and confluent mounds of parakeratosis with plasma, neutrophils, and lymphocytes. The overlying cornified layer shows parakeratosis and a scaly crust with neutrophils. (From Elder DE. *Lever's Histopathology of the Skin.* 11th ed. Wolters Kluwer Health; 2019:226. Kindle Edition.)

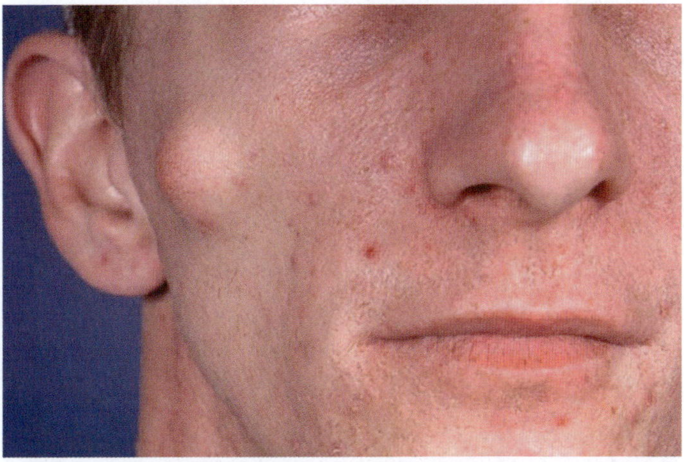

FIGURE 6-20 Epidermal cyst. The cyst distends the overlying skin of the cheek. (From Elder DE. *Lever's Histopathology of the Skin.* 11th ed. Wolters Kluwer Health; 2019:980. Kindle Edition.)

- **HIDROCYSTOMA**—a benign adenomatous cystic proliferation derived from the blocked ducts of apocrine sweat glands (apocrine hidrocystoma, aka cyst of Moll) or eccrine sweat glands (eccrine hidrocystoma) (Figure 6-34).[12,13,15]
- **HORN CYST**—a circumscribed, round, intraepidermal accumulation of keratin. Keratin-filled invaginations of the epidermis are referred to as "pseudo-horn cysts." Both horn cysts and pseudo-horn cysts are characteristic of seborrheic keratoses, although they may also be found in other neoplasms of the skin (Figures 6-22, 6-35, and 6-72).[6,10-13]

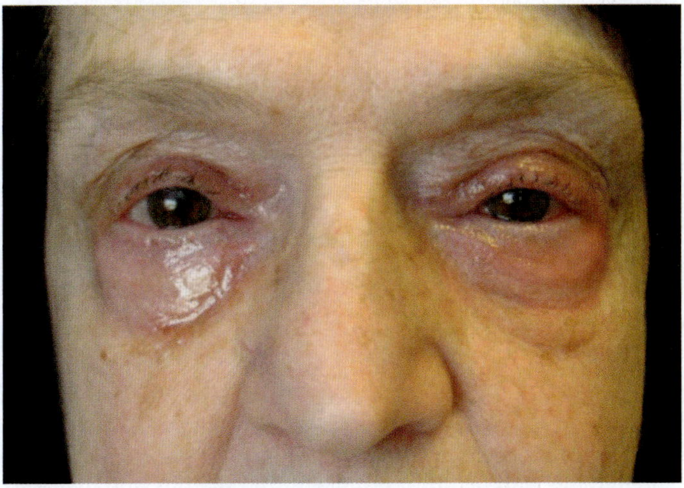

FIGURE 6-21 Allergic contact dermatitis from medicated eye drops. (From Bobonich M, Nolen M, Honaker J, DiRuggiero D. *Dermatology for Advanced Practice Clinicians.* 2nd ed. Wolters Kluwer Health; 2021:135. Kindle Edition.)

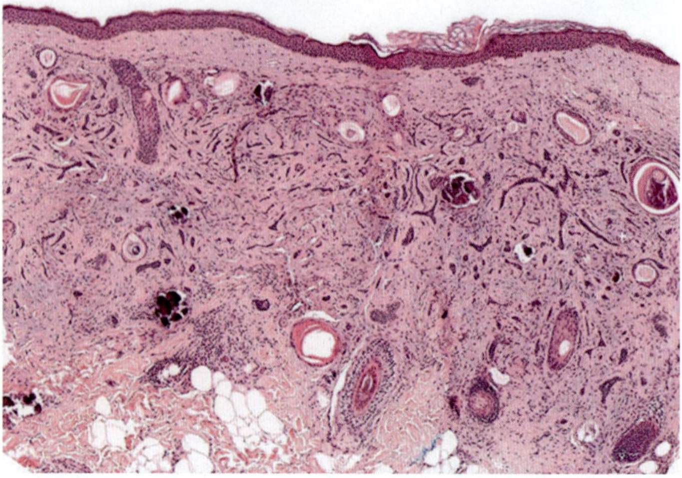

**FIGURE 6-22** Desmoplasia in a desmoplastic trichoepithelioma. Horn cysts and narrow strands of epithelial cells are embedded in a fibrous stroma. (From Elder DE. *Lever's Histopathology of the Skin.* 11th ed. Wolters Kluwer Health; 2019:1050. Kindle Edition.)

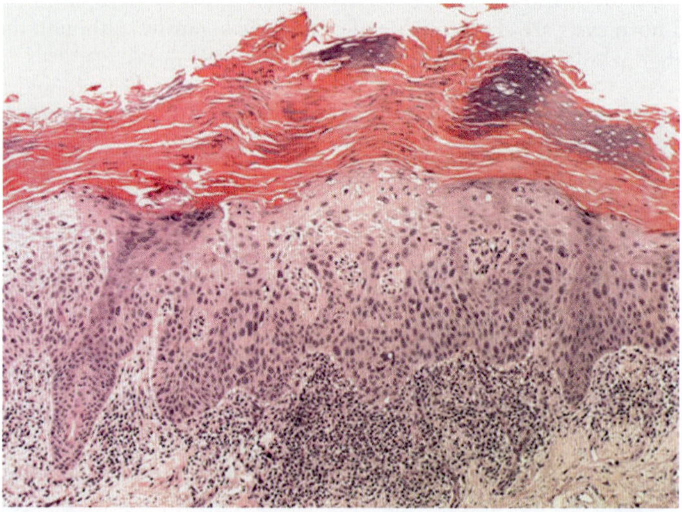

**FIGURE 6-23** Dysplasia in actinic keratosis. Actinic keratoses are essentially keratinocytic dysplasia. Tall columns of parakeratotic keratin alternate with bands of orthokeratotic keratin, with moderate atypia of the underlying keratinocytes. (From Elder DE. *Lever's Histopathology of the Skin.* 11th ed. Wolters Kluwer Health; 2019:988. Kindle Edition.)

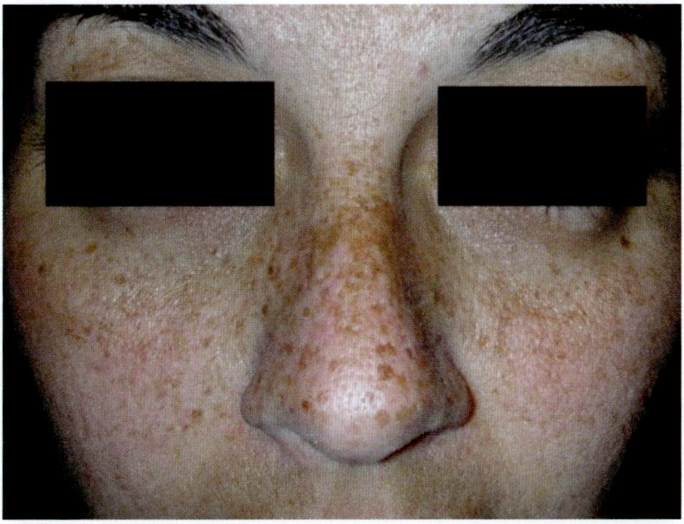

**FIGURE 6-24** Ephelides or common freckles result from UVR exposure and usually fade in the winter. (From Bobonich M, Nolen M, Honaker J, DiRuggiero D. *Dermatology for Advanced Practice Clinicians*. 2nd ed. Wolters Kluwer Health; 2021:38. Kindle Edition.)

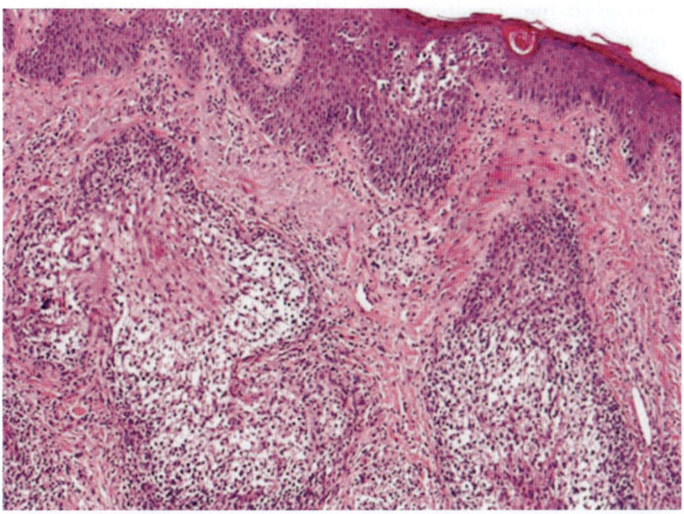

**FIGURE 6-25** Follicular mucinosis associated with folliculotropic mycosis fungoides. In addition to changes of follicular mucinosis, there is extensive folliculotropism of lymphocytes. Epidermotropism of large lymphocytes is also present. (From Elder DE. *Lever's Histopathology of the Skin.* 11th ed. Wolters Kluwer Health; 2019:555. Kindle Edition.)

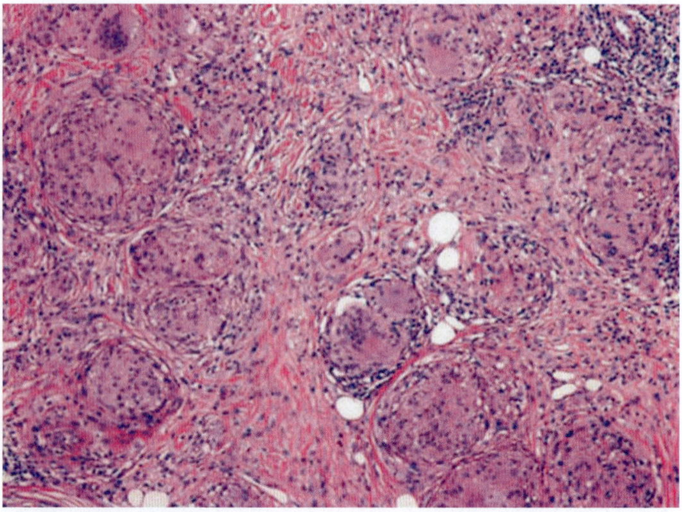

**FIGURE 6-26** Epithelioid cells in sarcoid. Well-circumscribed, roundish collections of epithelioid histiocytes, some multinucleated, with few lymphocytes. (From Elder DE. *Lever's Histopathology of the Skin.* 11th ed. Wolters Kluwer Health; 2019:438. Kindle Edition.)

- **HYPERKERATOSIS**—increased thickness of the epidermis's stratum corneum (horny layer). Hyperkeratosis may result from orthokeratosis, parakeratosis, or a combination of these two (Figures 6-36 and 6-58).[10,12,13]

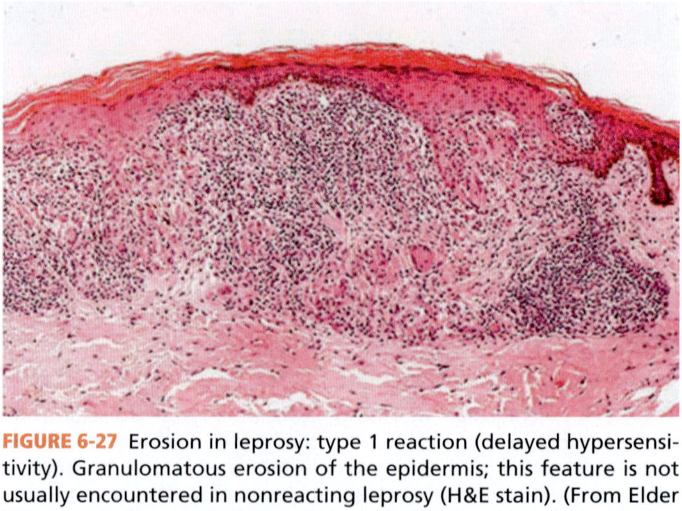

**FIGURE 6-27** Erosion in leprosy: type 1 reaction (delayed hypersensitivity). Granulomatous erosion of the epidermis; this feature is not usually encountered in nonreacting leprosy (H&E stain). (From Elder DE. *Lever's Histopathology of the Skin.* 11th ed. Wolters Kluwer Health; 2019:670. Kindle Edition.)

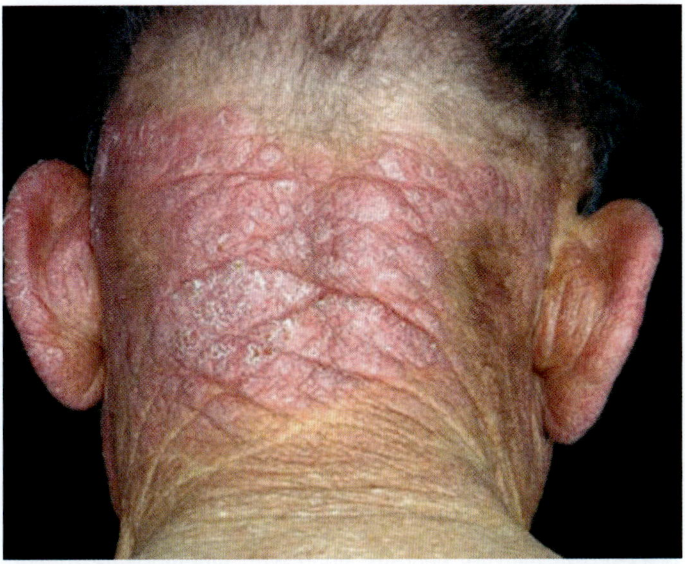

**FIGURE 6-28** Chronic actinic dermatitis. Extensive lichenification and excoriation. (From Elder DE. *Lever's Histopathology of the Skin*. 11th ed. Wolters Kluwer Health; 2019:399. Kindle Edition.)

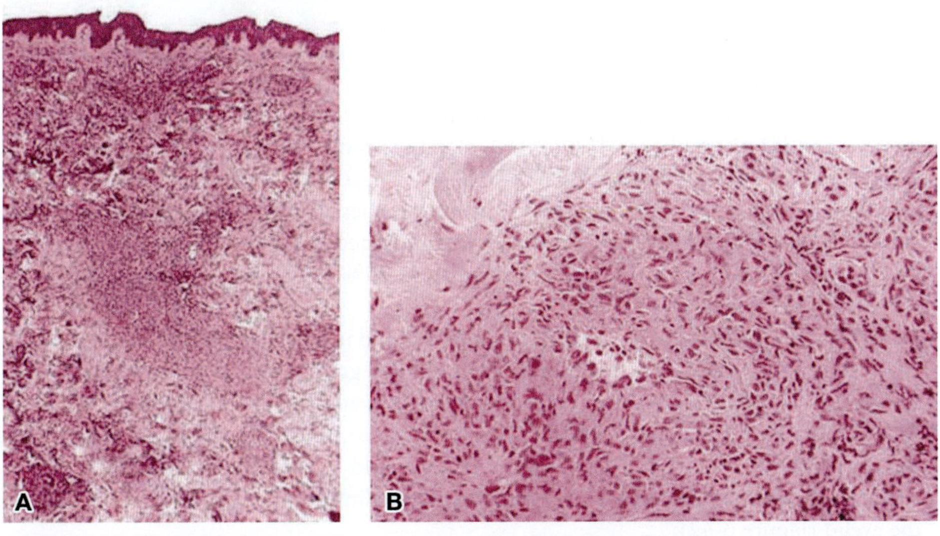


**FIGURE 6-29** Fibrinoid degeneration and granulomatous vasculitis. Note perivascular histiocytic/granulomatous infiltrate (**A**) and focal vascular damage with fibrinoid degeneration of the vessel wall (**B**). (From Elder DE. *Lever's Histopathology of the Skin.* 11th ed. Wolters Kluwer Health; 2019:249. Kindle Edition.)

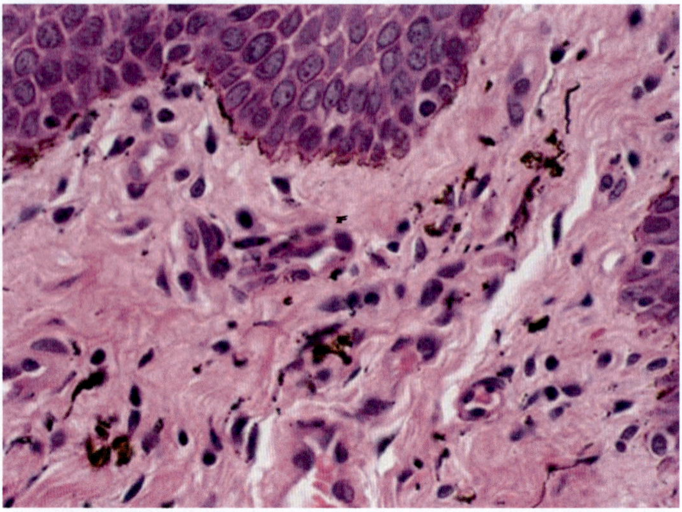

**FIGURE 6-30** Foreign-body giant cells in mercury deposition. Large, black-brown mercury deposits along with multinucleate foreign-body giant cells are seen in the papillary dermis and along the basement membrane in this case of traumatic mercury implantation in the buccal mucosa. (From Elder DE. *Lever's Histopathology of the Skin.* 11th ed. Wolters Kluwer Health; 2019:381. Kindle Edition.)

- **HYPERPLASIA**—a proliferation of cells (increase in cell number), which is reactive and not neoplastic (Figure 6-37).[12,13]
- **INFLAMMATION**—the result of the immune system reacting to stress. Inflammation manifests as swelling, pain, tenderness, redness, and heat. Inflammatory cell types include (1) neutrophils, seen in acute or early inflammation; (2) lymphocytes, seen in chronic inflammation; and (3) macrophages (histiocytes), seen in chronic inflammation (Figure 6-38).[10-13]
- **INVERTED FOLLICULAR KERATOSIS**—a benign tumor of the follicular infundibulum with the characteristic presence of squamous eddies (Figure 6-39).[12,13,16]
- **KERATOACATHOMA**—a well-differentiated cutaneous squamous cell carcinoma that may spontaneously regress. It may represent up to 30% of cutaneous squamous cell carcinoma cases (Figure 6-40).[11-13,17]
- **KERATOHYALIN**—darkly basophilic granules found in keratinocytes of the granular layer (stratum granulosum) of the epidermis. Keratohyalin granules form a matrix that cements cytokeratin tonofibrils, resulting in increased strength and stability (Figure 6-41).[6,12,13]
- **KOILOCYTES**—vacuolated keratinocytes with eccentrically placed, basophilic, shrunken nuclei surrounded by clear halos. Koilocytes are found in the upper spinous and granular cell layers of the epidermis in human papillomavirus infections such as verruca vulgaris of the eyelid (Figure 6-42).[12,13]
- **LANGHANS' GIANT CELLS**—multinucleated giant cells derived from the fusion of epithelioid cells (activated macrophages). They are large cells with nuclei arranged along the cell's periphery, forming an arc. Langhans' giant cells are nonspecific and may be seen in

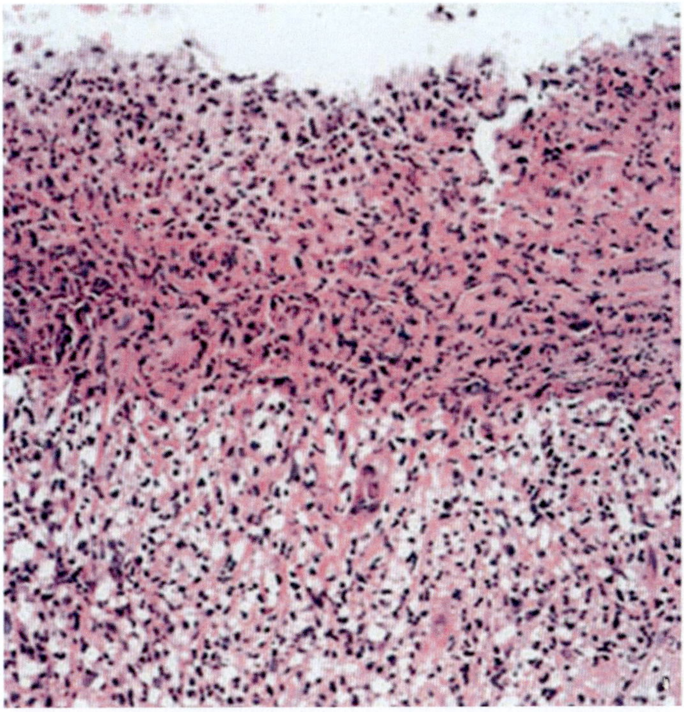

**FIGURE 6-31** Chancroid. Three-zone pattern of ulcer and inflammation: superficial necrotic zone, underlying granulation tissue, and deeper fibrosis with plasma cells (H&E stain). (From Elder DE. *Lever's Histopathology of the Skin.* 11th ed. Wolters Kluwer Health; 2019:699. Kindle Edition.)

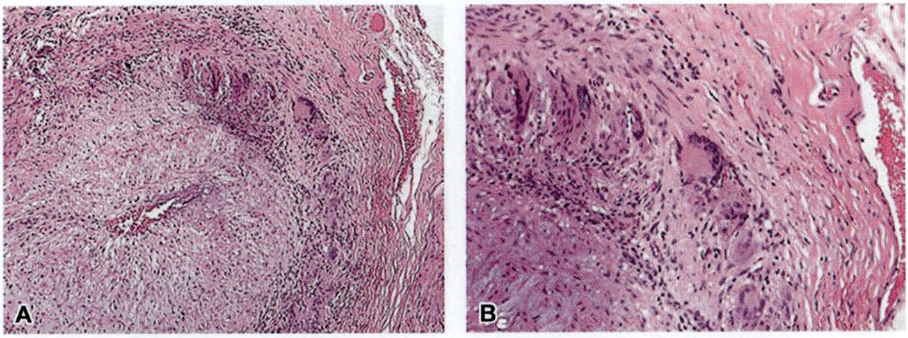


**FIGURE 6-32** Granulomatous inflammation in giant cell arteritis. **A** and **B**, Biopsy of the temporal artery shows a predominantly mononuclear cell infiltrate with a few giant cells in the region of the internal elastic lamina. (From Elder DE. *Lever's Histopathology of the Skin.* 11th ed. Wolters Kluwer Health; 2019:244. Kindle Edition.)

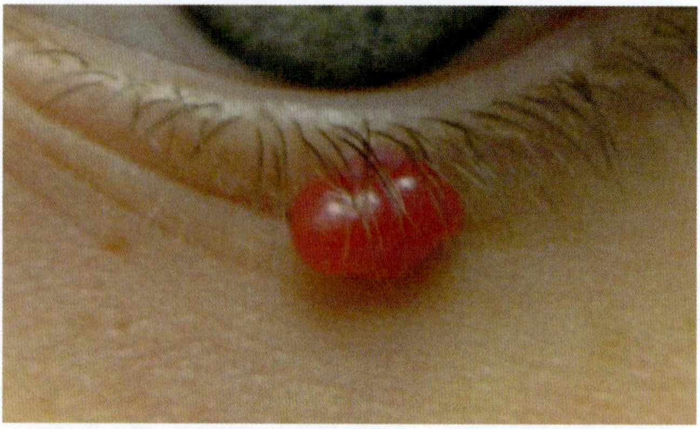

**FIGURE 6-33** Pyogenic granuloma. Pyogenic granuloma on lower eyelid margin. (Used with permission from Gru AA, Wick M. *Pediatric Dermatopathology and Dermatology*. Wolters Kluwer Health; 2018. Kindle Edition.)

immune-type granulomas (such as sarcoidosis and tuberculosis) and foreign-body granulomas (Figure 6-43).[12,13]

- **LICHENIFICATION**—(aka, lichenoid inflammation or lichenoid reaction pattern) refers to a dense band of lymphocytes clustered around the interface between the epidermis and dermis. Lichenoid inflammation is common to many dermatologic conditions, though only a few, such as erythema multiforme and graft-versus-host disease, are seen in the eyelids (Figures 6-19 and 6-44).[6,10,12,13]
- **MACULE**—a circumscribed, flat lesion with color change up to 1 cm in size that is not palpable (Figure 6-45).[12,13]

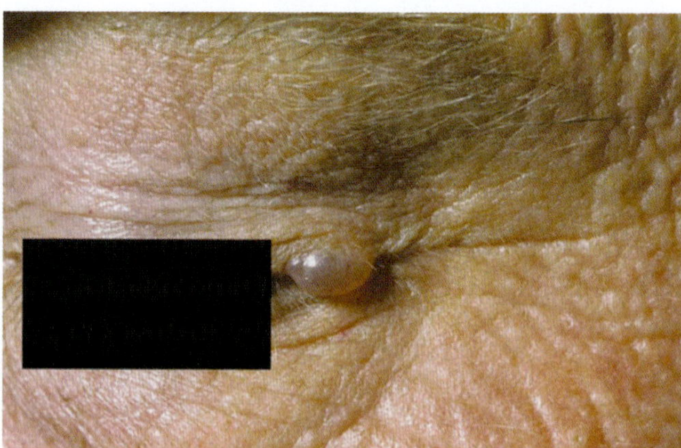

**FIGURE 6-34** Apocrine hidrocystoma. A translucent cystic lesion with a bluish hue is noted. (From Elder DE. *Lever's Histopathology of the Skin.* 11th ed. Wolters Kluwer Health; 2019:1071. Kindle Edition.)

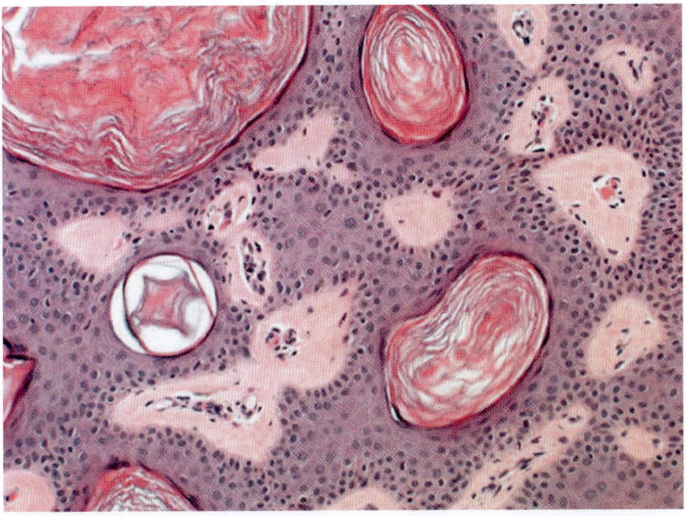

**FIGURE 6-35** Horn cysts in seborrheic keratosis. High magnification. Most cells have a basaloid appearance, with interspersed horn cysts filled with keratin. (From Elder DE. *Lever's Histopathology of the Skin.* 11th ed. Wolters Kluwer Health; 2019:975. Kindle Edition.)

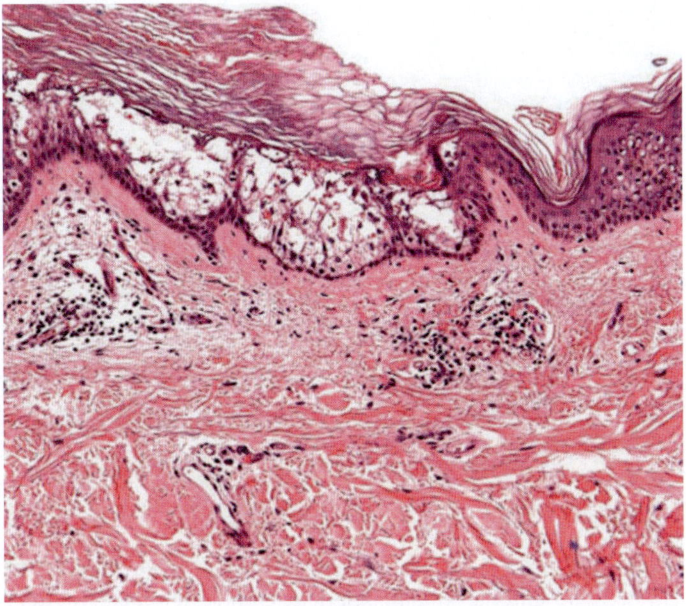

**FIGURE 6-36** Incidental (focal) epidermolytic hyperkeratosis is a common, nonspecific finding that may be seen in normal and especially sun-damaged skin. (From Elder DE. *Lever's Histopathology of the Skin.* 11th ed. Wolters Kluwer Health; 2019:65. Kindle Edition.)

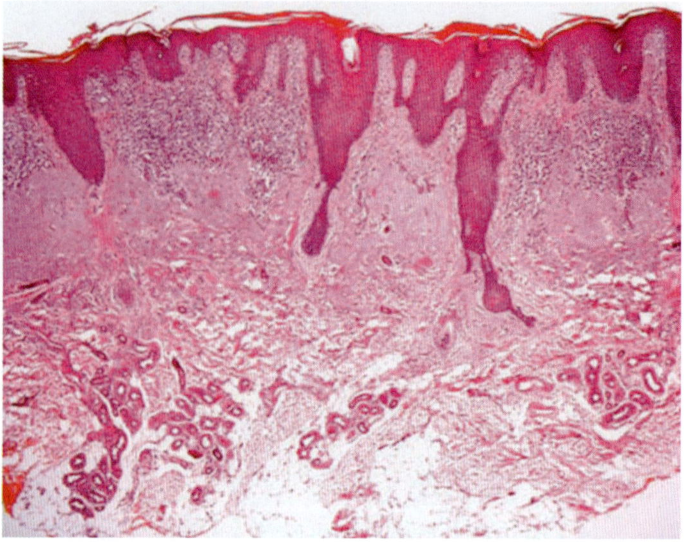

**FIGURE 6-37** Hyperplasia in chronic actinic dermatitis. The lesion presents prominent hyperplasia of the epidermis and the infundibular portion of hair follicles. (From Elder DE. *Lever's Histopathology of the Skin.* 11th ed. Wolters Kluwer Health; 2019:400. Kindle Edition.)

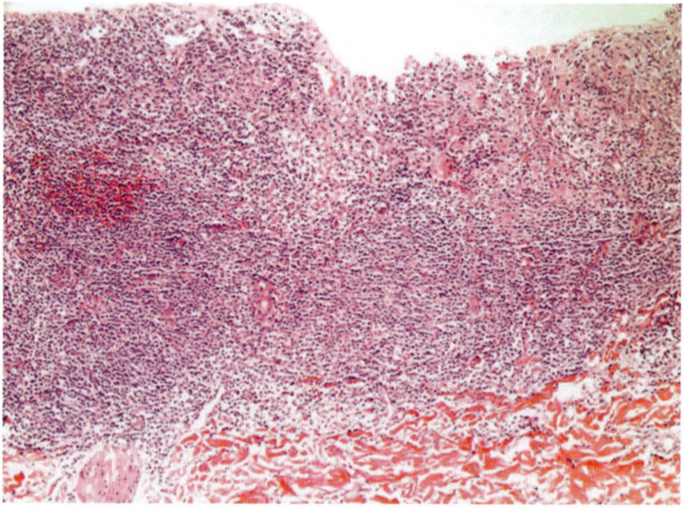

**FIGURE 6-38** Chronic inflammation in chronic leishmaniasis (CL). Low-power view of ulcerated lesion of CL with a dense mixed inflammatory infiltrate of histiocytes, lymphocytes, and plasma cells. (From Elder DE. *Lever's Histopathology of the Skin.* 11th ed. Wolters Kluwer Health; 2019:763. Kindle Edition.)

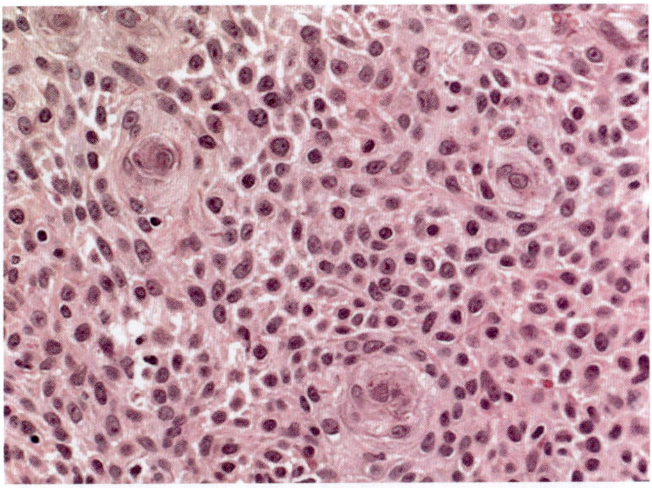

**FIGURE 6-39** Inverted follicular keratosis. Squamous eddies are present, composed of whorls of squamous cells. There is no substantial cytologic atypia. (From Elder DE. *Lever's Histopathology of the Skin.* 11th ed. Wolters Kluwer Health; 2019:976. Kindle Edition.)

- **MELANOMA (CUTANEOUS)**—a malignant melanocytic tumor arising from melanocytes in the skin. Accounts for the majority of deaths from skin cancer worldwide. Breslow's depth measurement is the most important prognostic factor (Figures 6-46 and 6-47).[11-13]
- **MELANOPHAGE**—a macrophage containing phagocytized melanin is referred to as a melanophage. Melanophages are seen in the dermis in inflammatory conditions affecting the epidermis and in neoplasms such as seborrheic keratosis, blue nevus, and melanomas (Figure 6-48).[12,13]

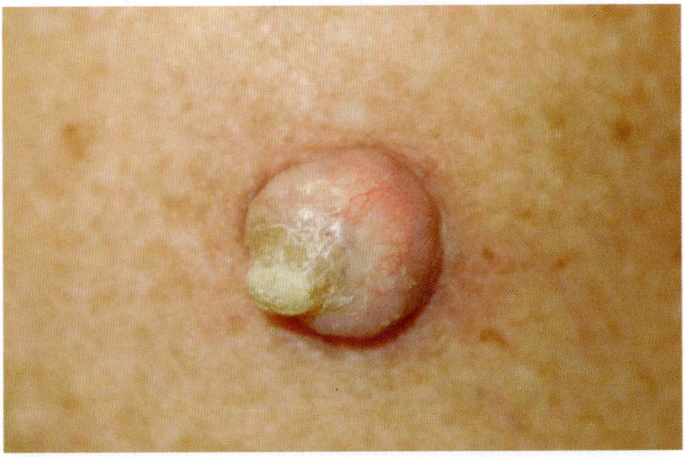

**FIGURE 6-40** Keratoacanthoma. The lesion is symmetric, with keratin protruding from its center. (From Elder DE. *Lever's Histopathology of the Skin.* 11th ed. Wolters Kluwer Health; 2019:1019. Kindle Edition.)

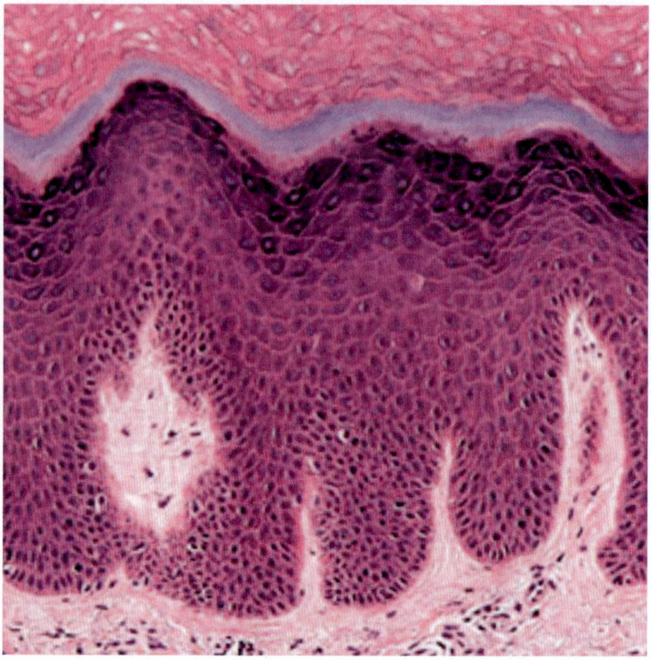

**FIGURE 6-41** Keratohyalin granules fill the darkly staining stratum granulosum directly below the bluish stratum lucidum in this section of acral skin. (From Elder DE. *Lever's Histopathology of the Skin.* 11th ed. Wolters Kluwer Health; 2019:11. Kindle Edition.)

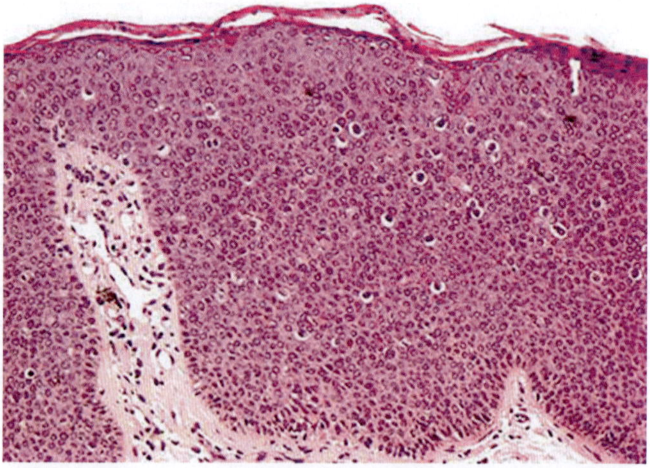

**FIGURE 6-42** Koilocytes in Bowenoid papulosis. The keratinocytic nuclei are crowded, and there is partial arrest of maturation. Mitoses are present above the basal layers, and the nuclei tend to be hyperchromatic and irregular, sometimes with nucleoli. (From Elder DE. *Lever's Histopathology of the Skin.* 11th ed. Wolters Kluwer Health; 2019:803. Kindle Edition.)

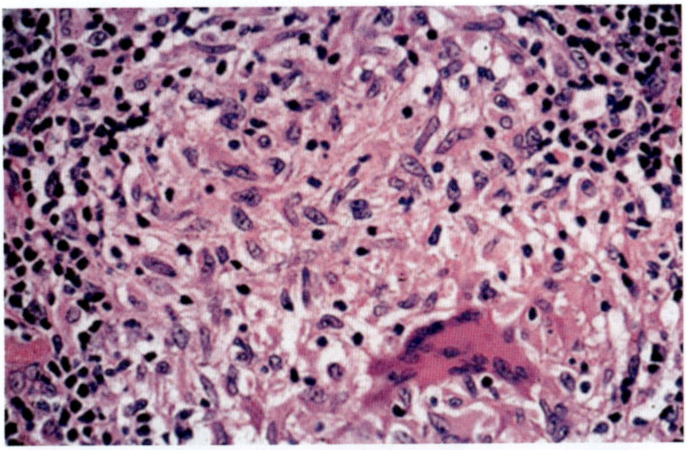

**FIGURE 6-43** Lupus vulgaris showing an epithelioid cell granuloma and Langhans' giant cell (H&E stain). (From Elder DE. *Lever's Histopathology of the Skin.* 11th ed. Wolters Kluwer Health; 2019:674. Kindle Edition.)

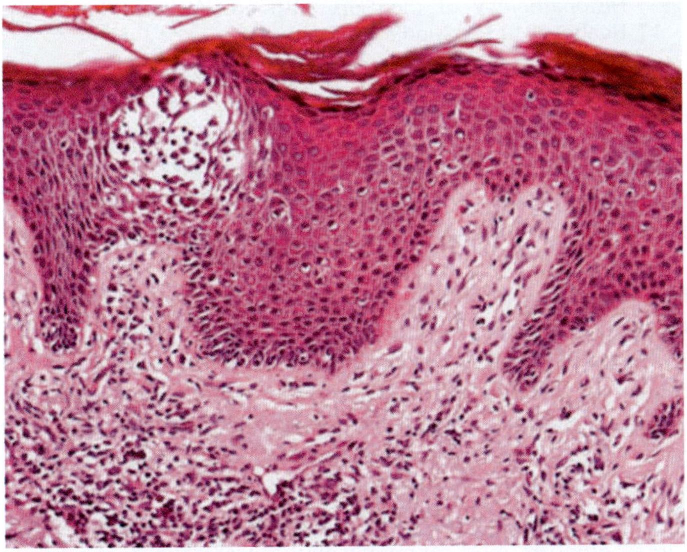

**FIGURE 6-44** Lichenification in chronic actinic dermatitis. Lichenification in association with prominent spongiotic changes and exocytosis of lymphocytes. (From Elder DE. *Lever's Histopathology of the Skin.* 11th ed. Wolters Kluwer Health; 2019:400. Kindle Edition.)

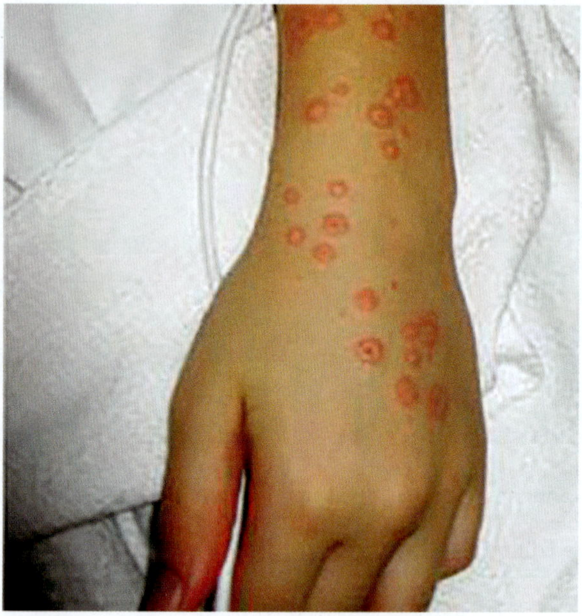

**FIGURE 6-45** Macules in erythema multiforme. Target lesions on the arm of a young boy. (From Elder DE. *Lever's Histopathology of the Skin.* 11th ed. Wolters Kluwer Health; 2019:313. Kindle Edition.)

- **MERKEL CELL CARCINOMA**—an extremely aggressive malignant neuroendocrine carcinoma primarily affecting the older adults (Caucasians older than 70 years old) and immunocompromised. It may present as an expanding violaceous nodule. Eighty percent are associated with Merkel cell polyomavirus, with a minority being UV mediated (Figure 6-49).[12,13,18]
- **METAPLASIA**—a change of cell type to a form that does not normally occur in the tissue in which it is found (Figure 6-50).[12,13]
- **METASTASIS**—malignant cells can spread distally through lymphatic vessels (lymphogenous dissemination) or blood vessels (hematogenous dissemination) to a distant organ and grow into tumors called metastases. Most malignant tumors spread both ways but prefer to spread one way more often. Carcinomas prefer lymphogenous dissemination, whereas sarcomas prefer hematogenous dissemination.[6,10]
- **MILIA**—(singular: milium) are benign subepidermal keratin cysts appearing as small white papules in various numbers, most commonly on the face (Figure 6-51).[12]
- **MYCOSIS FUNGOIDES**—peripheral T-cell lymphoma presenting as patches, plaques, tumors, and erythroderma. Biopsies show bandlike papillary dermal lymphoid infiltrates with background fibroplasia, lymphocytes tagging the junction, and migrating to the epidermis as single cells or groups termed Pautrier microabscesses (Figure 6-52).[12,13,19]

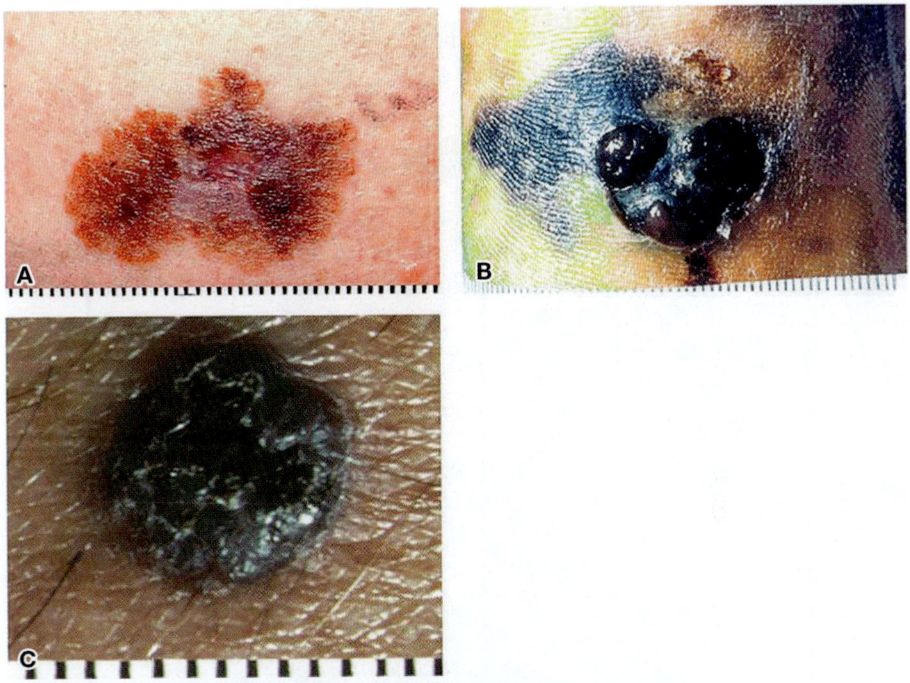


**FIGURE 6-46** **A,** Superficial spreading melanoma. The lesion is large and asymmetric, with an irregular border and variegated colors, including reddish-brown and focal areas of blue–black, as well as a focal grayish area of partial radial growth phase regression (near the middle of the lesion). **B,** Acral lentiginous melanoma, with extensive radial growth phase, partial regression of the radial growth phase, and a bulky ulcerated tumorigenic vertical growth phase nodule. **C,** Nodular melanoma. The focally ulcerated surface may present symptoms of bleeding and oozing, which are signs of relatively advanced melanoma. (From Elder DE. *Lever's Histopathology of the Skin.* 11th ed. Wolters Kluwer Health; 2019:905. Kindle Edition.)

- **MYXOID CHANGE**—in dermatopathology, refers to a mucoid, gelatinous consistency on gross examination and accumulation of extracellular blue-gray mucin on microscopic examination (Figure 6-53).[12,13]
- **NECROSIS**—the death of tissue (cells) by autolysis. Necrosis may be present in inflammation and neoplasms (Figure 6-54).[6,11-13]
- **NEOPLASM**—a *new growth* of indigenous cells not under normal physiologic control. It may be benign or malignant.[6]
- **NODULE**—a palpable, solid lesion greater than 10 mm in diameter (Figure 6-51).[12,13]
- **NEUROFIBROMA**—benign peripheral nerve sheath tumor with classic features, including Schwann cells and fibroblasts (Figure 6-55).[12,13]
- **NEVUS**—a congenital or acquired melanocytic proliferation (Figure 6-56).[10-13]
- **ORTHOKERATOSIS**—is an increased thickness of the horny layer (stratum corneum) by anucleate (i.e., normal appearing) cells. Orthokeratosis may be compact, laminated, or have a basket-weave configuration (Figures 6-23 and 6-57).[12]

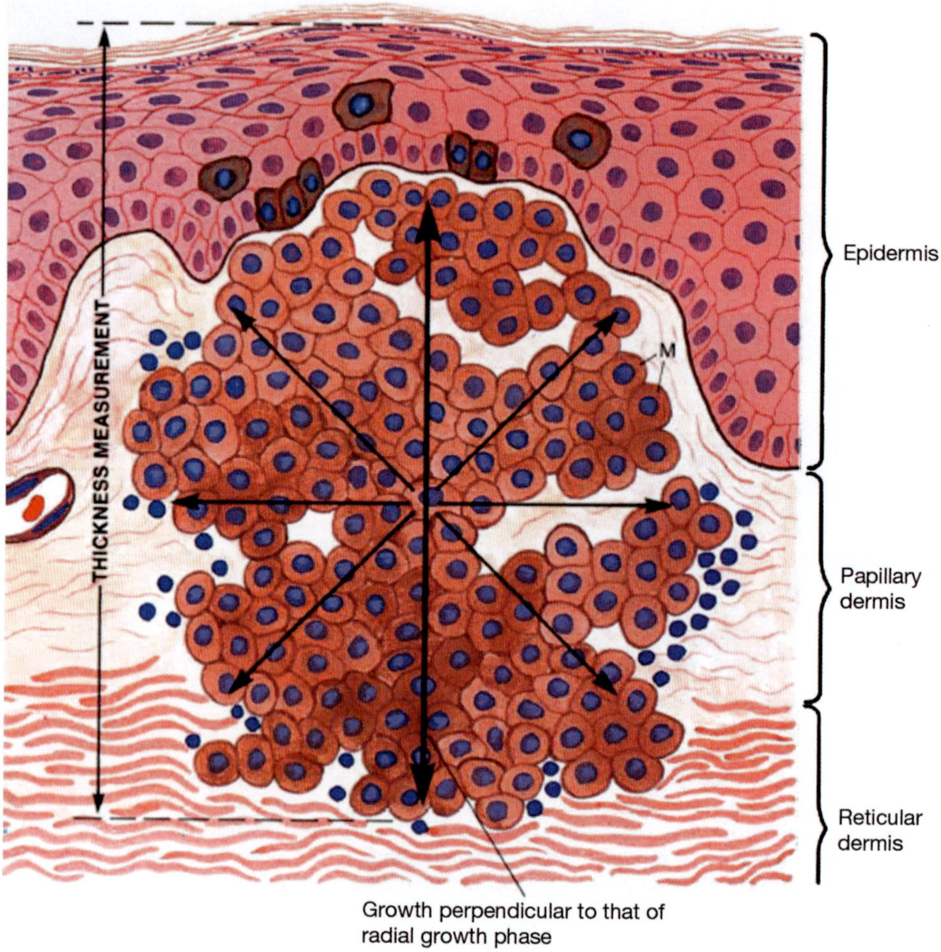


**FIGURE 6-47** Breslow's depth measurement of invasion by melanoma. (From Rubin R, Strayer DS, Rubin E. *Rubin's Pathology: Clinicopathologic Foundations of Medicine*. 6th ed. Wolters Kluwer Health | Lippincott Williams & Wilkins; 2019.)

- **PAPILLOMATOSIS**—is characterized histologically by abnormally elongated epidermis and papillary dermis, resulting in an irregular undulation of the epidermal surface. Papillomatosis is seen most in seborrheic keratosis and verruca vulgaris (Figure 6-58).[11-13]
- **PAPULE**—a solid or cystic raised spot on the skin that is less than 1 cm wide (Figures 6-59 and 6-77).[12,13]
- **PARAKERATOSIS**—is an increased thickness of the horny layer (stratum corneum) by nucleated cells. Parakeratosis represents a defect in cellular differentiation and is usually associated with a thinned or absent granular layer (Figures 6-62, 6-65, and 6-24).[10-13]

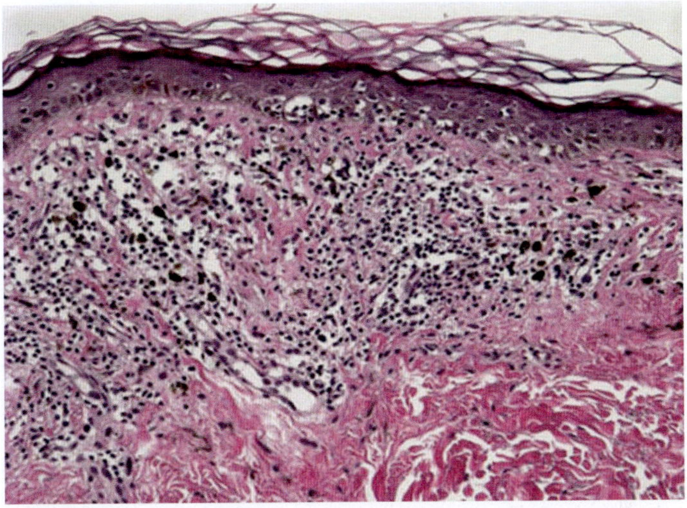

**FIGURE 6-48** Melanophages in a fixed drug eruption. This section shows the characteristic lichenoid lymphocytic infiltrate and abundant pigment incontinence with scattered melanophages. In addition, basal vacuolar alteration and dyskeratotic cells occur in the epidermis. (From Elder DE. *Lever's Histopathology of the Skin.* 11th ed. Wolters Kluwer Health; 2019:368. Kindle Edition.)

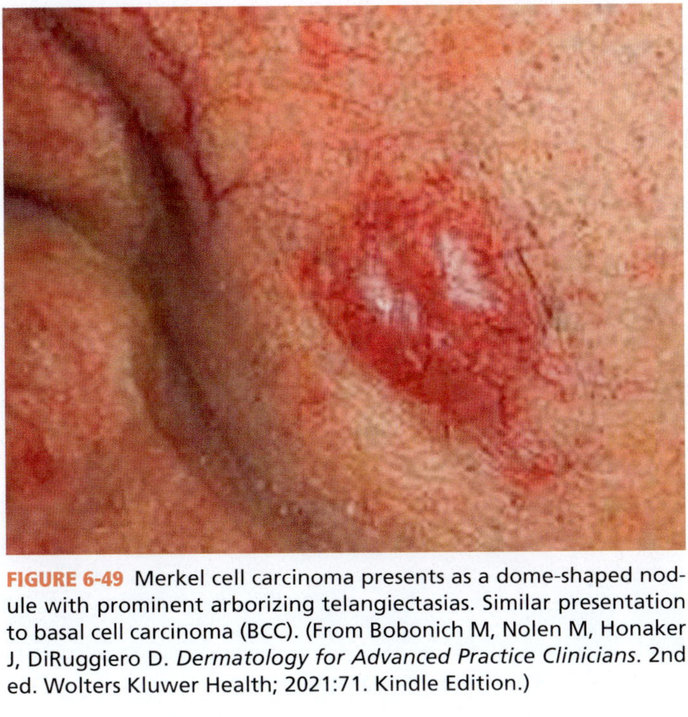

**FIGURE 6-49** Merkel cell carcinoma presents as a dome-shaped nodule with prominent arborizing telangiectasias. Similar presentation to basal cell carcinoma (BCC). (From Bobonich M, Nolen M, Honaker J, DiRuggiero D. *Dermatology for Advanced Practice Clinicians.* 2nd ed. Wolters Kluwer Health; 2021:71. Kindle Edition.)

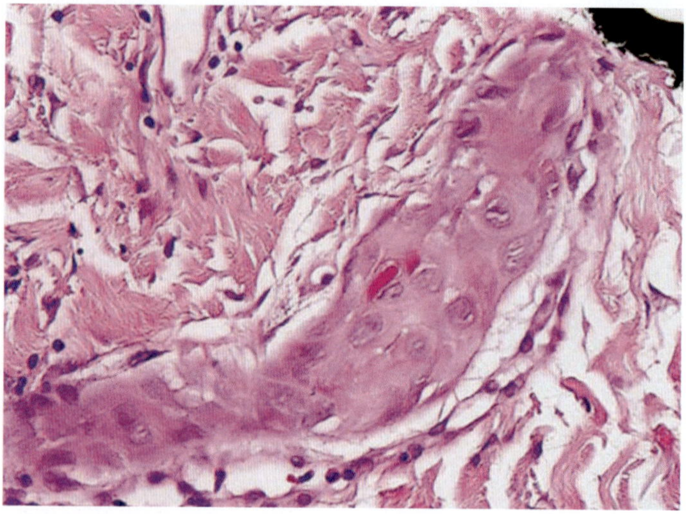

**FIGURE 6-50** Syringosquamous metaplasia. This eccrine duct is lined by squamoid cells with ample eosinophilic cytoplasm and large nuclei rather than the normal cuboidal cells. (From Elder DE. *Lever's Histopathology of the Skin.* 11th ed. Wolters Kluwer Health; 2019:383. Kindle Edition.)

- **PETECHIA**—a small bruise (hematoma) or blood collection in the skin smaller than 0.5 cm in diameter (Figure 6-60).[12]
- **PIGMENT INCONTINENCE**—refers to the release of melanin granules from the epidermis and its resulting deposition in the upper dermis, either free or within macrophages (melanophages) (Figure 6-50).[13,20]
- **PILOMATRIXOMA**—(aka pilomatricoma or calcified epithelioma of Malherbe). A benign neoplasm arising from hair matrix. A malignant variant (malignant pilomatrixoma) has been identified (Figure 6-61).[12,13]

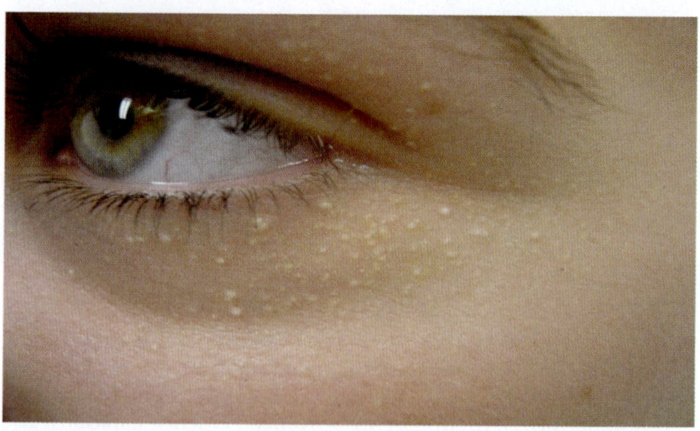

**FIGURE 6-51** Milia. (From NSU-OCO Archives.)

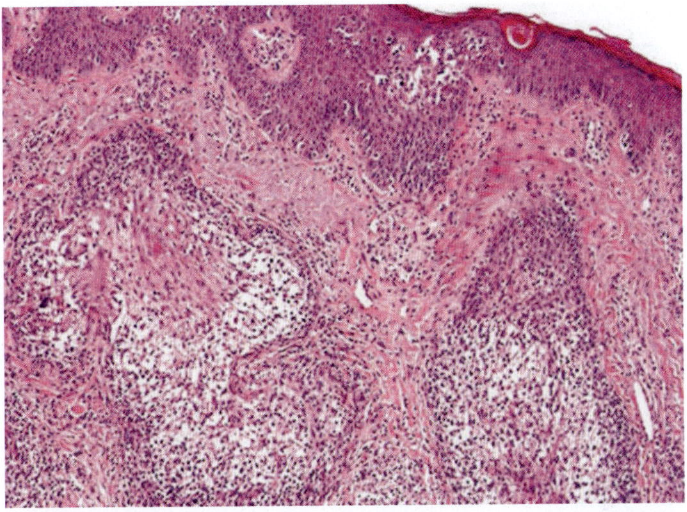

**FIGURE 6-52** Follicular mucinosis associated with folliculotropic mycosis fungoides. In addition to changes in follicular mucinosis, there is extensive folliculotropism of lymphocytes. Epidermotropism of large lymphocytes is also present. (From Elder DE. *Lever's Histopathology of the Skin.* 11th ed. Wolters Kluwer Health; 2019:555. Kindle Edition.)

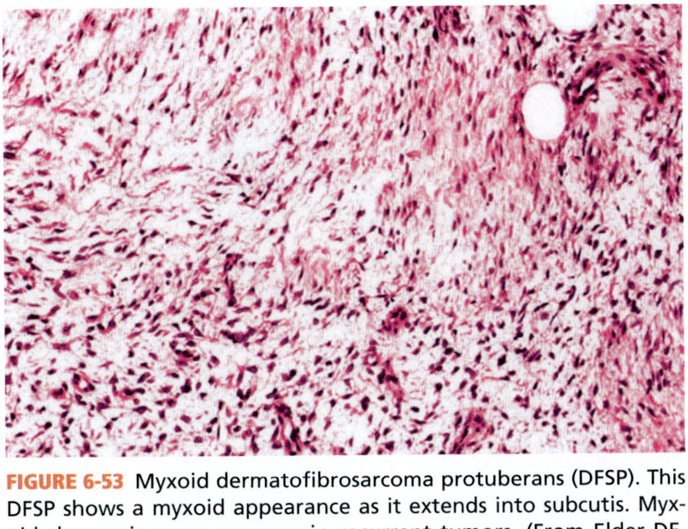

**FIGURE 6-53** Myxoid dermatofibrosarcoma protuberans (DFSP). This DFSP shows a myxoid appearance as it extends into subcutis. Myxoid change is more common in recurrent tumors. (From Elder DE. *Lever's Histopathology of the Skin.* 11th ed. Wolters Kluwer Health; 2019:1211. Kindle Edition.)

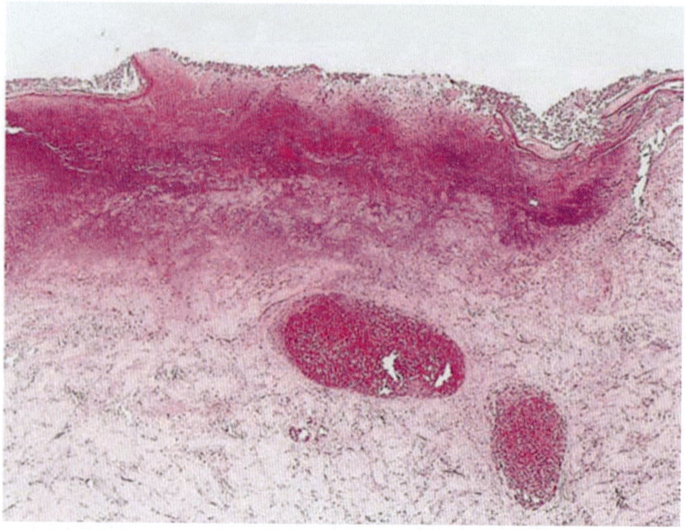

**FIGURE 6-54** Necrosis. *Rickettsia conorii* infection. Typical eschar necrosis of superficial dermis and epithelium. Note the absence of nuclei (H&E stain). (From Elder DE. *Lever's Histopathology of the Skin.* 11th ed. Wolters Kluwer Health; 2019:689. Kindle Edition.)

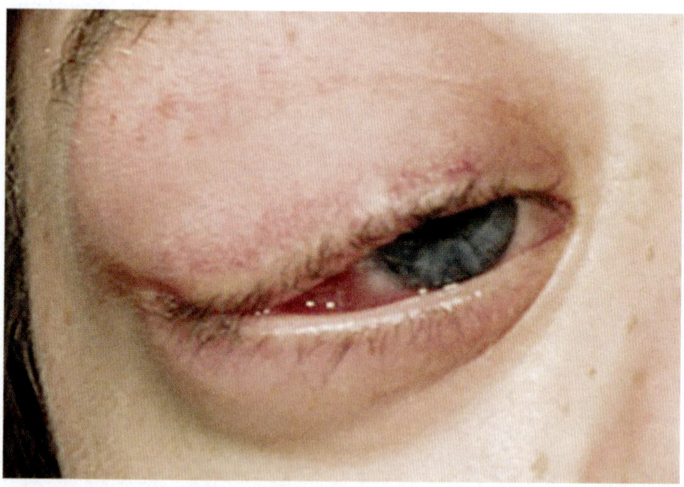

**FIGURE 6-55** Neurofibroma of the upper lid. (From NSU-OCO Archives).

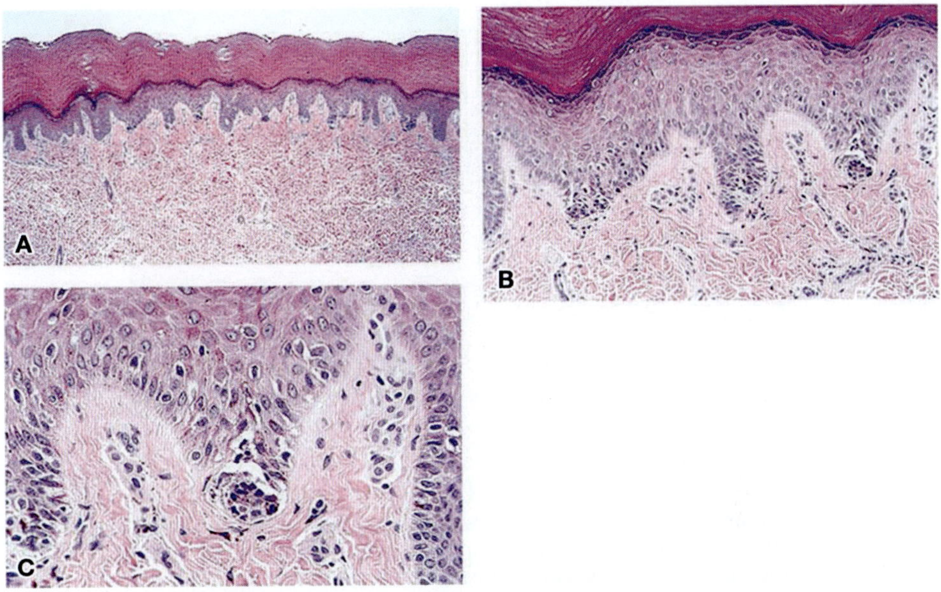

**FIGURE 6-56** Acral lentiginous nevus. **A,** The lesion is small, well circumscribed, and entirely contained within the biopsy specimen. **B,** Nests of nevoid to small epithelioid melanocytes predominate near the dermal–epidermal junction. They tend to be small, evenly spaced, and discrete. **C,** Although a few lesional cells may be present above the junction in a "pagetoid" pattern, there is no severe atypia or mitotic activity. (From Elder DE. *Lever's Histopathology of the Skin.* 11th ed. Wolters Kluwer Health; 2019:874. Kindle Edition.)

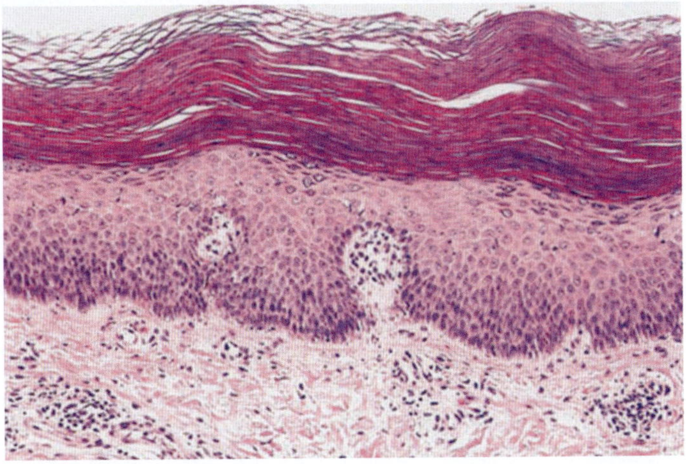

**FIGURE 6-57** Orthokeratosis in pityriasis rubra pilaris. Moderate acanthosis with short and broad rete ridges, focally thin granular layer, and alternating vertical and horizontal foci of orthokeratosis and parakeratosis. (From Elder DE. *Lever's Histopathology of the Skin.* 11th ed. Wolters Kluwer Health; 2019:225. Kindle Edition.)

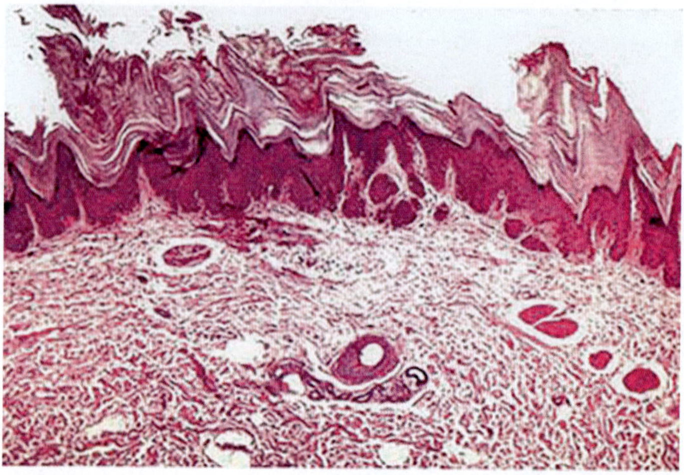

**FIGURE 6-58** A well-circumscribed lesion shows hyperkeratosis and papillomatosis. The papillomatosis is associated with elevations of the epidermis resembling church spires (original magnification ×100). (From Elder DE. *Lever's Histopathology of the Skin.* 11th ed. Wolters Kluwer Health; 2019:164. Kindle Edition.)

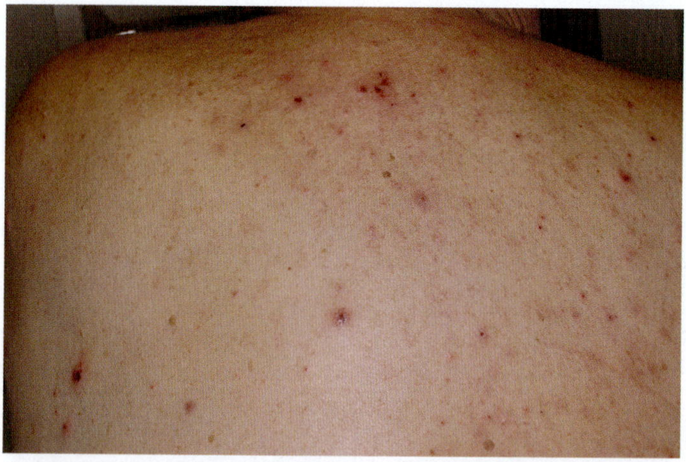

**FIGURE 6-59** Numerous intact erythematous papules and excoriated papules on the upper back. (Reprinted with permission from Gru AA, Schaffer A. *Hematopathology of the Skin*. 2nd ed. Wolters Kluwer; 2024:593; Figure 57-3.)

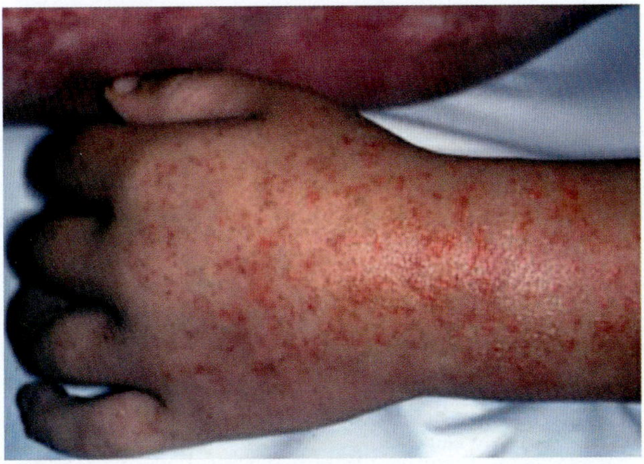

**FIGURE 6-60** Tiny skin hemorrhages (petechiae) in a child with thrombocytopenia. (From Bobonich M, Nolen M, Honaker J, DiRuggiero D. *Dermatology for Advanced Practice Clinicians.* 2nd ed. Wolters Kluwer Health; 2021:346. Kindle Edition.)

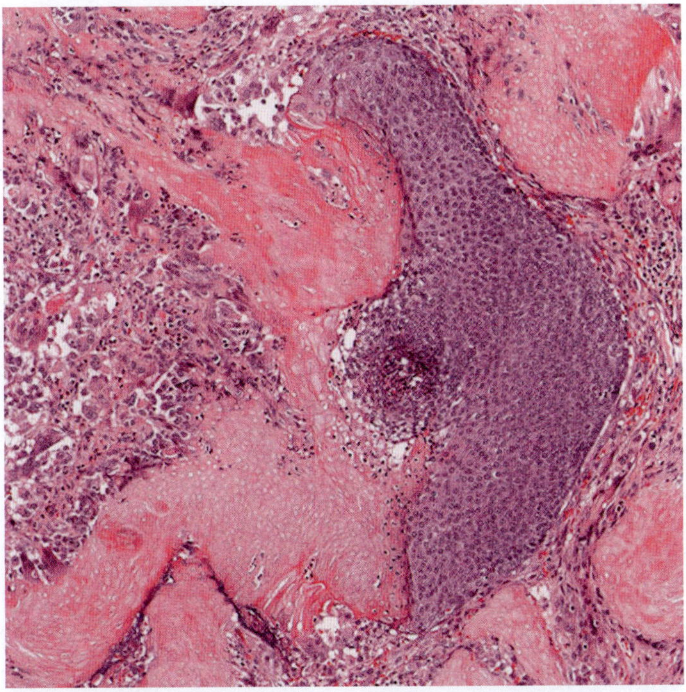

**FIGURE 6-61** Pilomatricoma. The tumor is often well circumscribed and composed of epithelial islands embedded in a cellular stroma. Two types of cells comprise the islands: basophilic cells and shadow cells. The basophilic cells resemble hair matrix cells. The shadow cells show a central unstained shadow at the site of the lost nucleus. In the center of the field, one can see the transformation of the basophilic cells into shadow cells. (From Elder DE. *Lever's Histopathology of the Skin.* 11th ed. Wolters Kluwer Health; 2019:1055. Kindle Edition.)

- **PLAQUE**—a well-defined raised flat-topped lesion (Figures 6-14, 6-21, and 6-62).[10-13]
- **POLYP**—a growth comprised of a head attached to a surface by a stalk (Figure 6-63).[12,13]
- **PSEUDOCARCINOMATOUS HYPERPLASIA**—is a histopathologic reaction pattern manifesting as irregular hyperplasia of the epidermis with prominent acanthotic down growth of the epidermis. Epidermal proliferation occurs in response to various stimuli, including chronic irritation, trauma, and dermal fungal infections (Figure 6-64).[12,21]
- **PURPURA**—cutaneous bleeding resulting in small petechia or large ecchymosis (Figure 6-65).[10-13]
- **PUSTULE**—a circumscribed raised area containing pus (Figure 6-66).[11-13]
- **SARCOMA**—a malignant neoplasm derived from mesenchymal tissues (Figure 6-67).[12,13]
- **SCALE**—accumulated dead epidermal cells resulting from an abnormal growth rate and decreased shedding (Figures 6-21 and 6-68).[12,13]
- **SCAR**—a dense collection of collagen fibers that form after an injury to the skin or other tissue (Figures 6-69 and 6-70).[10-13]
- **SEBACEOUS CELL CARCINOMA**—a non-melanocytic malignant neoplasm with sebaceous differentiation. Atypical sebaceous cells (sebocytes) can be well, moderately, or poorly differentiated—rare association with Muir-Torre syndrome.[10]
- **SEBORRHEIC KERATOSIS**—(aka basal cell papilloma) is a benign proliferation of immature keratinocytes, resulting in well-demarcated, round, or oval, flat-shaped macules (Figures 6-71 and 6-72).[6,10,12,13]
- **SHADOW CELLS**—(aka ghost cells) are pale, eosinophilic cells with a clear area in place of the nucleus, characteristic of pilomatrixoma (Figure 6-61).[12]
- **SOLAR ELASTOSIS** (actinic elastosis) is a condition associated with chronic UV damage superimposed on aging skin. It presents a yellowish thickened appearance to the skin, which is bumpy and covered with furrows—histologically, characterized by lightly basophilic, irregular, thickened elastic fibers in the dermis. Individual fibers are sometimes not evident, and there may be only an amorphous mass of lightly basophilic material in the dermis (Figure 6-73).[12]
- **SPONGIOSIS**—is intercellular edema between squamous cells of the epidermis that is characteristic of acute dermatitis and may lead to micro- and macrovesicles (spongiotic blisters). Intracellular edema may accompany severe spongiosis, resulting in the bursting of epidermal cells and the formation of multilocular bulla (Figure 6-74).[11,12]

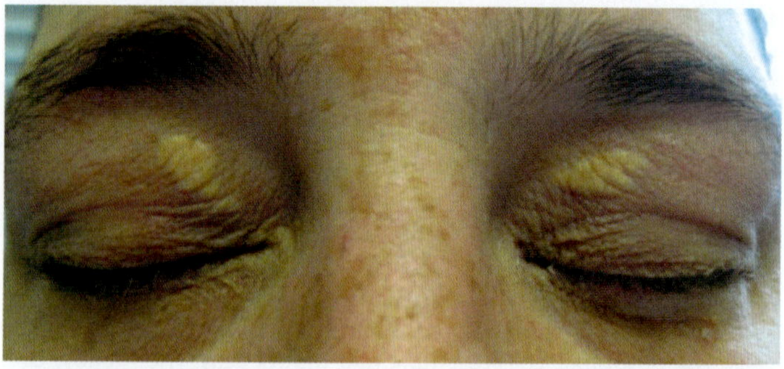

**FIGURE 6-62** Xanthelasmas presenting as yellowish plaques are often caused by a defect in lipid metabolism. (From Bobonich M, Nolen M, Honaker J, DiRuggiero D. *Dermatology for Advanced Practice Clinicians*. 2nd ed. Wolters Kluwer Health; 2021:88. Kindle Edition.)

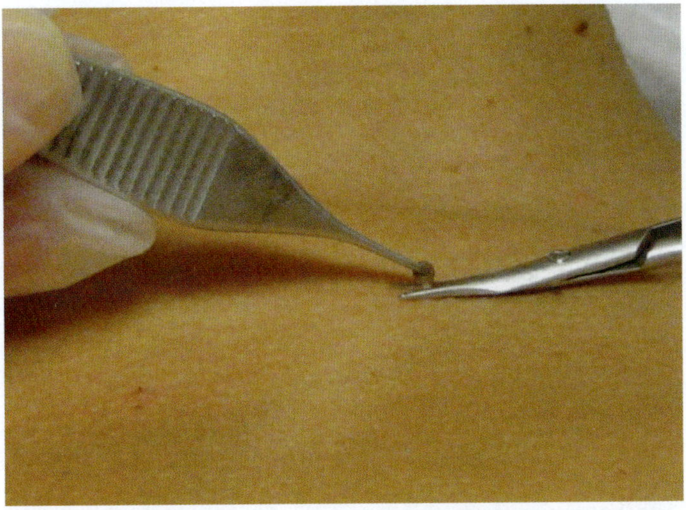

**FIGURE 6-63** Snip excision of a fibroepithelial polyp (skin tag). (From Bobonich M, Nolen M, Honaker J, DiRuggiero D. *Dermatology for Advanced Practice Clinicians*. 2nd ed. Wolters Kluwer Health; 2021:542. Kindle Edition.)

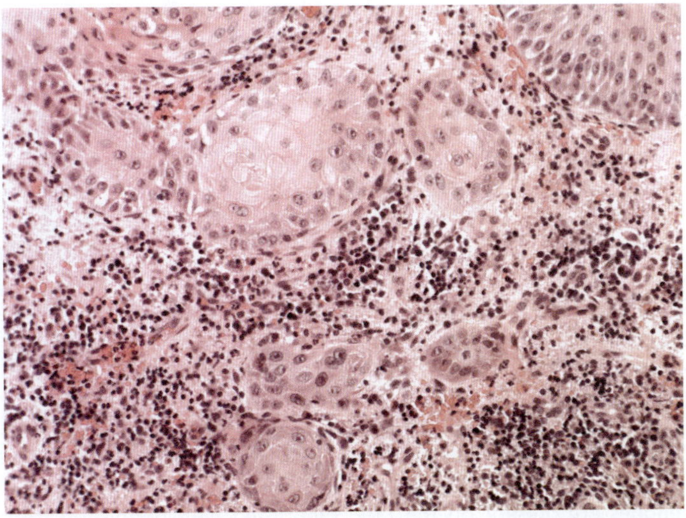

**FIGURE 6-64** Pseudocarcinomatous hyperplasia. This curetting specimen shows a proliferative squamous lesion without substantial atypia and mimicking an invasive lesion. (Reprinted with permission from Elder DE. *Lever's Histopathology of the Skin*. 11th ed. Wolters Kluwer; 2015:1005; Figure 29-69.)

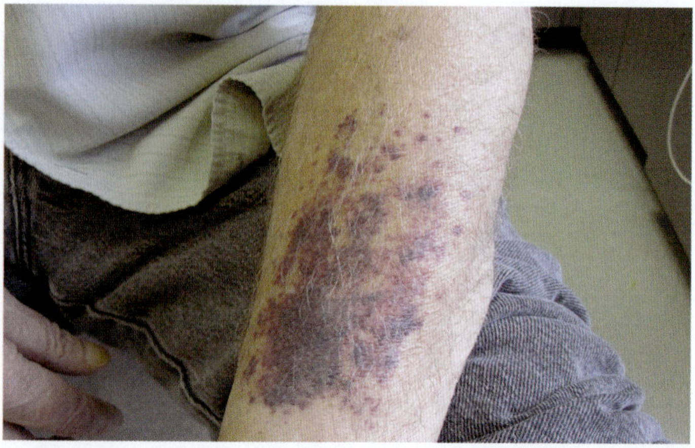

**FIGURE 6-65** Actinic purpura. Senile, or actinic, purpura. Ecchymoses are present on the dorsal forearms in this elderly man. (Reprinted with permission from *Goodheart HP, Gonzalez ME. Goodheart's Same-Site Differential Diagnosis*. 2nd ed. Wolters Kluwer; 2023:166; Figure 13-14.)

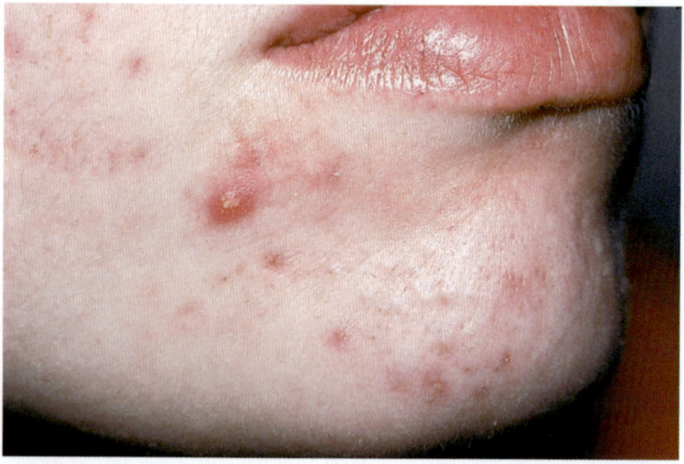

**FIGURE 6-66** Acne. Inflammatory papules, pustules, and closed comedones are present on the face. (Reprinted with permission from Nath J. *Programmed Learning Approach to Medical Terminology*. 3rd ed. Wolters Kluwer; 2019:59; Figure 2-9.)

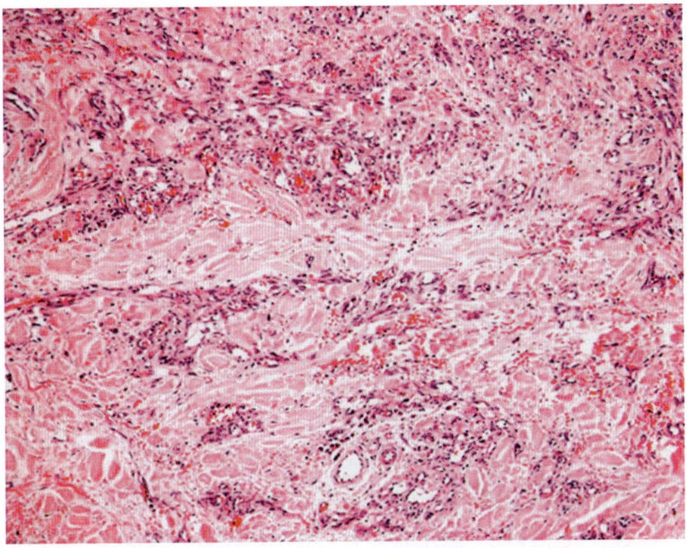

**FIGURE 6-67** Well-differentiated angiosarcoma. Irregular and congested vascular channels are infiltrating between collagen bundles. (From Elder DE. *Lever's Histopathology of the Skin.* 11th ed. Wolters Kluwer Health; 2019:1289. Kindle Edition.)

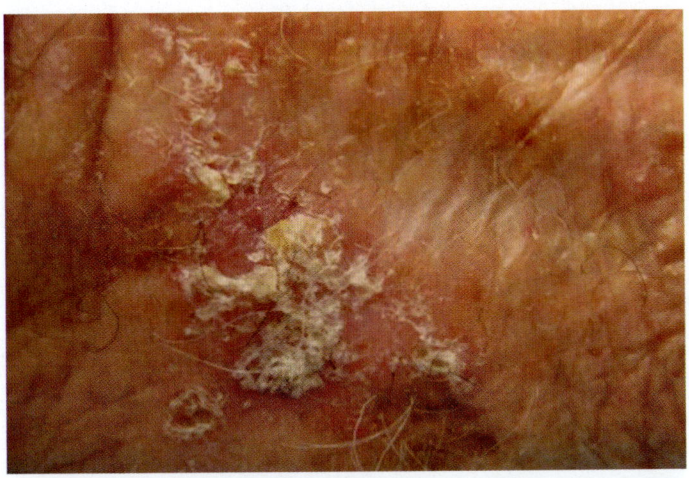

**FIGURE 6-68** Squamous cell carcinoma in situ presents an irregularly shaped erythematous thin plaque with a thick scale. (From Bobonich Margaret, Nolen M, Honaker J, DiRuggiero D. *Dermatology for Advanced Practice Clinicians.* 2nd ed. Wolters Kluwer Health; 2021:61. Kindle Edition.)

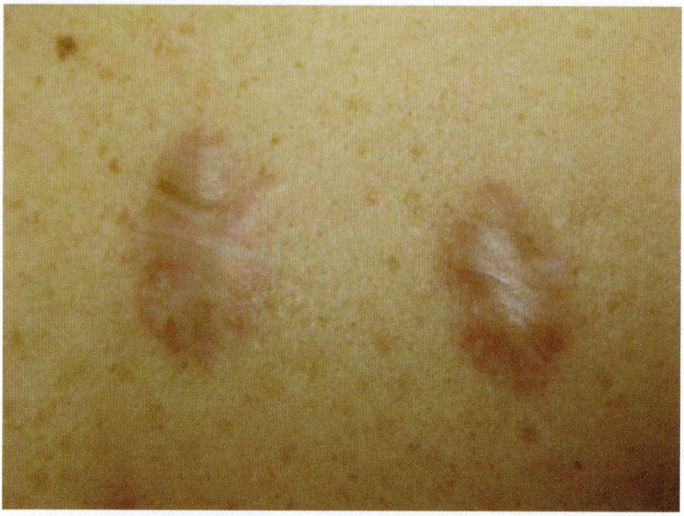

**FIGURE 6-69** Hypertrophic scars are thickened scars that do not exceed the wound border. (From Bobonich M, Nolen M, Honaker J, DiRuggiero D. *Dermatology for Advanced Practice Clinicians*. 2nd ed. Wolters Kluwer Health; 2021:85. Kindle Edition.)

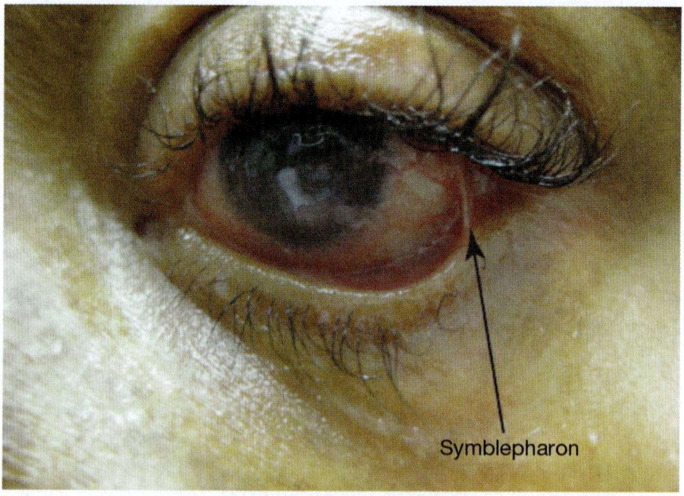


**FIGURE 6-70** Erosions in ocular mucous membrane pemphigoid heal with scarring or symblepharon. (From Bobonich M, Nolen M, Honaker J, DiRuggiero D. *Dermatology for Advanced Practice Clinicians*. Wolters Kluwer Health; 2021:325. Kindle Edition.)

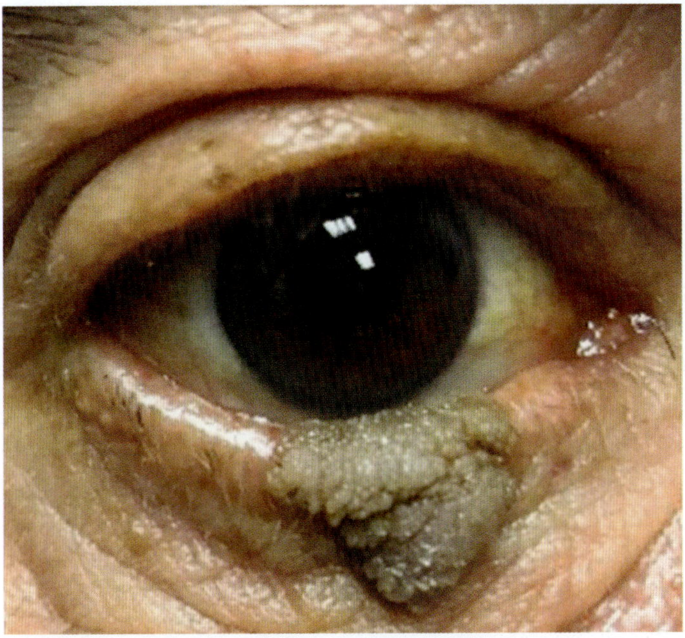

FIGURE 6-71 Seborrheic keratosis eyelid. (From Bobonich M, Nolen Mary, Honaker J, DiRuggiero D. *Dermatology for Advanced Practice Clinicians*. Wolters Kluwer Health; 2021:78. Kindle Edition.)

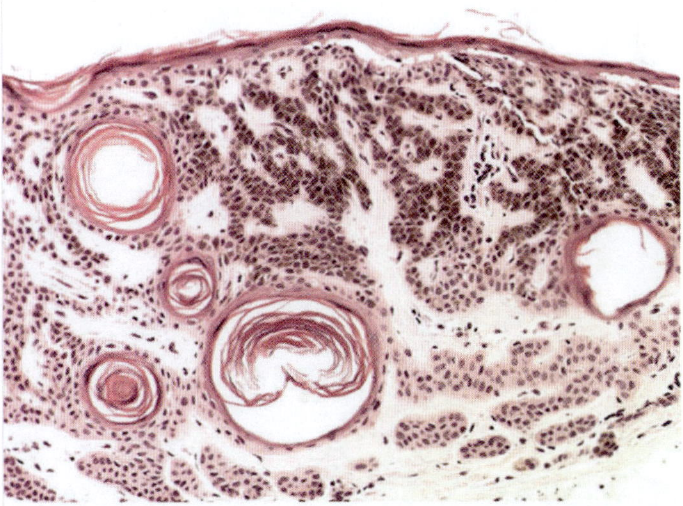

FIGURE 6-72 Pigmented seborrheic keratosis. Thin interwoven cords of basaloid cells show cytoplasmic melanin pigmentation and horn cysts. (From Elder DE. *Lever's Histopathology of the Skin.* 11th ed. Wolters Kluwer Health; 2019:975. Kindle Edition.)

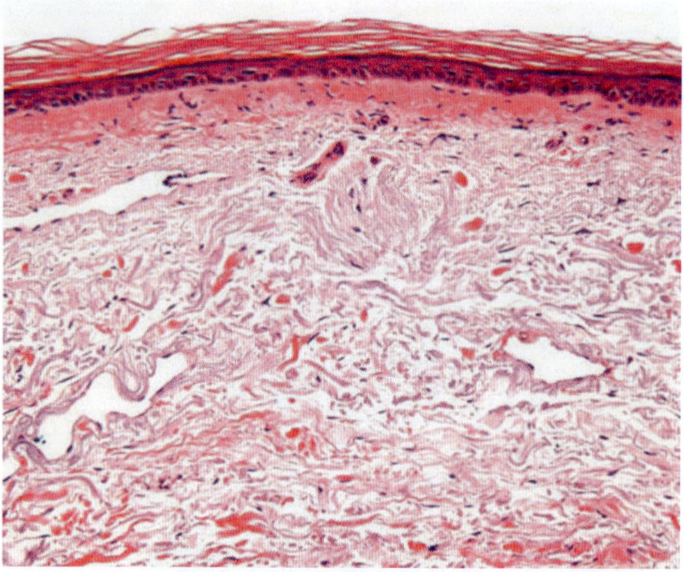

**FIGURE 6-73** Solar (actinic) elastosis. Changes associated with skin aging include a thinner epidermis with a flattened dermal–epidermal junction and telangiectatic dermal vessels associated with marked solar elastosis in the form of bluish-gray fibers, the latter related to chronic sun damage. (From Elder DE. *Lever's Histopathology of the Skin.* 11th ed. Wolters Kluwer Health; 2019:61. Kindle Edition.)

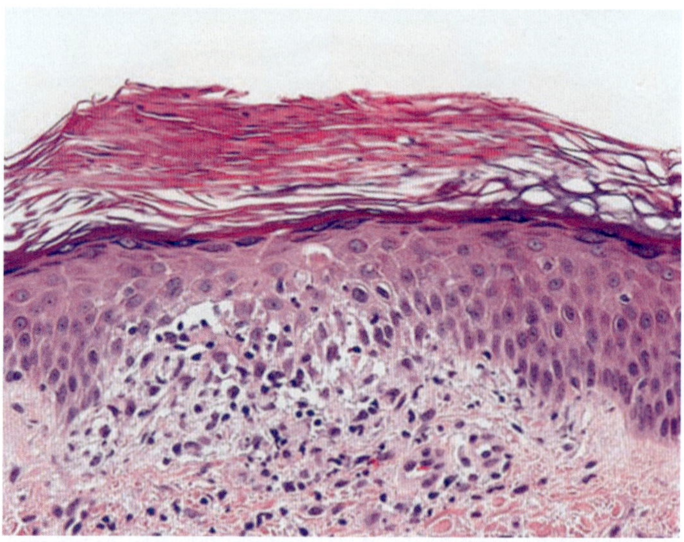

**FIGURE 6-74** Spongiosis in lichen striatus. A closer view shows an infiltrate of lymphocytes and histiocytes, exocytosis of lymphocytes, acanthosis, spongiosis, and focal parakeratosis. (From Elder DE. *Lever's Histopathology of the Skin.* 11th ed. Wolters Kluwer Health; 2019:223. Kindle Edition.)

- **SQUAMOUS CELL CARCINOMA (CUTANEOUS)**—cutaneous squamous cell carcinoma is a non-melanocytic malignancy of epidermal keratinocytes that may display variable degrees of differentiation and cytologic features (Figures 6-15 and 6-75).[12,13,22]
- **SQUAMOUS EDDIES**—are whorled onionskin-like foci of brightly eosinophilic keratinocytes. They are a typical feature of irritated seborrheic keratoses (Figure 6-39).[12]
- **SUPPURATION**—acute inflammation characterized by infiltration of neutrophils at the microscopic level and pus at the gross level (Figure 6-76).[12]
- **TELANGIECTASIA**—small, dilated blood vessels visible on the skin (Figure 6-77).[10,12,13]
- **TOUTON GIANT CELLS**—are multinucleated giant cells derived from the fusion of epithelioid cells (activated macrophages). They have a ring of nuclei surrounding eosinophilic nonvacuolated cytoplasm centrally and lipid-filled foamy cytoplasm peripherally. They are characteristic of xanthogranulomas and xanthelasmas (Figure 6-78).[12]
- **TUMOR**—a mass or lump attributed to a neoplasm, hyperplasia, distention, swelling, or anything that causes a local increase in volume.[6]
- **ULCER** (skin)—a focal full-thickness loss of the skin due to injury, poor circulation, or pressure (Figure 6-77).[12,13]
- **VESICLE**—a small blister (area of acantholysis), less than 0.5 cm in diameter (Figure 6-79).[13]
- **WHEAL**—a superficial dermal swelling (Figure 6-80).[13]
- **XANTHELASMA**—benign lesion(s) appearing as yellow plaques typically within the medial canthal area consisting of large, pale, fat-laden histiocytes within the dermis (Figures 6-62 and 6-81).[12,13,23]

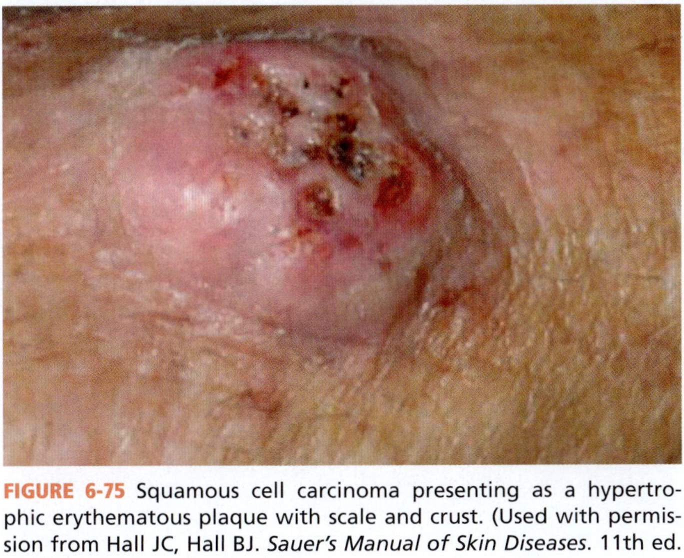

**FIGURE 6-75** Squamous cell carcinoma presenting as a hypertrophic erythematous plaque with scale and crust. (Used with permission from Hall JC, Hall BJ. *Sauer's Manual of Skin Diseases*. 11th ed. Wolters Kluwer Health; 2017.)

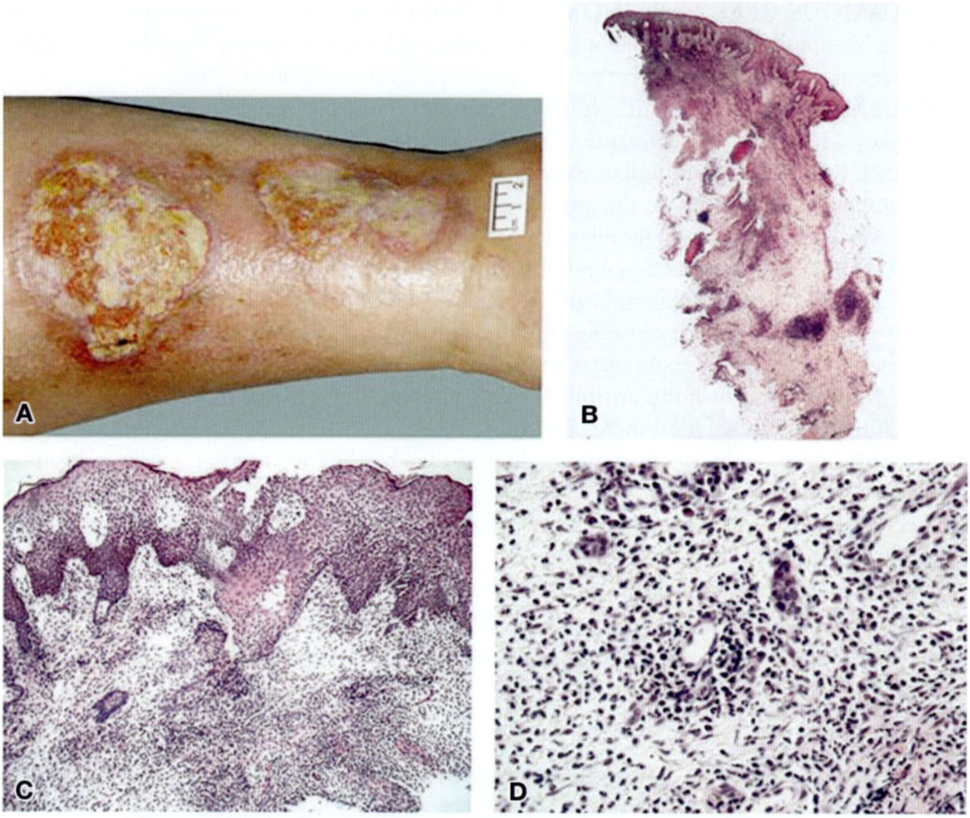

**FIGURE 6-76** Suppuration in pyoderma gangrenosum. **A,** Superficial ulcers with central suppurative exudate and a peripheral raised and slightly undermined border. **B,** Punch biopsy from the edge of an ulcer shows a mixed inflammatory infiltrate spanning the dermis and the panniculus. The infiltrate is deeper and more extensive than that in classic Sweet syndrome. **C,** A mixed inflammatory infiltrate in the dermis with spongiosis of the epidermis at the edge of the ulcer. **D,** Neutrophils and lymphocytes surround a vessel, but there is no frank vasculitis. (From Elder DE. *Lever's Histopathology of the Skin.* 11th ed. Wolters Kluwer Health; 2019:263. Kindle Edition.)

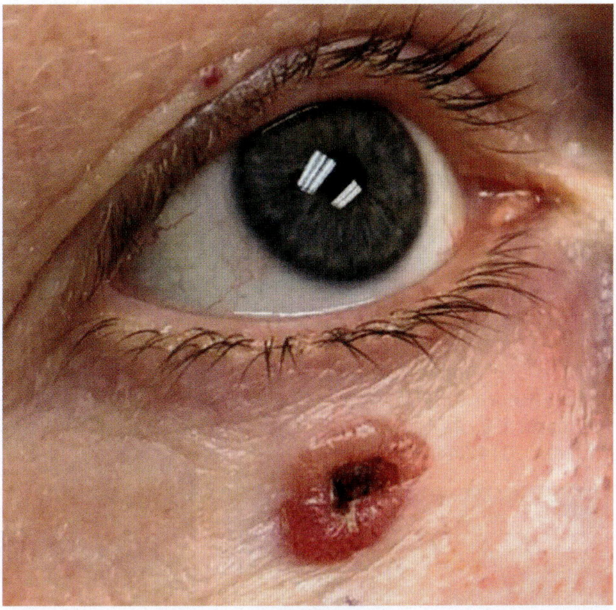

**FIGURE 6-77** Basal cell carcinoma presenting as ulcerative papules with central crusted depression, rolled border, and arborizing telangiectasias on the rim. (From Bobonich M, Nolen M, Honaker J, DiRuggiero D. *Dermatology for Advanced Practice Clinicians*. 2nd ed. Wolters Kluwer Health; 2021:68. Kindle Edition.)

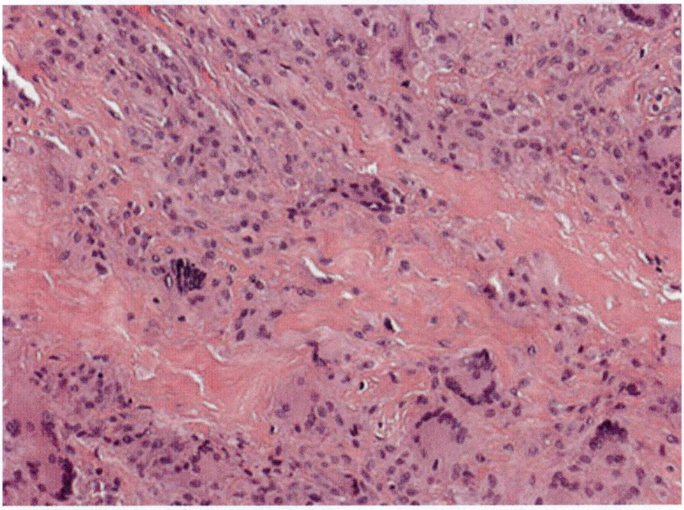

**FIGURE 6-78** Necrobiotic xanthogranuloma showing numerous bizarre foreign-body and Touton giant cells and extensive necrobiosis (blurring and loss of collagen bundles). (From Elder DE. *Lever's Histopathology of the Skin.* 11th ed. Wolters Kluwer Health; 2019:834. Kindle Edition.)

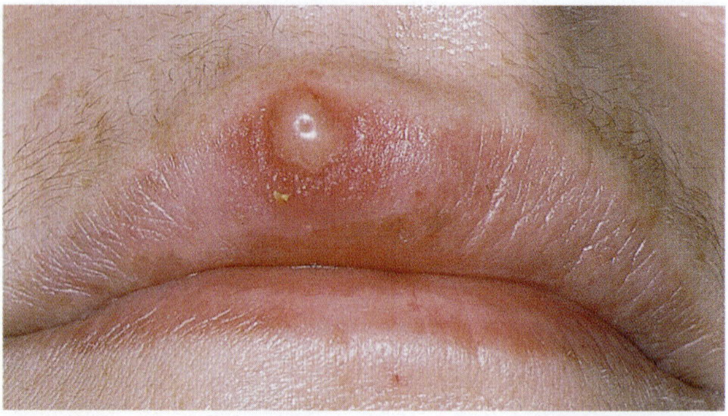

**FIGURE 6-79** Vesicle. A vesicle is a small blister filled with fluid. (Reprinted with permission from Nield-Gehrig JS, Wilmann DE. *Patient Assessment Tutorials*. 3rd ed. Wolters Kluwer; 2014:344; Figure 11-23.)

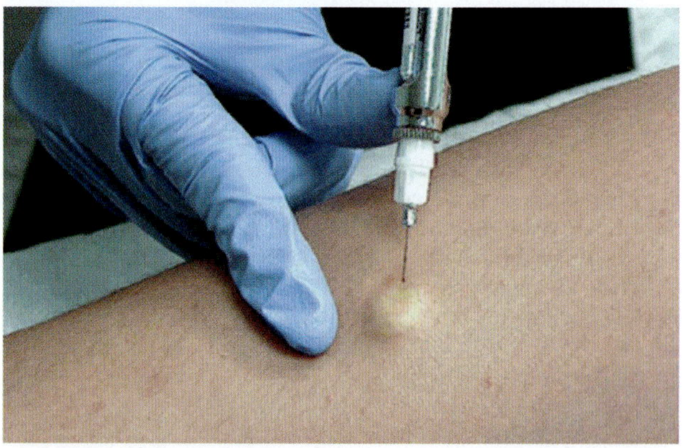

**FIGURE 6-80** Injection of local anesthetic using a 30G needle that produces a wheal under the lesion for biopsy. (From Bobonich M, Nolen M, Honaker J, DiRuggiero D. *Dermatology for Advanced Practice Clinicians*. Wolters Kluwer Health; 2021:540. Kindle Edition.)

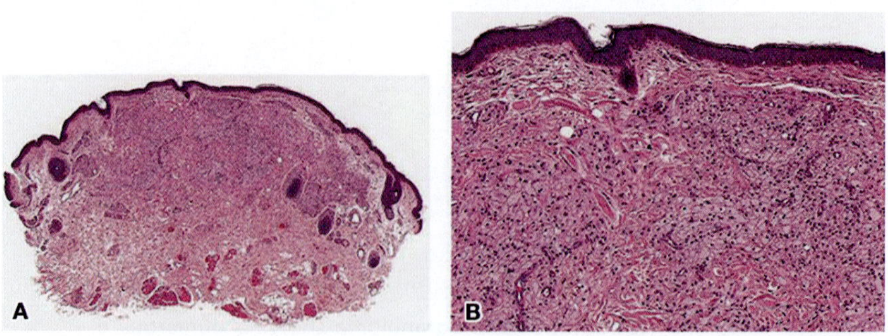


**FIGURE 6-81** Xanthelasma. **A,** The thin epidermis and muscle fibers at the base are a clue to the eyelid location. **B,** Lobules of foamy cells in this location allow the specific diagnosis of xanthelasmas. (From Elder DE. *Lever's Histopathology of the Skin.* 11th ed. Wolters Kluwer Health; 2019:833. Kindle Edition.)

# REFERENCES


1. Greenwood JD, Merry SP, Boswell CL. Skin biopsy techniques. *Prim Care.* 2022;49(1):1-22.
2. Sadeghipour A, Babaheidarian P. Making formalin-fixed, paraffin embedded blocks. *Methods Mol Biol.* 2019;1897:253-268.
3. Buesa RJ. Histology without formalin? *Ann Diagn Pathol.* 2008;12(6):387-396.
4. Stratman EJ, Elston DM, Miller SJ. Skin biopsy: identifying and overcoming errors in the skin biopsy pathway. *J Am Acad Dermatol.* 2016;74(1):19-25.
5. Elston DM, Stratman EJ, Miller SJ. Skin biopsy: biopsy issues in specific diseases [published correction appears in *J Am Acad Dermatol.* 2016 Oct;75(4):854]. *J Am Acad Dermatol.* 2016;74(1):1-16; quiz 17-18. doi:10.1016/j.jaad.2015.06.033.
6. Dinulos JG, *Habif's Clinical Dermatology: A Color Guide to Diagnosis and Therapy.* 7th ed. Elsevier; 2022.
7. Seshadri D, Kumaran MS, Kanwar AJ. Acantholysis revisited: back to basics. *Indian J Dermatol Venereol Leprol.* 2013;79(1):120-126.
8. Hirt PA, Castillo DE, Yosipovitch G, Keri JE. Skin changes in the obese patient. *J Am Acad Dermatol.* 2019;81(5):1037-1057.
9. Deka AC, Dutta AM, Sarma PC, Baruah KC. Solar elastosis in conjunctival squamous cell neoplasm. *Indian J Cancer.* 2014;51(3):245-246.
10. Wolf K, *Fitzpatrick's Color Atlas and Synopsis of Clinical Dermatology.* 8th ed. McGraw Hill; 2017.
11. Tadrous PJ. *Diagnostic Criteria Handbook in Histopathology: A Surgical Pathology Vade Mecum.* 1st ed. John Wiley & Sons; 2008.
12. Elder DE. *Lever's Histopathology of the Skin.* 11th ed. Wolters Kluwer Health. 2015. Kindle Edition.
13. Bobonich M, Nolen M, Honaker J, DiRuggiero D. *Dermatology for Advanced Practice Clinicians.* 2nd ed. Wolters Kluwer Health; 2021. Kindle Edition.
14. Anderson JM, Rodriguez A, Chang DT. Foreign body reaction to biomaterials. *Semin Immunol.* 2008;20(2):86-100.
15. Cape HT, Mukit FA, Mukit M, et al. Apocrine hidrocystoma of the upper eyelid. *Eplasty.* 2022;22:ic13.
16. Karadag AS, Ozlu E, Uzuncakmak TK, et al. Inverted follicular keratosis successfully treated with imiquimod. *Indian Dermatol Online J.* 2016;7(3):177-179.
17. Kwiek B, Schwartz RA. Keratoacanthoma (KA): an update and review. *J Am Acad Dermatol.* 2016;74(6):1220-1233.
18. Becker JC, Stang A, DeCaprio JA, et al. Merkel cell carcinoma. *Nat Rev Dis Primers.* 2017;3:17077.
19. Kamijo H, Miyagaki T. Mycosis fungoides and Sézary syndrome: updates and review of current therapy. *Curr Treat Options Oncol.* 2021;22(2):10.
20. Cramer SF, Salgado CM, Reyes-Múgica M. A study of dermal melanophages in childhood nevi. Reassessing so-called "pigment incontinence". *J Cutan Pathol.* 2020;47(9):809-814.
21. Grunwald MH, Lee JY, Ackerman AB. Pseudocarcinomatous hyperplasia. *Am J Dermatopathol.* 1988;10(2):95-103.
22. Waldman A, Schmults C. Cutaneous squamous cell carcinoma. *Hematol Oncol Clin North Am.* 2019;33(1):1-12.
23. Parkes ML, Waller TS. Xanthelasma palpebrarum. *Laryngoscope.* 1984;94(9):1238-1240.

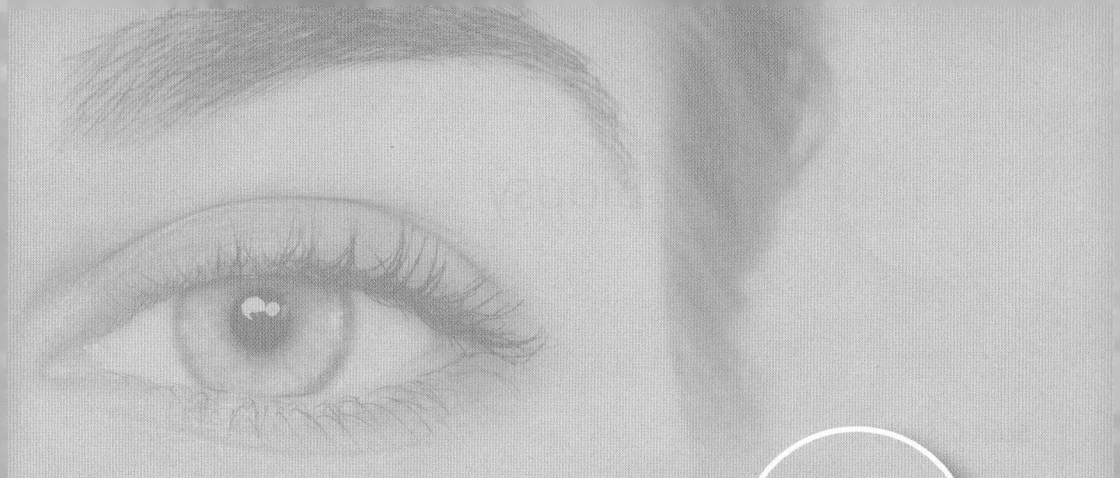

# SECTION 3

# Lids, Lashes, and Adnexa

# 7 Eyelid Biopsy

**Scott C. Sigler**

One of the most overlooked sections of the eight-part eye exam is the external examination. The external exam consists of evaluation of the face and periocular area: paying close attention to the lid position, lash line, and globe position, and noting any unusual lesions or growths on the lids. Proptosis, face palsy, dermatochalasis, lagophthalmos, and brow ptosis should be noted, as well as lid malposition like ptosis, ectropion, and entropion. If a lid lesion is identified and the decision is made for excisional or incisional biopsy, the examiner needs to be comfortable in performing this procedure.

Lid lesions are very common, especially in the older population. Fortunately, 85% to 90% of eyelid lesions are benign. They can be unsightly, but rarely uncomfortable. If large, they can cause lid malposition or obstruction in the visual field. The examining clinician should be aware of the characteristics seen in malignant tumors. A patient's history may also cause a clinician to be more suspicious for skin cancer. Some of the most significant signs and symptoms of eyelid lesion malignancy are:

- Loss of lashes associated with the lesion
- Distorted architecture of the lid
- Increased or changing pigmentation
- White, pearly surface
- Ulcerated center
- History of bleeding from the lesion
- History of chronic blepharitis/conjunctivitis on one side only
- Any history of skin cancer of the face or lids

A patient may request a lesion to be removed. This may be due to the appearance of the lesion, interference with makeup, itching or bleeding, or obstructing the patient's vision or visual field. Some patients may present with a concern that the lesion is a skin cancer. The examiner may recommend a lesion be removed due to a concern for possible malignancy. **No clinician can tell for sure whether a lesion is benign or malignant without a histopathologic examination under the microscope to identify the lesion and cells.** Many a clinician has been wrong about the nature of a skin lesion in the past. Both benign and malignant lesions are usually slow growing. However, there are some lesions like seborrheic keratosis, cysts, and papillomas that have a distinct appearance under the slit lamp, and the patient can be assured the lesion is benign. Congenital nevi of the lid can grow rapidly during puberty, pregnancy, or when the patient's hormones have changed quickly. Benign lesions can start to accumulate pigment and become darker with age. It is recommended that any lesion that is suspicious be sent in formalin to a pathology laboratory along with clinical information for histopathologic identification. The patient needs to be aware that there may be a pathology processing fee as well as a pathologist charge for reading the specimen. Medicare and most insurances will pay these fees. Some insurances require precertification before removing a lesion in the office. Check with the patient's insurance provider to be sure.

The anatomical position of the eyelid lesion will dictate the best approach for the examiner to proceed. The three main areas are **lid margin** (Figure 7-1), **lash line** (Figure 7-2), **and periocular lid lesions** (not involving the lash line or lashes) (Figure 7-3A and B). Lid lesion biopsies can be divided into **excisional, shave or incisional, and punch biopsy**. Excisional biopsy involves removing the *whole* lesion completely. Incisional biopsy involves removing *some* of the lesions, leaving tumor or abnormal cells behind. If the lesion is being cut flush with the surrounding remaining skin, that is a shave biopsy. The clinician is aware that some cells of the lesion are most likely still present to avoid causing a defect in the lid or excessive loss of lashes. A punch biopsy can be either an excisional or incisional biopsy, depending on the size of the lesion and the punch diameter and size. The decision to do an excisional, incisional, shave, or punch biopsy depends on the location and size of the area to be biopsied and the level of concern for malignancy.

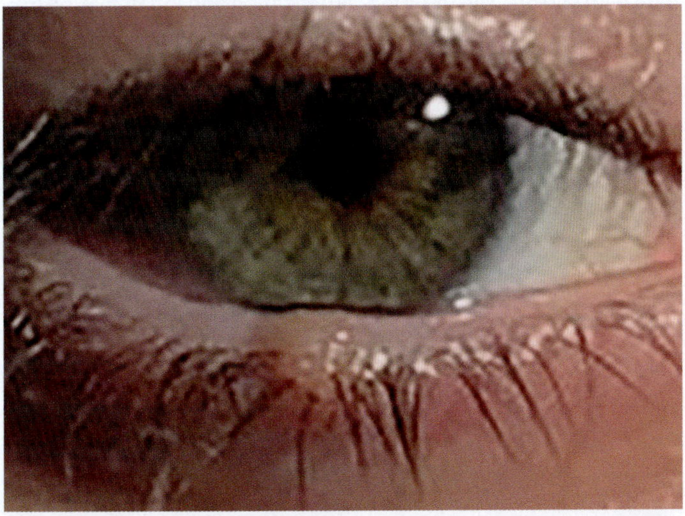

**FIGURE 7-1** Lid margin lesion. The patient noticed that the lesion has grown since she has been pregnant. Diagnosis is most likely congenital nevus, changing because of hormonal changes. If she wants it removed, recommendation would be a shave biopsy with possible use of a chalazion clamp. This should be performed after the patient has delivered and is no longer nursing. It might return over many years, but the clinician should avoid leaving a noticeable notch or divot in the eyelid margin.

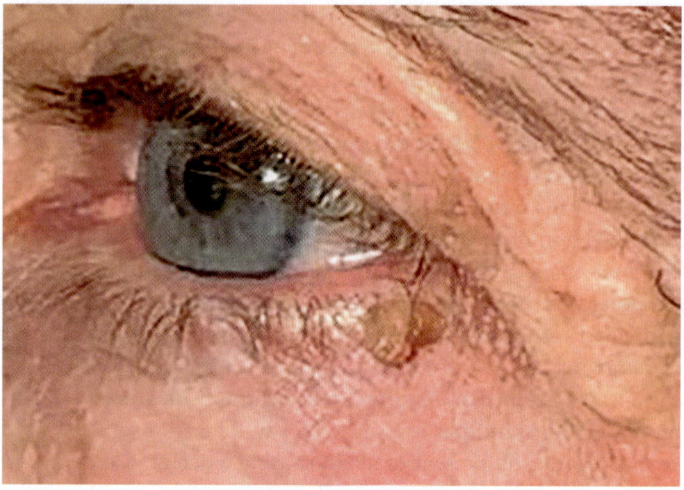

**FIGURE 7-2** This is a pedunculated lesion, most likely a seborrheic keratosis or papilloma along the lash line. Recommendation would be an excisional or incisional biopsy with cautious cauterization to avoid injuring lash follicles. The majority or even all the mass can be removed by pulling up on the lesion with forceps and cutting at the base with scissors. The resulting cauterization and inflammation may destroy any remaining cells of the lesion. Let the patient know there will be a scab that will need to heal. No sutures should be needed.

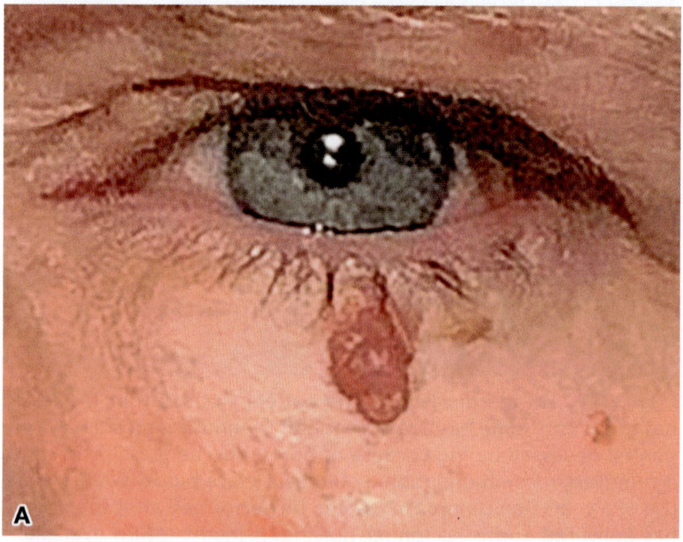


**FIGURE 7-3** **A** and **B**, This patient presents with a slightly pigmented lesion of the periocular skin. Recommend removal by excision with biopsy sent to pathology for diagnosis: scissors or blade could be used and may need sutures to close the defect. Final pathology report was seborrheic keratosis.

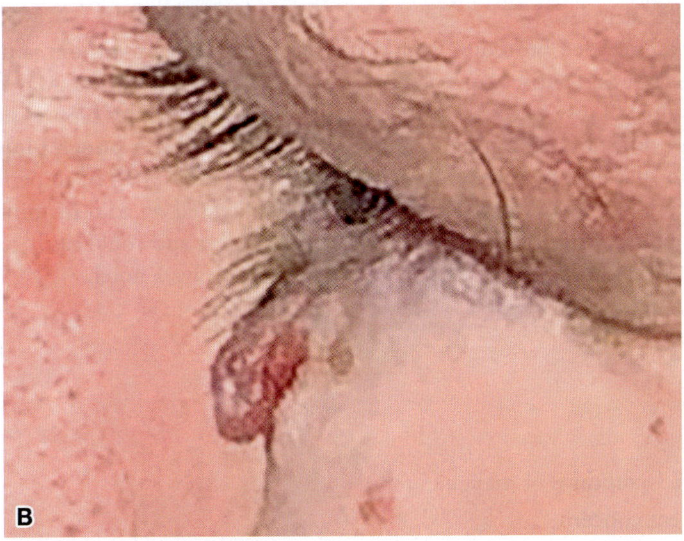


**FIGURE 7-3** *(continued)*

- **Lid margin** lesions
  A **shave biopsy** is recommended for these lesions. Being too aggressive with removing the lesion or cauterizing too much to stop bleeding can leave a notch in the lid. If there is a concern for malignancy, the specimen is sent in formalin to a pathology laboratory. If the lesion is reported back as malignant, the recommendation would be for the patient to be referred to an oculoplastics specialist and to have more surgery to be sure all the tumor cells are gone. The goal of the specialist would be to remove the remaining tumor cells and confirm under the microscope that the margins were clear and then to repair the lid in such a way that there is no notch and the lid is cosmetically pleasing to the patient. If there is no concern for malignancy, the specimen is discarded in a medically appropriate way. If the clinician is too aggressive, a notch can occur. However, if the patient has a notched lid that is obvious in exchange for a benign lesion, then the patient is not happy, which can make the doctor unhappy as well. It is best to inform the patient that you will remove the lesion and make the tissue flush with the lid margin. Benign lesions rarely grow back enough to be noticed again. But if that happens and the lesion returns, the patient may need to have a full-thickness lid resection by a specialist to be sure there are no cells left. That would be the safest and most cosmetically pleasing way to remove every cell of the benign lesion and not to leave a lid notch. Most of the time, the benign lesion will not return if the examiner gets most of the lesion.
- **Lash line** lesions
  The recommended procedure would be a **shave biopsy, either excisional or incisional**. The patient needs to be aware that in removing the lesion, some lashes may be lost. This is not a huge problem in the lower lid, but can be obvious in the upper lid, especially in female patients. The goal is to take as much of the lesion the examiner can without damaging too many lash follicles. Some lesions of the lash line can be grasped with the forceps and lifted and the entire base cut and cauterized, thus removing the entire lesion. Some can only be debulked (incisional) without losing lash follicles.

- **Periocular skin** lesions
  The recommended procedure would be **excisional** with or without suture closure. If the lesion is large and entire removal may cause the lid to pull down or away from the eye, then an incisional biopsy to get a diagnosis may be appropriate. This biopsy is removing some of the tissue, but not attempting to remove the lesion totally. A **punch biopsy** can be used in the periocular area to remove a small lesion totally (excisional) or to perform an incisional biopsy for diagnosis. A punch biopsy should *not* be used on a lid margin and is rarely used on a lash line lesion. The biopsy leaves a circular defect and could easily cut deeper than the clinician would desire on the lid margin and would leave a notch.

## INDICATIONS

### Key Indications

- Signs/symptoms of malignancy
- Patient concern
- Future eyelid malposition if there is growth
- Lesion location
- Any lesion with loss of lashes, change of eyelid architecture, bleeding, ulceration, increasing pigmentation, rapid growth
- Patient has irritation, visual obstruction, concern for malignancy
- Lesion that causes lid malposition due to size or location
- Lesion location is such that growth in the future may cause a problem for the patient. It is easier to remove a small lesion than when it has grown and may then need more aggressive surgery to close the skin/muscle defect.

The most common reason for a lid biopsy in the office is to remove a lid lesion that is bothering the patient in some way. The patient may see it in the mirror, experience irritation, or find it unsightly. Occasionally, the examiner will notice a lesion that the patient has not even known was there. Any suspicious characteristics, such as those that were discussed previously, warrant a biopsy to identify whether the lesion is benign or malignant.

## CONTRAINDICATIONS

### Key Contraindications

- Allergy
- History of bleeding
- History of vasovagal episode
- Chronic oxygen use
- Patient unable to lay flat

- Allergy to any local anesthetic or supplies to be used, including latex if latex-free supplies not available
- History of bleeding. Many patients are on medications that thin the blood. Usually, biopsies can be performed safely in the office even if the patient remains on their blood thinners. Epinephrine in the local anesthetic will constrict blood vessels in the area after 10 to 15 minutes of being injected and help control bleeding. However, if there is a history of bleeding disorder or perfuse bleeding when the patient gets a cut or is nicked, the clinician may want to refer the patient to a specialist for further treatment. If it is desired for the patient to stop a blood-thinning medication prior to the biopsy, medical clearance from the patient's doctor is indicated.
- History of vasovagal episode with fainting at the sight of needles or minor procedures
- Patient is on chronic oxygen and not able to be off for even a short period of time. (Supplemental oxygen is flammable with cautery use.)
- History of the patient being intolerant of lying flat or slightly reclined

## INFORMED CONSENT CONSIDERATIONS

Informed consent with the patient's signature and witnessed by someone other than the patient is essential before this procedure. The patient should be aware of what other options are available besides a lid biopsy in the office today:

- **Alternative options** besides biopsy include:
  - Return on a separate date in the future that is more convenient for the patient to have the biopsy.
  - Observe the lesion for growth or changes, and schedule a return appointment in 6 months.
  - Referral to an eyelid surgeon for opinion and treatment
  - Topical treatment with antibiotic and/or steroid ointment to see if the lesion responds. The clinician's medical judgment may determine whether this will or will not be effective.

Informed consent should have a description of the procedure in simple words for nonmedical individuals to understand. For example, "This procedure is a lid biopsy to remove either in part or completely an abnormal growth on the eyelid. If indicated, the lesion may be sent to pathology for identification." On the form, an explanation of the procedure should be included verbally or in writing, with possible risks and benefits listed verbally *and* in written form.

The clinician might say, "Once in a reclined position, a drop of topical anesthetic will be placed in the eye closest to the eyelid lesion to be removed. The area will be cleaned with either povidone–iodine antiseptic or other antiseptic solution to help prevent infection.

An injection will be given in the eyelid near the lesion, which will numb the lid so the rest of the procedure will not hurt. **The discomfort from the injection will last about 10 seconds.** There will be burning and some discomfort during those 10 seconds. The lesion will be biopsied, and the oozing stopped with a cautery. The cautery can have unusual or sometimes unpleasant smell, like burnt hair or protein. If indicated, sutures may be used to close the area, but usually there will be a scab that has to heal over the next week or so. You may swell and bruise that can last up to 2 weeks, but usually resolves within a few days."

## RISKS/BENEFITS

**Key Risks**

- Bleeding
- Ulceration
- Infection
- Eyelash loss
- Scarring or distortion of lid anatomy
- Recurrence of lesion
- Additional surgery if pathology identifies malignancy

Removal of the lesion is usually the desired benefit. Another benefit might be to get a diagnosis that would dictate whether any further treatment is needed.

Risks and complications inherent to a lid biopsy include, but are not limited to, bleeding, infection, lash loss, eye irritation, distortion of the lid anatomy, recurrence, allergic reaction to local anesthetic, ophthalmic ointment or supplies, burn to the skin or lashes, scarring, and injury to the eye (extremely rare). Temporary decrease in vision due to lid edema or ophthalmic ointment may occur. Permanent vision loss is incredibly rare with this procedure. Additional surgery by a specialist may be indicated if the lesion is a malignancy.

If a biopsy is being sent, the patient should be aware that it will take about a week to get a result back from the pathologist. Let the patient know that your office will call the patient and inform them of the results. If it is a skin cancer, you will refer them to an eyelid surgeon for complete removal of the tumor and reconstruction. Reassure the patient that **90% of lid lesions are benign**. Of the 10% that are malignant, by far the majority of malignancies are basal cell carcinomas that usually do not spread through the bloodstream and can be completely treated in most cases, especially if diagnosed early.

The counseling clinician should not only obtain a signature and witness of the consent form but feel confident that the patient understands. Consent is obtained with communication between the clinician and the patient. The form is just a legal document confirming and recording what has already happened in the office between the two parties. The chart should document that the patient has been counseled on the nature of the procedure, the risks, benefits, and alternatives to the procedure. The expected results have been discussed.

## PREOPERATIVE CARE

It is important to document the specific location of the lesion on the eyelids, either by a **photograph or a diagram**. If a photograph is performed, the CPT code for external photography is **92285**. Documentation of the lesion is important in that if the lesion is malignant, it helps the eyelid specialist know where the biopsy was taken. Usually, the patient waits a period after the biopsy to be seen and the site may have healed, showing little evidence of a procedure.

Also, if the lesion is benign, the patient may return with another lesion and think it is a recurrence of the same lesion, but documentation may show it is a new lesion. It also may support why the lesion was removed. If the patient opts for observing the lesion, a photograph allows comparison for the return visit.

Having the patient place ice to the lid will help decrease the discomfort of the injection. Some offices use a numbing cream like topical lidocaine, but that usually takes 15 minutes or more to take effect.

Many patients are on aspirin or some blood thinners. In fact, few patients older than 60 years are not on some sort of blood-thinning medicines: aspirin, nonsteroidal anti-inflammatories, clopidogrel (Plavix), warfarin (Coumadin), apixaban (Eliquis), and so on. Biopsies can be performed on these patients without taking them off their blood-thinning medicines, which were prescribed to prevent the worsening of health issues. If there is a concern, refer the patient to a specialist or obtain medical clearance for the patient to be off the concerning medication prior to the biopsy.

## Supplies (Figures 7-4 and 7-5)

- Topical anesthetic for the eye (proparacaine 0.5% or tetracaine 0.5%)
- Nonsterile or sterile surgical marking pen—fine point
- 3-mL syringes
- 30- to 32-gauge needle
- Larger gauge needle to draw up local anesthetic
- (8–27 gauge) or sterile cap made for drawing local anesthetic from the bottle
- 1% lidocaine with 1:100,000 epinephrine
- Sterile nonlatex surgical gloves in appropriate size
- Povidone–iodine antiseptic swabs or solution pads (do not use povidone–iodine scrub around the eyes.)
- Sterile 4 × 4 gauge pads
- Sterile cotton tip applicators
- Sterile scissors (e.g., Westcott or Vannes)
- Sterile forceps with teeth (e.g., 0.5 or Bishop Harman forceps)
- Sterile needle driver (e.g., Castroviejo)
- High-temperature 2,200-degree battery cautery (e.g., brand Bovie) or something for hemostasis
- Suture if needed (5-0 fast absorbing gut is usually the best to have in office.)
- Disposable No. 10, No. 11, or No. 15 surgical blade and handle
- Punch biopsy tool (Recommend a 2- to 3-mm diameter cutting circle for eyelids.)
- Small chalazion clamp
- Pathology specimen containers with formalin and pathology request sheets with identification labels
- Autoclave to clean instruments and sealed bags or trays in which to store sterilized instruments
- Good lighting to perform the procedure
- A chair that will recline the patient to almost supine, but with head higher than the heart and feet. (Reverse Trendelenburg: foot down, head up supine position)

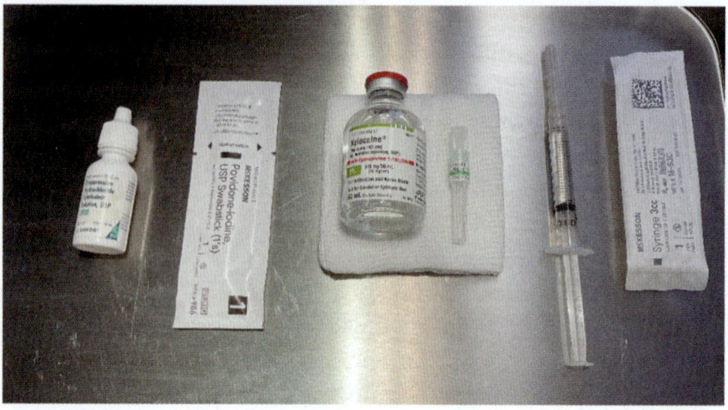


**FIGURE 7-4** Preoperative supplies: Presented are the items needed for local injection and for cleaning the biopsy area. Topical anesthetic eye drops, povidone–iodine swab sticks, 1% lidocaine with 1:100,000 epinephrine, a 30-gauge needle, and a 3-mL syringe shown here. For most office-based lid biopsies, only 1 to 2 mL of local anesthetic is required.

Prior to the procedure, the local anesthetic is drawn up into the 3-mL syringe with a large bore needle or from the sterile cap on the bottle. If the 30-gauge needle is used to draw the local anesthetic, the tip will dull and be harder to go through the patient's skin on injection. The top of the bottle should be wiped with an alcohol pad first. The mayo tray or workspace needs to be prepared with a sterile sheet covering below and the instruments placed out using a sterile

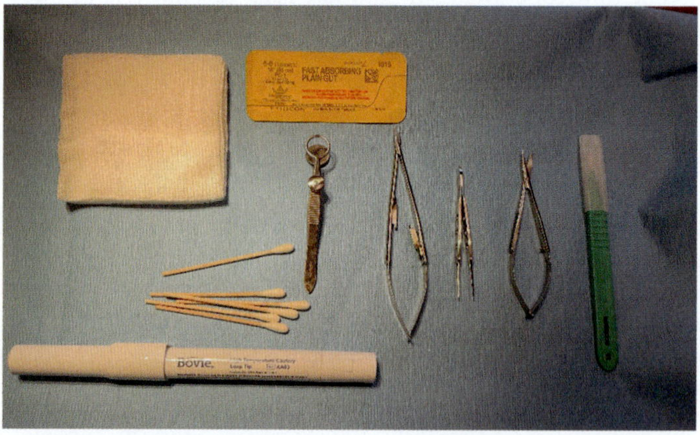


**FIGURE 7-5** Procedure supplies and instruments: Supplies shown include sterile 4 × 4 gauze pads, sterile cotton-tipped applicators, small chalazion clamp, 5-0 fast absorbing gut suture, needle driver, forceps, scissors, and disposable No. 15 surgical scalpel placed on a sterile field. Also seen in the left lower corner is a disposable battery-operated handheld cautery. Most lid biopsies in the office do not need a suture, a needle driver, a chalazion clamp, or a surgical blade and handle.

technique. The sterile wrap around the instruments can serve as the sterile cover base on which to place any other supplies. Also, cotton applicators, gauze pads, and cautery should be opened and placed sterilely. If there is uncertainty whether suture will be used, have it ready, but not opened until sure it is needed. It is the most expensive disposable supply used in office-based lid biopsies.

The method to clean the area needs to be made available. Some pour povidone–iodine solution onto gauze pads on the sterile field to use for cleaning. Others use prepackaged povidone–iodine swab sticks or pads. The benefit of this is that the area can be prepped using nonsterile gloves holding just the handle of the swab, using only one pair of sterile gloves for the biopsy itself. This reduces overhead because sterile gloves are more expensive.

Once the area is clean, the procedure can begin.

# PROCEDURE

## Excisional Biopsy: Complete Lesion Removal

The lesion has been identified to be biopsied and has been documented. The patient has been informed of the risks, benefits, and alternatives of the procedure. The consent has been signed and witnessed. Excisional biopsy is recommended for non-lid margin lesions (Figure 7-6). It can be performed on lash line lesion; however, it may cause loss of lashes. It is usually recommended for periocular areas of the lids, away from lashes or margins.

1. Area to perform the procedure has been prepared with appropriate supplies and equipment as described earlier.
2. Patient is brought to the procedure chair. The patient is informed the chair will be moved back into a reclined position. Be sure the patient is comfortable to be here for a few minutes. Some patients will need a pillow placed under their knees to take pressure off their back.
3. If the lesion is small or flat, the clinician may want to mark it with a surgical marker. Sometimes after the local anesthetic is given, it is hard to identify the growth.
4. Topical anesthetic drop placed in the eye that is on the same side of the lesion.
5. Ice or numbing cream can be applied. Either can take a few minutes to be effective. Ice works quicker than the numbing cream usually. (Some offices purchase logo-branded small circular ice packs that can be reused by the patient. It also is advertising for the office.)
6. Surgical lamp or light is adjusted to give maximal lighting. The patient should be warned that a bright light is about to shine, ask them to please keep their eye closed without squeezing the lids.
7. The clinician or technician puts on a set of gloves and preps the area with povidone–iodine swabs or solution. Povidone–iodine scrub is more toxic to the eye and should not be used around the eye. The sterile swabs can be opened and used with nonsterile gloves. If alcohol is used, it must be allowed to dry completely prior to using a cautery. Alcohol is flammable and if not allowed to dry can cause a fire and burn the patient or clinician. Alcohol is colorless, and the area that was prepped cannot easily be identified whereas povidone–iodine has a yellowish color and allows the clinician to know what areas have been treated.
8. The clinician informs the patient that they will feel an initial stick and a burning sensation. Ask the patient to try not to move or squeeze the eyelids closed. Squeezing can increase bruising from the injection. The patient needs to be aware that the discomfort will only

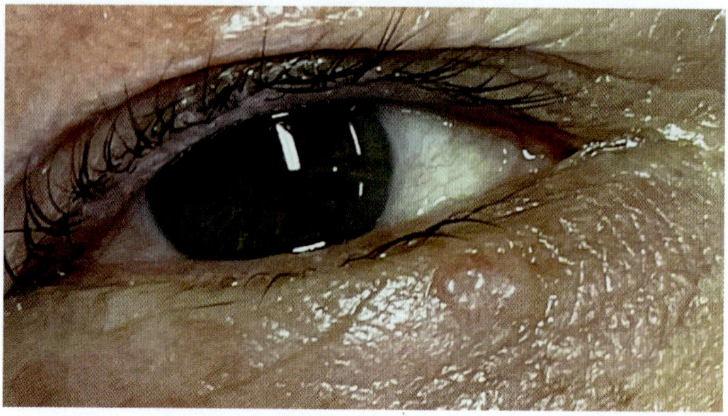

**FIGURE 7-6** The patient is a 56-year-old male with a 6-month history of a lesion of the right lower lid. He reports no pain or bleeding. He has no history of previous trauma or skin cancer. He would like it removed. He is on 81 mg of aspirin a day. He has no known drug allergies. Clinically, the lesion is slightly raised and is about 5 mm in size. There is no ulcer or especially concerning features. It is in the periocular area, with no lash line or margin involvement. It is unclear clinically whether this is a benign or malignant lesion. The lesion has a slightly pearly appearance on the edges. Differential diagnosis would be benign seborrheic keratosis, papilloma, nevus, or a malignancy like basal cell carcinoma. Recommendation is an excisional biopsy to remove the entire identifiable lesion with closure with sutures due to the size with pathologic diagnosis. A shave biopsy might be acceptable as well if the specimen is still sent to pathology. There appears to be enough lax skin to remove the lesion without causing the lid to pull down. The specimen was sent to pathology. The patient underwent an excisional biopsy without complications. The final pathologic report was basal cell carcinoma with one margin not entirely cleared of malignant cells. The patient was referred to an eyelid specialist for additional surgery with microscopic confirmation of clear margins with no remaining tumor cells. This is immediately followed by eyelid reconstruction.

last about 10 seconds. The doctor injects with the entry site right next to the lesion but allows the tip of the needle to go just below the lesion. The local anesthetic is given slowly over 10 seconds. The area under and on either side of the lesion should balloon up. Injecting slowly hurts the patient less than injecting fast. The needle and syringe are removed and placed sterilely on the field in case more is needed later.

9. Using a toothed forceps, the lesion is grasped and elevated. If it is small, the mass can be excised using a scissor around the base, being sure that the incision is in normal tissue below the elevated mass. It is always best to make incisions of the eyelid along the skin tension lines. The skin tension lines are the natural lines of passive tension of the skin and underlying muscle. For example, a horizontal incision is preferred to a vertical one on the eyelid. It will heal better and have less chance of a significant scar. If a scalpel is used, an elliptical incision is made along the skin tension lines to remove the mass with some surrounding normal tissue.

10. After the lesion is removed, it is set aside on the sterile field either to be discarded or placed in a formalin specimen container.
11. Hemostasis is obtained to stop any bleeding. Some type of thermal cauterization is needed in the office. The high-temperature battery cautery is a perfect instrument to stop bleeding in the office. It is relatively inexpensive. Bipolar instruments also work well but are much more expensive to have in the office. Remember that no supplemental oxygen can be on the field. If near the lash line, be careful of the cautery in its proximity to them. False lashes are also a potential fire hazard.
12. Cauterization shrinks the surrounding tissue, making the defect smaller and will kill most remaining cells. Inflammation alone from the procedure can also kill some of the abnormal cells. Most defects can granulate in over a few weeks, without leaving a significant scar. If sutures are required, use the suture and suture holder to close with interrupted stitches spaced evenly. A 2-loop, 1-loop, 1-loop throw is usually adequate to tie the suture. The 5-0 fast absorbing gut suture usually dissolves in 2 weeks. If permanent suture is used like 6-0 nylon, it should be removed in 7 to 10 days.
13. If the specimen is being sent for pathologic examination, be sure the specimen container is labeled with the appropriate sticker from the pathology sheet as well as the biohazard bag. Place the specimen in the sealed and labeled container into the also labeled, biohazard bag and seal the bag closed. The specimen sheet should be filled out by the office with all pertinent information. The clinician should fill out which lid was biopsied and any pertinent history to help the pathologist. The specimen is now ready to be sent to the pathology laboratory. Most laboratories either will pick up the specimen or have an address where the specimen can be mailed.

## Incisional Biopsy: Partial Lesion Removal

The initial procedure follows steps 1 to 8 as listed earlier under excisional biopsy. With an incisional biopsy, the goal is not to remove every cell of the lesion. The goal might be to remove a portion of the lesion to obtain a histopathologic diagnosis. Once a diagnosis is made, a treatment plan can be recommended. Another reason for an incisional biopsy is to debulk a benign lesion without interrupting the normal architecture or position of the lid. There are two different types of incisional biopsy: **shave and punch**.

## Incisional Biopsy: Shave Biopsy (Figure 7-7A and B)

This is recommended if the lesion is raised on the lid margin or is a raised lesion along the lash line. The goal is to remove the mass flush with the surrounding normal tissue and to not leave a divot or hollow area. Tissue can still be obtained for diagnosis if needed. The examiner is aware that some remaining cells of the growth may remain, although postprocedure inflammation or cauterization may destroy any remaining cells. This is less invasive than an excisional biopsy and causes less anatomical defects to the lid.

1. Steps 1 to 8 as listed earlier under excisional.
2. If it is a lid margin lesion, a scalpel or scissors is used to cut off the lesion flush with the margin. The tissue is grasped with a forceps. If the lesion is hard to grasp, a chalazion clamp

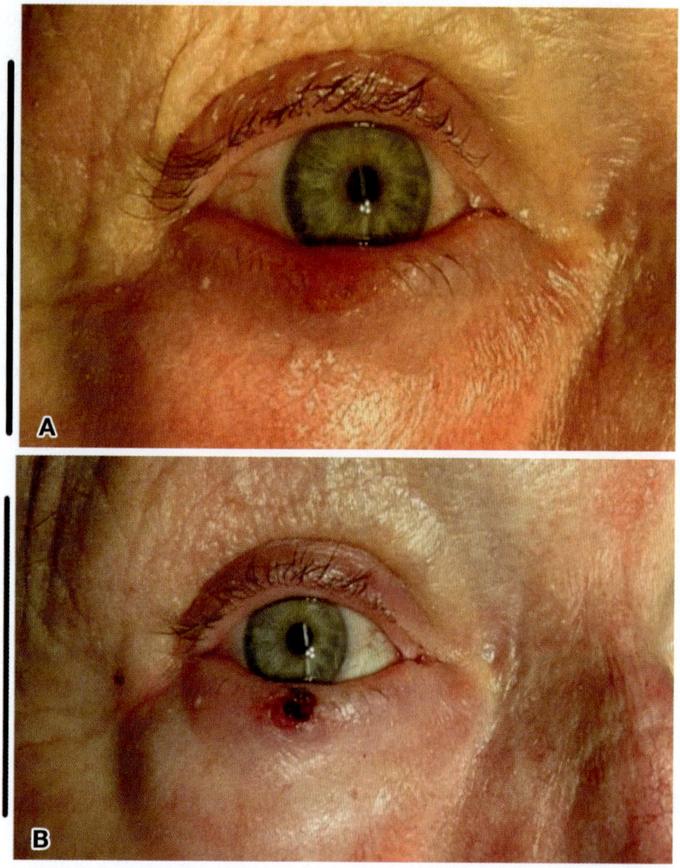

FIGURE 7-7 **A** and **B**, The right lower lid of this patient has an erythematous, scaly, slightly raised lesion with lash loss. A shave biopsy of the lash line lesion is recommended, and the specimen should be sent to pathology to rule out malignancy. Differential diagnosis includes old chalazion with inflammation, seborrheic keratosis, basal cell carcinoma, and squamous cell carcinoma. The loss of lashes makes it more suspicious to be a malignant lesion. The scab will heal over the next 2 weeks. Erythromycin ophthalmic ointment at bedtime for a week usually will prevent any complications due to infection.

comes in handy. Clamp the lid with the back plate on the palpebral conjunctiva side. Use a blade to cut the lesion up against the metal plate. The specimen is sent to pathology or discarded appropriately.

3. Hemostasis is obtained with the cautery or thermal unit available. Sparing use of the thermal energy is recommended to reduce notch formation for lid margin lesions. If the chalazion clamp is in place, cauterize them with the protection of the eye with the metal shield back of the clamp.
4. Sutures are not used with shave biopsies.

## Incisional Biopsy: Punch Biopsy

A punch biopsy is a type of incisional biopsy, **although it can be an excisional biopsy if the lesion is smaller than the diameter of the punch tool available.** A 2- to 3-mm punch biopsy tool is recommended on the eyelid. If it is used for diagnosis of a possible malignancy, the area biopsied should be at the outer edge of the lesion and not in a necrotic center. A small sample is taken and then examined under a microscope by a pathologist. Punch biopsies are rarely performed on the lid margin. The defect is a complete circle and results in lid notching. It works well with periocular lesions: small (excisional) or large (incisional for diagnosis). Punch biopsy tools come in different sizes. The end of the tool has a sharp metal circle. The end is placed on the skin, and the clinician gently rotates it clockwise and counterclockwise, pushing down with a little pressure to cut the skin. Usually, the biopsy is about 3 to 4 mm in depth. The doctor needs to remember that the eyelid skin is the thinnest in the body and that care must be observed to not go too deep into the tissue.

1. Steps 1 to 8 as listed earlier under excisional.
2. The punch biopsy tool has been placed on the sterile field. It is grasped by the handle and placed on the skin that is to be biopsied. If excisional, the punch surrounds the lesion.
3. The tip is flush with the skin. The doctor rotates clockwise and counterclockwise with slight pressure. The tool is removed, and the specimen is grasped with a forceps and elevated. The base of the biopsy will need to be cut with scissors.
4. Hemostasis is obtained with thermal cautery energy.
5. Sutures are not used with a punch biopsy.

# POSTOPERATIVE CARE/COMANAGEMENT (FOLLOW-UP SCHEDULE)

### Key Postoperative Considerations

- Topical ophthalmic antibiotic, once or twice daily for 1 week
- Ice on and off to decrease swelling
- Watch for signs of infection

After the procedure, the face is cleaned, removing the cleaning solution and any blood. The skin area is dried.

1. A topical ophthalmic antibiotic is recommended at least once or twice a day for the first week. Erythromycin ophthalmic ointment is inexpensive and covers many skin infections and is therefore often used. If available, place it on the patient before correcting the chair to the sitting position.
2. Have the patient wait a few moments in the sitting position to be sure they feel good before allowing them to get up and walk. Less stable patients may need assistance.
3. Makeup over the scab or incision/sutures is avoided until the area heals. This is usually 2 weeks. Makeup can be worn on the face away from the area, but the patient must be careful in removing the makeup so as not to rub harshly the biopsied area.

4. Ice on and off the first day can help decrease swelling.
5. Oral antibiotics are only indicated if the patient's health history makes them more prone to infections.
6. The patient needs to be aware that there may be a bruise or swelling that can take up to 2 weeks to go away.
7. Avoid rubbing the eyelids or pulling on the lids. Sometimes the area can itch as it is healing.
8. Signs to be aware of: increased redness or swelling, discharge, increasing pain, and bleeding that cannot be controlled with ice and pressure on the lid. No lifting over 10 pounds or bending over at the waist for a week if a patient is having some problems with oozing or bleeding. Most patients can resume all normal activities that day, including lifting and bending.
9. Follow-up is not needed for most biopsies. Patient should know to call if they have any concerns.

## POTENTIAL COMPLICATIONS AND THEIR TREATMENT

### Key Potential Complications

- Postoperative infection
- Persistent bleeding
- Scar or lid notch formation
- Lash loss

The most common complication of an eyelid biopsy is **infection**. If an infection occurs, oral cephalexin 500 mg three times a day or oral clindamycin 300 mg three times a day treats most postoperative cellulitis. Be sure to ask the patient if they are allergic to any medications. Sometimes patients are very lax in filling out paperwork for eye doctors, thinking that general medical information is not important for the eye doctor.

Patients may present after the procedure with **bleeding**, especially those on blood thinners or with poorly controlled hypertension. Usually, bleeding can be controlled with ice and tamponade. Pressure is not to be placed on the eye, but on the eyelid area. Sometimes additional cauterization is required. Usually, local anesthetic is injected first followed by cauterization. If it cannot be controlled, the patient may need to be referred to a specialist or to the emergency room. This is a rare occurrence.

As the area heals, the patient may be dissatisfied with the **scar or a lid margin notch.** Allow at least 3 months for the area to heal. Occasionally, a steroid ophthalmic ointment can be of benefit for undesirable scars. Avoid using scar-reducing creams or gels that are not approved to be used around the eye. Having a photograph of the lesion is helpful to remind the patient what the lid looked like before the removal of the lesion. If this does not satisfy the patient, refer to a specialist. If the scar is causing lid malposition, refer to an oculoplastics specialist.

**Lash loss** in the area can be a complication. The patient should be made aware that this is a possibility. Occasionally, lash-growing products like bimatoprost (Latisse) can help if there are any functioning lash follicles left.

## VIDEOS OF PROCEDURES

**Video 7-1**—Excisional biopsy: lash line and periocular lesions. Excisional biopsy: This patient has two lesions to be removed, a lateral exophytic lesion away from the eyelid margin and a medial lid margin lesion close to the inferior punctum. Informed consent was already obtained, and the form was signed and witnessed. The patient was placed in a supine position, and topical anesthetic ophthalmic drops were placed in the eye. An ice pack was placed on the lid for 2 to 3 minutes. The periocular area was cleaned with the povidone–iodine solution. Local anesthetic was injected into the lid using a 30-gauge needle around both lesions. Using a toothed forceps in one hand, the lesion is grasped, and the base is cut using a Westcott scissors in the other hand. The base of the lesion is then cauterized with a handheld high-temperature battery cautery. The lesion has been excised.

**Video 7-2**—Incisional biopsy/shave: lid margin using chalazion clamp. Lid margin/shave biopsy: This patient has a flat, pigmented lesion of the upper eyelid. Consent was obtained, and the form was signed and witnessed. An ice pack was placed on the lid for 2 to 3 minutes. The area was cleaned with a povidone–iodine solution after topical ophthalmic anesthetic drops were placed in the eye. Local anesthetic was injected into the area of the lesion using a 30-gauge needle. A chalazion clamp is placed to protect the eye and to help with hemostasis. The lesion is incised at the edge of the lesion with a scalpel, and the lesion is shaved off the margin. Because some residual tissue is still attached, the clamp is removed and a toothed forceps is used to grasp the lesion. The Westcott scissors are used to cut the lesion completely off the lid. Hemostasis is obtained with a handheld high-temperature battery cautery with great care not to cause a notch or divot in the eyelid margin. The specimen was sent for histopathologic diagnosis.

**Video 7-3**—Shave excision of eyelid skin lesion using a No. 11 surgical blade under local anesthesia. (Video courtesy of Leonid Skorin, Jr. and Scott A. Bauer.)

**Video 7-4**—Excision of actinic keratosis eyelid skin lesion under local anesthesia. (Video courtesy of Leonid Skorin, Jr. and Kynndyl Giannonatti.)

**Video 7-5**—Excision of seborrheic keratosis, maxillary skin lesion under local anesthesia. (Video courtesy of Leonid Skorin, Jr. and Kynndyl Giannonatti.)

**Video 7-6**—Excision of squamous papilloma, medial canthus. Healing by secondary intention. (Video courtesy of Leonid Skorin, Jr. and Andrew Krein.)

**Video 7.7**—Shave excision of eyelid margin lesion using a No. 11 surgical blade under local anesthesia. (Video courtesy of Leonid Skorin, Jr. and Laura Goemann.)

## EFFICACY

The ability to obtain an accurate histopathologic diagnosis is very high with incisional or excisional biopsy. Because incisional biopsy has slightly more accuracy than a punch biopsy, it is recommended over a punch biopsy in an atypical lesion.

The reoccurrence rate is low with an excisional biopsied lesion where the margins are clear of any irregular or atypical cells. However, as stated previously, the goal of removing a benign lesion is to remove as much as possible of the abnormal cells without distorting the anatomy or causing a noticeable change to the lid or lid position. Therefore, the incidence of reoccurrence of benign lesions is higher in a shave biopsied lid lesion than in an excisional biopsied lesion.

## CODING/BILLING

**CPT code: 67840**—In this procedure, the clinician excises a diseased or damaged area from the eyelid, excluding a chalazion. If necessary, they close the wound with sutures. (Lesion may or may not be sent to pathology for identification). Used for **Excisional biopsy** which may include punch biopsy if the goal is to remove the entire lesion. If not sent to the pathologist, this is the code to use for all non-lid margin lesions including lash line lesions.
**CPT code: 67810**—The clinician takes a sample of suspicious area on the skin of the eyelid or its edges. The specimen is submitted to a laboratory for analysis to determine its nature. Used for **incisional biopsy: shave or punch**. This can be used for shave biopsy of the lid margin if the specimen is sent to pathology for identification. This can be for lid margin, lash line, and periocular lesions.
**CPT code: 67850**—The clinician destroys a small lesion of the **lid margin**, no larger than 1 cm, on the area between the front lid edge and back edge of any of the four lids of the eye. From the definition, this code does not appear to include specimens that need to be sent to pathology.
**Office exam: CPT per level of examination**—Some insurance carriers will not pay for both the office visit and lesion removal on the same day unless there are other ocular disease or conditions listed and addressed; for example, cataracts, dermatochalasis, and refractive error.
**Photography: 92285**—External ocular photography documents the medical progress of the external eye and ocular adnexa. Photographs record conditions and pathology of the adnexa, external eye, and anterior segment more accurately than charting notes or drawings. They are used to track changes in patient's abnormal conditions over time.

Common ICD-10 codes that support these procedures include the following:

- **D23.1 (benign neoplasm of eyelid)**—This can be further delineated by D23.111 right upper lid, D23.112 right lower lid, D23.121 left upper lid, and D23.122 left lower lid.
- **D49.2 (neoplasm of unspecified behavior of the skin)**.
- **C44.10 (malignant neoplasm of the eyelid)**—This can also be delineated for which particular lid has the lesion, C44.1021 right upper lid, C44.1022 right lower lid, C44.1091 left upper lid, and C44.1092 left lower lid.

## SUGGESTED READINGS

1. Spaeth GL. *Ophthalmic Surgery: Principles and Practice*. 2nd ed. W.B. Saunders Co; 1990:591-606.
2. Dortzbach RK. *Ophthalmic Plastic Surgery: Prevention and Management of Complications*. Raven Press; 1994:111-123.
3. Nerad JA. *Oculoplastic Surgery: The Requisites In Ophthalmology*. Mosby; 2001:254-281.
4. American Academy of Ophthalmology. Classification of eyelid disorders. In: *Basic and Clinical Science Course, Section 7: Oculofacial Plastic and Orbital Surgery*. American Academy of Ophthalmology; 2020-2021:187-228.
5. Manuel-Deprez M. Clinicopathological feature of eyelid skin tumors. A retrospective study of 5504 cases and review of literature. *Am J Dermatopathol*. 2009;31(3):256-262.

# 8 Radiofrequency for Lesion Removal, Trichiasis Ablation, and Punctal Occlusion

Nate Lighthizer • Komal Patel • Cole Sutherland • Matthew Bills

## BACKGROUND

Radiofrequency (RF) is an approachable surgical technique for the ophthalmic clinician, providing a minimally invasive and safe surgical option, with a relatively quick learning curve.[1] RF has its historical roots in electrocautery, which involves passing current through a resistive material at the end of an electrode. The resistive material creates heat, causing the tip of the electrocautery unit to heat up. Electrocautery is useful for coagulation and tissue destruction but can cause significant lateral tissue damage. RF surgery instead involves passing an electrical current through the body, with the targeted tissue acting as the resistive material.[2]

RF surgery passes electricity through the body to cause changes to the targeted tissue. Normally, when electricity enters the body, it causes nerve cells to depolarize, resulting in muscular contraction.[2] This effect is maximum at frequencies less than 100 kHz.[2] RF surgery employs higher frequencies of over 200 kHz to avoid stimulating nerve or muscle fibers in humans. This avoids the risks of electrocution or unwanted neuromuscular contraction.[2] Modern electrosurgery devices have a frequency on the order of 3.8 MHz, causing no concern for unwanted neuromuscular stimulation.[3]

Electrical resistance is the force that impedes electrical flow through a material.[4] Resistance occurs in radiosurgery when the current created by the RF unit is passed through the tip of the electrode and into the target tissue. The tissue resists the current flow, and intracellular heat is created. The amount of intracellular heat depends on the waveform being produced by the RF unit as well as the targeted tissue. High resistivity tissue (such as dry skin) creates more intracellular heat, whereas low resistivity tissue (such as moist skin) creates significantly less intracellular heat.[2,3] Fully rectified, high-frequency cutting waveforms produce the least amount of intracellular heat. When applied with an electrode, the cutting waveform creates intracellular heat, causing individual cells to vaporize. With partially rectified or coagulation waveforms, more lateral heat is created, causing a coagulatory effect.[2] Thus, the optimal conditions for minimal lateral damage are moist skin, with a cutting waveform.[2,3,5]

## WAVEFORMS/RADIOFREQUENCY UNIT SETTINGS

Choosing an appropriate setting for the procedure being performed is a critical first step before beginning any RF procedure. The main ophthalmic setting options are as follows:

- Setting 1—"Cutting mode," most commonly used for lesion removal.
- Setting 2—"Blended mode," useful for combined destruction and coagulation.
- Setting 3—"Coagulation mode," used to cauterize or coagulate bleeding tissue.

Modern RF surgery units have three or four different waveform outputs, which constitute the different surgical settings and therefore the ultimate effect on the targeted tissue. Waveforms are described by their degree of rectification and filtration, in other words, the processing that has been performed by the RF unit to change the radio waves to produce the desired effect (Figure 8-1).

Rectification is the conversion of alternating current (AC) electricity that is commonly available from North American power outlets to direct current (DC) electricity.[6] DC current causes sustained cell depolarization that results in cell death. AC current causes cells to depolarize and repolarize, and at high frequencies produces heat.[2] RF surgery exploits the degree that each waveform is rectified to alter the desired effect on the tissue.

Cutting mode, or setting #1 on most RF units, consists of a continuous sine wave current. This sine wave current at high frequency produces very little lateral heat, and therefore the least amount of collateral tissue damage. This waveform is focused and produces an almost pure cutting effect on tissue. Cutting waveforms are fully filtered and rectified. Setting #1 is used for incision into tissue, shave excisions, and lesion removal.

Coagulation mode, or setting #3 on most RF units, results from a dampened waveform. This waveform pulses electricity, with the waveforms reducing in amplitude over time. There are intermittent periods of no current in between each pulse. This creates lateral tissue and heat damage, not penetrating as deep into the target tissue as the cutting mode. In combination, this provides coagulatory effects on the tissue. Coagulation mode uses a partially rectified current. Setting #3 is useful for cauterization of bloody surgical fields, removal of vascular lesions like capillary hemangiomas, or destruction of hair follicles in RF trichiasis surgery.

Blend mode, or setting #2 on most RF units, is a mix between cutting and coagulation mode. The waveform is fully rectified and continuous but exhibits the "dampening" effects of coagulation mode. The result is a waveform with diminishing amplitudes, but no intermittent pauses in currents. This waveform combines the properties of cutting and coagulation, resulting in a "best of both worlds" scenario for bloodless incisions.

Fulguration or electrodesiccation uses the same dampened, alternating waveform as setting #3 coagulation, but the voltage and current are modified to create heat/sparks that cause tissue destruction. In contrast to the other three waveforms, the electrode in fulguration does not contact the skin, relying on sparks to jump from the electrode to the target tissue causing the tissue to burn. This causes a wider area of tissue damage. Fulguration has limited ophthalmic indications, given the delicacy of the eyelids and periocular tissue. Most RF instruments do not come with a fulguration setting.

| | Waveform | Use | Oscilloscope configuration |
|---|---|---|---|
| 1 | Fully filtered and fully rectified | Cutting | 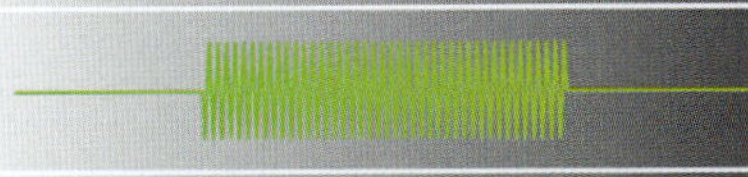 |
| 2 | Fully rectified | Cutting and coagulation | 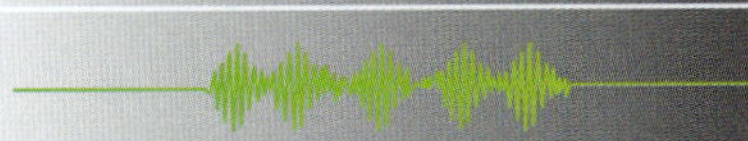 |
| 3 | Partially rectified | Haemostasis | 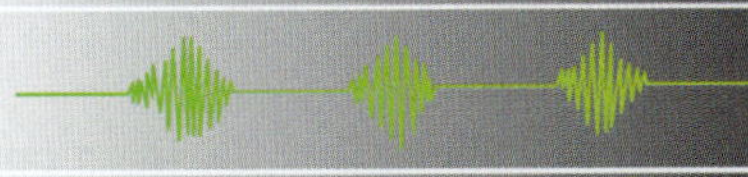 |
| 4 | Markedly damped (spark gap) | Fulguration and electrodesiccation | 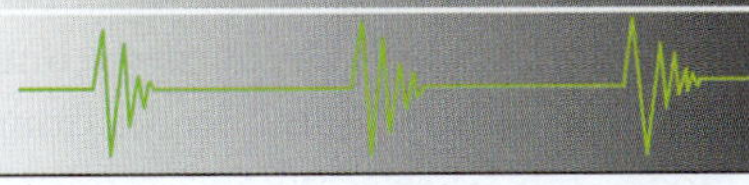 |

**FIGURE 8-1** An example of the waveforms used in radiofrequency surgery. The top waveform is cutting, with a high frequency continuous sine pattern. The second waveform is blended mode, with a continuous dampened pattern. The third waveform is coagulation, with the dampened, interrupted pattern. The bottom waveform is fulgeration, which also displays the damped, interrupted pattern, but with less voltage than the coagulation waveform. (From Brown JS. Minor Surgery: A Text and Atlas. 4th ed. Arnold; 2000.)

## Equipment List

- RF unit
- Electrode tips—disposable
- Scratch pad—cleaning
- 0.12 forceps toothed
- 0.12 forceps nontoothed
- Corneal shields—plastic, nonconducting
- 18-gauge needles
- 27-gauge 1″ needles
- 30-gauge ½″ needles
- 3- or 5-mL syringes
- Lidocaine 1% or 0.5% with epinephrine 1:200,000
- Lidocaine 4% (topical)—to anesthetize mucous membranes
- Ophthalmic 5% povidone–iodine (Betadine)
- Povidone–iodine (Betadine) 10% skin swab sticks
- Gauze
- Cotton tip applicators
- Alcohol swabs
- Sterile saline
- Eye spear sponges (Weck-Cel)
- Ophthalmic antibiotic ointment
- Magnification—surgical loupes or surgical microscope
- Autoclave

## Components of the RF Surgical Unit

- RF unit
- Handpiece
- Electrode tips
- Antennae
- Foot pedals
- Smoke evacuation unit

RF surgical units consist of the main power unit that generates the radio waves necessary for surgery. The power unit has ports to connect the antenna, monopolar or bipolar electrodes, and the foot pedal control unit. On the front of the main unit, the different modes and powers for said modes can be selected and modified. When activated, the unit will emit a different high-pitch sound depending on the mode that has been chosen. On some units, the volume of this sound can be adjusted.

The monopolar handpiece plugs into the main power generator of the RF machine. The electrode tips can be swapped for different surgical indications. Most handpieces have cut, blend, and coagulation activation buttons built into the handle. Two examples of RF units are pictured in Figures 8-2 and 8-3.

The antenna plugs into the main power generator of the RF machine. It does not function as a true grounding electrode but acts to concentrate the radio waves and improve cutting function. Although the antenna does not need to be physically in contact with the patient, incision with RF is more efficient when the antenna is closer to the site of surgery.[3] An example of an antenna is pictured in Figure 8-4.

Foot activation pedals are a convenient way to activate the RF machine without requiring additional dexterity from the clinician. When compared to handpiece activation, foot pedals

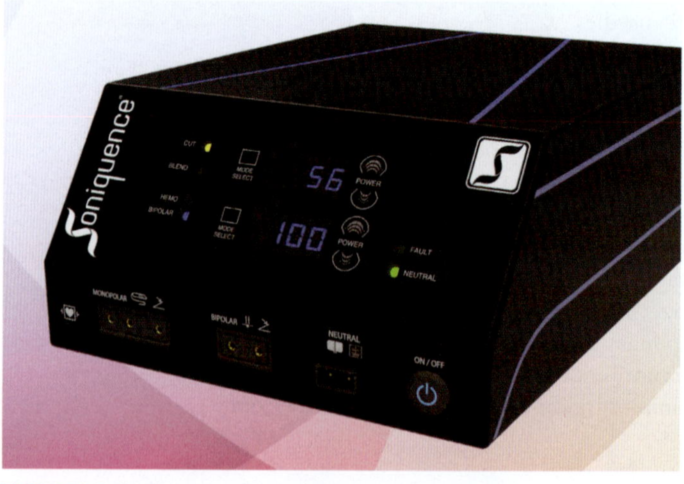


**FIGURE 8-2** Soniquence SmoothWave i100 radiofrequency device.

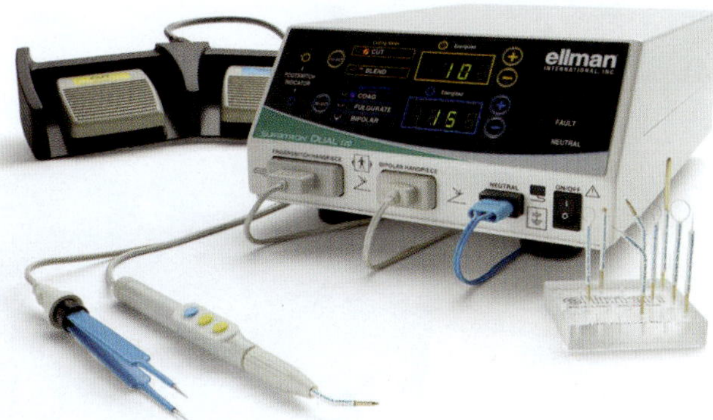


**FIGURE 8-3** Ellman Surgitron Dual EMC 90 radiofrequency device.

are easy to press and do not require any additional force to be put on the RF handpiece. This helps in avoiding any unnecessary pressure that can lead to adverse effects when performing RF surgery. Foot pedals plug into the main RF unit. Typically, there are two pedals: one that activates the "cut" and "blend" modes and one that activates the coagulation mode. An example of these pedals is pictured in Figure 8-5.

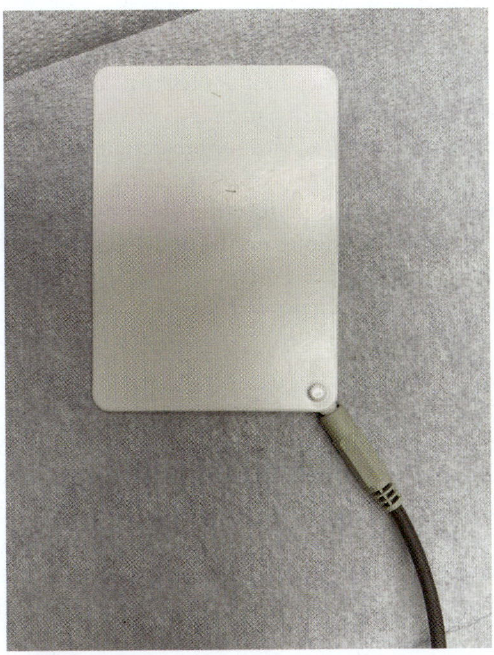

**FIGURE 8-4** An example of a radiofrequency antennae/passive electrode.

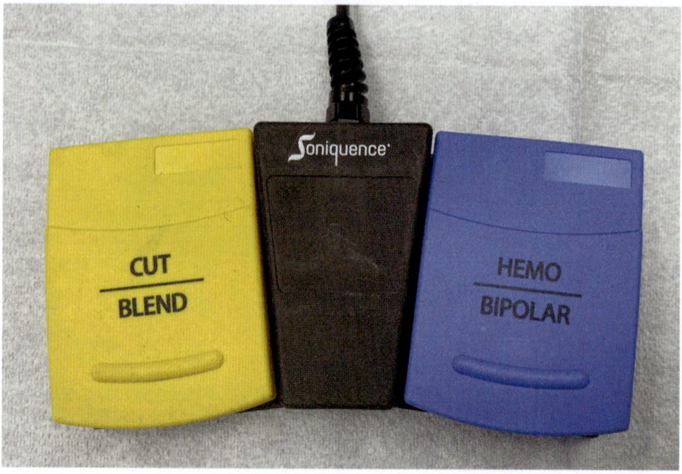


FIGURE 8-5 An example of radiofrequency (RF) unit foot pedals. The foot pedals can be used to activate the RF instrument. On the left (yellow) pedal, setting #1 and #2 are activated separately or one at a time. On the right (blue) pedal, setting #3 is activated.

## POWER SETTINGS

The power settings of the radiofrequency unit are relative, as they do not represent a specific number of watts or correlate between different brands of surgical units. In general, the power ranges on a surgical unit from 0 to 60+. Most ophthalmic procedures can be completed at a power setting of approximately 10 to 15. The power setting is adjusted according to the lesion being removed or the procedure that is performed. The power settings should initially be set at a lower setting and increased depending on the tissue response, following the principle of minimal power for desired surgical effect. Power settings for cutting mode, coagulation mode, and blend mode can all be adjusted independently.

## ELECTRODE TYPES

Electrodes can be further broken down based on their shape and polarity. Electrodes are classified as either bipolar or monopolar. Bipolar electrodes are rarely used in ophthalmic surgery and are generally used for cauterization. Forceps are the most common bipolar electrode (Figure 8-6), where each tip of the forceps is an electric pole. Radio waves travel from one tip of the forceps to the other, and any tissue between the forceps tips in the surgical field is cauterized. This cauterization is very local and can be useful to stop individual bleeding vessels in surgery.

Monopolar electrodes are the more common electrode type found in ophthalmic surgery. Radio waves travel from the monopolar probe through the body and are focused by

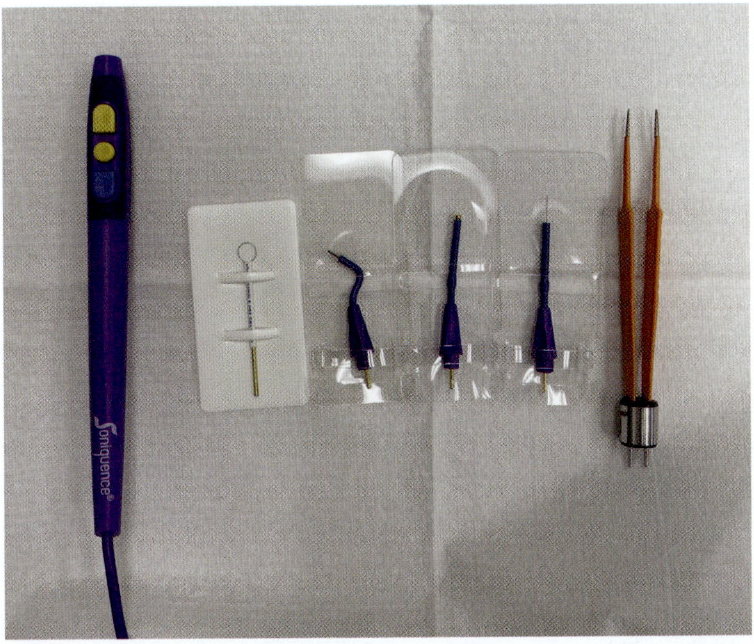


**FIGURE 8-6** Common electrodes used for radiofrequency surgery. From left: radiofrequency (RF) handpiece with buttons for settings #1 and 2 (yellow), setting #3 (blue); small loop electrode; pin/"bent tip" electrode; ball electrode; fine wire electrode; bipolar forceps electrode.

the antenna plate placed near the patient. It is important to place the antenna close to the surgical field, for optimal tissue response. The antenna does not need to be directly contacting the patient and is most often placed under the patient's back as they are reclined prior to surgery.

There are several different electrode tips that can be inserted into the monopolar handpiece that is most commonly used for ophthalmic surgery. Figure 8-6 depicts a variety of commonly used electrode tips. The most versatile and commonly used tip is the pin (aka "bent tip") electrode. This electrode can be used to perform shave excisions by lightly touching the lesion to be removed with the electrode perpendicular to the skin. Loop electrodes can also be used for shave excisions, using the distal end of the loop to cut into the tissue. Loop electrodes are also popular for pedunculated lesions. Straight wire electrode tips are used for ablation of hair follicles in trichiasis surgery or for making fine incisions into cysts or other tissue. Ball electrodes are useful for coagulation or removal of capillary hemangiomas.

## SMOKE EVACUATOR

An essential part of the radiofrequency surgical unit is a smoke evacuation device. RF surgery produces fumes that contain the water contents of vaporized cells.[7] The fumes have been shown to retain viral and bacterial loads, including human papilloma virus (HPV), human immunodeficiency virus (HIV), and mycobacterium tuberculosis.[8] The fumes are also noxious and unpleasant for both the patient and the doctor. Removal of the fumes is a necessary step for any radiofrequency procedure. The tube of the smoke evacuation unit should produce suction and be positioned such that the fumes created are sucked away from a patient's nose. The tube should be placed as close as possible to the surgery site, without interfering with the clinician's mobility or field of view.

## TROUBLESHOOTING

Under proper conditions, the electrode should pass through tissue with little resistance, and minimal to no pressure being applied (e.g., like a hot knife through butter). Minimal to no pressure should be used when applying an electrode to tissue. Several factors can contribute to this not being the case. Some of the most common tissue interactions that the doctor may encounter and tips for troubleshooting them are as follows:

- Electrode is dragging/sticking when attempting to pass it through the tissue. Although common, this can be troubleshot in a stepwise manner. First, clean the tip of the electrode with a scratch pad or gauze. If the electrode is still dragging, clean the surgical site with a wet cotton-tipped applicator to remove carbonized tissue. Ensure that the targeted tissue is sufficiently wet by rubbing a wet cotton-tipped applicator on the surgical site. As a last resort (after performing the steps mentioned earlier), increase the power by one or two units until the electrode no longer drags through the tissue.
- Electrode is sparking or producing excessive amounts of smoke when it comes into contact with the tissue. In this case, the power settings of the radiofrequency unit are likely set too high. There is too much energy being focused at the tip of the electrode, causing sparks to fly from the electrode to the surrounding tissue. Power settings should be turned down to avoid causing unnecessary tissue damage.
- If bleeding occurs, pressure with surgical gauze or a sterile cotton-tipped applicator can be applied. Coagulation with setting #3 will also slow and stop any bleeding in the surgical field but should be used cautiously to avoid excessive tissue damage or scarring.

## MAGNIFICATION

When performing ophthalmic procedures, magnification can prove useful for visualizing fine details on the eyelid and the actual lesions being removed. A surgical microscope or surgical loupes are recommended to increase visualization in these delicate areas. Surgical loupes typically come in 1.5× to 3.5× magnification powers. Surgical loupes often have built-in lights to properly illuminate the surgical field (Figure 8-7). Keep in mind that in general, the higher the magnification power, the closer the working distance required to have a clear view. This will vary depending on the type and brand of surgical loupe used. Surgical loupes that rely on angular magnification will allow increased magnification while maintaining a larger working

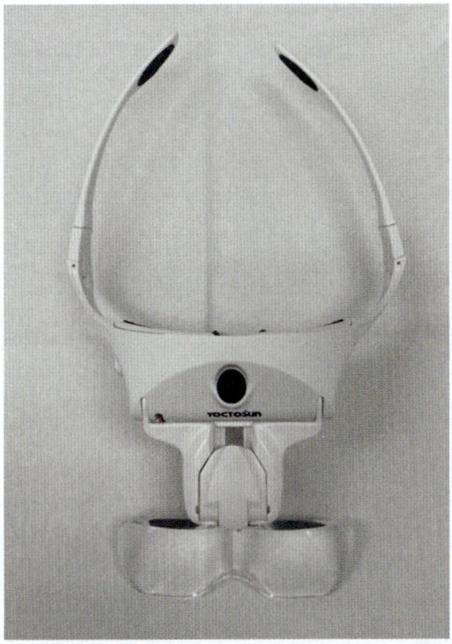

**FIGURE 8-7** An example of glass-mounted surgical loupes with a built-in illumination system.

distance. Surgical microscopes are larger and more expensive but come with the benefit of being able to record the procedure being performed if a camera is attached to the microscope. Surgical microscopes rely on angular magnification as opposed to relative distance magnification (for surgical loupes) and therefore can achieve a clear surgical field at most working distances. This can prove beneficial for doctor and patient comfort during the procedure. Surgical microscopes are significantly more expensive and take up more space than head-mounted surgical loupes, ultimately making them an impractical solution for many clinicians in an office-based setting.

## MOIST WOUND HEALING

Promoting good wound healing is an important aspect of patient care following RF surgery. Creating an incision, removing a skin lesion, or ablating eyelash follicles creates a wound or opening in the skin, which leads to an increased risk of infection. Doctors should apply an antibiotic ointment to the wound at the conclusion of surgery.[3] The antibiotic's main purpose is to keep the wound moist, which decreases the risk of scarring by preventing the wound from drying up.[3,9] Should an antibiotic ointment be unavailable or contraindicated due to allergy, bland petroleum-based ointments have been shown to be equally effective for wound healing.[10]

# RADIOFREQUENCY INDICATIONS

**Key Indications**

- Removal of benign or suspected benign ocular adnexal and eyelid lesions such as papillomas, cysts, seborrheic keratosis, capillary hemangiomas, nevi, and so on.
- Permanent punctal closure
- Eyelash follicle ablation in trichiasis or distichiasis
- Incisions during blepharoplasty, ptosis repair, or other ocular surgeries

RF surgery is a quick and effective surgical option for periocular incisions or lesion removal on the eyelid or ocular adnexa. RF surgery has many advantages when compared to traditional scalpel surgery, offering an easy setup process and a minimally bloody surgical field. RF surgery can be useful in the removal of skin tags, papillomas, and cysts in the ocular adnexa. RF is an effective option for permanent punctal occlusion and eyelash follicle ablation in trichiasis. RF can also be used as an effective tool for incision into the skin during ocular surgeries such as blepharoplasty or ptosis repair.

# RADIOFREQUENCY CONTRAINDICATIONS

**Key Contraindications**

- Suspected malignant lesion
- Cardiac pacemaker, defibrillator, or other implantable cardiac device (relative contraindication)
- Anesthetic allergy
- Patient unable to cooperate, hold still, or lie flat

The most significant contraindication for RF lesion removal is a lesion with suspicion or concern of malignancy. As such, any lesion that requires a biopsy should not be removed with RF surgery.

Characteristics of suspicious lesions include:

- Smooth, pearl-like, or nodular lesions
- Round lesions with central ulceration
- Madarosis on or surrounding the lesion
- Increase/change in size or shape of the lesion over time
- Lesion distorting the regular eyelid architecture
- Lesions with abnormal vasculature

The most common eyelid malignancies are basal cell carcinoma and squamous cell carcinoma. Basal cell carcinomas account for approximately 90% of eyelid malignancies in the

United States and Western countries.[11] Squamous cell carcinoma is the second most common eyelid malignancy but represents less than 5% of eyelid malignancies overall.[11] If suspected, these lesions should be biopsied or removed with unchanged margins. Margins of excised tissue play an important role in histopathologic evaluation of lesions to determine whether they are malignant or benign.[1,5] RF causes very little lateral damage to surrounding tissue, but destroys the edge tissue, making histopathology difficult.[1] Thus, suspicious lesions are an absolute contraindication for RF surgery.

Other contraindications to radiofrequency surgery are largely relative and are generally left up to clinician discretion. The presence of a cardiac pacemaker or other implantable cardiac device (ICD) has theoretically been considered a contraindication to radiofrequency surgery in the past.[12] This assumption was largely based on the theory of high-frequency radio waves from the surgical unit interfering with the radio waves emitted by the implantable cardiac pacemaker. Adverse interactions with pacemakers or ICDs have been reported as rare, especially when radiofrequency surgery is being performed dermatologically.[12,13] Advances in shielding technology have also been hypothesized to lead to a decrease in concern for interference with pacemakers or ICDs.[1,3,12]

Although not a true contraindication for radiosurgery, allergies to lidocaine or epinephrine could disqualify patients for radiosurgery procedures. These are the two most common medications used for local anesthesia and vasoconstriction while performing RF surgery. Epinephrine helps to blanch blood vessels and minimize bleeding during surgery.[14] Although advantageous, epinephrine is not an absolute requirement for RF surgery and can be excluded should the patient be allergic. Local anesthetic is a requirement for RF surgery, which makes an allergy to lidocaine an absolute contraindication unless an alternative anesthetic is available.

Lastly, radiofrequency surgery requires a level of cooperation and compliance from the patient. They must be able to remain still during injections and surgery procedures. The eye is a delicate organ, and radiofrequency has the potential to inflict a significant amount of damage to the globe if the patient is unable to remain relatively still and moves in an unpredictable way. Patients who cannot lie flat on their back on a surgical procedure table for approximately 20 to 30 minutes can also be poor candidates. Doctors should be selective with their choice of patients for radiofrequency surgery and be upfront with their patients on the requirements to stay still during the procedure.

# RADIOFREQUENCY FOR LESION REMOVAL

## Indications

**Key Indications**

- Papillomas/skin tags
- Nevi (unquestionably benign)
- Verruca
- Molluscum contagiosum
- Dermatosis papulosis nigra

- Seborrheic keratoses
- Capillary hemangiomas
- Xanthelasma
- Actinic keratoses
- Basal cell carcinoma
- Squamous cell carcinoma

RF surgery is a versatile technology that can be used for the removal of any benign lesion as well as actinic keratoses and basal and squamous cell carcinomas.[2] Although it can theoretically be used for biopsy of lesions, this is discouraged. The cutting mode will leave very little tissue damage to the edges of the cut, but it will destroy the edge tissue, making it impossible to determine if the full lesion was removed should the malignant tissue extend to the margin.[1,5] Under no circumstances should radiofrequency surgery be used if there is suspicion of melanoma for the same reasons.[1]

## CONTRAINDICATIONS

### Key Contraindications

- Suspicion of melanoma
- Biopsies (relative contraindication)
- Pacemakers (relative contraindication)
- Patient unable to cooperate, hold still, or lie flat

As previously noted, suspicion of melanoma is an absolute contraindication; tissue damage at the incision margin will prevent accurate biopsy results, preventing pathology from determining if the lesion was fully excised.[1] Biopsy is otherwise a relative contraindication due to the damage done at incision margins by radiofrequency surgery.[1,5]

Pacemakers are a relative contraindication. Although modern pacemakers are shielded (and hence theoretically impervious to electromagnetic interference), there is always a danger that the shielding is malfunctional or the pacemaker is of a nonshielded variety.[1,3,5,12] All of the lesions indicated earlier have alternative treatments for removal; however, should radiofrequency surgery still be deemed the best option, reasonable precautions include placing the antenna well away from the heart, activating the device intermittently, and avoiding the use of cut mode (relying on blend instead). Potential complications include pacemaker reprogramming, skipped beats, asystole, bradycardia, and tachycardia.[12]

# PREOPERATIVE PREPARATION

## Key Preparation and Instrumentation

- Blood pressure and pulse measurement
- Informed consent obtained
- Preoperative photographs of the lesion taken
- Radiofrequency unit
- Appropriate electrodes (pin electrode, loop electrode)
- Electrode cleaning pad
- Smoke evacuator
- Surgical loupes (or surgical microscope)
- Sterile surgical gloves
- Sterile surgical drapes
- Ophthalmic topical anesthetic (e.g., proparacaine 0.5%, tetracaine 0.5%)
- Alcohol swab
- 2- to 3-mL 0.5% or 1% lidocaine (usually with epinephrine) in a 3-mL syringe with a 27- to 30-gauge needle
- 10% povidone–iodine (Betadine) swab stick
- Surgical hair cap
- Sterile gauze pads
- Cotton-tipped applicators (~10–15)
- Sterile saline
- Sterile fluid reservoir
- Ophthalmic antibiotic ointment
- 0.12 toothed forceps
- Wescott scissors
- Needle driver (usually not needed)
- Sutures (usually not needed)

Before beginning the procedure, blood pressure and pulse should be checked to ensure no significant, uncontrolled hypertension is present. Patients at or near hypertensive crisis should be better controlled before surgery to reduce the risk of surgical complications both during and after surgery.

Instruments should be placed on a sterile surgical drape on a clean Mayo tray (Figure 8-8), then covered in another sterile drape. Ophthalmic topical anesthetic can be nonsterile and

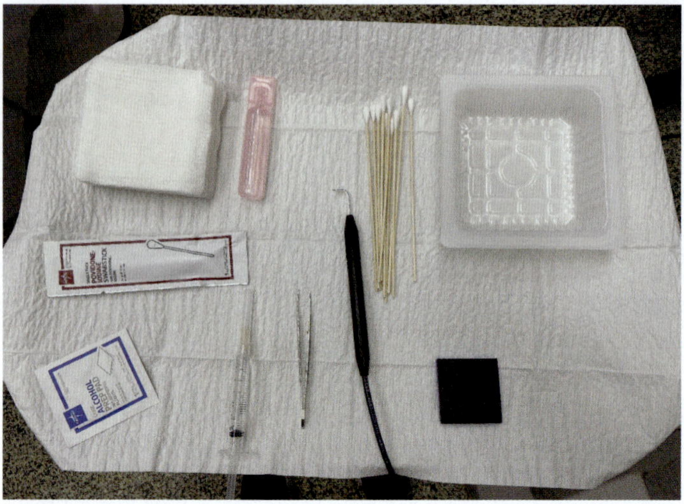


**FIGURE 8-8** The Mayo stand setup for lesion removal is pictured. The radiofrequency handpiece is pictured with the pin/"bent tip" electrode, in black. A tube of sterile saline and a container for it are present, as well as cotton-tipped applicators, gauze pads, disinfectants (an alcohol swab and povidone–iodine [Betadine]), fine-toothed forceps, lidocaine 1% with epinephrine, and an electrode cleaning pad. For large lesions, sutures and a needle driver may be added to the tray if closure with sutures is anticipated to be needed.

off to the side, as it is used for patient comfort before creating an aseptic procedure field. There are multiple styles of radiofrequency units, and all are relatively similar; clinician preference and cost are the primary determinants in selection. For both the Soniquence and Ellman units, a starting power of 10 to 12 is recommended on setting #1 "cut." Other units may have different power levels; clinicians should begin by practicing on a beef steak to determine what settings work best for their unit.[1] Experience also plays a role in determining what setting to be used; clinical judgment must be utilized.

A smoke evacuator is critical. RF vaporizes tissue, which creates extremely unpleasant (and long lasting) odors. Although smoke evacuation does not completely remove the smell, it will be significantly reduced and should not permeate the surgical room for any length of time.[1] In addition to smell, intact HPV DNA has been found in smoke plumes.[15] Theoretically, this could also affect any viral DNA, but there has been no recorded evidence of infection from radiosurgery smoke.[7]

Electrode tips come in a variety of styles (Figure 8-9), and the styles needed will vary depending on the application. For general lesion removal around the adnexa, a pin electrode is recommended. This electrode has excellent ergonomics for a touch-and-off procedure when tissue vaporization is desired, but can also be used for cutting should a lesion need to be debulked first, such as a pedunculated papilloma or a skin tag. It is also large enough to use for coagulation should the need arise.

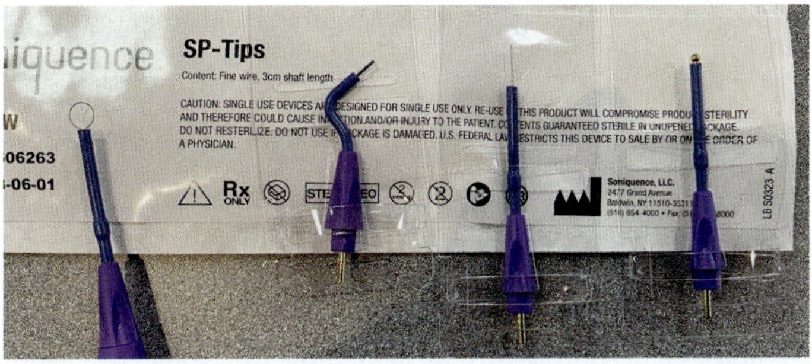


**FIGURE 8-9** Radiofrequency electrodes from left to right: Loop electrode, pin electrode, fine wire electrode, and ball electrode.

Many practitioners use the loop electrode for general treatment (e.g., not specifically around the ocular adnexa).[3,5] When used on pedunculated lesions, the loop can be placed around the lesion and activated before pulling through the stalk; the loop can then be used for feathering the remaining portions of the lesion. The challenge is that because no resistance is felt, the clinician can easily go too deep; therefore, caution is required.[3] These loops come in a variety of sizes and shapes depending on what size and technique are needed.

The ball electrode is excellent for coagulation of bleeding vessels, but should never be used for cutting. It is also excellent for the treatment of capillary hemangiomas, as they are treated through coagulation.[1]

There should be a method of cleaning electrodes present. Even when using sterile electrodes, char will build up during the procedure, which will prevent efficient lesion removal. To remedy this, the electrode can be cleaned during the procedure by either scraping it along an electrode cleaning pad or placing the electrode in a damp piece of gauze and activating it momentarily before wiping away the char.[3]

Ophthalmic topical anesthetic, alcohol and povidone–iodine (Betadine) swab sticks, and lidocaine with epinephrine injections are used for patient preparation. For lesions where epinephrine would be contraindicated, such as capillary hemangiomas, epinephrine should be avoided. There will also be lesions where direct anesthetic injection is not feasible; in these cases, 4% lidocaine can be used topically with an eye spear sponge (Weck-Cel) for application. Lidocaine is only contraindicated in patients with true amide allergies, and epinephrine has no absolute contraindications. Relative contraindications include vascular abnormalities, such as hypertension and diabetes, hypersensitivity to sympathomimetics, or narrow-angle glaucoma.[14,16] However, one double-blind, placebo-controlled study showed that among patients without hypertension, exposure to epinephrine versus a placebo produced no changes in systolic or diastolic blood pressure, mean arterial pressure, or heart rate.[17]

Patients need not be taken off of blood thinners for radiofrequency surgery. If bleeding is a significant concern, the blend mode can be used to coagulate as surgery is performed.[3]

A sterile fluid reservoir should be filled with saline, and cotton tip applicators should be laid to the side or placed in the saline to soak. Often the simplest (and cheapest) sterile reservoir is the plastic case from which sterile gauze is removed (see the bottom left portion of Figure 8-8). Cotton tip applicators may be replaced with sterile gauze pads if needed. These are used to wipe char off of the patient as the procedure is performed and to rewet the lesion, which allows the radiofrequency unit to be more effective and efficient.[3] Cotton tip applicators carry the added benefits of being easier to maneuver in a crowded surgical field with forceps and electrodes, as well as being less likely to drip excess saline on the patient (and thus increasing patient comfort).

The patient's hair should be placed in a surgical hair cap. This ensures that no loose hairs enter the surgical field. The patient should be laid back for comfort and reduction of movement. Reclining the patient to the full supine position also allows the clinician to sit comfortably during the procedure. The antenna should be placed behind the patient and near the surgical site.[5] It does not, however, need to be directly behind the site—often placing the plate behind the shoulder is sufficient. Although the beginning settings vary by unit, clinical experience has shown that on setting #1 "cut," a power of 10 to 12 is generally sufficient on most common models. If unsure of what setting to use, prepare by experimenting on beef steak.[1] The ideal power setting for cut mode is one where the electrode cuts smoothly with no resistance, like a hot knife through butter.[3] Experience with individual units will lead to tailoring the beginning settings. If using a foot pedal to activate the electrode, it should be placed in an easily accessible location, but care must be taken that it will not be activated accidentally.[5]

Ophthalmic antibiotic ointment should be prepared so it can be placed on the surgical site immediately after the procedure is done. Although most periocular lesions will not require sutures, clinical judgment must be used to determine if they should be immediately on hand. Because unforeseen circumstances may arise, they should be nearby in a readily accessible location should they be required. Similarly, Westcott scissors may be required for some lesions, and therefore should be nearby for all procedures should they be needed.

# PROCEDURAL TECHNIQUE

**Key Procedural Points**

- Select the appropriate waveform/setting and power, usually setting #1 "cut," power 10 to 12.
- Instill ophthalmic topical anesthetic (e.g., proparacaine 0.5%) eyedrops in both eyes to eliminate blink reflex.
- Alcohol swab area around the lesion to prep for injection
- Inject the anesthetic, usually lidocaine 0.5% or 1% with epinephrine 1:200,000.
- Disinfect with a 10% povidone–iodine (Betadine) swab stick.
- Remove the lesion with radiofrequency electrode (usually bent tip electrode or loop electrode) in small passes to prevent excessive depth.
- Excise the lesion fully.
- Feather edges to make lesion removal area smooth and flush with the surrounding skin.
- Suture (if needed)
- Apply ophthalmic antibiotic ointment

Before beginning, ensure that the correct waveform has been selected. For general lesion removal, the cut setting should be used; this setting has a small amount of coagulation occurring (90% cutting, 10% coagulation), which limits bleeding but still allows for smooth cutting through lesions. Blend mode (50% cutting, 50% coagulation) can be used on significantly vascularized tissue to maintain a clear field, but because of the increased coagulation would cause significantly higher damage to adjacent tissue. Other modes should be avoided in lesion removal. If there is significant bleeding during or after lesion removal, coagulation mode (10% cutting, 90% coagulation) can be used for hemostasis.[3]

The process for radiofrequency lesion removal typically involves a number of steps for general lesions in the adnexal region.

1. Ophthalmic topical anesthetic is given in both eyes to reduce blink response.
2. The lesion and area immediately adjacent are wiped with an alcohol swab, starting from the lesion and circling outward.
3. The patient is injected with 0.5% or 1% lidocaine, often in combination with epinephrine. Typically, 0.5 to 1.0 mL or less is enough to fully anesthetize the area; the exact dose will depend on the size of the lesion. It must be remembered that it will take several minutes to reach full effect. Epinephrine should not be used on a capillary hemangioma, as it will make assessing the proper endpoint difficult. For lesions directly on the lid margin or on the conjunctiva, in addition to injectable lidocaine, 4% lidocaine can be placed on an eye spear sponge (Weck-Cel) and placed directly on the conjunctiva in the area of the lesion. It should be held for approximately 30 to 60 seconds to ensure full anesthesia.
4. The lesion is swabbed with a 10% povidone–iodine (Betadine) swab stick, which is allowed to rest for approximately 1 to 3 minutes to reach full effect before the excess is sponged off with gauze.
5. The lesion should be pinched with fine-toothed forceps to establish that anesthesia has reached full effect. The patient may feel the sensation of touching or pressure, but no pain, pinching, or sharpness should be felt.
6. Once the patient is fully anesthetized, removal can begin. Ensure that the smoke evacuator is in a position where it is as close as possible to the lesion without compromising the view. It should be as close as possible to the procedure site and should be placed so as to draw the smoke away from the patient's nose.[5]

Start by wetting the lesion with saline. This allows for improved action by the electrode. Begin on setting #1 cut, power approximately 10 to 12 (for most common units) and utilize the appropriate electrode. The clinician should position themselves comfortably with the hand carrying the electrode braced on the patient's face for stability. This ensures that if the patient moves, the electrode moves with them, reducing the risk of unintentional laceration.[1] The lesion can be touched with the electrode without activation until comfortable that the view and positioning are sufficiently clear and comfortable to begin. Electrodes can then be activated either by foot pedal or by button on the handpiece, and should be activated before touching the lesion; activation of electrode while in contact with the lesion inhibits current flow, leading to poor results when cutting.[5]

For small lesions, a "touch-and-off" approach can be used—simply touch the lesion momentarily, vaporizing a small amount of tissue, and immediately pull the electrode away. This allows for tissue vaporization to occur at a slow and steady pace and reduces the risk of cutting too deeply. Remember that radiofrequency surgery causes no tissue resistance, so any movement can cause significant damage if not done carefully. Whenever not actively removing the lesion, the electrodes should be deactivated by releasing the foot pedal or buttons on the handpiece. If using the touch-and-off method, proceed until the lesion has been fully excised, and the tissue underneath is flush with the surrounding skin (Figure 8-10A-D). For pedunculated lesions, the lesion can be lifted with forceps and the stalk can be cut using the loop or pin electrode (Figures 8-11A-C and 8-12A-D). This maximizes efficiency and leads to shorter procedures. With experience, raised lesions can be shaved down using radiofrequency surgery units. Care should be taken to shave small amounts at a time, as the lack of resistance in radiosurgery can easily lead to cutting too deep. In any case, when the lesion has been fully excised, the edges should then be "feathered" by lightly brushing the edges of the removed lesion toward the center, perpendicular to the circumference of lesion removal. This promotes smoother healing and reduces the likelihood of scarring.[1,3,5] The majority of periorbital lesions

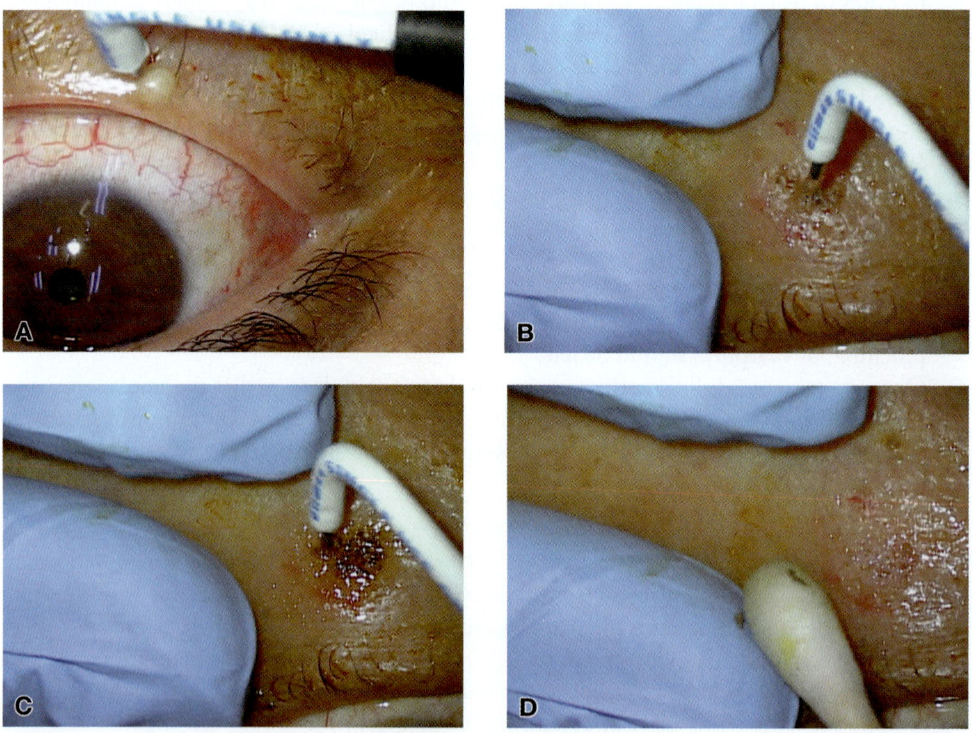


**FIGURE 8-10** **A,** Radiofrequency pin electrode (aka bent tip electrode) about to be used to incise into a cyst of Zeiss. **B,** Radiofrequency pin electrode (aka bent tip electrode) about to be used to vaporize and remove a seborrheic keratosis. **C,** Radiofrequency pin electrode (aka bent tip electrode) being used to vaporize a seborrheic keratosis. Note the charring or "carbonized tissue" that will develop during lesion removal with RF. Also, note the perpendicular orientation of the "bent tip" electrode to the skin. **D,** Nearing the end of the removal of this seborrheic keratosis with RF. Utilization of a cotton-tipped applicator with sterile saline is being done to wipe away the "carbonized tissue." This is an important step throughout the RF lesion removal process.

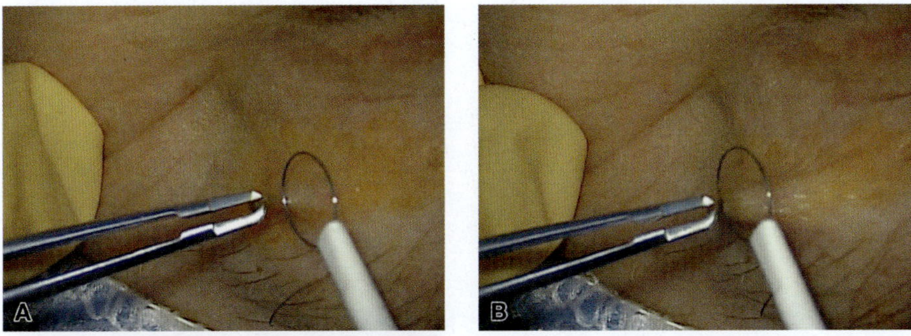

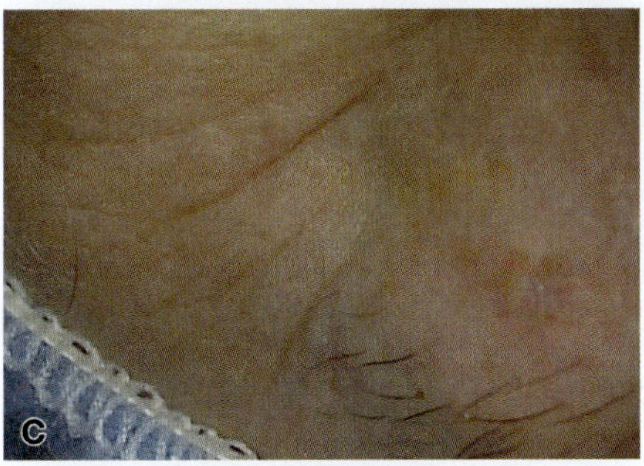

**FIGURE 8-11** **A,** Radiofrequency loop electrode about to be used to remove a squamous papilloma. **B,** Radiofrequency loop electrode being used to take off the papilloma through the stalk of the lesion. **C,** Immediate postoperative appearance after the lesion removal. Note complete removal of the lesion.

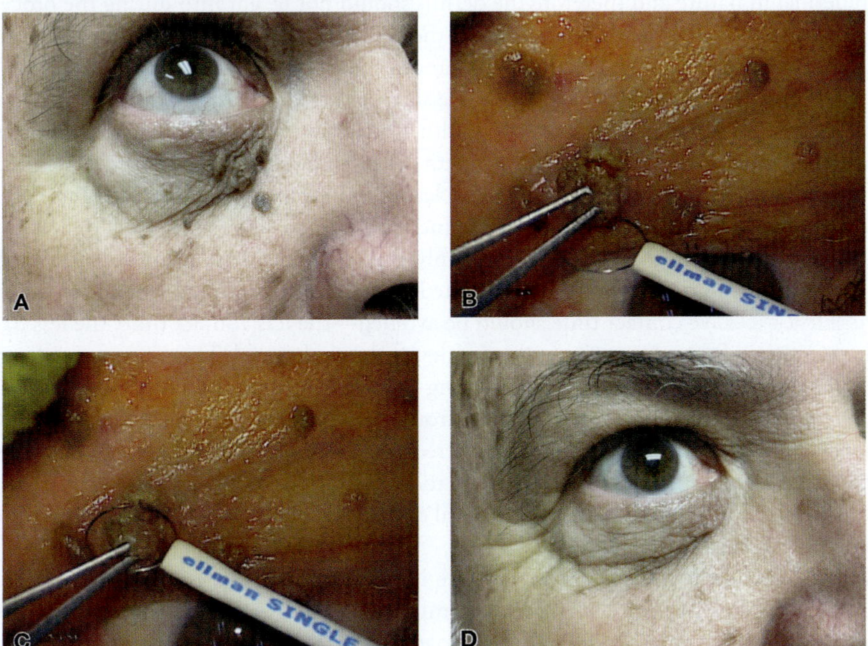


**FIGURE 8-12** **A,** Viral papillomas and verruca on a patient's right lower eyelid. **B,** Radiofrequency loop electrode and toothed forceps starting a pass through a lesion to remove a large portion of this verruca. **C,** Radiofrequency loop electrode and toothed forceps finishing the pass through the lesion. Note a large portion of the lesion has been removed. **D,** Postoperative appearance showing complete resolution.

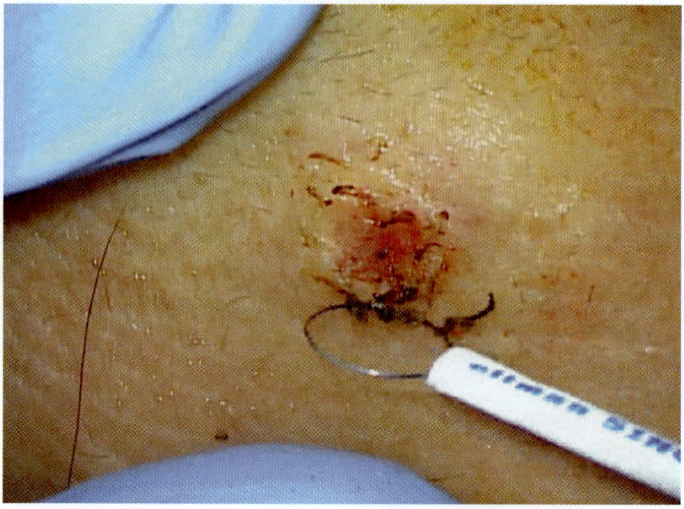

**FIGURE 8-13** Radiofrequency removal of a compound nevus with the loop electrode on setting #1 cut power 12. Note the carbonized tissue that can develop during a radiofrequency lesion removal. This can easily be cleared with a cotton-tipped applicator.

are epidermal in nature and therefore the dermis should not be cut into during the procedure, thus preventing scarring.[18] However, should the lesion be deeper, removal can be continued until the lesion is fully excised. During the procedure, char will build up on the tissue being removed (Figure 8-13). As this occurs, the site should be gently scrubbed with either gauze or a cotton-tipped applicator moistened with saline. This improves electrode contact removal as well as remoistens the area for further treatment. Char will also develop on the electrode itself. This can be cleaned off by using a disposable cleaning block or simply wrapping the end of the electrode in moist gauze and activating it momentarily.[3]

Although radiosurgery primarily affects only the touched tissue, because it is a vaporization process, surrounding tissue can be affected. To minimize this risk, several steps must be taken.[1] First, excessive contact time should be avoided—the less contact time, the less damage to adjacent tissue. Second, appropriate power levels should be used. The minimum power level that will smoothly cut tissue without catching or dragging should be utilized. Third, larger electrodes will also cause more damage to surrounding tissue; hence, the ball electrode would be inappropriate for incision. Fourth, the correct waveform should be selected. Finally, tissue resistance is a factor in the amount of damage to adjacent tissue—the drier a tissue is, the more difficult it will be to cut and the more collateral damage is likely to occur. This can be remedied by regularly moistening the lesion.

When the lesion is fully removed, if there is significant bleeding pressure with gauze or a cotton tip applicator for a few seconds to minutes is often effective in stopping bleeding. If bleeding persists, gentle cautery using coagulation mode can be used. Depending on which electrode was used for cutting, an alternative electrode may need to be used; the ball electrode is particularly effective.[3] Once bleeding has been staunched, apply ophthalmic antibiotic ointment to the lesion. If necessary, sutures can be used to close the wound; however, this will be uncommon for general lesion removal. Should they be necessary, interrupted sutures are often the simplest and most effective option, as few (1-5) sutures are typically needed.

## CAPILLARY HEMANGIOMA

Treatment of capillary hemangiomas differs significantly from typical lesion removal with the radiofrequency unit. Anesthesia can proceed as usual, with the exception that epinephrine should not be used to prevent blanching of the lesion leading to undertreatment. To begin, utilize a ball electrode on setting #3 "coagulation," with power approximately 8 to 10. The electrode should be activated and placed in direct contact with the hemangioma for a moment before pulling off. This slight "tap tap" motion on and off of the hemangioma should be repeated until the hemangioma turns white. The electrode should then be removed and the area wiped with a cotton-tipped applicator to remove the white tissue on the surface of the hemangioma. Often times this will then reveal an underlying red area still present. This means the bottom half of the hemangioma still remains, and treatment to that area needs to continue. The procedure is repeated until the hemangioma area turns black, and there is no red tissue remaining (Figure 8-14).[1] This ensures that the blood vessels comprising the lesion have been coagulated enough to not return.

## TROUBLESHOOTING

When performing radiofrequency surgery, challenges may arise that would not do so with traditional surgical approaches. Some of the possible challenges as well as their remedies are as follows:[1,3,5]

- Sparking
  - Power too high; turn down power setting 2 to 3 points
- Electrode catching and not cutting smoothly
  - Ensure the lesion and electrode tip are both clear of char; reclean both.
  - Remoisten the surgery site.
  - Move more slowly through the tissue.
  - Only after trying these should the power level be turned up, and only incrementally by 1 to 2 points until a smooth cut is achieved.
  - If challenges continue, check that the antenna is plugged in and placed in the correct position.
- Excessive tissue damage
  - Minimize contact time.
  - Lower power level.
  - Check settings (cut vs. coagulation vs. blend).
  - Increase moisture on the lesion.

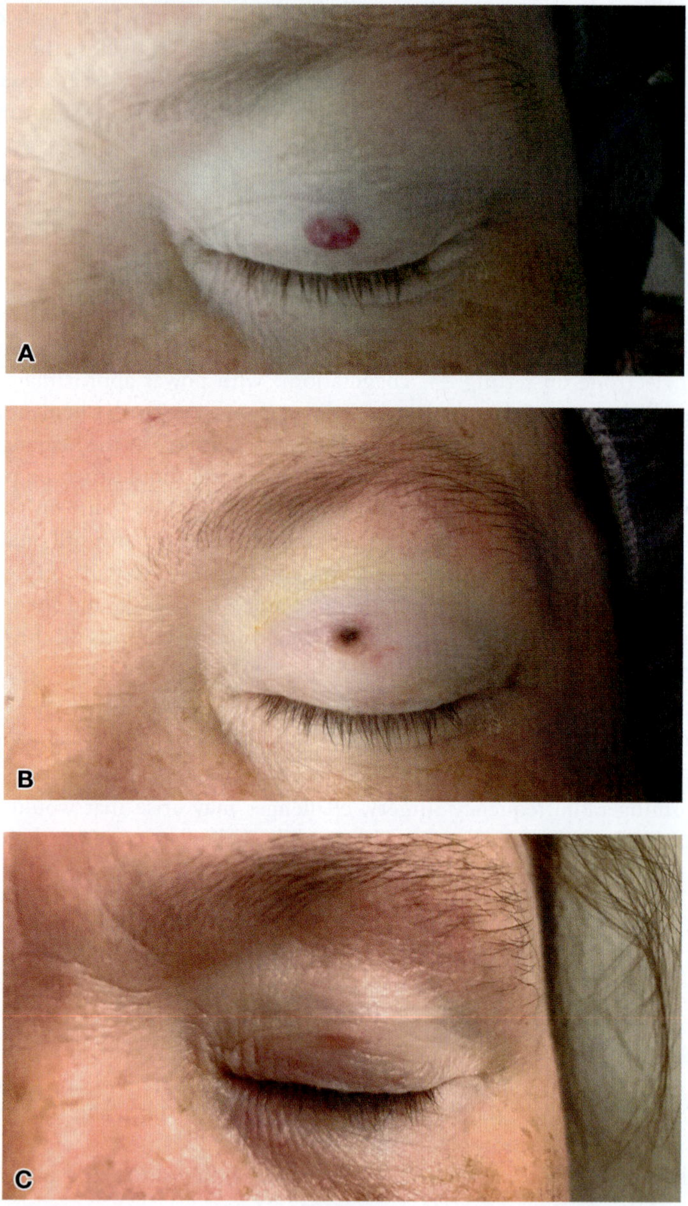


**FIGURE 8-14** **A,** Preoperative appearance of a capillary hemangioma. **B,** Immediate postoperative appearance of a capillary hemangioma with a radiofrequency device. We used setting #3 coagulation. Note the now black color of the hemangioma. That indicates this vascular lesion has been fully ablated. **C,** Two-week postoperative appearance. The area is healing nicely and showing resolution of the hemangioma.

# POSTOPERATIVE CARE

## Key Postoperative Care

- Blood pressure and pulse measured postoperatively to ensure no elevation was seen
- Ophthalmic antibiotic ointment three times a day (TID) for 1 week
- Follow-up visit as needed depending on lesion size, lesion location, clinician preference

Following the procedure, the patient should be raised to a sitting position (if the procedure was performed lying down). The patient should be allowed to rest comfortably with legs hanging for a short time to ensure no orthostatic hypotension has occurred. Blood pressure should be checked again, following which the patient should be given ophthalmic antibiotic ointment to be used TID for 1 week. (Erythromycin ophthalmic is a common drug of choice.) Patients should be educated that keeping the wound clean and moist will improve healing times and reduce the likelihood of scarring.[3]

Return to clinic instructions will vary with the significance of the surgical procedure, whether or not further treatment will be required, and whether sutures were used. More severe procedures, those requiring a second round of treatment, and those with sutures should be scheduled back; however, most benign "lump and bump" removals around the eyelids are minor and will require no follow-up unless problems develop. As with any procedure, patients should be educated on the signs and symptoms of infection, including redness, significant swelling, pain, fever, and drainage, and to return to clinic immediately should any of these occur.

## Potential Complications and Management

### Key Complications

- Excessively deep cutting
- Destruction of tissue to be biopsied
- Pacemaker malfunction
- Burns
- Scarring
- Recurrence of lesion
- Misdiagnosis of lesion (removing a pigmented lesion that is actually melanoma)
- Postoperative pain, bleeding, or infection
- Spreading of infection
- Broken electrode wires
- Incorrect use of technology
- Fire

Although there are many possible complications of radiofrequency surgery, most are rare. To reduce the chances of complications, a clinician who is new to the technology should practice first on patient models, such as steak.[1] This provides a realistic simulation of the procedure and will prevent the more common mistakes, from which many of the complications may arise.

An excessively deep cut is a great risk for a clinician transitioning from traditional cutting methods to radiofrequency surgery. Unlike the scalpel, there is no tissue resistance when the machine is used properly, removing much of the tactile response from surgery. Deep excision also increases the risk of scars, bleeding, and pain after the procedure.[1] Before beginning the procedure, the clinician should also check to ensure that the correct settings have been applied.[5]

Another simple mistake that can easily be avoided is the incorrect use of the technology. Often these units are operated by foot pedals and have two separate pedals to activate different settings or modes. Pressing the incorrect pedal can lead to tissue damage from incorrect mode selection.

Because of the destructive nature of radiofrequency surgery, some risks are inherently higher than traditional bladed surgery. Even cutting mode has 10% coagulation, leading to a very minute amount of tissue damage peripherally. If the settings are incorrect (e.g., using blend rather than cut, having the power setting too high, etc.), burns and tissue destruction are more likely. This is of particular concern for tissue to be biopsied, as it can make it difficult to tell if the margins of the lesions are clear from pathology. As such, caution should be taken when performing biopsies, and alternative methods should be considered.[1,5] Additionally, because radiofrequency surgery has some aspect to coagulation, there is less initial bleeding; however, wounds can seep more blood than they would with traditional surgery, as initial minimal coagulation during the procedure can break over time. Patients should be educated on this risk.[5] RF surgery also has the potential for sparking (typically when the power settings are too high), and thus a potential for ignition of flammable materials is possible.[5] The most common concern in most offices will be alcohol cleanser. Simply ensuring the cleanser has fully dried, and using the correct settings will make this risk negligible.[5]

Clinicians should inspect electrodes before use, ensuring they are using sterile equipment for each surgery and that no damage has occurred to the electrodes or wires.[5] This is of particular concern if electrodes are being reused.

Other complications are universal to surgery. Infection is a risk any time the skin is broken, and universal precautions should be taken. Cutting too deep can lead to scarring, pain, or excessive bleeding. Any misdiagnosed malignant lesion has the potential for long-term harm to a patient, which must be carefully considered when pigmented lesions are removed. Practicing caution during surgery can minimize the risk of any of these universal complications.

## VIDEOS OF PROCEDURES

**Video 8-1**—Papilloma removal. Not shown in the video is the area being prepped with an alcohol swab and 10% povidone–iodine (Betadine), as well as approximately 0.3 to 0.4 mL of lidocaine 0.5% with epinephrine injected around the skin tag to provide proper anesthesia. A 0.12-mm toothed forceps is used to grasp the top half of the lesion to enable an efficient removal of the lesion at its base. A radiofrequency loop electrode is used on setting #1 cut, power 10 to remove the lesion near its base. The same loop electrode is then used to gently feather the lesion down until it is smooth and flush with the surrounding skin and completely remove the papilloma. Note the cotton-tipped applicator soaked in sterile saline is used to help wipe away carbonized tissue during the removal process. The papilloma was completely excised, and the patient was thrilled with the outcome. (Video courtesy of Nate Lighthizer.)

**Video 8-2**—Seborrheic keratosis (SK) removal. Not shown in the video are the areas being prepped with an alcohol swab prior to the injections. Shown in the video are multiple subcutaneous injections of lidocaine 0.5% with epinephrine being performed around multiple SK lesions to provide anesthesia. The injections are performed with a 30-gauge ½" needle on a 3-mL syringe with a total of less than 1 mL of anesthetic used to anesthetize all the lesions. The areas are then prepped with a 10% povidone–iodine (Betadine) swab stick. A 0.12-mm toothed forceps is used to pinch the areas to ensure appropriate anesthesia is achieved. A radiofrequency pin electrode (aka "bent tip" electrode) is used on setting #1 cut, power 10 to vaporize and completely remove the multiple SKs. When removing the lesions on or near the eyelid margin, note how the eyelid is pulled away from the globe as much as possible. Also note a cotton-tipped applicator soaked in sterile saline is used to remove carbonized tissue during the lesion removal and following the lesion removal. Erythromycin ophthalmic antibiotic ointment is applied to the surgical sites. (Video courtesy of Nate Lighthizer.)

**Video 8-3**—Verruca removal. Not shown in the video are the areas being prepped with an alcohol swab prior to the injections. Shown in the video is a subcutaneous injection of lidocaine 0.5% with epinephrine being performed around the large viral papilloma lesion to provide proper anesthesia. The injections are performed with a 30-gauge ½" needle on a 3-mL syringe with a total of less than 1 mL of anesthetic used to anesthetize all the lesions. The areas are then prepped with a 10% povidone–iodine (Betadine) swab stick. A 0.12-mm toothed forceps is used to pinch the areas to ensure appropriate anesthesia is achieved. A radiofrequency loop electrode is used on setting #1 cut, power 14 to remove and biopsy a portion of the suspected viral papilloma. Note the first pass through the lesion the area becomes white, indicating the tissue has been heated up too much. The tissue specimen is "fried" and would not be useful for a biopsy reading. That initial piece of tissue was placed in the biohazard container. A second pass through the lesion on a lower power of 10 nicely removed a portion of the lesion to be put in the biopsy specimen container. The biopsy report came back as a squamous papilloma, likely verruca. Because the multiple lesions had been present for many years, and our index of suspicion was very low for malignancy, the rest of the lesions were removed with the loop electrode. Note a cotton-tipped applicator soaked in sterile saline is used to remove carbonized tissue during the lesion removals and following the lesion removals. Erythromycin ophthalmic antibiotic ointment is applied to the surgical sites (not shown in the video). See Figure 8-12A-D for preoperative, perioperative, and postoperative photographs. (Video courtesy of Nate Lighthizer.)

**Video 8-4**—Cyst of Zeis, seborrheic keratosis, and papilloma removal. Not shown in the video are the areas being prepped with an alcohol swab and 10% povidone–iodine (Betadine), as well as approximately 0.6 to 0.7 mL of lidocaine 0.5% with epinephrine injected around the lesions to provide proper anesthesia. A radiofrequency pin electrode (aka "bent tip" electrode) is used on setting #1 cut, power 10 to vaporize and completely remove the papilloma. The pin electrode is then used to incise into the cyst of Zeis, followed by a 0.12-mm toothed forceps and cotton-tipped applicator used to drain the contents of the cyst. A Westcott scissors and nontoothed forceps are then used to excise the remaining capsule. The incision is left to heal by secondary intention. Finally, the pin electrode is used on setting #1 cut, power 10 to vaporize and completely remove the seborrheic keratosis. Note a cotton-tipped applicator soaked in sterile saline is used to remove carbonized tissue during the lesion removal and following the lesion removal. Erythromycin ophthalmic antibiotic ointment is applied to the surgical sites. See Figure 8-16A–C for preoperative, immediate postoperative, and one-month postoperative photos, respectively. (Video courtesy of Nate Lighthizer.)

## EFFICACY

There are few articles on the efficacy of radiofrequency surgery for ocular lesion removal. However, what is available shows good results. One study looked in part at recurrence rates among various eyelid tumors, both benign and malignant, and found a 0.54% rate of recurrence for benign tumors and a 12.7% recurrence rate for malignant tumors;

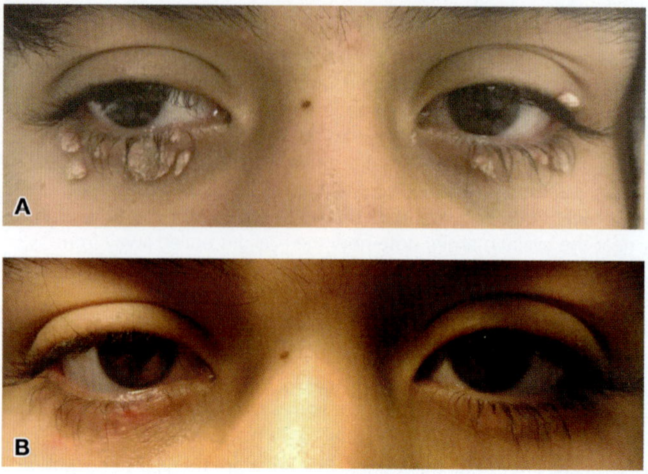

FIGURE 8-15 **A,** Preoperative appearance of a young male patient with extensive verruca on three eyelids. **B,** Postoperative appearance 10 days after all the verruca were removed with a radiofrequency device.

however, the removal method was not specified.[19] Overall, clinical experience has shown radiofrequency surgery to be a superbly effective and efficient procedure for removing periocular lesions with a low side effect profile and a low recurrence rate (Figures 8-15A, B and 8-16A-C).

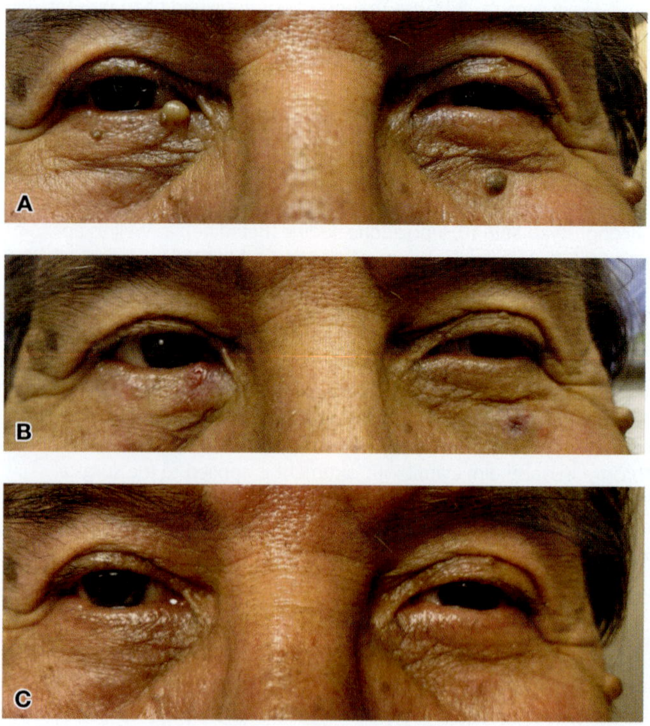

FIGURE 8-16 **A,** Preoperative appearance of a male patient with a cyst of Zeis, small papilloma, and seborrheic keratosis. **B,** Immediate postoperative appearance after removal with a radiofrequency device. **C,** One-month postoperative appearance after removal with a radiofrequency device. Note complete resolution.

# CODING/BILLING AND MODIFIERS

## Key CPT Codes

- **11102**—Tangential biopsy of skin, single lesion
  - **11103**—Each separate/additional lesion after the first; code each additional lesion biopsied separately.
- **11106**—Incisional biopsy of skin, including closure if needed, single lesion
  - **11107**—Each separate/additional lesion after the first; code each additional lesion biopsied separately.
- **11200**—Removal of skin tags, multiple fibrocutaneous tags, any area; up to and including 15 lesions
  - **11201**—Removal of each additional 10 lesions; may be billed multiple times as needed
- **1144X**—Excision, other benign lesions including margins, except skin tag (unless listed elsewhere), face, ears, eyelids, nose, lips, mucous membrane
  - 0—lesion 0.5 cm or less
  - 1—lesion 0.6 to 1.0 cm
  - 2—lesion 1.1 to 2.0 cm
  - 3—lesion 2.1 to 3.0 cm
  - 4—lesion 3.1 to 4.0 cm
  - 6—lesion larger than 4.0 cm
- **17000**—Destruction of premalignant lesion (e.g., actinic keratoses); first lesion
  - **17003**—Second through 14th lesion; list each separately in addition to the code for the initial lesion.
  - **17004**—15 or more lesions; standalone code (not to be used with 17000 or 17003)
- **17106**—Destruction of cutaneous vascular proliferative lesion (e.g., capillary hemangioma) less than 10 $cm^2$
- **1711X**—Destruction of benign lesions other than skin tags or cutaneous vascular proliferative lesions
  - 0—up to 14 lesions
  - 1—15 or more lesions
- **67810**—Incisional biopsy of eyelid skin including lid margin
- **67840**—Excision of lesion of eyelid (except chalazion) without closure or with simple direct closure

There are no special codes specifically for radiofrequency surgery; as such, general surgical codes can be used.

Biopsy codes include 11102/3, 11106/7, and 67810. When the eyelid margin is involved, the 67810 code should be used; otherwise, 11102 is used for the initial lesion if the shave technique is used, and 11103 for each additional lesion removed at that appointment with the shave technique. If multiple, nonmargin lesions are biopsied, both 11102 and 11103 should be coded. For example, if three lesions were removed for biopsy, the clinician could code 11102, 11103, and an additional 11103 for the third lesion. The same holds true for 11106/7, the difference being that 11106 is used for the initial incision biopsy, and 11107 is used for additional incision biopsies. Should radiofrequency be used for incision and shave biopsies at the same appointment, the codes can be combined. For example, a shave and incision biopsy of two separate lesions could be coded as 11102 for the shave, and 11107 for the additional incision.[20]

Multiple codes exist for the destruction of lesions, depending on the type of lesion being destroyed. For premalignant lesions, 17000 is used for the initial lesion. 17003 is used for each additional lesion until the 14th lesion; with 15 or more lesions, 17004 should be coded. For example, for three lesions, the clinician should code 17000 once and 17003 twice. If the patient had 16 lesions, only 17004 should be coded. For vascular lesions, size is the main concern. Any significantly sized lesion should not be treated with radiofrequency surgery; laser treatments are more effective for larger lesions. If a vascular lesion is treated with radiofrequency surgery, 17106 is coded for any lesion less than 10 $cm^2$. Finally, destruction of benign lesions has only two codes, based on the number destroyed. If the number is 14 or less, 17110 should be coded; 15 or more, 17111.[20]

Lesion excision is the third group of codes. For skin tag removal, the 11200 code is used for up to 15 lesions. If there are more than 15 skin tags are removed, 11201 covers an additional 10 lesions and can be used as often as needed. If a patient were to have 28 tags removed, the clinician would code 11200, 11201, and a second 11201. If the lesion is anything besides a skin tag, the codes 1144X or 67840 can be used. The decision for which code should be used is based on the lesion depth. For lesions that involve only the skin, the 1144X codes should be used, with the X varying based on lesion size; for 67840, the lesion should involve deeper tissues.[20]

Global periods vary based on the code; see the following table for more information on specific periods for specific codes.[21]

| CODE | GLOBAL PERIOD |
|---|---|
| 11102/3 | Day of procedure |
| 11106/7 | Day of procedure |
| 11200/1 | 10 days |
| 1144X | 10 days |
| 1700X | 10 days |
| 17106 | 90 days |
| 1711X | 10 days |
| 67810 | 10 days |
| 67840 | 10 days |

## TRICHIASIS MANAGEMENT

Epilation of misdirected eyelashes is routinely used in eye care to help alleviate patient symptoms from trichiasis. This temporary treatment typically requires frequent repeating every 4 to 6 weeks.[22,23] A permanent treatment method involves the use of electrosurgery to cause follicular destruction.[3] RF is used to selectively ablate the root of eyelash follicles without side effects caused by electrocautery on the eyelid.

## INDICATIONS

### Key Indications

- Primary trichiasis
- Secondary trichiasis
- Distichiasis
- Entropion (spastic, involutional, cicatricial, congenital)

Trichiasis is a condition characterized by misdirected eyelashes toward the globe. It may result in corneal or conjunctival abrasion, chronic ocular surface disease, and ulceration in more severe cases.[24] Patient symptoms may vary but most report pain, irritation, epiphora, and foreign-body sensation.[25] It can be classified as primary trichiasis or secondary trichiasis. In primary trichiasis, the eyelid margin is normally positioned, but the eyelash follicles are misaligned causing eyelashes to be misdirected towards the globe. Primary trichiasis may occur due to severe blepharitis, recurrent chalazia, tumors, herpes zoster ophthalmicus, eyelid trauma, or previous surgery.[22] In secondary trichiasis, the eyelash follicles are aligned normally, but the eyelid margin is rotated inward, such as in entropion, causing eyelashes to contact the globe.[24] Secondary trichiasis is caused by entropion associated with eyelid laxity, retractor disinsertion, or posterior lamellar contraction, as seen in conditions such as cicatricial ocular pemphigoid, Stevens–Johnson syndrome, trachoma, or chemical burns.[3,24]

The average eyelash depth is approximately 1.8 mm in the upper eyelid and 1.0 mm in the lower eyelid.[23] Accordingly, follicular coagulation needs to be performed 2.4 mm into the eyelid margin on the upper eyelid and 1.4 mm in the lower eyelid.[3] There is no age predilection for trichiasis, although it typically occurs in older age and is more commonly seen in females.[26]

Distichiasis is characterized by one or more extra rows of eyelashes located within the tarsus and growing behind the normal row of eyelashes at the meibomian gland orifices.[24,25] This condition may be congenital or acquired. The cilia, although aligned normally, commonly result in globe touch due to their more posterior origination requiring treatment.

When associated with entropion, efforts should be made to correct the underlying condition before performing eyelash ablation. If entropion surgery cannot be performed or trichiasis remains after surgery, radiofrequency ablation can be performed.

Irritation, discomfort, pain, and vision changes are all symptoms that patients may complain of with trichiasis and distichiasis. These symptoms in addition to signs of ocular surface disease and ineffectiveness of eyelash epilation are key indications for undergoing eyelash ablation with radiofrequency.

# CONTRAINDICATIONS

## Key Contraindications

- Electronic implants (e.g., cardiac pacemaker, defibrillator)
- Flammable fumes or liquids (e.g., oxygen, alcohol)
- Patient unable to cooperate, hold still, or lie flat
- Active herpetic infection
- Allergies to anesthetics or medications (e.g., lidocaine, epinephrine, erythromycin)

The contraindications involved with trichiasis ablation with radiofrequency surgery involve the cautionary approach exercised when using radiofrequency devices. RF devices when used with cardiac pacemakers can cause asystole and tachycardia, and thus should be avoided in these patients.[1,27] If alternative treatments are not an option, the grounding plate can be placed away from the heart and the lowest power setting can be used. Flammable fumes such as oxygen are contraindicated due to flame risk. Trichiasis ablation can be a timely procedure depending on the number of eyelashes that need to be removed, thus patients should be comfortable lying flat on their back for at least 15 to 30 minutes. Any active herpetic infection should be treated prior to surgery.[3] Caution should be taken to avoid or use alternative medications or anesthesia in the case of anesthetic allergy.

# PREOPERATIVE PREPARATION

## Key Preoperative Considerations

- Photographs of trichiasis with offending eyelashes
- Consent form
- Visual acuity
- Blood pressure measurement
- Pulse measurement
- Ophthalmic topical anesthetic (e.g., proparacaine, tetracaine) instilled

## Instrumentation (Figure 8-17)

1. Ophthalmic topical anesthetic (e.g., proparacaine, tetracaine)
2. 70% isopropyl alcohol prep pad
3. Local anesthesia (0.5%, 1%, or 2% lidocaine with epinephrine 1:100,000 or 1:200,000)
4. 4% topical lidocaine
5. 10% povidone–iodine (Betadine) swab stick (optional)

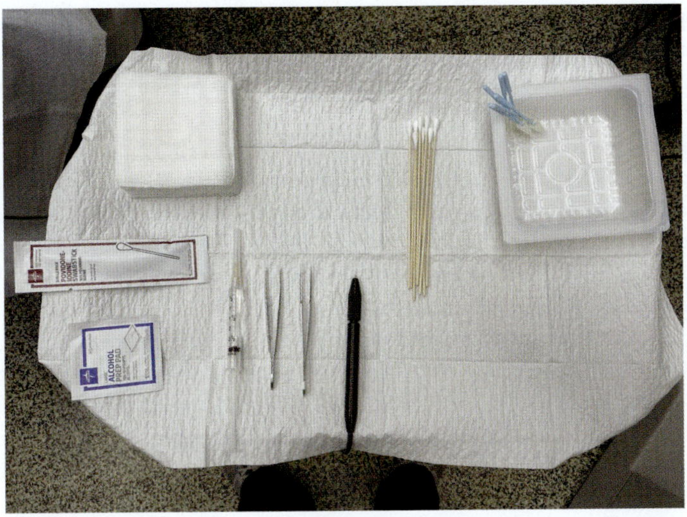


**FIGURE 8-17** Instrument tray showing the proper instruments used for radiofrequency ablation of trichiasis.

6. 30-gauge needle (1/2″ length)
7. 18-gauge needle to draw up anesthetic medication from vial—staff often performs prior to the procedure.
8. 3- or 5-mL syringe
9. Cotton-tipped applicators
10. Gauze
11. Sterile saline
12. Eye spear sponges (Weck-Cel)
13. Surgical gloves
14. RF unit (Soniquence i100 or Ellman Surgitron Dual EMC 90)
15. Fine wire electrode (Soniquence) or microinsulated needle electrode (Ellman)
16. 0.12-mm toothed forceps or jewelers forceps
17. Ophthalmic antibiotic ointment (e.g., 0.5% erythromycin ophthalmic ointment)
18. Magnification: surgical microscope or ophthalmic loupes

## RADIOFREQUENCY SETTINGS

Setting 3: coagulate/hemostasis (10% cutting, 90% coagulation)—power 3 to 6

## PROCEDURE

1. Place the patient in supine position with the grounding plate/passive electrode of the radiofrequency unit underneath the patient's back or shoulder area.
2. Set up the surgical microscope or loupes.

3. Instill topical anesthetic (proparacaine, tetracaine) into both eyes to minimize reflex lacrimation, the blink reflex, and keep the patient comfortable during the procedure.
4. Use an alcohol prep pad to clean around the skin and eyelashes where anesthetic will be injected.
5. Use a 30-gauge needle with bevel up to inject anesthesia (0.5%, 1%, or 2% lidocaine with epinephrine 1:100,000 or 1:200,000) subcutaneously at a 10° to 15° angle adjacent to the eyelid margin where eyelashes will be treated. Avoid injecting toward the globe or directly into the eyelid margin. Continue to inject as the needle is withdrawn to form a small bolus of anesthetic either directly below the offending lashes (if on the lower eyelid) or directly above the offending lashes (if on the upper eyelid).
6. A gauze pad or cotton-tipped applicator can be used to massage the anesthesia into the area.
7. Use a 10% povidone–iodine (Betadine) swab stick to clean the ocular adnexal area and eyelashes to maintain asepsis. Povidone–iodine should remain on the skin for 1 to 3 minutes. This is an optional step depending on the treating clinician's preference.
8. Use the forceps to test the area for proper anesthesia. The patient is asked if they feel any pain or pinching. Pressure sensation is expected.
9. If inadequate anesthesia is present on the eyelid margin, which commonly occurs, apply two eye spear sponges (Weck-Cel) soaked in 4% topical lidocaine directly onto the offending eyelashes and eyelid margin. Hold each on the eyelid for approximately 30 to 60 seconds. Always ensure the patient is fully anesthetized before performing the procedure.
10. Turn on the smoke evacuator and place it as close to the operative site as possible, no further than 2 cm.[3]
11. Partially evert the eyelid to visualize the offending eyelashes and to keep the eyelid margin away from the globe.
12. Align the microinsulated needle electrode or fine wire electrode down the shaft of the offending eyelash. The electrode should be inserted adjacent to the eyelash to the base of the follicle. This is approximately 2.4 mm for the upper eyelid and 1.4 mm for the lower eyelid. It is important to match the orientation of the electrode with the orientation of the offending eyelash (Figures 8-18A, B and 8-19A-E).

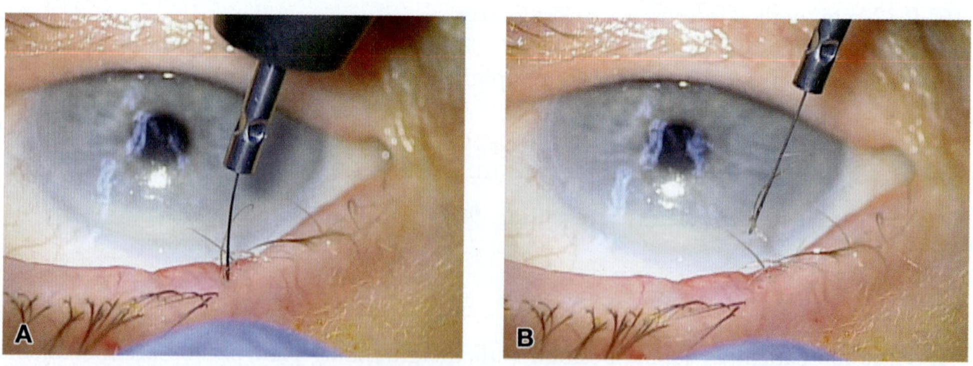


**FIGURE 8-18** **A,** Insertion of the needle electrode down to the follicle. Note the correct orientation of the electrode matching the orientation of the follicle. **B,** Ideal endpoint during radiofrequency ablation of aberrant eyelashes. Note the eyelash has stuck to the probe indicating coagulation of the follicle.

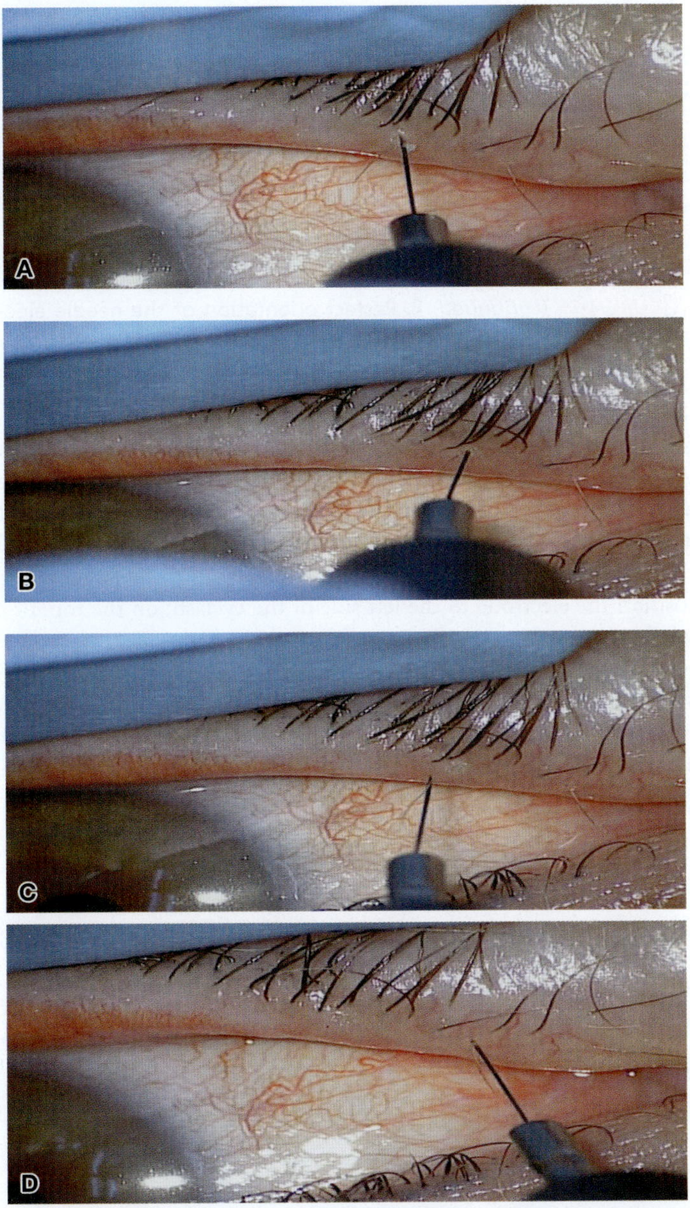


FIGURE 8-19 **A,** Note the poor angle of the needle electrode compared to the eyelash. Multiple attempts to coagulate the eyelash were unsuccessful. **B,** Changing the orientation of the needle electrode to better match the orientation of the eyelash leads to success in coagulating the follicle. **C,** Changing the orientation of the needle electrode to better match the orientation of the eyelash leads to success in coagulating the follicle. Note the eyelash stuck to the electrode. **D,** Perfect orientation of the needle electrode on the second offending lash leads to coagulation of the eyelash follicle on the first attempt.

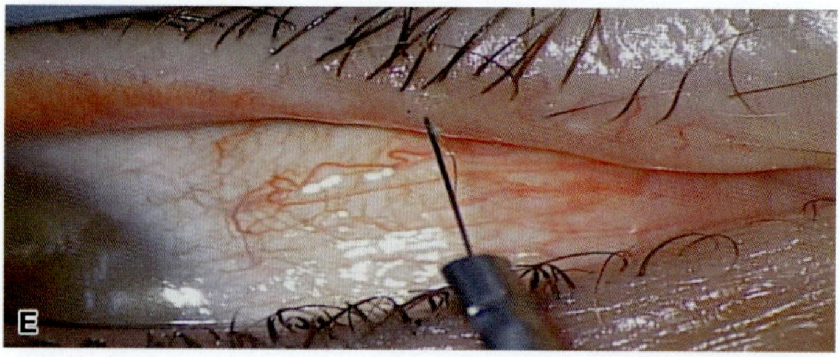

FIGURE 8-19 (*continued*) **E,** Perfect orientation of the needle electrode leads to coagulation of the eyelash follicle on the first attempt.

13. Once in the hair follicle, the foot pedal is pressed for 1 to 2 seconds on setting 3 (coagulate/hemostasis) at a starting power of 3. A successful removal is when the eyelash comes out on the electrode.[3,28] Multiple attempts are often required to successfully get the eyelash to stick to the electrode. If multiple attempts are required, it is encouraged to go around the lash when treating. For example, if the electrode is on the right side of the eyelash and multiple attempts fail to coagulate the follicle and remove the lash, subsequent attempts should position the electrode to the left side of the eyelash, on the top, or on the bottom of the eyelash.
14. If the eyelash is not sticking to the electrode after several attempts (5–10), use forceps to gently pull on the eyelash to see if it removes with ease (Figure 8-20). If a tugging sensation is felt, coagulate again. No resistance should be felt upon removing the eyelash, indicating a successful ablation.[29]

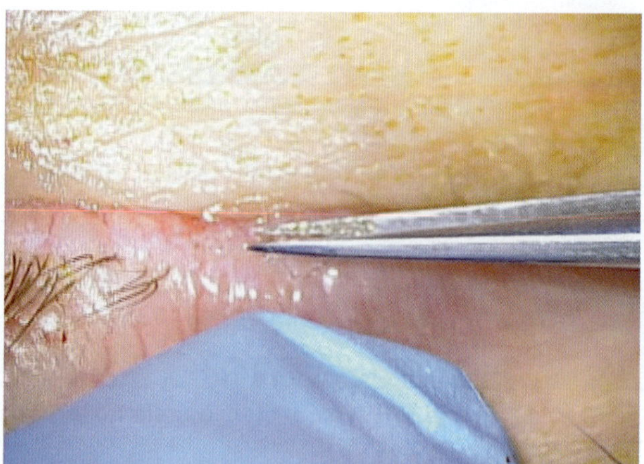

FIGURE 8-20 If after several (5-10) attempts with the needle electrode the eyelash does not stick to the probe, it is advisable to grab the eyelash with the forceps. The follicle may have been coagulated but just didn't stick to the probe.

15. Repeat this process until all offending eyelashes have been removed.
16. Apply erythromycin 0.5% ophthalmic ointment to the eyelid margin.
17. No bandages or patches are needed at the conclusion of the procedure.
18. Measure blood pressure and pulse.

## POSTOPERATIVE CARE/COMANAGEMENT (FOLLOW-UP SCHEDULE)

### Key Postoperative Considerations

- Documentation and operative report
- Blood pressure measurement
- Pulse measurement
- Erythromycin 0.5% ophthalmic ointment
- Follow-up in 1 to 2 months

An operative report should be completed after every procedure that describes the steps taken to perform the procedure. Blood pressure and pulse are measured at the conclusion of the procedure due to the injection of epinephrine. An antibiotic ointment is used three times a day for 7 days to prevent infection and aid healing.[29] A 1- to 2-month follow-up appointment is typically booked to assess the success of treatment and to determine whether retreatment is needed. Follow-up prior to 1 month likely will not yield final conclusions as to whether the eyelash will recur or not. The patient is advised to return sooner if signs and symptoms of infection arise.

## POTENTIAL COMPLICATIONS AND THEIR TREATMENT

### Key Potential Complications

- Recurrence
- Redness
- Bruising
- Infection
- Scarring
- Eyelid notching
- Madarosis
- Hyperpigmentation or hypopigmentation
- Hazard to the globe
- Activation of herpes zoster ophthalmicus

Recurrence of eyelash growth is always a possibility as radiofrequency ablation is not 100% effective. RF surgery can be repeated two to three months after initial treatment.[24] Redness and bruising are temporary during the postoperative phase and will self-resolve once completely healed. Bruising may occur from injection of anesthesia and typically resolves within a week. Infection is rare and prevented with the antibiotic ointment that is prescribed postoperatively. If infection were to occur, topical or oral antibiotics can be used to treat the infection. Eyelid complications including notching and scarring are more common with electrocautery than radiofrequency, although can occur if the depth of the electrode is excessive or if the radiofrequency power setting is too high.[3] Due to the proximity of the eyelid margin to the globe, accidental injury to the eye may occur. One study found a complication rate of 14% after radiofrequency ablation. These complications included eyelid notching, madarosis, progressive entropion, and hyperpigmentation.[30] Another study, using a smaller group size, found faint hypopigmentation in 8.3% of patients and eyelid notching in 16.6% of patients.[30] Activation of herpes zoster has also been reported after radiofrequency eyelash ablation.[3]

## VIDEOS OF PROCEDURES

**Video 8-5**—Radiofrequency ablation of trichiasis. Not shown in this video is the area being prepped with an alcohol swab, along with a subcutaneous injection of lidocaine 0.5% with epinephrine being placed just below the offending lower eyelid lashes. A surgical spear sponge (Weck-Cel) is also soaked with 4% topical lidocaine and placed right on the offending lashes to provide an additional layer of anesthesia. Shown in the video, a microinsulated electrode is used on setting #3 coagulation/hemostasis, power 3 to coagulate one of the lashes. Note a few failed attempts where the lash did not come out. Changing the orientation of the handpiece so the angle of the electrode matched the angle of the eyelash was the key to coagulating the follicle, which is shown when the eyelash and follicle stick to the probe. The end of the video shows a preoperative appearance of the eyelashes before removal and an 8-week postoperative visit. All seven offending lashes (only one removal shown in this video) were permanently removed, and the patient's symptoms were completely resolved. Video courtesy of Nate Lighthizer.

**Video 8-6**—"A Tale of Two Lashes"—radiofrequency ablation of trichiasis. Not shown in this video is the area being prepped with an alcohol swab, along with a subcutaneous injection of lidocaine 0.5% with epinephrine being placed just below the offending lower eyelid lashes. Shown in this video is a surgical spear sponge (Weck-Cel) soaked with 4% topical lidocaine being placed right on the offending lashes to provide an additional layer of anesthesia. A microinsulated electrode is being used on setting #3 coagulation/hemostasis, power 3. Note for the first eyelash, 8 to 10 attempts are made to coagulate the follicle without success. The angle of the probe is not perfectly matching the angle of the eyelash, which likely is contributing to the unsuccessful attempts. Finally, after better matching the angle of the electrode with the angle of the eyelash, the desired endpoint of the eyelash sticking to the probe occurs. For the second eyelash, the angle of the eyelash was perfectly angled so the electrode could easily match the orientation of the lash, and on the first attempt the desired endpoint occurs. Truly a tale of two lashes, with the first taking 8 to 10 attempts to get it, and the second eyelash only taking one attempt. Even with a very good alignment of the electrode with the lash, it can often take multiple attempts for the lash to stick to the electrode. Not shown is erythromycin ophthalmic antibiotic ointment being applied to the surgical sites after all of the offending eyelashes have been removed. (Video courtesy of Nate Lighthizer.)

**Video 8-7**—Radiofrequency ablation of trichiasis. Not shown in this video is the area being prepped with an alcohol swab, along with a subcutaneous injection of lidocaine 0.5% with epinephrine being placed just above the offending upper eyelid lashes. A microinsulated electrode is being used on setting #3 coagulation/hemostasis, power 3. Shown here are numerous lashes being removed with the desired endpoint of the eyelash and follicle sticking to the electrode immediately after the foot pedal is pressed. At the very end of the video, one small offending lash would not stick to the electrode after repeated attempts. In that scenario, it is acceptable to utilize a nontoothed forceps to grasp the lash and give it a very gentle tug. If the lash comes out smooth as silk, that is the second most desirous endpoint and likely indicates that the follicle has been coagulated. (Video courtesy of Komal Patel and Nate Lighthizer.)

## EFFICACY

The prognosis after trichiasis ablation in cases related to trauma or nonprogressive scarring is usually good. Chronic progressive inflammatory disorders such as ocular cicatricial pemphigoid often have recurrence, thus are harder to permanently treat.[26] One study found that the overall success rate of radiofrequency ablation was 65% after one treatment and 100% after two or three treatments (Figure 8-21A, B).[31]

One group sought to compare the efficacy of argon laser versus radiofrequency in treating trichiasis. A total of 100 patients were included, with 472 eyelashes (82.4%) successfully treated with radiofrequency and 383 eyelashes (62.9%) successfully treated with argon laser.[32] Complications including eyelid notching occurred in four cases, three of which were treated with radiofrequency, although this was not statistically significant. Overall, they found that radiofrequency was superior to argon laser in treating the central upper and lower eyelids.[32]

Another study examined radiofrequency ablation as a new treatment option for trichiasis using a radiofrequency device (Ellman Surgitron). They concluded that single treatment success rate for the 30 eyelids treated was 67%.[33] Complications involved recurrence in eight patients, eyelid notching in two patients, and granuloma formation in 1 patient. Overall, they demonstrated radiofrequency ablation with the Ellman unit to be an effective treatment option for localized trichiasis.[33]

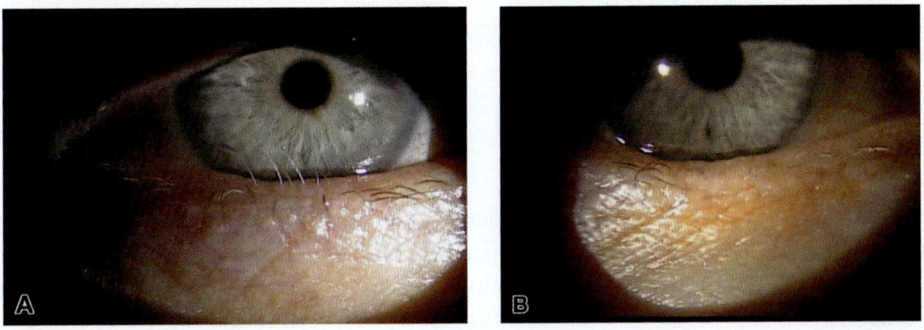


**FIGURE 8-21 A,** Preoperative photograph before treatment. Note the six offending distichiasis lashes. **B,** Two-month follow-up visit post radiofrequency trichiasis ablation. Note the complete removal of all six lashes with no recurrence. Patient symptoms were completely gone.

# CODING/BILLING

## Key CPT Codes

- **CPT code 67825**—Correction of trichiasis; epilation by other than forceps (e.g., by electrosurgery, cryotherapy, laser surgery)
- **CPT code 67825** has a 10-day postoperative global period.
  Common ICD-10 codes that support this procedure include the following:

- **H02.051 (trichiasis without entropion right upper eyelid)**
- **H02.052 (trichiasis without entropion right lower eyelid)**
- **H02.053 (trichiasis without entropion right eye, unspecified eyelid)**
- **H02.054 (trichiasis without entropion left upper eyelid)**
- **H02.055 (trichiasis without entropion left lower eyelid)**
- **H02.056 (trichiasis without entropion left eye, unspecified eyelid)**
- **H02.059 (trichiasis without entropion unspecified eye, unspecified eyelid)**
- **Q10.3 (Distichiasis) (Other congenital malformations of eyelid)**
- **H02.001 to H02.009 (Unspecified entropion)**
- **H02.011 to H02.019 (Cicatricial entropion)**
- **H02.021 to H02.029 (Mechanical entropion)**
- **H02.031 to H02.039 (Senile entropion)**
- **H02.041 to H02.049 (Spastic entropion)**

# PUNCTAL OCCLUSION

## Indications

**Key Indications**

- Dry eye disease
- Success with temporary punctal plugs and failure of, or contraindication to, permanent punctal plugs
- Significant corneal disease

RF punctal occlusion is indicated in patients with ocular surface disease where an increase in tear volume may provide a therapeutic effect.[34-36] The most common indication is aqueous deficient dry eye.[34,36] Other indications include significant corneal diseases such as recurrent corneal erosions, superficial keratitis, and corneal ulcers.[36,37] In order for the patient to be a good candidate for permanent RF punctal occlusion, patients should undergo a trial with temporary punctal plugs.[37] Good candidates for permanent punctal plugs or permanent punctal occlusion will demonstrate improvement in their symptoms and objective signs of dry eye disease 1 to 2 weeks following insertion. Permanent punctal plugs should then be attempted unless contraindicated due to allergy or cost.[37] Patients should have a history of punctal plug extrusion or other failure of these permanent punctal plugs. Once this has been demonstrated, good candidates can proceed with RF punctal occlusion.

## CONTRAINDICATIONS

### Key Contraindications

- Nasolacrimal infection (dacryocystitis)
- Significant inflammation of the ocular surface or eyelids
- Epiphora
- Allergy to local anesthetics
- Pacemakers (relative contraindication)

In patients who have a current nasolacrimal infection or significant inflammation of the ocular surface and adnexa, punctal occlusion should be delayed until the condition can be resolved with a course of treatment. Upon resolution, provided they have no other contraindications, these patients may continue with the procedure.

As with temporary punctal occlusion, patients with epiphora are poor candidates for RF punctal occlusion, as permanently occluding their puncta will decrease the lacrimal systems' drainage capacity further compounding their condition.

Patients with allergies to lidocaine are contraindicated, as lidocaine is the topical and local anesthetic of choice for RF procedures. If alternative local and topical anesthetic options are available, the procedure may be performed. Pacemakers are a relative contraindication, as there is some theoretical and anecdotal evidence of electromagnetic interference reprogramming pacemakers during radiofrequency surgery.[12] Advances in pacemaker shielding technology, in conjunction with the low coagulation power and short activation burst required for punctal occlusion, make pacemakers only a relative contraindication, generally left up to the doctor's discretion.

## PREOPERATIVE PREPARATION

### Key Preoperative Considerations

- Slit-lamp examination to assess indications and contraindications
- Blood pressure and pulse measurement
- Informed consent obtained
- Preoperative photographs of the area taken
- Radiofrequency unit
- Microincision electrode or Chedly punctal occlusion electrode (Figure 8-22A, B)
- Surgical loupes (or surgical microscope)
- Sterile surgical gloves

- Ophthalmic topical anesthetic (e.g., proparacaine, tetracaine) instilled
- Alcohol swab
- 2- to 3-mL 0.5% or 1% lidocaine (usually with epinephrine) in a 3-mL syringe with a 27- to 30-gauge needle
- Topical 4% lidocaine
- Eye spear sponges (Weck-Cel)
- 10% povidone–iodine (Betadine) swab stick
- Surgical hair cap
- Sterile gauze pads
- Cotton-tipped applicators (~10–15)
- Sterile saline
- Sterile fluid reservoir (often the empty gauze container)
- 0.12-mm toothed forceps
- Puncta can be dilated with a punctal dilator for ease of probe insertion.

An example of the Mayo stand setup for radiofrequency surgery punctal occlusion is pictured in Figure 8-23.

Prior to the procedure, a careful slit-lamp examination should be performed. The ocular surface should be assessed to determine the level of dry eye disease and the current level of inflammation. The puncta should be visualized and examined for any signs of current infection. Applying slight pressure to the puncta can help reveal any discharge indicative of a current dacryocystitis.

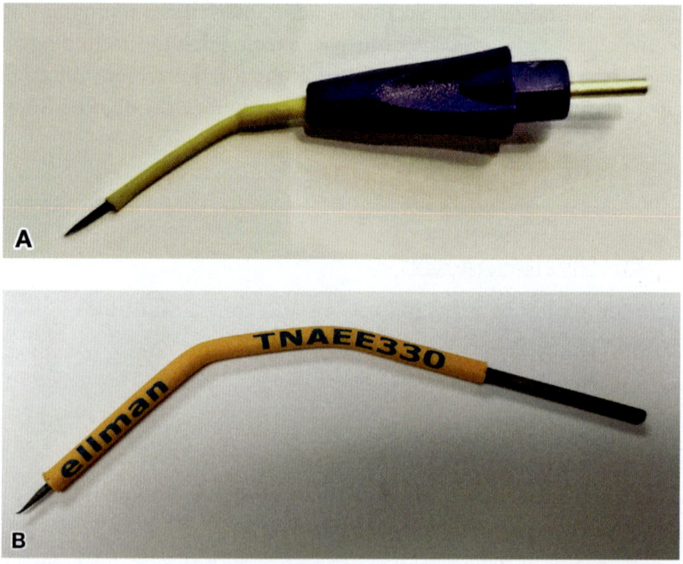


**FIGURE 8-22** **A,** Microincision electrode used for radiofrequency punctal occlusion. **B,** Chedly punctal occlusion electrode used for radiofrequency punctal occlusion.

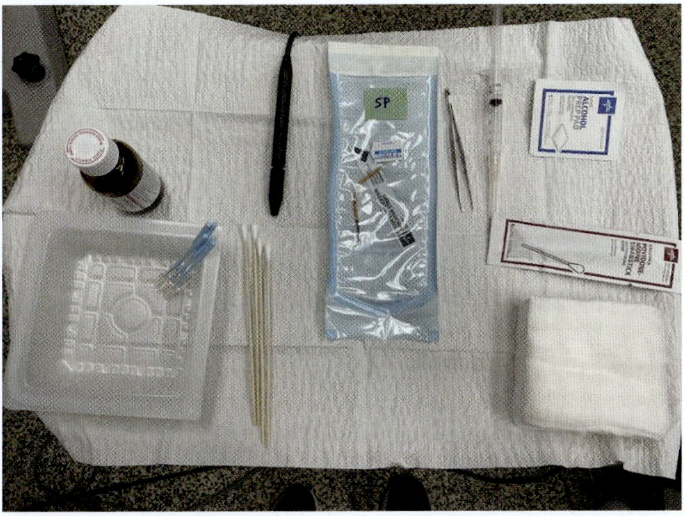


**FIGURE 8-23** The Mayo stand setup for radiofrequency punctual occlusion is pictured. Eye spear sponges (Weck-Cel) sponges are pictured, soaking in a sterile fluid reservoir filled with 1 mL of topical 4% lidocaine. The Chedly punctal occlusion electrode is pictured next to the handle of the radiofrequency surgical unit, in black. Also pictured are cotton-tipped applicators, gauze pads, disinfectants (an alcohol swab and povidone–iodine [Betadine]), and fine-toothed forceps.

The puncta on which the procedure will be performed should be dilated with a punctal dilating tool. This will allow easier insertion of the RF electrode into the puncta.

Smoke evacuation is not indicated for punctal occlusion, as there should be very little fumes produced from the coagulation of the punctum. As such, the smoke evacuation unit that is required in other RF surgeries is not indicated.

## PROCEDURE

### Key Procedural Points

- Select setting #3 "coagulation/hemostasis," power of 3 to 4.
- Preoperative topical ophthalmic anesthetic instilled
- Disinfect and anesthetize punctum (topically) and surrounding area (local injection).
- Cauterize/coagulate punctum until blanching is observed.

Before beginning the punctal occlusion procedure, ensure that the correct waveform (coagulation, setting #3) has been selected. Setting #3 is an almost completely coagulatory setting. This will allow scar tissue to form, blocking the punctum. It is best to avoid setting #1 (cut) or setting #2 (blend), as unintended cutting through the skin of the puncta may occur. Confirm the puncta or punctum on which you are going to perform the procedure.

1. Instill ophthalmic topical anesthetic into each eye. This is an important first step to limit any irritation of reflexive movements from the patient during the procedure.
2. Next, the area where local anesthetic is to be injected is cleaned. If using a subcutaneous injection (injecting the anesthetic externally through the skin, which is the preferred injection route), clean the injection site with an alcohol swab. If injecting anesthetic through the conjunctiva (subconjunctival injection), instill 1 drop of Betadine and let sit in the eye for 30 seconds. Rinse thoroughly with preservative-free saline before proceeding, as Betadine can be a significant irritant to a patient's eye if not rinsed out.
3. Next, inject subcutaneously 0.2 to 0.4 mL of 0.5% or 1% lidocaine with epinephrine into the nasal portion of the eyelid. This should be sufficient to provide local anesthesia for the procedure. Care should be taken not to inject too close to the lid margin. Injecting the anesthetic away from the lid margin and rolling the bolus of anesthetic toward the lid margin with a cotton-tipped applicator is the preferred method.
4. Topical anesthetic may be required for sufficient anesthesia. If required, soak an eye spear sponge (Weck-Cel) in topical 4% lidocaine, in a sterile container. Hold a soaked sponge on the puncta for 30 seconds and repeat with a second sponge.
5. Wipe the puncta and surrounding lid margin/lashes with a topical 10% povidone–iodine (Betadine) swab stick. Do so in a circular motion, starting on the puncta and wiping in an outward fashion. Allow to sit for approximately 1 to 3 minutes to reach full sterilization effect. Dab the excess off with gauze.
6. Test for proper anesthesia with the toothed forceps. Pinch around the punctum and lid margin, in multiple different spots. Ask the patient whether they can feel any sharpness or pinching. Feeling pressure or the sensation of lid manipulation is common, but the patient should not be able to feel any sharpness or pain.
7. When local anesthesia has been achieved, begin with punctal occlusion. If the puncta is not wide enough for the electrode to be inserted, use a punctal dilator to widen the opening.
8. Evert the lower lid, and insert the microincision electrode or Chedly punctal occlusion electrode 2 to 3 mm into the punctal opening. Using short bursts of coagulation, hold the electrode in the puncta and pulse the RF unit. You will see the area around the puncta start to blanch. The proper end point for permanent punctal occlusion is the blanching of the punctal opening and surrounding tissue (Figure 8-24A, B).
9. Repeat with the other puncta, as desired.

## POSTOPERATIVE CARE

### Key Postoperative care

- Ophthalmic antibiotic ointment TID for 1 week
- Postoperative blood pressure and pulse measurements
- 1- to 2-week follow-up visit to assess for efficacy, improvement in symptoms, and any potential complications

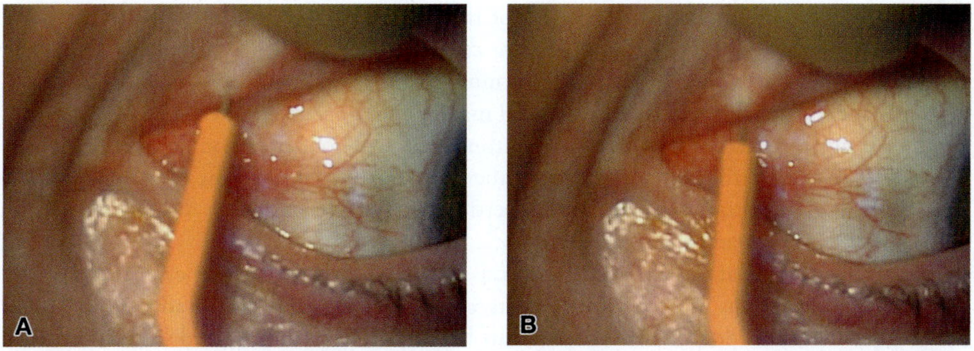


**FIGURE 8-24** **A,** Radiofrequency surgical closure of a puncta. A Chedly punctal occlusion electrode is inserted in the puncta on setting #3 coagulation, power 3 to coagulate and close the puncta permanently. Note that as this is the start of the procedure, the puncta is still open. **B,** Radiofrequency surgical closure of a puncta. Now that the procedure is complete, note the closed and cauterized puncta with the correct blanched appearance.

Once the procedure has been completed, apply an ophthalmic antibiotic ointment to the occluded punctum with a sterile cotton-tipped applicator. Patients should be given or prescribed an antibiotic ointment to use TID for a week and educated on the importance of keeping the surgical area clean and moist to reduce healing time. Postoperative blood pressure should be obtained as local epinephrine was used.

Follow-up schedule will vary depending on the severity of the condition. Acute conditions such as superficial keratitis will require a shorter follow-up time, whereas chronic conditions like ocular surface disease may follow up on a less routine basis. Punctal patency can be assessed at follow-up to determine whether the puncta were effectively occluded, and additional therapy can be considered.

# POTENTIAL COMPLICATIONS AND MANAGEMENT

## Key Complications

- Excessive coagulation
- Inadvertent damage to the lid margin
- Pacemaker malfunction
- Incomplete occlusion
- Postoperative infection

Excessive coagulation leading to scarring of the lid margin can result from erroneous placement of the RF electrode, excessive treatment exceeding the proper endpoint, and using a power setting that is too high.[1] Care should be taken to avoid improper placement by choosing the correct electrode tip based on the size of the puncta and dilating the puncta to ensure electrode fit if needed. Proper training and a conservative approach of using the minimum necessary energy for the desired effect can minimize clinician errors.[1]

Inadvertent damage to the punctum or lid margin could occur should the incorrect setting on the RF unit be selected by pressing the wrong foot pedal or button on the RF handpiece. Blend and cutting settings are activated by the same foot pedal, whereas coagulation uses a separate pedal. Activating the blend or cut setting could cause laceration and/or inadvertent damage to the puncta and surrounding tissue.[5]

Pacemaker complications are rare, for reasons described earlier. Should they occur, the most common manifestations include skipped beats, asystole, tachycardia, and bradycardia.[12]

Postoperative infection risk is low and can be prevented with proper disinfection, using sterile surgical instruments, and proper use and application of topical ophthalmic antibiotic ointment during healing.[3]

## VIDEO OF PROCEDURE

**Video 8-8**—Radiofrequency permanent closure of a puncta. The patient was a dry eye patient successfully treated with punctal plugs; however, the plugs repeatedly kept falling out. Not shown in this video is the area being prepped with an alcohol swab. Also not shown in the video is the area just below and lateral to the puncta being anesthetized with a local injection of lidocaine 0.5% with epinephrine. Approximately 0.2 to 0.3 mL of lidocaine were used; 4% topical lidocaine soaked in a surgical spear sponge (Weck-Cel) is held directly on the puncta to further assist in numbing the area. Shown in the video is the use of a Chedly punctal occlusion electrode being inserted in the puncta on setting #3 coagulation/hemostasis, power 3 to coagulate and close the puncta permanently. Note at the start of the procedure the puncta is still open, and at the conclusion of the procedure the mucosa of the puncta has been coagulated and brought together to close the puncta. The white donut-shaped blanched appearance of the puncta at the conclusion of the procedure is the desired endpoint. (Video courtesy of Nate Lighthizer.)

# EFFICACY

Studies on the efficacy of surgical punctal occlusion by radiofrequency are limited. Punctal occlusion by thermocautery has been shown to be effective, reducing symptoms, ocular surface staining, tear breakup time, and Schirmer's test.[37] Efficacy data for temporary punctal plugs, which work on a similar principle to RF punctal occlusion, are very well established. Punctal plugs have been shown to decrease symptoms, frequency of ocular lubricants, and corneal fluorescein staining.[35] Permanent punctal occlusion by other surgical methods has also been described as effective.[34]

# CODING/BILLING AND MODIFIERS

## Key CPT Codes

- **68760**—Closure of the lacrimal punctum
  - Global period is 10 days.
  - If a bilateral procedure is performed, use a modifier (−50).

CPT code 68760 covers the closure of the lacrimal puncta by thermocauterization, ligation, or laser surgery. Although RF is not true thermocauterization, the procedure is billed under this code.

Medicare-established ICD-10 codes that support CPT code 68760 as medically necessary are listed as follows.

| ICD-10 CODE | DIAGNOSIS |
|---|---|
| H16.001–H16.009 | Corneal ulcer |
| H16.101–H16.109 | Superficial keratitis without conjunctivitis |
| H16.121–H16.129 | Filamentary keratitis |
| H16.201–H16.219 | Certain types of keratoconjunctivitis |
| H18.831–H18.839 | Recurrent erosion of the cornea |
| H04.121–H04.129 | Dry eye syndrome of lacrimal glands |
| H16.221–H16.229 | Keratoconjunctivitis sicca |

# REFERENCES


1. Hainer BL. Electrosurgery for the skin. *Am Fam Physician.* 2002;66:1259-1266.
2. Bolotin D, Alam M. Electrosurgery. In: Robinson JK, Hanke DW, Siegel DM, et al, eds. *Surgery of the Skin: Procedural Dermatology*. Elsevier; 2015.
3. Fowler G. *Pfenninger and Fowler's Procedures for Primary Care*. Elsevier; 2020.
4. Tenny KM, Keenaghan M. Ohms law. In: *StatPearls* [Internet]. StatPearls Publishing; 2022.
5. Brown JS. *Minor Surgery: A Text and Atlas*. 4th ed. Arnold; 2000.
6. Hemour S, Wu K. Radio-frequency rectifier for electromagnetic energy harvesting: development path and future outlook. *Proc IEEE.* 2014;102:1667-1691.
7. O'Grady KF, Easty AC. Electrosurgery smoke: hazards and protection. *J Clin Eng.* 1996;21:149-155.
8. Chowdhury KK, Meftahuzzaman SM, Rickta D, Chowdhury TK, Chowdhury BB, Ireen ST. Electrosurgical smoke: a real concern. *Mymensingh Med J.* 2011;20:507-512.
9. Junker JPE, Kamel RA, Caterson EJ, Eriksson E. Clinical impact upon wound healing and inflammation in moist, wet, and dry environments. *Adv Wound Care (New Rochelle).* 2013;2:348-356.
10. Draelos ZD, Rizer RL, Trookman NS. A comparison of postprocedural wound care treatments: do antibiotic-based ointments improve outcomes? *J Am Acad Dermatol.* 2011;64:S23-S29.
11. Rana H, Stokkermans TJ, Purt B, Chou E. Malignant eyelid lesions. In: *StatPearls [Internet]* StatPearls Publishing; 2022.
12. El-Gamal HM, Dufresne RG, Saddler K. Electrosurgery, pacemakers and ICDs: a survey of precautions and complications experienced by cutaneous surgeons. *Dermatol Surg.* 2001;27:385-390.
13. Weyer C, Siegle RJ, Eng GGP. Investigation of hyfrecators and their in vitro interference with implantable cardiac devices. *Dermatol Surg.* 2012;38:1843-1848.
14. Dalal R, Grujic D. Epinephrine. In: *StatPearls [Internet]*. StatPearls Publishing; 2022.
15. Garden JM, O'Banion MK, Shelnitz LS, et al. Papillomavirus in the vapor of carbon dioxide laser-treated verrucae. *JAMA.* 1988;259:1199-1202.
16. Achar S, Kundu S. Principles of office anesthesia: part I. Infiltrative anesthesia. *Am Fam Physician.* 2002;66:91-94.
17. Bellew SD, Johnson KL, Nichols MD, Kummer T. Effect of intranasal vasoconstrictors on blood pressure: a randomized, double-blind, placebo-controlled trial. *J Emerg Med.* 2018;55:455-464.
18. Pe'er J. Pathology of eyelid tumors. *Indian J Ophthalmol.* 2016;64:177-190.

19. Sendul SY, Akpolat C, Yilmaz Z, Eryilmaz OT, Guven D, Kabukcuoglu F. Clinical and pathological diagnosis and comparison of benign and malignant eyelid tumors. *J Fr Ophtalmol.* 2021;44:537-543.
20. American Medical Association. *CPT 2021 Professional Edition*. Optuminsight Inc; 2020.
21. Jurisdiction M Part B. Global Surgery Calculator. Accessed November 22, 2022. https://palmettogba.com/palmetto/jmb.nsf/DID/LSR6L6TMZC.
22. Bowling B, Kanski JJ. *Kanski's Clinical Ophthalmology: A Systematic Approach*. 8th ed. Elsevier; 2016:135-136.
23. Cohen AJ, Burkat CN. *Oculofacial, Orbital, and Lacrimal Surgery: A Compendium*. Springer International Publishing; 2019.
24. Dutton JJ, Waldrop TG. *Atlas of Oculoplastic and Orbital Surgery*. 2nd ed. Wolters Kluwer; 2019.
25. Onofrey BE, Skorin L Jr, Holdeman NR. *Ocular Therapeutics Handbook: A Clinical Manual.* 3rd ed. Lippincott Williams & Wilkins; 2012.
26. Penne RB. *Color Atlas and Synopsis of Clinical Ophthalmology: Oculoplastics*. 3rd ed. Wolters Kluwer; 2019.
27. Robinson JK. *Surgery of the Skin: Procedural Dermatology*. 3rd ed. Elsevier; 2015.
28. Older JJ. Review: the value of radiosurgery in oculoplastics. *Ophthalmic Plast Reconstr Surg*; 2002;18(3):214-218.
29. Levine MR, Allen RC. *Manual of Oculoplastic Surgery*. 5th ed. Springer; 2018.
30. Sakarya Y, Sakarya R, Yildihm A. Electrolysis treatment of trichiasis by using ultra-fine needle. *Eur J Ophthalmol.* 2010;20:664-668.
31. Kirkwood BJ, Kirkwood RA. Trichiasis: characteristics and management options. *Insight.* 2011;36(2):5-9.
32. Salour H, Rafati N, Falahi MR, Aletaha M. A comparison of argon laser and radiofrequency in trichiasis treatment. *Ophthalmic Plast Reconstr Surg.* 2011;27:313-316.
33. Kezirian GM. Treatment of localized trichiasis with radiosurgery. *Ophthalmic Plast Reconstr Surg.* 1993;9:260-266.
34. Liu D, Sadhan Y. Surgical punctal occlusion: a prospective study. *Br J Ophthalmol.* 2002;86:1031-1034.
35. Ervin A-M, Wojciechowski R, Schein O. Punctal occlusion for dry eye syndrome. *Cochrane Database Syst Rev.* 2010;CD006775.
36. Best A-L, Labetoulle M, Legrand M, M'Garrech M, Barreau E, Rousseau A. Punctal and canalicular plugs: indications, efficacy and safety. *J Fr Ophtalmol.* 2019;42:e95-e104.
37. Ohba E, Dogru M, Hosaka E, et al. Surgical punctal occlusion with a high heat-energy releasing cautery device for severe dry eye with recurrent punctal plug extrusion. *Am J Ophthalmol.* 2011;151:483-487.e1.

# 9 Cyst Removal

**Komal Patel • Leonid Skorin, Jr**

Cysts of the eyelid are often encountered in eye care. These include cysts of Moll, being the most commonly encountered cyst,[1] and others such as eccrine hidrocystomas, cysts of Zeis, and epidermal inclusion cysts. Identification and differences between these cysts are outlined later. Patients often elect to remove these lesions due to cosmetic concerns or symptoms of irritation, itching, and discomfort. Surgical removal via excision with blade and radiofrequency will be discussed in this chapter.

## INDICATIONS

**Key Indications**

- Cyst of Moll/apocrine hidrocystoma/cystadenoma/sudoriferous cyst
- Eccrine hidrocystoma
- Cyst of Zeis
- Epidermal inclusion cyst/epidermoid cyst/epidermal cyst/infundibular cyst/keratin cyst

### Cyst of Moll

Cysts of Moll, also known as, apocrine hidrocystoma, cystadenoma, or sudoriferous cyst, are a common type of benign eyelid cyst.[2-4] They are nontender lesions that develop due to a blockage of apocrine sweat glands on the eyelid margin associated with eyelash hair follicles.[2,3] Presenting as round, dome-shaped, translucent nodules that transilluminate, they are typically filled with a clear fluid, but may manifest with a blue color in deeper lesions (Figures 9-1 and 9-2).[1,4] Cysts of Moll are usually 1 to 3 mm in diameter, but can be as large as 10 to 15 mm.[1,2] These cysts usually develop in adults between the ages of 30 to 70 years and do not have a sex or race predilection.[5,6] Differential diagnoses for apocrine hidrocystomas include eccrine hidrocystomas, cyst of Zeis, and cystic basal cell carcinoma.[5,6] Multiple bilateral apocrine cystadenomas may be associated with Schopf–Schulz–Passarge syndrome, an ectodermal dysplasia syndrome.[7] This autosomal recessive condition is characterized by bilateral apocrine cystadenomas, hypodontia, palmar-plantar hyperkeratosis, and onychodystrophy.[8]

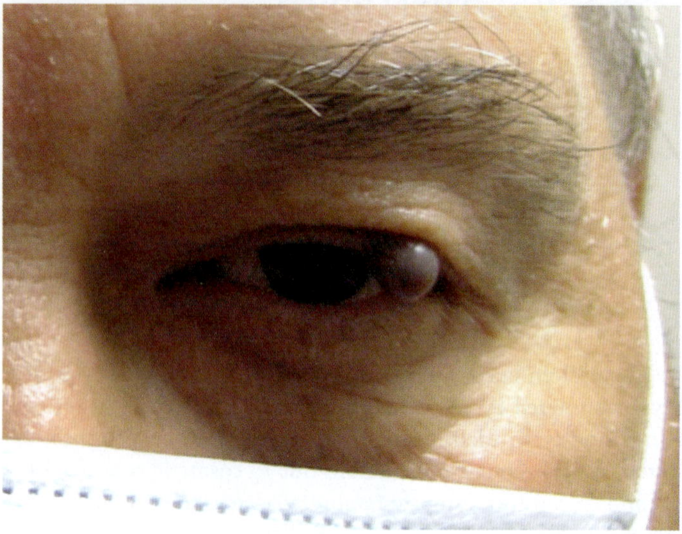

**FIGURE 9-1** Cyst of Moll (apocrine hidrocystoma) on the left upper eyelid.

## Eccrine Hidrocystoma

Eccrine hidrocystomas are clinically very similar to apocrine hidrocystomas. This ductal retention cyst develops in water-producing sweat glands, also known as eccrine glands. Eccrine hidrocystomas are benign, clear, fluid-filled lesions ranging in size from 4 to 10 mm. They typically occur in adults and are much less common than apocrine hidrocystomas.[2,7] Whereas

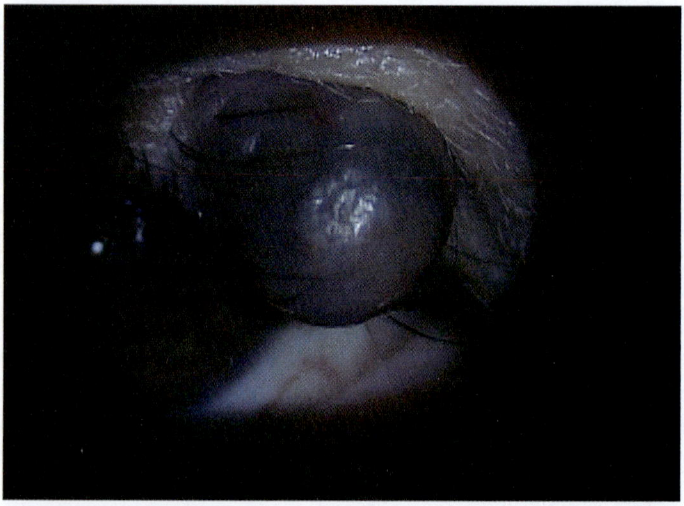

**FIGURE 9-2** Magnified view of the same cyst of Moll (apocrine hidrocystoma) on the left upper eyelid.

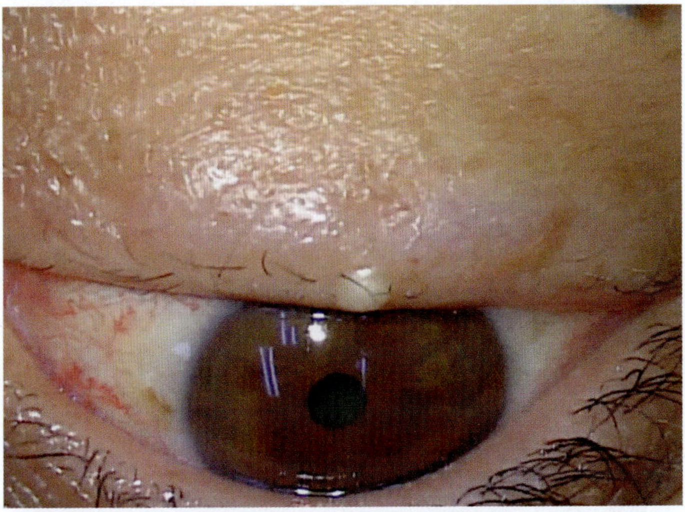

FIGURE 9-3 Cyst of Zeis on the right lower eyelid.

cysts of Moll occur along the eyelid margin, eccrine hidrocystomas occur in the pretarsal and preseptal skin a few millimeters away from the eyelid margin.[7]

## Cyst of Zeis

Cysts of Zeis occur due to blocked sebaceous glands associated with hair follicles, also known as glands of Zeis, on the eyelid margin.[1,3] They present as round, nontranslucent, defined lesions filled with oily, yellow sebum (Figure 9-3). As opposed to cysts of Moll, these do not transilluminate.[4]

## Epidermal Inclusion Cyst

Epidermal inclusion cysts are also known as epidermoid cyst, epidermal cyst, infundibular cyst, keratin cyst, and inclusion cysts.[2,9] This benign subcutaneous cyst presents as an elevated, round, smooth, white, or skin-colored lesion that does not transilluminate as it is filled with keratin (Figure 9-4).[2,3] They are typically 3 to 8 mm in diameter.[1] Most inclusion cysts occur

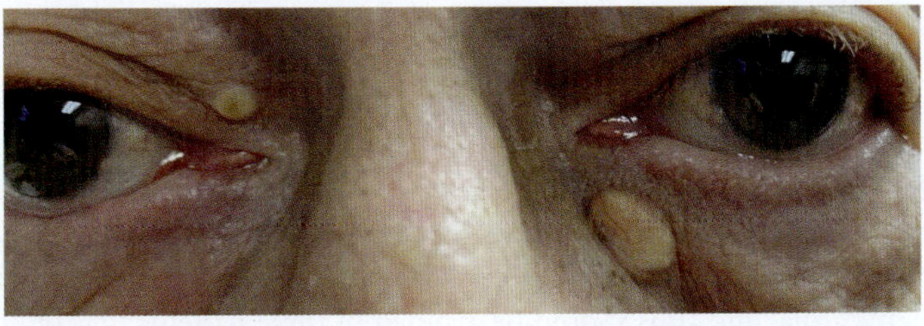

FIGURE 9-4 Patient with epidermal inclusion cysts on the right upper eyelid and left lower eyelid.

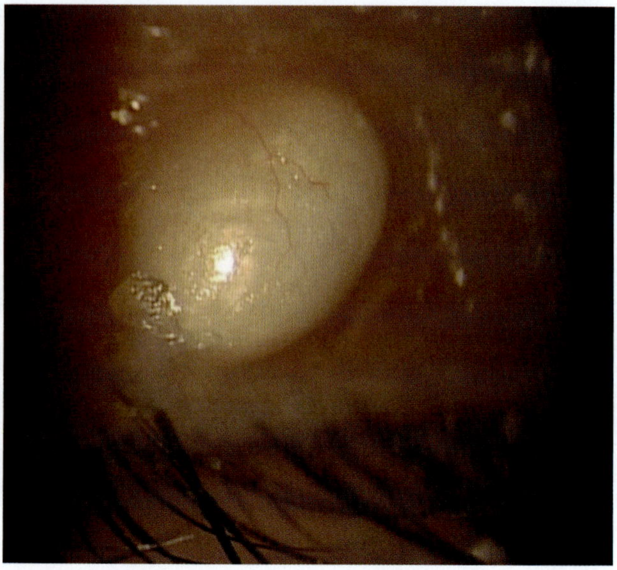

**FIGURE 9-5** Magnified view of an epidermal inclusion cyst. Notice the blood vessels overlying the cyst. These are normal anatomical vessels.

due to the implantation of the epidermis into the dermis as a result of injury or surgery.[3,7] Inclusion cysts may also occur at the infundibulum of hair follicles due to blockage of the orifice.[5,9] Telangiectatic vessels may be seen on the surface of these cysts (Figure 9-5).[1]

## CONTRAINDICATIONS

### Key Contraindications

- Electronic implants (e.g., cardiac pacemaker, defibrillator) (if using radiofrequency)
- Flammable fumes or liquids (e.g., oxygen, alcohol) (if using radiofrequency)
- Unable to lay on back for prolonged periods
- Allergies to anesthetics or medications (e.g., lidocaine, epinephrine, povidone–iodine, erythromycin)
- Lesion to be treated is malignant.

There are few contraindications to the removal of eyelid cysts if not using a radiofrequency device. The contraindications listed involve the cautionary approach exercised when using radiofrequency units. Radiofrequency devices when used with cardiac pacemakers can cause asystole and tachycardia, and thus should be avoided in these patients.[10,11] If alternative treatments are not an option, the grounding plate can be placed away from the heart and the lowest power setting can be used. The cut mode (setting 1) should be avoided as it holds the highest risk of complications such as pacemaker dysfunction.[10] Flammable fumes such as oxygen are contraindicated due to flame risk.[11] Lesion removals do not take an extensive amount of time, but when preparation time is included, patients should be comfortable lying down on their back for at least 15 to 30 minutes. Caution should be taken to avoid or use alternative medications or anesthesia in the case of allergy. If there is any suspicion that the cyst may be malignant, a biopsy should be performed prior to removal.

## PREOPERATIVE PREPARATION

- Photographs of the cyst
- Consent form
- Visual acuity
- Blood pressure measurement
- Pulse measurement

Blood pressure and pulse must be checked prior to the procedure if epinephrine is being injected with lidocaine for local anesthesia. Epinephrine is used because of its vasoconstrictive properties and ability to prolong the duration of action of anesthesia due to its slower absorption.[12] Potential complications from epinephrine include tachycardia, tremor, premature ventricular contraction, apprehension, or excessive bleeding if blood pressure is elevated. Allergic reactions to lidocaine are generally rare, but can present with rash, hives, edema, dyspnea, tachycardia, and hypotension.[12]

### Instrumentation (Figure 9-6)

1. Ophthalmic topical anesthetic (e.g., proparacaine, tetracaine)
2. 70% isopropyl alcohol prep pad
3. Local anesthesia (0.5%, 1%, or 2% lidocaine with or without epinephrine 1:100,000 or 1:200,000)
4. 4% topical lidocaine
5. 10% povidone–iodine (Betadine) swab sticks
6. 30-gauge needle (1/2″ length)
7. 3- or 5-mL syringe
8. Cotton-tipped applicators
9. Gauze pad
10. Sterile saline
11. Eye spear sponges (Weck-Cel)
12. Sandpaper pad
13. Surgical gloves
14. Surgical skin marker
15. Radiofrequency unit (Ellman Surgitron Dual EMC 90)
16. Bent tip electrode
17. 0.12-mm toothed or nontoothed forceps or jewelers forceps
18. #11 or #15 surgical blade (scalpel)
19. Vannas or Westcott tenotomy scissors (curved or straight—clinician preference)

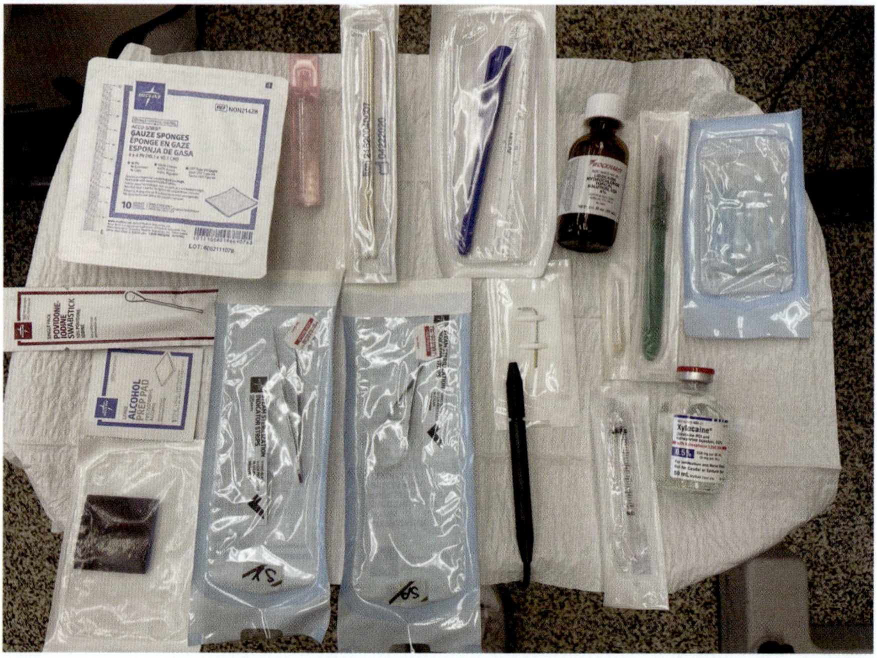

**FIGURE 9-6** Surgical tray with instruments needed for removal: 70% isopropyl alcohol prep pad, 0.5% lidocaine with 1:200,000 epinephrine, 4% topical lidocaine, 10% povidone–iodine (Betadine) swab stick, 30-gauge needle, 3-mL syringe, cotton-tipped applicators, gauze pads, sterile saline, eye spear sponges (Weck-Cel), sandpaper pad, surgical skin marker, toothed forceps, #15 blade scalpel, Westcott tenotomy scissors, radiofrequency bent tip electrode.

20. Erythromycin 0.5% ophthalmic ointment
21. Sterile fenestrated surgical drape (optional)
22. Magnification: surgical microscope or ophthalmic loupes
23. Sterile gloves
24. Face mask
25. 6-0 silk, Vicryl, or nylon suture for skin closure of larger excisions

## RADIOFREQUENCY SETTINGS

These settings are specific to the radiofrequency device being used. The settings outlined below are for the Ellman Surgitron Dual EMC 90 or the Soniquence SmoothWave i100. Setting 1 (cut) is used to open the cyst wall. Settings 1 (cut) and 2 (blend) can be used once the cystic contents are removed to traumatize the cyst capsule. Setting 2 (blend) or setting 3 (coagulate) can be used to aid with hemostasis in cases of bleeding.

Setting 1: cut (90% cutting, 10% coagulation)—power 10 to 15
Setting 2: blend (50% cutting, 50% coagulation)—power 10 to 15
Setting 3: coagulation (90% coagulation, 10% cutting)—power 8 to 10

## PROCEDURE

Definitive treatment for eyelid cysts involves complete surgical excision of the cyst and capsule. This is the best practice to prevent recurrence. Surgical removal should be performed when the cyst is not inflamed or infected. Removal of eyelid cysts with a radiofrequency unit (Ellman Surgitron Dual EMC 90) is discussed below. This is a nontraumatic method for removal using high-frequency radio waves to cut and coagulate tissue, with clean vaporization and minimal thermal damage, outlining its safety, effectiveness, and ease of use.[13,14]

1. Place the patient in supine position with the grounding plate of the radiofrequency unit underneath the patient's back.
2. Set up the surgical microscope or loupes.
3. The surgeon should maintain aseptic technique via the use of sterile gloves and a face mask.
4. Instill topical anesthetic (proparacaine, tetracaine) into both eyes to minimize reflex lacrimation, and keep the patient comfortable during the procedure.
5. A sterile fenestrated surgical drape can be placed over the patient's face to expose only the treatment zone.
6. Use an alcohol prep pad to clean around the lesion and skin where the anesthetic will be injected.
7. A skin marker can be used to mark the border of the cyst.
8. Use a 30-gauge needle with bevel up to inject anesthesia (0.5%, 1%, or 2% lidocaine with epinephrine 1:100,000 or 1:200,000) subcutaneously at a 10° to 15° angle around the cyst, not directly into the cyst (Figure 9-7). A bolus should be seen where the anesthesia was injected. Continue to inject as the needle is withdrawn. If additional anesthesia is needed, the patient will feel less pain if you inject in an area that was already anesthetized. Ensure that needle placement does not occur through the skin marker so as not to drag marker ink into the injection site.
9. A gauze pad or cotton-tipped applicator can be used to massage the anesthetic into the area.
10. Use a 10% povidone–iodine (Betadine) swab stick to clean the lesion surface, ocular adnexal area, and eyelashes to maintain asepsis. Povidone–iodine should remain on the skin for 3 minutes.
11. Use a piece of gauze to remove any excess povidone–iodine if needed. Use caution to not wipe from uncleaned skin onto clean skin.
12. Use the forceps to test the area to ensure it is anesthetized. The patient is asked if they feel any pain or pinching. Pressure sensation is expected.
13. If the patient is not adequately anesthetized, inject more anesthesia around the cyst. Always ensure the lesion is fully anesthetized before performing the procedure.
14. If the cyst is near the eyelid margin, a few Weck-Cel sponges soaked in 4% topical lidocaine can be applied directly onto the cyst and eyelid margin. Hold each sponge on the eyelid for approximately 30 to 60 seconds; 4% topical lidocaine should never be injected.
15. Turn on the smoke evacuator that comes with the radiofrequency unit, and place it as close to the operative site as possible; no further than 2 cm.[10]
16. Use a cotton-tipped applicator to moisten the lesion with sterile saline.

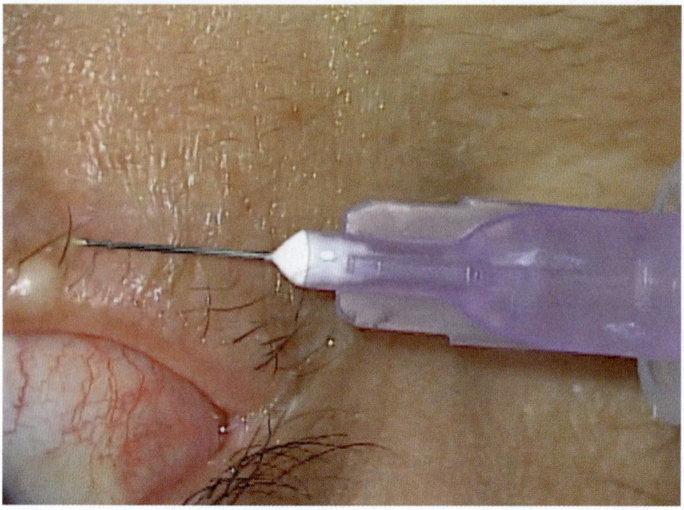

**FIGURE 9-7** Cyst of Zeis (sebaceous cyst) being injected with lidocaine with epinephrine prior to removal.

17. Press down on the foot pedal and use a bent tip electrode held perpendicularly to the cyst to make a linear opening in the superior cyst wall (Figure 9-8).[13] A #11 or #15 blade scalpel may also be used to create this incision. Caution should be taken to incise along minimal skin tension lines to optimize cosmetic results.
18. After every few passes with the bent tip, moisten the lesion with sterile saline. This also functions to remove hyperkeratotic tissue from the skin. Buildup of tissue on the bent tip can hinder adequate vaporization. Use sandpaper to clean the bent tip as needed.

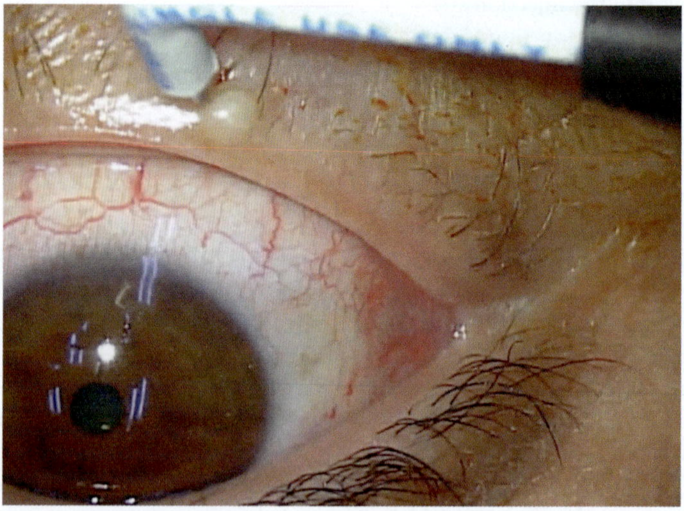

**FIGURE 9-8** Radiofrequency pin electrode about to be used to incise into a cyst of Zeis.

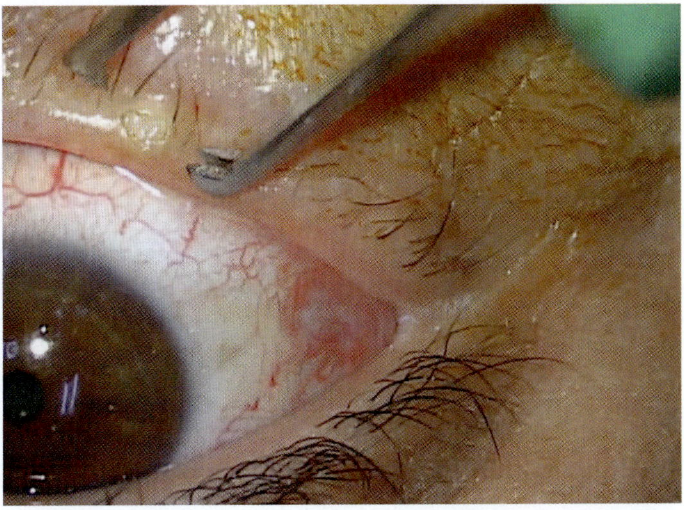

FIGURE 9-9 Toothed forceps being put into position to squeeze the bottom half of the cyst to remove the contents of the cyst.

19. Use the Westcott scissors to excise the entire cyst and capsule (Figures 9-9 to 9-11). For a fluid-filled cyst, the contents may be released if the capsule is ruptured.
20. Once the cystic contents and capsule are removed, the radiofrequency unit placed on setting #1 (cut) or setting #2 (cut and coagulate) may be used to further traumatize the capsule to avoid recurrence. Toothed or nontoothed forceps can also be used to remove the remaining contents of the capsule lining or sack (Figures 9-12 and 9-13).

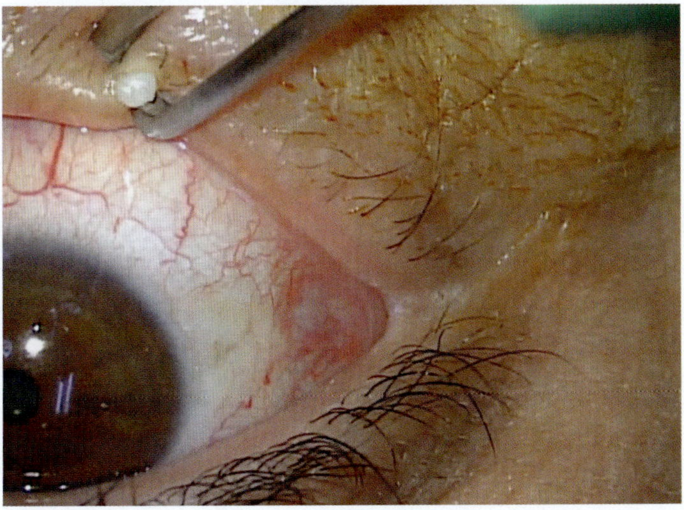

FIGURE 9-10 Toothed forceps being used to help remove sebaceous material within the cyst.

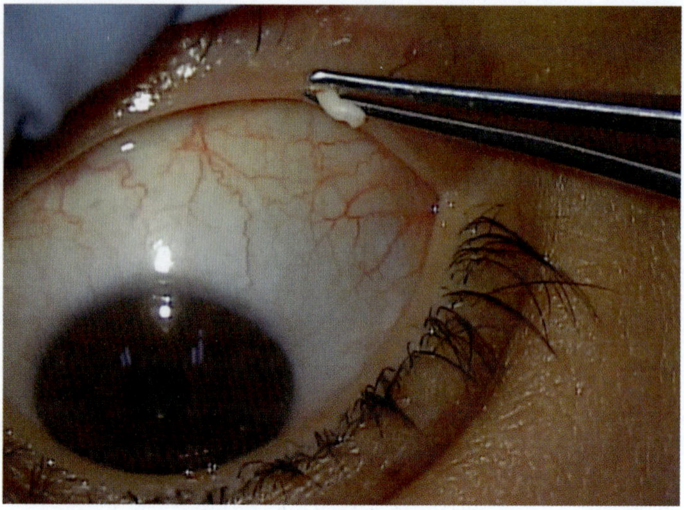

**FIGURE 9-11** Nontoothed forceps being used to remove sebaceous "cheesy" material within a cyst of Zeis (sebaceous cyst).

21. Postoperative bleeding is minimal and can be controlled with direct pressure using gauze, cotton-tipped applicators, or coagulation (setting 2 or 3) on the radiofrequency unit.[14]
22. Apply erythromycin 0.5% ophthalmic ointment to the lesion removal site.
23. No bandages or patches are needed at the conclusion of the procedure. Sutures may be used for larger cyst excisions.
24. Measure blood pressure and pulse.

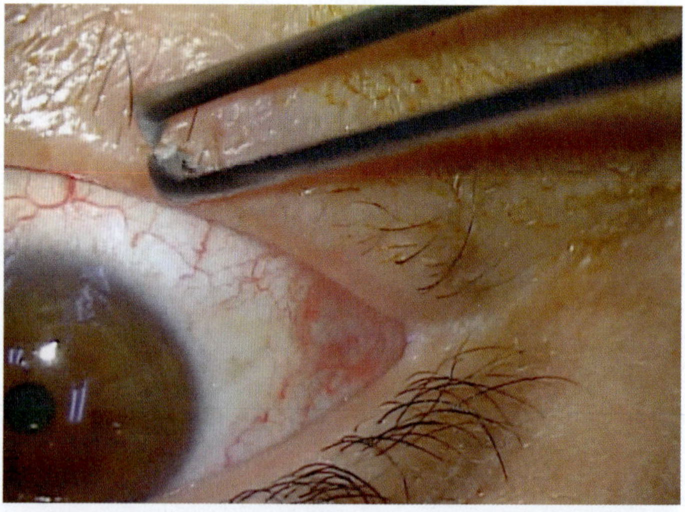

**FIGURE 9-12** Toothed forceps being used to grasp small remaining contents of the capsular lining or sack.

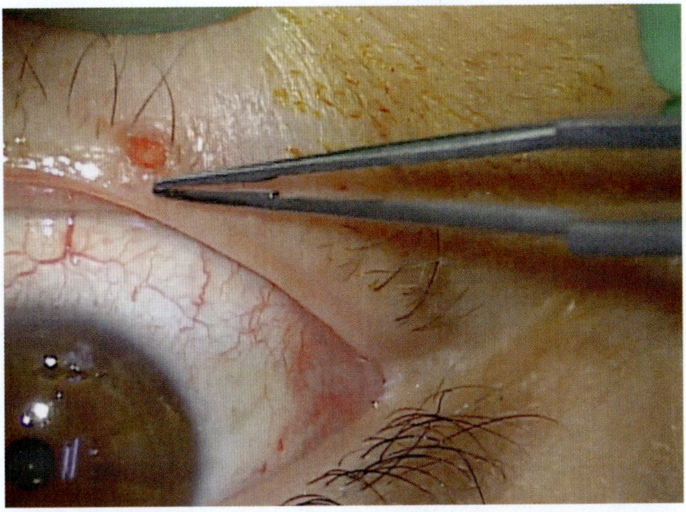

**FIGURE 9-13** Fine nontoothed forceps can also be used to grasp small remaining remnants of the capsule. In this photo, the cyst removal is complete. Notice the final appearance of the cyst. No white lining or capsule is left, indicating complete removal.

In those cases where excision of the cyst is performed without the radiofrequency unit, a surgical blade (usually #11 blade) and either Vannas or Westcott scissors can be used (Figures 9-14 to 9-16). Appropriate local anesthesia and sterile prepping should be performed as described previously. A #11 surgical blade is used to make a skin incision directly adjacent to the cyst (Figure 9-17). For smaller cysts, Vannas scissors can be used to simply excise the complete cyst including its capsule. Toothed forceps are used to grasp the cut edge of the skin to help expose the underlying cyst. The toothed forceps are then used to grasp the cyst and its capsule while the cyst is excised (Figure 9-18). All specimens should be collected and sent

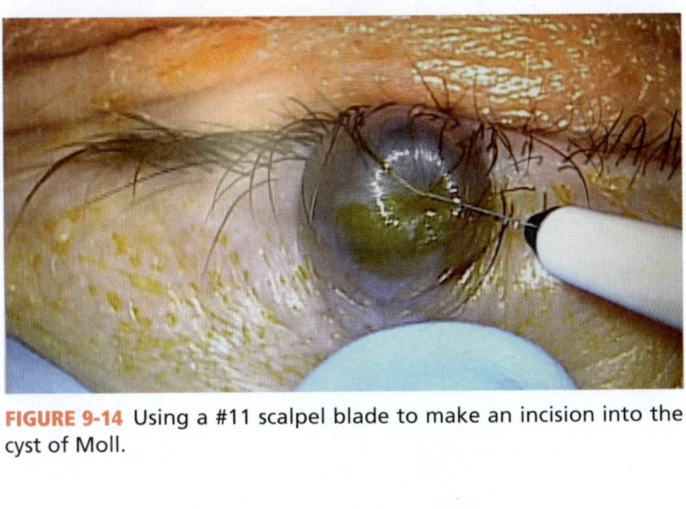

**FIGURE 9-14** Using a #11 scalpel blade to make an incision into the cyst of Moll.

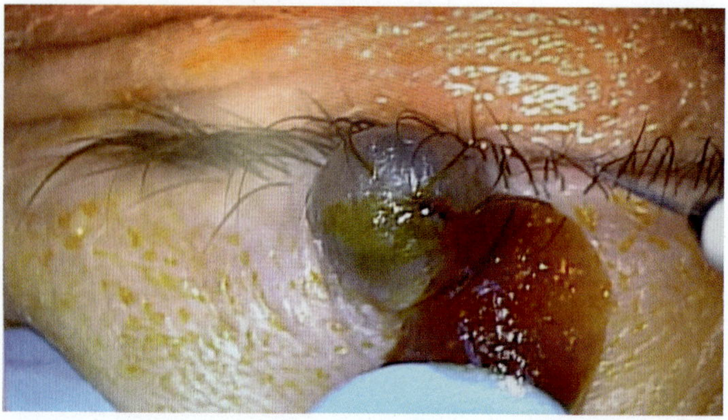

**FIGURE 9-15** Notice upon making a small incision, the cyst immediately drained fluid. The cyst was then drained, and the capsule and surrounding skin were excised and biopsied.

**Diagnosis:**
Left upper eyelid, skin shave biopsy:
Hidrocystoma, benign.
No evidence of malignancy

**FIGURE 9-16** The biopsy report came back with a cyst of Moll (hidrocystoma) as expected.

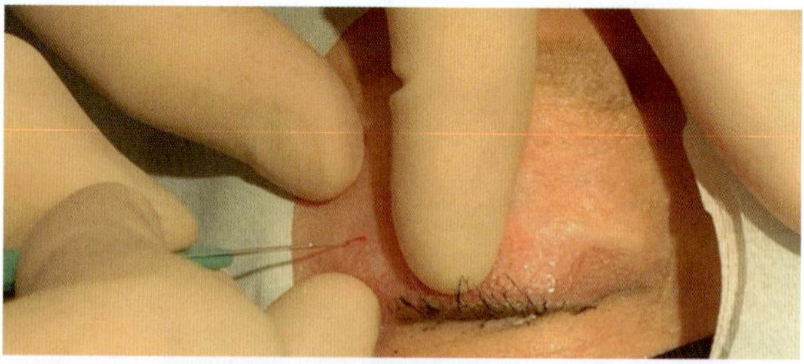

**FIGURE 9-17** Incision being made with a #11 scalpel blade to gain access to the eccrine hidrocystoma.

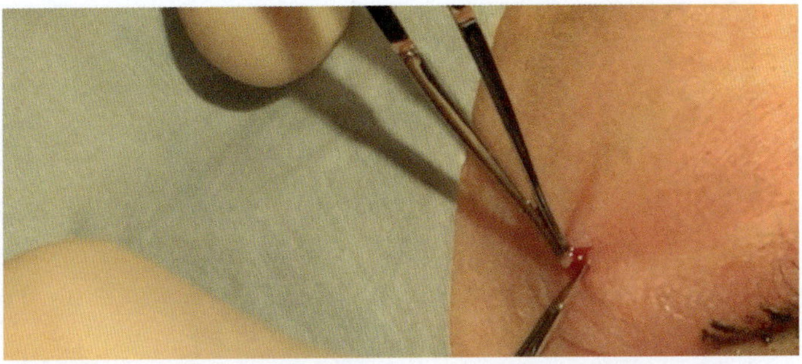

**FIGURE 9-18** After the hidrocystoma drained during the incision, toothed forceps and Westcott scissors are used to excise the cyst capsule.

to pathology for final histopathologic analysis. Handheld battery-operated cautery is used for hemostasis. After hemostasis is accomplished, the ophthalmic antibiotic ointment is applied to the surgical site. These small excision sites can be left to heal by secondary intention.

For larger cysts, blunt-tip Westcott tenotomy scissors are more useful. After the initial skin incision is made adjacent to the cyst with the #11 surgical blade, the skin edge is grasped gently with toothed forceps to help expose the underlying cyst. The blunt-tip Westcott tenotomy scissors are then used to do blunt dissection of the connective tissue around the cyst and its capsule (Figures 9-19 and 9-20). Final sharp excision of any remaining connective tissue can be performed once the complete intact cyst and its surrounding capsule have been isolated. Care should be taken not to rupture the cyst. If the cyst and its capsule are removed intact, then recurrence will not occur (Figure 9-21). If the capsule is punctured during the excision, some of the capsule may be retained and recurrence of the cyst is possible. All specimens should be collected and sent to pathology for final histopathologic analysis. Handheld battery-operated cautery is used for hemostasis. For these larger excisions, 6-0 silk, Vicryl, or nylon suture should be used to close the incision in an interrupted fashion (Figure 9-22). Ophthalmic antibiotic ointment is applied to the surgical site.

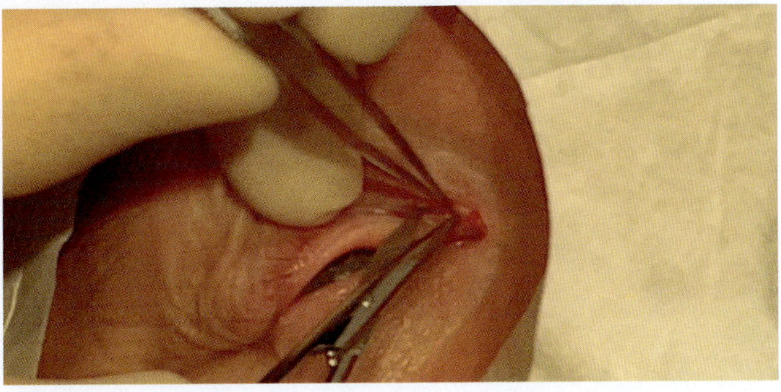

**FIGURE 9-19** Following the incision, Westcott scissors being used for blunt dissection to separate connective tissue from the cyst.

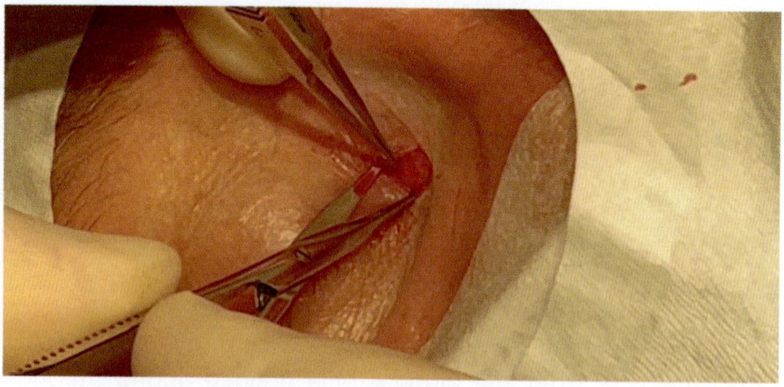

**FIGURE 9-20** Blunt dissection continues of surrounding connective tissue underneath the cyst to free the cyst.

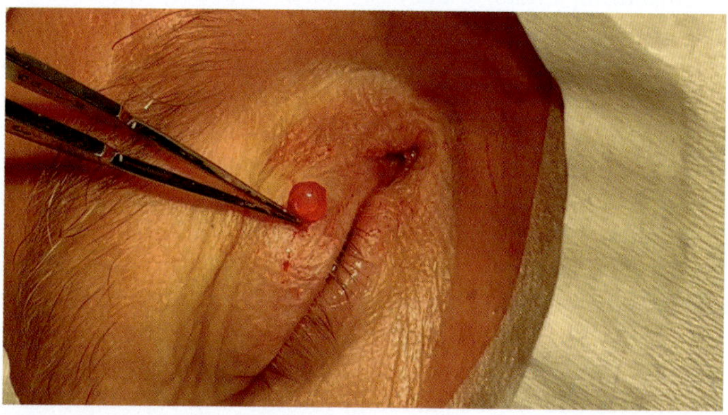

**FIGURE 9-21** The "holy grail" of cyst of Moll removal. The cyst was removed in one complete piece with the capsule intact.

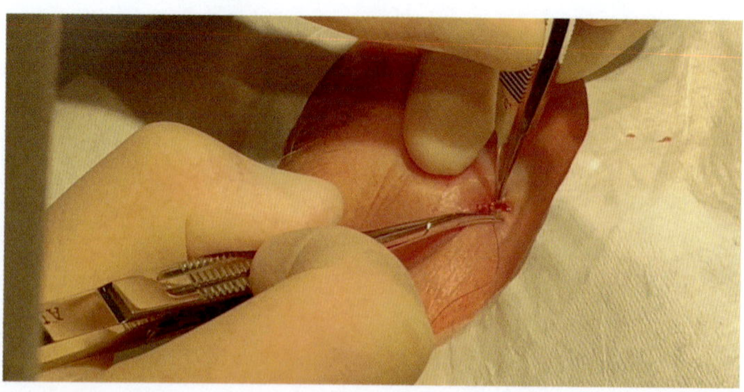

**FIGURE 9-22** Suture being placed to close the incision. Three sutures were required to completely close the surgical wound.

## POSTOPERATIVE CARE/COMANAGEMENT (FOLLOW-UP SCHEDULE)

- Documentation and operative report
- Blood pressure measurement
- Pulse measurement
- Erythromycin 0.5% ophthalmic ointment
- Follow-up is not necessary but can be booked 1 month postoperatively.
- If sutures were used to close the surgical site, the patient should return in 1 week for suture removal, and the ophthalmic antibiotic ointment is continued for another 2 to 3 days after the sutures are removed.

An operative report should be completed after every procedure. Blood pressure and pulse are measured at the conclusion of the procedure due to the injection of epinephrine. Erythromycin 0.5% ophthalmic ointment is applied two to three times a day for 1 week to the cyst removal site to prevent infection and aid healing, as moist healing leads to minimal scarring.[10] No follow-up appointments are typically needed if sutures were not used to close the surgical site, unless symptoms arise or in the case of cyst recurrence. If sutures were used, the patient should return in 1 week for suture removal. The ophthalmic antibiotic ointment is continued for another 2 to 3 days after the sutures are removed.

## POTENTIAL COMPLICATIONS AND THEIR TREATMENT

### Key Potential Complications

- Recurrence
- Redness
- Bruising
- Itching
- Infection
- Scarring

In cases of recurrence, surgical removal can be redone after complete healing. Removing the entirety of the cyst capsule is key to avoid recurrence. Redness, bruising, and itching are temporary during the postoperative phase and will self-resolve once complete healing has occurred. Bruising may occur from injection of anesthesia and typically resolves within a week. Infection is prevented with the antibiotic ointment that is prescribed postoperatively. If infection were to occur, topical or oral antibiotics can be used to treat the infection.[15] Scarring is rare with radiofrequency but may occur if the excision is too deep.[10]

## VIDEOS OF PROCEDURES

**Video 9-1**—Incision is made over the hidrocystoma with a #11 surgical blade. Toothed forceps and Vannas scissors are used to undermine and excise the hidrocystoma. Cautery is applied for hemostasis. The incision is left to heal by secondary intention. Erythromycin ophthalmic antibiotic ointment is applied to the surgical site. (Video courtesy Leonid Skorin, Jr., and Lucas J. Asfeld.)

**Video 9-2**—Incision is made over the cyst of Moll with a #11 surgical blade. Toothed forceps and blunt-tip curved Wescott tenotomy scissors are used for blunt dissection and excision of the intact cyst of Moll. Cautery is applied for hemostasis. The incision is closed with multiple interrupted 6-0 Vicryl sutures. Erythromycin ophthalmic antibiotic ointment is applied to the surgical site. (Video courtesy Leonid Skorin, Jr., and Tyler Clairmont.)

**Video 9-3**—Cyst of Zeis removal. The cyst and area around the cyst were prepped with an alcohol swab and 10% povidone–iodine (Betadine). The area just below the cyst is injected with approximately 0.4 to 0.5 mL of lidocaine 0.5% with epinephrine, taking care not to inject directly into or through the lid margin. A cotton-tipped applicator is used to massage the anesthetic toward the cyst. A radiofrequency pin electrode (aka "bent tip" electrode) is used on setting #1 cut, power 12 to make a small incision into the cyst. The contents of the cyst are drained, and the capsule is removed with the combination of both toothed and nontoothed forceps. Once the cyst is completely drained, the same pin electrode is used on setting #2 blend, power 12 to touch the base of the cyst to help ensure that any deep capsular contents are coagulated. This step is done to help minimize the chance of recurrence. The incision is left to heal by secondary intention. Erythromycin ophthalmic antibiotic ointment is applied to the surgical site. (Video courtesy of Nate Lighthizer.)

**Video 9-4**—Hidrocystoma drainage, biopsy, and removal. Not shown in the video is the area being prepped with an alcohol swab and 10% povidone–iodine (Betadine), as well as approximately 0.4 to 0.5 mL of lidocaine 0.5% with epinephrine injected around the cyst to provide proper anesthesia. In the video, a feather blade is used to incise into the cyst, and immediate drainage of fluid is seen. A large cotton-tipped applicator is used to soak up much of the fluid, as well as push on and squeeze the cyst to drain it as much as possible. Not shown in the video is a 0.12-mm toothed forceps and a Westcott scissors being used to excise the capsular contents and remainder of the cyst which were put in a biopsy container. The biopsy report came back with a cyst of Moll (hidrocystoma) as expected (see Figure 9-16). (Video courtesy of Nate Lighthizer.)

**Video 9-5**—Cyst of Zeis, seborrheic keratosis, and papilloma removal. Not shown in the video are the areas being prepped with an alcohol swab and 10% povidone–iodine (Betadine), as well as approximately 0.6 to 0.7 mL of lidocaine 0.5% with epinephrine injected around the lesions to provide proper anesthesia. A radiofrequency pin electrode (aka "bent tip" electrode) is used on setting #1 cut, power 10 to vaporize and completely remove the papilloma. The pin electrode is then used to incise into the cyst of Zeis, followed by a 0.12-mm toothed forceps and cotton-tipped applicator used to drain the contents of the cyst. A Westcott scissors and nontoothed forceps are then used to excise the remaining capsule. The incision is left to heal by secondary intention. Finally, the pin electrode is used on setting #1 cut, power 10 to vaporize and completely remove the seborrheic keratosis. Note that a cotton-tipped applicator soaked in sterile saline is used to remove carbonized tissue during the lesion removal and following the lesion removal. Erythromycin ophthalmic antibiotic ointment is applied to the surgical sites. See Figure 8-16A-C for preoperative, immediate postoperative, and 1-month postoperative photos, respectively. (Video courtesy of Nate Lighthizer.)

## EFFICACY

One systemic review compared the efficacy of various hidrocystoma treatments and found that destructive surgical procedures had the greatest efficacy for solitary cysts over skin-directed therapies, systemic medical therapies, or a combination of therapies.[16] The surgical procedures examined included incision and drainage, electrosurgery, carbon dioxide laser, diode laser, cryotherapy, and excision. Destructive surgical procedures had a response rate of 92.9% and a recurrence rate of 10.8%. Excision was shown to be the most efficacious for solitary hidrocystomas, with a recurrence rate of only 4.7%. Only three cysts were treated with electrosurgery. These cysts showed a 100% response rate, and one had recurrence 9 months after treatment.[16]

Another case report studied the efficacy of electrosurgery and excision in treating apocrine hidrocystomas. Researchers found that electrosurgery was a safe, simple, and cosmetically favorable treatment modality over excision.[17] They concluded that cysts less than 1 cm in size be treated with electrosurgery and cysts larger than 1 cm with excision. In the cysts removed via electrosurgery, no scarring was noticeable at the 1-year follow-up and recurrence occurred 9 months after removal.[17] These studies lend support that radiofrequency and excision are beneficial and cosmetically pleasing therapies for apocrine hidrocystomas. Recurrence can be minimized by removing the entire cyst capsule.

## CODING/BILLING

- **CPT code 67840**—Excision of lesion of eyelid (except chalazion) without closure or with simple direct closure
- **CPT code 67850**—Excision and destruction procedures on the eyelids
- Both **CPT code 67840** and **CPT code 67850** have a 10-day postoperative global period.
- Cyst removals for cosmesis are not paid by insurance carriers. Proper documentation listing a functional complaint must be listed in the chief complaint for insurance reimbursement.

Common ICD-10 codes that support this procedure include the following:

- **H02.821** (cysts of right upper eyelid)
- **H02.822** (cysts of right lower eyelid)
- **H02.823** (cysts of right eye, unspecified eyelid)
- **H02.824** (cysts of left upper eyelid)
- **H02.825** (cysts of left lower eyelid)
- **H02.826** (cysts of left eye, unspecified eyelid)
- **H02.829** (cysts of unspecified eye, unspecified eyelid)

## REFERENCES

1. Nerad JA. *Techniques in Ophthalmic Plastic Surgery: A Personal Tutorial.* 2nd ed. Elsevier; 2021:419-463.
2. Pe'er J. Pathology of eyelid tumors. *Indian J Ophthalmol.* 2016;64(3):177-190.
3. Bowling B, Kanski JJ. *Kanski's Clinical Ophthalmology: A Systematic Approach.* 8th ed. Elsevier; 2016:3-6.
4. Sun MT. Huang S, Huilgol SC, Selva D. Eyelid lesions in general practice. *Aust J Gen Pract.* 2019;48(8):509-514.

5. Penne RB. *Color Atlas and Synopsis of Clinical Ophthalmology: Oculoplastics.* 3rd ed. Wolters Kluwer; 2019:1-23.
6. Sarabi K, Khachemoune A. Hidrocystomas—a brief review. *MedGenMed.* 2006;8(3):57.
7. Nema HV, Nema N. *Ocular Tumors.* Springer; 2021.
8. Albert DM, Azar DT, Miller JW, Young LH. *Albert and Jakobiec's Principles and Practice of Ophthalmology.* 4th ed. Springer; 2022:5861-5902.
9. Hoang VT, Trinh CT, Nguyen CH, et al. Overview of epidermoid cyst. *Eur J Radiol Open.* 2019;6:291-301.
10. Fowler G. *Pfenninger and Fowler's Procedures for Primary Care.* Elsevier; 2020:170-178.
11. Robinson JK. *Surgery of the Skin: Procedural Dermatology.* 3rd ed. Elsevier; 2015:134-149.
12. Dutton JJ, Waldrop TG. *Atlas of Oculoplastic and Orbital Surgery.* 2nd ed. Wolters Kluwer; 2018:4-5.
13. Chiarello SE. Radiovaporization: radiofrequency cutting current to vaporize and sculpt skin lesions. *Dermatol Surg.* 2003;29(7):755-758.
14. Eshraghi B, Torabi HR, Kasaie A, Rajabi MT. The use of a radiofrequency unit for excisional biopsy of eyelid papillomas. *Ophthalmic Plast Reconstr Surg.* 2010;26(6):448-449.
15. Botting J, Schofield J. *Brown's Skin and Minor Surgery: A Text and Colour Atlas.* 5th ed. CRC Press; 2020:330.
16. Trischman T, Scott JF. Comparative efficacy of hidrocystoma treatments: a systematic review. *J Cutan Med Surg.* 2020;24(5):474-480.
17. Gupta S, Handa U, Handa S, Mohan H. The efficacy of electrosurgery and excision in treating patients with multiple apocrine hidrocystomas. *Dermatol Surg.* 2001;27(4):382-384.

# 10 Bichloracetic Acid Treatment

**Andrew W. Krein • Leonid Skorin, Jr**

Bichloracetic acid, also known as dichloroacetic acid, has been used as a chemical cauterant in medicine for many years. Bichloracetic acid is a colorless solution with a highly acidic pH, enabling it to act as an effective cauterizing agent.[1] The employment of chemical cautery has many uses in medicine, including the treatment of in-grown toenails, seborrheic keratosis, xanthomas, and corns.[2] In eye care, it is focused on the treatment of benign lesions such as xanthelasma, papilloma, and seborrheic keratosis.[3] The presence of cosmetically displeasing ocular adnexal growths has led many patients to pursue medical intervention to remove blemishes. The use of bichloracetic acid can be a valuable asset for an in-office procedure that carries less risks than other traditional surgical techniques. Selecting the proper patient, as well as educating them on the risks of the procedure, is an imperative step in the process of treatment.

## INDICATIONS

### Key Indications

- Xanthelasma palpebrarum
- Papilloma
- Seborrheic keratosis

The common use for bichloracetic acid in eye care is for removal of benign lesions in the periocular region.[2] Xanthelasma, papillomas, and seborrheic keratoses are the most common lesions that present in the periocular region.[4] Xanthelasma palpebrarum, known more simply as xanthelasma, are soft, nontender, benign yellow growths within the cutaneous surface and are asymptomatic (Figure 10-1).[2,5] Commonly, the yellow xanthelasma plaques will present in the inner canthus areas of both upper and lower eyelids.[6] Xanthelasma can occur in a patient of any age, race, or sex; however, more commonly presenting in the fourth or fifth decade of life.[2,3] There is also a higher predilection for it to present in females.[3] In an individual who presents with xanthelasma under the fourth decade of life, it is necessary to perform a cholesterol panel to rule out hereditary or dietary hyperlipemic conditions.[2,7] Although rare, systemic abnormalities associated with xanthelasma include types IIA, IIB, and III lipoprotein disorders, hypercholesterolemic xanthomatosis, mixed hyperlipidemia type IV, biliary obstruction,

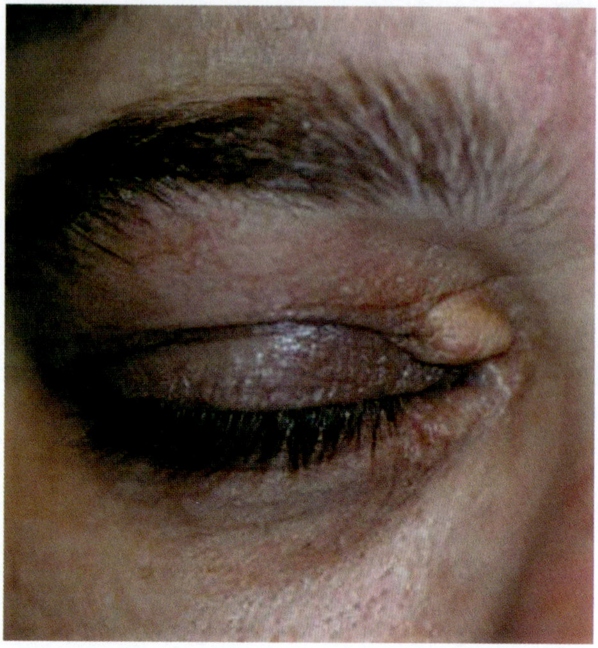

**FIGURE 10-1** Xanthelasma located on medial canthal area of the right upper eyelid.

apolipoprotein E phenotypes, and in association with Schneider crystalline corneal dystrophy.[5] Histologic analysis will reveal an epidermis that is uninvolved or flattened, and a dermis layer packed with diffuse deposits of foamy histiocytic cells.[7] There is an absence of inflammation or fibrosis.[7] Xanthelasma plaques are effectively removed with bichloracetic acid due to their relatively flat contour.[6,7] Papillomas, commonly known as skin tags, are the most common benign eyelid lesion.[3] These lesions can occur anywhere in the ocular adnexal region. A papilloma is a finger-like projection with a central fibrovascular pedunculation.[8] Histologically, these benign lesions show a hyperplasia of the squamous epithelium.[9,10] In cases where the papilloma is overtly elevated, a traditional snip excision may be warranted. Seborrheic keratosis lesions are another common benign periocular growth. Seborrheic keratosis has a predilection for the eyelid and forehead.[11] These lesions have a classical "stuck-on" appearance.[11] They present in various shades from black to light brown and have a wart-like texture.[12] Typically, they become more numerous as the patient ages. They have no gender predilection. Individuals with lighter skin tones, especially less than Fitzpatrick skin type III, are more susceptible to seborrheic keratosis.[12] Seborrheic keratosis is a noncancerous propagation of immature keratinocytes.[11] These proliferations are usually slow growing and maintain a delineated border.[11] If the patient presents with an eruption of new seborrheic keratosis lesions, it may be an ominous sign of a gastrointestinal or pulmonary malignancy and is known as the Leser–Trélat sign.[13]

# CONTRAINDICATIONS

**Key Contraindications**

- Fitzpatrick skin types V and VI
- Contact with conjunctiva or other mucous membrane
- Lesion to be treated is malignant

Contraindications for bichloracetic acid treatment are few; however, they are intrinsically important to note. Individuals with a melanin-rich complexion are contraindicated for this procedure. The bichloracetic acid will rapidly penetrate the cutaneous layer and act in a keratolytic manner, causing a disruption in the melanin complex.[3] The Fitzpatrick skin type scale as seen in Table 10-1 is a good indicator of suitable candidates.[14] Types V and VI are a contraindication to this procedure. The V and VI skin types have higher amounts of epidermal melanin, which causes a lighter flesh-like appearance to the skin after it heals.[2] Once the treated area heals, there is a very prominent incongruity between that and the surrounding skin in types V and VI.

Location of the lesion is also extremely important due to the highly corrosive nature of the acid. Care should be taken to avoid contact with any mucous membranes such as the

**TABLE 10-1 FITZPATRICK SKIN TYPE SCALE**

| FITZPATRICK SKIN TYPE | SKIN COLOR BEFORE SUN EXPOSURE | EYE COLOR | HAIR COLOR | SUN REACTION |
|---|---|---|---|---|
| Skin type I | Ivory | Light blue, light gray, or light green | Red or light blonde | Skin always freckles, always burns and peels often, and never tans |
| Skin type II | Fair or pale | Blue, gray, or green | Blonde | Skin usually freckles, burns and peels often, and rarely tans |
| Skin type III | Fair to beige, with golden undertones | Hazel or light brown | Dark blonde or light brown | Skin usually freckles, burns and peels often, and rarely tans |
| Skin type IV | Olive or light brown | Dark brown | Dark brown | Doesn't really freckle, burns rarely, and tans often |
| Skin type V | Dark brown | Dark brown to black | Dark brown to black | Rarely freckles, almost never burns, and always tans |
| Skin type VI | Deeply pigmented dark brown to darkest brown | Brownish black | Black | Never freckles, never burns, and always tans darkly |

Courtesy of McGee SR, Stonecipher K. Intense pulsed light therapy. In: Freisberg L, Lighthizer N, Skorin L, Stonecipher K, Zimmerman AB, eds. *The Ophthalmic Laser Handbook*. Wolters Kluwer; 2021:373.

conjunctiva. The preparation for treatment requires the acid to be sequestered by a thick layer of petroleum jelly spanning 2 to 3 mm beyond the outside border of the lesion. Therefore, if this border cannot be maintained and begins to invade a mucous membrane such as the conjunctiva, it is advised to seek a different procedural route.

If there is any suspicion that the lesion is of a malignant nature, the practitioner should elect to biopsy the tissue. When a benign finding is confirmed, and the patient fulfills the adequate requirements, the practitioner may proceed with bichloracetic acid treatment.

## PREOPERATIVE PREPARATION

### Instrumentation

1. Ophthalmic topical anesthetic (e.g., tetracaine 0.5%, proparacaine 0.5%)
2. Petroleum jelly
3. Cotton-tipped applicators
4. Bichloracetic acid
5. 3″ wooden applicator sticks
6. Sterile fenestrated surgical drape
7. Surgical gloves
8. Magnification: ophthalmic loupes/slit lamp

## PROCEDURE

1. Appropriate consent should be obtained and photodocumentation of the lesion performed.
2. Before beginning the procedure, topical anesthetic is applied to both eyes to prevent reflex lacrimation.
   i. Lacrimation may lead to tears draining into the treatment zone.
3. Positioning:
   i. If using a slit lamp, position the patient to ensure a comfortable height.
   ii. If using ophthalmic loupes, place the patient in a supine position at a comfortable working level for the practitioner.
4. Apply a sterile fenestrated surgical drape over the patient's face to expose only the treatment zone.
   i. Bichloracetic acid acts as a cauterizing agent to the bacterial flora in the treatment zone; therefore, there is no further prophylactic preoperative steps that many other periocular surgeries require.
5. Using a cotton-tipped applicator, apply petroleum jelly to the border of the lesion that extends 2 to 3 mm beyond the lesion.
   i. A precise border around the plaque is imperative, as the petroleum jelly will act as a barrier to the bichloracetic acid. If the petroleum jelly invades the treatment zone of the lesion, the acid will not reach the cutaneous layer due to the impermeable nature of the petroleum jelly.

ii. If the petroleum jelly invades the treatment zone, take a clean cotton-tipped applicator and wipe away the excess petroleum jelly.
iii. Once the lesion(s) are adequately sequestered, prepare the bichloracetic acid wooden applicator stick.

6. Transfer the acid into a small glass vial using the dropper.
7. Take the wooden applicator stick and dip only the tapered tip into the bichloracetic acid.
   i. Saturate the tip of the applicator with acid.
   ii. Ensure the shaft of the wooden applicator stick is not dripping acid by holding the stick slightly above the fluid in the glass vial.
8. Once the wooden applicator stick is prepared with acid, slowly begin to spot treat the xanthelasma plaque (or other benign lesion) by touching the tip of the applicator to the lesion (Figure 10-2).
   i. Tell the patient that they may feel a slight burning or tingling sensation as the area is treated and for a short period following the procedure.
   ii. As the cauterization begins, you will notice the treated area turning to an ashy-white hue, known as a "fried-egg" appearance (Figure 10-3). This indicates that the area has been deleted of any viable vasculature. This causes the treatment area to become necrotic.
   iii. Once the hallmark "fried-egg" appearance is achieved, treatment with the acid is complete.
9. Following cauterization, remove the petroleum jelly using a fresh cotton-tipped applicator.
10. Treatment is complete.

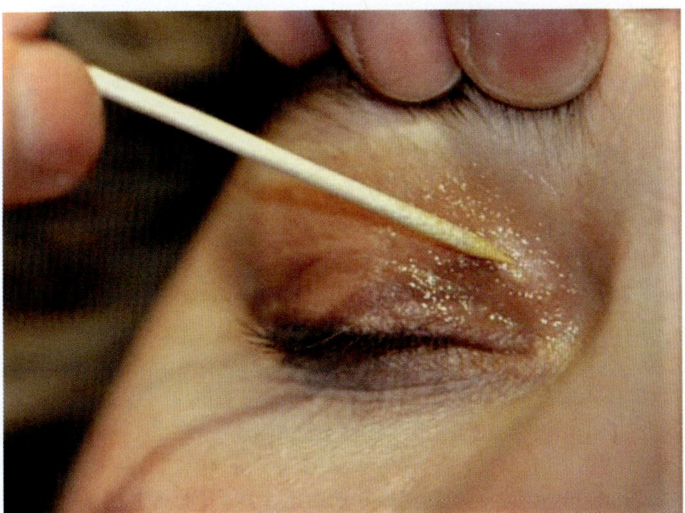

**FIGURE 10-2** Application of bichloracetic acid using wooden applicator stick to xanthelasma surface.

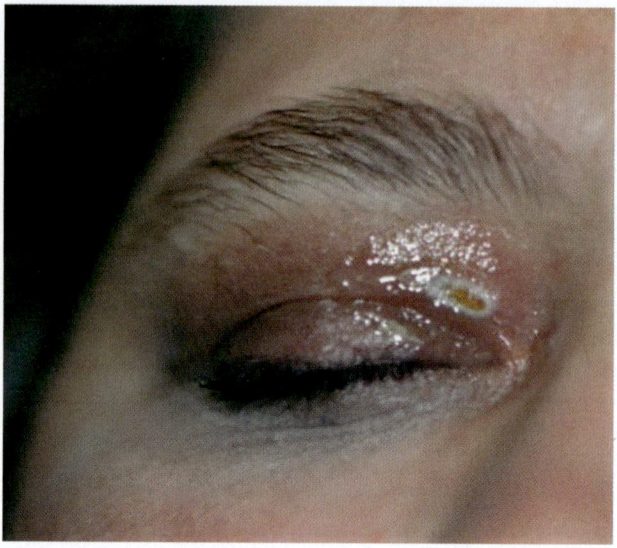

**FIGURE 10-3** Immediately after bichloracetic acid treatment, the xanthelasma takes on a "fried-egg" appearance.

# POSTOPERATIVE CARE/COMANAGEMENT (FOLLOW-UP SCHEDULE)

## Key Postoperative Considerations

- No prophylactic treatment is necessary; however, tobramycin/dexamethasone ointment can be applied TID for 1 week
- Over-the-counter analgesics such as ibuprofen or acetaminophen as necessary
- Recheck in 1 week, 2 weeks, and then 1 month postoperatively
- Apply sunscreen on the area to avoid sunburn.

Postoperative management is quite simple for treatment with bichloracetic acid. The acid cauterizes the local flora as well as potential pathogens, mitigating the risk for infection.[2] However, some clinicians use a steroid/antibiotic ointment to mitigate inflammation and infection.[3] A recommendation is for tobramycin/dexamethasone ointment (TobraDex) to be used on the lesion site TID for 7 days.[3,4] Minimal postoperative pain is incurred by the patient; however, they may experience a slight tingling or warmth around the treatment zone. Some patients may benefit from over-the-counter analgesics such as ibuprofen or acetaminophen. The follow-up schedule for patients is 1 week, 2 weeks, and then 1 month postoperatively. During the healing process, the patient will notice the treatment zone becoming darker and scabbing over, which is known as eschar formation (Figure 10-4).[2,3] Around 2 weeks postoperatively, the

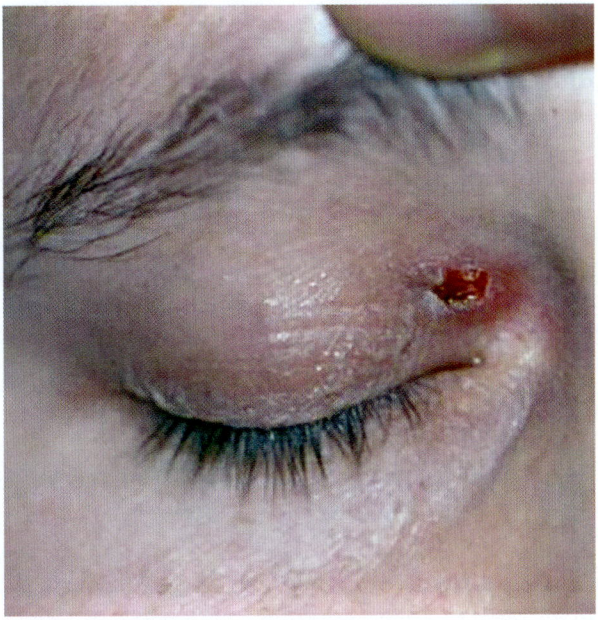

**FIGURE 10-4** One week postoperatively: Eschar present as treatment area heals.

eschar will debride itself naturally and leave behind healthy pink tissue that will transition to the patient's natural skin type. When the eschar sheds, revealing fresh skin, it may be advisable to recommend sunscreen on the area to avoid any sunburn.

## POTENTIAL COMPLICATIONS AND THEIR TREATMENTS

**Key Potential Complications**

- Skin discoloration
- Inadvertent treatment of normal tissue
- Undertreatment of lesion

Risks as well as complications of chemical cautery are few, however, impactful. The main risk that is encountered with the treatment of bichloracetic acid is skin discoloration.[2,15] In some instances, typically those patients higher on the Fitzpatrick scale, they can have areas of discoloration that does not match the surrounding skin following treatment. The acid disrupts the complexion of the skin, and this is why the selective nature of choosing patients is imperative. The other main risk associated with this modality is the potential for aberrant treatment. If the practitioner is not precise with their treatment, areas of surrounding normal tissue may undergo unnecessary cauterization. In these instances, the patient should be cared for with the usual postoperative treatment and follow-up schedule as listed earlier.[2] Undertreatment can also occur. This usually happens when some of the petroleum jelly bleeds over the area to be treated. This is identified by the patient and clinician later into the postoperative follow-up period. This requires retreatment to the untreated area. The clinician should warn the patient about this possibly happening beforehand and reassure the patient that a simple "touch-up" will rectify this issue if it was to occur.

## VIDEOS OF PROCEDURES

**Video 10-1**—Bichloracetic acid treatment (chemical cauterization). Petroleum jelly is applied with a cotton-tipped applicator to protect normal tissue. The bichloracetic acid is applied to the xanthelasma using a wooden applicator stick. Note that only the tip of the stick needs to be soaked with the bichloracetic acid. Note the tissue change to a "fried-egg" appearance as the acid is applied. The petroleum jelly is removed with a cotton-tipped applicator. (Video courtesy of Leonid Skorin, Jr., and Dessie Westall.)

**Video 10-2**—Bichloracetic acid treatment (chemical cauterization). Petroleum jelly is applied with a cotton-tipped applicator to protect normal tissue. The bichloracetic acid is applied to the xanthelasma using a wooden applicator stick. Note that only the tip of the stick needs to be soaked with the bichloracetic acid. Note the tissue change to a "fried-egg" appearance as the acid is applied. The petroleum jelly is removed with a cotton-tipped applicator. (Video courtesy of Leonid Skorin, Jr., and Andrew Krein.)

**Video 10-3**—Bichloracetic acid treatment (chemical cauterization). Petroleum jelly is applied using a cotton-tipped applicator to protect normal tissue. The bichloracetic acid is applied to the xanthelasma using a wooden applicator stick. Note that only the tip of the stick needs to be soaked with the bichloracetic acid. Note the tissue change to a "fried-egg" appearance as the acid is applied. The petroleum jelly is removed with a cotton-tipped applicator. (Video courtesy of Leonid Skorin, Jr., and Andrew Krein.)

## EFFICACY

Bichloracetic acid treatment is a very effective treatment modality. The efficacy of bichloracetic acid on xanthelasma palpebrarum has shown complete resolution in 85% of initial treatments.[15] After a 5-year longitudinal study of those same individuals, it was shown to have an efficacy of 72%.[15] The patients who required additional treatments after 5 years were shown to also have hyperlipidemia.[2,15] This modality is an easily repeatable procedure. If during the follow-up period the patient has any remnants of the lesion remaining, simply reapply the treatment to the persisting tissue as listed in the above procedure steps.[3]

## CODING/BILLING

**CPT code: 17250**—chemical cauterization of granulation tissue (proud flesh, sinus, or fistula). Is not to be used with removal or excision codes for the same lesion.

Common ICD-10 codes that support chemical cauterization include the following:

- **D23.10** (other benign neoplasm of skin of unspecified eyelid, including canthus)
- **D23.11** (other benign neoplasm of skin of right eyelid, including canthus)

- **D23.12** (other benign neoplasm of skin of left eyelid, including canthus)
- **D36.9** (benign neoplasm, unspecified site)
- **H02.60** (xanthelasma of unspecified eye, unspecified eyelid)
- **H02.61** (xanthelasma of right upper eyelid)
- **H02.62** (xanthelasma of right lower eyelid)
- **H02.63** (xanthelasma of right eye, unspecified eyelid)
- **H02.64** (xanthelasma of left upper eyelid)
- **H02.65** (xanthelasma of left lower eyelid)
- **H02.66** (xanthelasma of left eye, unspecified eyelid)
- **L82.0** (inflamed seborrheic keratosis)
- **L82.1** (other seborrheic keratosis)

## REFERENCES

1. IARC Working Group on the Evaluation of Carcinogenic Risks to Humans. Dichloroacetic acid. In: *Trichloroethylene, Tetrachloroethylene, and Some Other Chlorinated Agents*. International Agency for Research on Cancer; 2014. (IARC Monographs on the Evaluation of Carcinogenic Risks to Humans, No. 106.) https://www.ncbi.nlm.nih.gov/books/NBK294278/
2. Westall D, Skorin L. Spot remover. *Review of Optometry.* Accessed September 4, 2022. https://www.reviewofoptometry.com/article/spot-remover/
3. Kabat A, Sowka J. Kill 'em with chemicals. *Review of Optometry*. Accessed August 12, 2022. https://www.reviewofoptometry.com/article/kill-em-with-chemicals
4. Skorin L, Myint S. Eyelid and adnexal lesions. In: Onofrey B, Skorin L, Holdeman NR, eds. *Ocular Therapeutics Handbook: A Clinical Manual.* 4th ed. Wolters Kluwer; 2020:657-660.
5. Ostler HB, Maibach HI, Hoke AW, Schwab IR. *Diseases of the Eye & Skin: A Color Atlas*. Lippincott Williams & Wilkins; 2004:151-169.
6. Laftah Z, Al-Niaimi F. Xanthelasma: an update on treatment modalities. *J Cutan Aesthet Surg*. 2018;11:1-6.
7. Griffith DG, Salasche SJ, Clemons DE. *Cutaneous Abnormalities of the Eyelid and Face: An Atlas with Histopathology*. McGraw-Hill; 1987:147-158.
8. Pariser RJ. Benign neoplasms of the skin. *Med Clin North Am*. 1998;82(6):1285-1307, v-vi.
9. Pathology Residency and Fellowship Program. Squamous papilloma. Brown University. Accessed September 1, 2022. https://www.brown.edu/academics/biomed/departments/pathology/residency/digital-pathology-library/head-and-neck/oral-cavity-tonsils-and-neck/squamous-papilloma
10. Dutton JJ, Gayre GS, Proia AD. *Diagnostic Atlas of Common Eyelid Diseases*. CRC Press; 2007:225-226.
11. Choi JW, Park YW, Byun SY, Youn SW. Differentiation of benign pigmented skin lesions with the aid of computer image analysis: a novel approach. *Ann Dermatol.* 2013;25(3):340-347. doi:10.5021/AD.2013.25.3.340
12. Braun RP, Ludwig S, Marghoob AA. Differential diagnosis of seborrheic keratosis: clinical and dermoscopic features. *J Drugs Dermatol.* 2017;16(9):835-842.
13. Narala A, Cohen S, Narala S, et al. Cutaneous T-cell lymphoma-associated Leser-Trélat sign: report and world literature review. *Dermatol Online J*. 2017;23(1):4-5. doi:10.5070/D3231033672
14. McGee SR, Stonecipher K. Intense pulsed light therapy. In: Freisberg L, Lighthizer N, Skorin L, Stonecipher K, Zimmerman AB, eds. *The Ophthalmic Laser Handbook*. Wolters Kluwer; 2021:371-391.
15. Haygood LJ, Bennett JD, Brodell RT. Treatment of xanthelasma palpebrarum with bichloracetic acid. *Am Soc Dermatol Surg*. 1998;24:1027-1031.

# 11 Chalazion Management

Nate Lighthizer • Komal Patel

A chalazion is a benign, rigid, nonpainful, noninfectious, granulomatous lesion caused by obstruction of a meibomian gland or gland of Zeis.[1] These lipogranulomatous inflammatory lesions are filled with lipid deposits made up of epithelioid cells, multinucleated giant cells, and lymphocytes.[2,3] A pseudocapsule made of connective tissue usually forms around the lesion.[4] They present as round, enlarging nodules on the upper or lower tarsal plate (Figure 11-1). Chalazia typically occur after internal or external hordeola, which are infections of the meibomian gland and gland of Zeis, respectively.[5] There is no age or sex predilection, although they commonly occur in patients with chronic blepharitis and ocular rosacea.[6] Common clinical signs seen in association include eyelid margin telangiectasia, erythema, and eyelash debris.[7] A recurrent chalazion should be biopsied to rule out malignancies such as sebaceous gland carcinoma.[2,5]

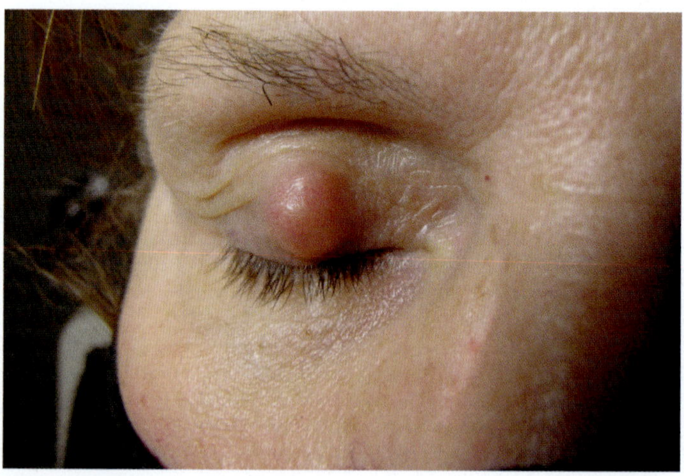

**FIGURE 11-1** Large chalazion.

# INDICATIONS

**Key Indications**

- Clinically significant chalazia

Treatment options for chalazia range from conservative to more aggressive. Treatment choice depends on a variety of factors including patient preference, doctor preference, size of the chalazia, and chronicity of the chalazion. These include warm compresses with or without oral antibiotics, intense pulsed light (IPL) therapy, steroid injection, and incision and curettage (I&C).

## Warm Compresses and Doxycycline

Warm compresses should be applied to the affected lid for 10 to 15 minutes four or more times per day with lid massage.[8] Most chalazia resolve within 1 month with these conservative measures, with a success rate ranging between 29% and 80%.[9] One study found a resolution rate of 46% after 3 weeks of hot compresses.[10] If the chalazion is draining, topical ophthalmic antibiotics such as bacitracin or erythromycin ointment can be applied twice a day for 1 to 2 weeks.[8] Doxycycline hyclate or monohydrate 50 to 100 mg by mouth once or twice a day for 4 to 6 weeks (or longer as needed) can also be considered due to its antibacterial and anti-inflammatory effects.[2,8] Both doxycycline hyclate or monohydrate can be used as they vary in their bioavailability and absorption, but are both equally effective.[11]

## Intense Pulsed Light Therapy

IPL therapy can be used to treat rosacea, meibomian gland dysfunction, and Demodex blepharitis in association with dry eye disease. The same IPL settings for meibomian gland dysfunction can be used for a chalazion. Two passes tragus to tragus and on the upper eyelids, with 2 to 3 additional pulses directly on the chalazion, should be performed. Laser-grade corneal shields must be used as the pulses are delivered approximately 2 mm away from the eyelash line.[12]

One study examining IPL therapy for the treatment of chalazia found that a combined treatment of IPL protocol for meibomian gland dysfunction with IPL applied directly to the eyelids showed 96.15% efficacy in treating chalazia. An average of 2.07 ± 0.97 IPL sessions were needed for complete resolution.[13] No adverse effects were observed in this study. These researchers outlined that IPL applied directly to the eyelids is a safe and effective treatment for chalazia, in addition to treating meibomian gland dysfunction and dry eye disease.[13]

See the supplemental reading section, located at the end of this chapter, for a detailed.

## Steroid Injection

Steroid injection of chalazia should be considered if more conservative options fail or if it is patient preference for treatment. Injection of 0.2 to 1.0 mL of triamcinolone acetonide suspension 40 mg/mL (Kenalog-40) is the treatment of choice, although Kenalog-10 can also be used. One study found Kenalog-40 to be more effective than Kenalog-10 in the treatment of chalazion; however, Kenalog-10 was associated with fewer complications including elevated intraocular pressure and yellow deposits due to steroid use.[14] For some anesthetic effect, 1:1 of triamcinolone acetonide and lidocaine with epinephrine can be used.[2] Steroid injection is a good treatment option for chalazia near the lacrimal punctum and can resolve a chalazion in a little over 2 weeks.[9]

### Incision and Curettage

When more conservative therapies or steroid injection fail to resolve a chalazion, surgical intervention with I&C can be considered. This is a procedure that drains the contents of the chalazion and more likely avoids recurrence as the entire lesion and capsule are removed.

## STEROID INJECTION

### Indications

**Key Indications**

- Chalazion

Cosmesis, discomfort, and ptosis are all possible reasons why patients opt to have a chalazion removed. Steroid injection works particularly well for smaller chalazia and those that are not suitable for surgical intervention due to location, such as close to the lacrimal punctum, eyelid margin, or temporal canthus.

## CONTRAINDICATIONS

**Key Contraindications**

- Darkly pigmented skin
- Suspected malignant lesions
- Allergies to medications (e.g., triamcinolone acetonide, lidocaine, and epinephrine)

Contraindications to chalazion injection involve common precautions with steroid use. Steroids may cause skin hypopigmentation, thus injection should be avoided in Fitzpatrick skin types V and VI.[6] If there is any suspicion that the lesion may be malignant, for example, in cases of chronic, unilateral chalazion in the same location, a biopsy should be performed prior to removal.[6] Caution should be taken to avoid steroid use, or use alternative medications or anesthesia, in the case of steroid allergy. Caution should also be exercised in patients with glaucoma or steroid responders, as case reports have outlined an elevation of intraocular pressure after periocular steroid injection.[14]

# PREOPERATIVE PREPARATION

## Key Preoperative Considerations

- Photographs of the chalazion need to be documented and on file.
- Consent form that includes the patient's symptoms and alternatives to the chosen treatment
- Visual acuity
- Blood pressure measurement
- Pulse measurement
- Instrumentation preparation

The preoperative preparation for this procedure is straightforward. The patient should be seated at the procedure chair, with the following instrumentation placed within arm's reach:

## Instrumentation

1. Ophthalmic topical anesthetic (e.g., proparacaine and tetracaine)
2. 70% isopropyl alcohol prep pad
3. Local anesthesia (0.5%, 1%, or 2% lidocaine with epinephrine 1:100,000 or 1:200,000) (optional)
4. 18-gauge needle to draw up steroid medication from the vial
5. 25- or 27-gauge needle (1/2″ or 1″ length) to inject into chalazion (avoid using a 30- or 32-gauge needle as it may be too small to push the steroid medication through.)
6. 1- or 3-mL syringe
7. Cotton-tipped applicators
8. Triamcinolone acetonide (Kenalog-40 or Kenalog-10)
9. Magnification: surgical microscope or ophthalmic loupes (optional)

# PROCEDURE

## Key Procedural Points

- Optional placement of corneal shield to protect the globe
- Sterile technique
- Needle injection away from the globe
- Patient placement at the discretion of the practitioner

## Procedural Steps

1. Using an 18-gauge needle, withdraw approximately 1 to 2 mL of triamcinolone acetonide into a 1- or 3-mL syringe. If anesthesia is being used, draw up 1:1 of lidocaine with epinephrine and triamcinolone acetonide.
2. Discard the 18-gauge needle in a sharps container, and add a 25- or 27-gauge needle to the syringe.
3. Ensure the steroid is well suspended before injection.
4. Set up the surgical microscope or loupes if needed. The procedure can also be done without magnification, depending on the practitioner's comfort.
5. Instill topical anesthetic (proparacaine, tetracaine) into both eyes to minimize reflex lacrimation, the blink reflex, and keep the patient comfortable during the procedure.
6. Use an alcohol prep pad to clean the lesion, ocular adnexal area, and eyelashes.
7. Use a 25- or 27-gauge needle with bevel up and inject an intralesional steroid injection into the chalazion. Prior to injecting the medication, it is advised to slightly pull back on the syringe plunger to ensure the needle is not in a blood vessel. If unable to inject directly into the chalazion, surround the chalazion with steroid using an extralesional injection.[15] A bolus should be seen around the chalazion. Some degree of resistance is often felt as the medication is injected due to the nature of the encapsulated chalazion. Continue to inject as the needle is withdrawn (Figures 11-2 and 11-3).
8. Bleeding is minimal but if it occurs, hold direct pressure with a cotton-tipped applicator.
9. No bandages, patches, or medications are needed at the conclusion of the procedure.

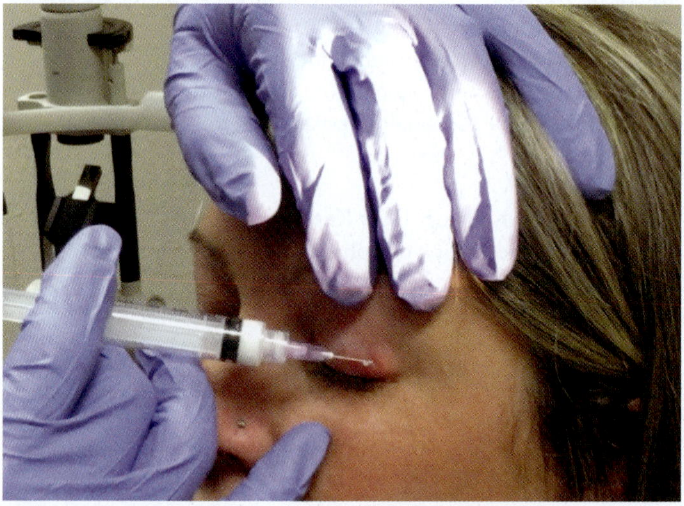

**FIGURE 11-2** Preparing to perform an intralesional triamcinolone steroid injection for a chalazion. A 27-gauge needle on a 3-mL syringe is being used.

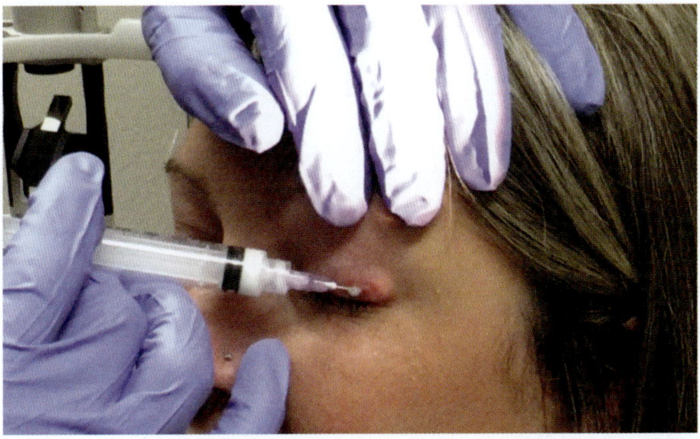

**FIGURE 11-3** Intralesional steroid injection being performed. The needle has been inserted inside the chalazion capsule, and steroid has been injected. Notice the area is already slightly turning white as you can see the white steroid medicine injected.

# POSTOPERATIVE CARE/COMANAGEMENT (FOLLOW-UP SCHEDULE)

## Key Postoperative Considerations

- Documentation and operative report
- Blood pressure measurement
- Pulse measurement
- Continue warm compresses and eyelid massage 3 days after injection two to three times a day (optional).
- Follow-up in 1 month

An operative report should be completed after every procedure that describes the steps taken to perform the procedure. Blood pressure and pulse are measured at the conclusion of the procedure if epinephrine was injected. A 1-month follow-up appointment is typically scheduled. This is to examine for resolution of the chalazion and to determine if additional treatment is needed. Two to three steroid injections are sometimes needed for larger chalazia. If chalazia fail to resolve with steroid injection, an I&C can be considered as the next treatment of choice. All patients should be educated to return to the clinic sooner if signs or symptoms of infection arise. Warm compresses with eyelid massage can be resumed 3 days after steroid injection as a supplemental therapy to aid resolution, although this is not required.

## POTENTIAL COMPLICATIONS AND THEIR TREATMENT

### Key Potential Complications

- Local skin hypopigmentation
- Skin fat atrophy
- Skin necrosis
- Infection
- Recurrence
- Increased intraocular pressure or steroid-induced glaucoma
- Subcapsular or traumatic cataract
- Retinal vascular occlusion

Steroid injections can lead to skin depigmentation, fat atrophy, or skin necrosis at the injection site, more so in darker skin tones. These may resolve anywhere from 7 to 12 months after injection, although may be permanent.[6,16] Infection can be treated with oral antibiotics. Recurrence or nonresolving chalazia may be retreated with steroid injection or treated with I&C. Caution should be taken if malignancy is a suspicion. Periocular steroid injection may lead to the formation of subcapsular cataracts or traumatic cataracts if the crystalline lens is penetrated by the needle during injection.[17-19] Elevation of intraocular pressure can also occur, especially with multiple steroid injections, which although rare, could lead to steroid-induced glaucoma.[14,17,18] In rare cases, intravascular injections may lead to retrograde infiltration, which could lead to a central retinal artery or vein occlusion.[8] Two case reports have outlined individual patients who had a retinal and choroidal vascular occlusion after periocular injection of corticosteroid.[20,21] This can be avoided by injecting with low pressure to minimize the retrograde arterial flow of steroid particles or by aspirating the needle and syringe to ensure it is not in a blood vessel.[6]

## EFFICACY

Overall, the success rate of one steroid injection for a chalazion is approximately 80%.[2] A second injection can be given 1 to 4 weeks later in cases of nonresolution. One study compared the success rates of I&C versus steroid injection for the treatment of chalazia and found that the range of success rates after one steroid injection was 8.7% to 86.7%.[22] After two injections, the success rate was 0% to 53.8%. In comparison, the success rates for one I&C were 60.0% to 92.0% and 83.3% to 100% for two I&Cs.[22] Another group concluded that chalazia that are nonresponsive to two or three steroid injections would benefit from an I&C.[23]

## VIDEO OF PROCEDURE

**Video 11-1**—In this video, a chalazia is injected with 0.2 to 0.3 mL of Kenalog-40 into the left upper eyelid. Notice multiple injections are done into the chalazia to puncture and penetrate through the capsule numerous times. Care is taken to ensure as much steroid medicine is inside the chalazia, as well as surrounding the chalazia with steroid medicine. Slight pressure with a gauze or a cotton tip applicator can be applied after the injection to aid in hemostasis.

# INCISION AND CURETTAGE

## Indications

### Key Indications

- Clinically significant chalazion that is large, chronic, or has been unresponsive to other therapies

Cosmesis, discomfort, and ptosis are all possible reasons why patients opt to have a chalazion removed. Practitioners may consider I&C as initial therapy for larger chalazia or after ineffectiveness of all other therapies. Patient preference may also dictate performing an I&C earlier in the treatment paradigm.

# CONTRAINDICATIONS

### Key Contraindications

- Electronic implants (e.g., cardiac pacemaker, defibrillator)—if using radiofrequency
- Flammable fumes or liquids (e.g., oxygen, alcohol)—if using radiofrequency
- Unable to lie flat on their back for prolonged periods
- Allergies to anesthetics or medications (e.g., lidocaine, epinephrine, povidone–iodine, tobramycin, and dexamethasone)
- Suspected malignant lesions

There are few contraindications to a chalazion I&C if not using a radiofrequency device. The first two contraindications listed involve the same cautions that should be taken when using radiofrequency units. Radiofrequency devices when used with cardiac pacemakers can cause asystole and tachycardia and thus should be avoided in these patients.[24,25] If alternative treatments are not an option, the grounding plate can be placed away from the heart and the lowest power setting can be used. The cut mode (setting 1) should be avoided as it holds the highest risk of complications. Flammable fumes such as oxygen are contraindicated due to flame risk. I&C does not take an extensive amount of time, but when preparation time is included, patients should be comfortable lying flat on their back for at least 15 to 30 minutes. Caution should be taken to avoid or use alternative medications or anesthesia in the case of allergy. If there is any suspicion that the lesion may be malignant, for example, in cases of chronic, unilateral chalazion in the same location, a biopsy should be performed prior to removal.[6] If a steroid is going to be injected during or at the end of the I&C, the same precautions as listed in the "Steroid Injection" section should be exercised.

## PREOPERATIVE PREPARATION

**Key Preoperative Considerations**

- Photographs of the chalazion need to be documented and on file.
- Consent form that includes the patient's symptoms and alternatives to the chosen treatment
- Visual acuity
- Blood pressure measurement
- Pulse measurement
- Instrumentation preparation

The preoperative preparation for this procedure is straightforward. The patient should be seated in the supine position at the procedure chair, with the following instrumentation placed within arm's reach:

### Instrumentation (Figure 11-4)

1. Ophthalmic topical anesthetic (e.g., proparacaine and tetracaine)
2. 70% isopropyl alcohol prep pad
3. Local anesthesia (0.5%, 1%, or 2% lidocaine with epinephrine 1:100,000 or 1:200,000)
4. 4% topical lidocaine
5. 10% povidone–iodine (Betadine) swab sticks
6. Ophthalmic 5% povidone–iodine (Betadine)
7. 18-gauge needle to draw up anesthetic
8. 30-gauge needle (1/2″ length) to inject anesthetic
9. 3- or 5-mL syringe
10. Cotton-tipped applicators
11. Gauze
12. Sterile saline
13. Weck-Cel sponges
14. Radiofrequency unit (Ellman Surgitron Dual EMC 90 or Soniquence i100) (optional)
15. Fine wire electrode
16. Chalazion clamps: small, medium, and large sizes
17. Chalazion curettes: varying sizes
18. Westcott tenotomy scissors, blunt or sharp tip

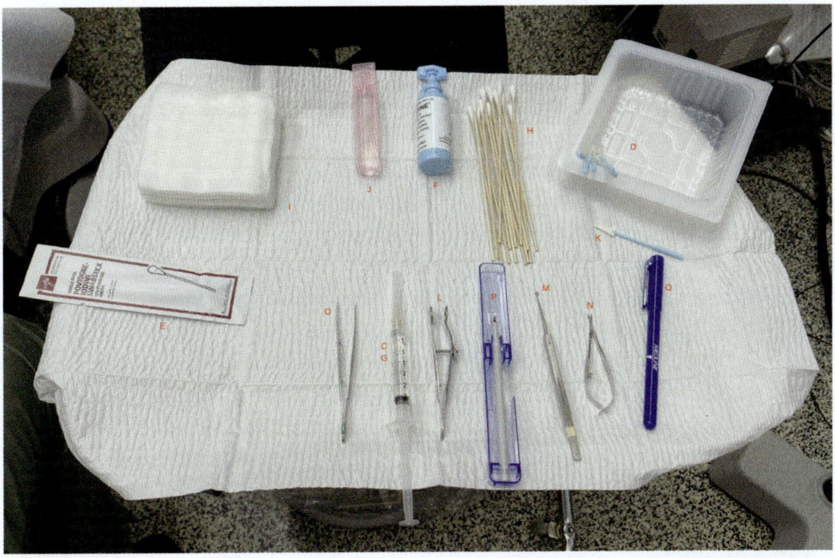

**FIGURE 11-4** Surgical tray with instrumentation needed for I&C. **A,** Ophthalmic proparacaine 0.5% (not pictured on tray), (**B**) alcohol prep pad (not pictured on tray), (**C**) 0.5% lidocaine with 1:200,000 epinephrine, (**D**) 4% topical lidocaine (sitting in the empty gauze tub with Weck-Cel sponges soaking in it), (**E**) 10% povidone-iodine (Betadine) swab sticks, (**F**) ophthalmic 5% povidone-iodine (Betadine), (**G**) 30G needle on 3-mL syringe, (**H**) cotton-tipped applicators, (**I**) gauze, (**J**) sterile saline, (**K**) Weck-Cel sponges, (**L**) chalazion clamp, (**M**) chalazion curettes, (**N**) Westcott tenotomy scissors, (**O**) toothed forceps, (**P**) blade scalpel, (**Q**) surgical skin marker, (**R**) antibiotic/steroid ointment (e.g., tobramycin 0.3%/dexamethasone 0.1%) (not pictured on tray).

19. #11 or #15 blade scalpel
20. 0.12-mm toothed forceps or jewelers forceps
21. Ophthalmic antibiotic/steroid ointment (e.g., tobramycin 0.3%/dexamethasone 0.1%)
22. Magnification: surgical microscope or ophthalmic loupes

# PROCEDURE

## Key Procedural Points

- **Radiofrequency settings (if using RF during the procedure that is optional)**
  Setting 1: cut (90% cutting, 10% coagulation)—power 10 to 15
  Setting 2: blend (50% cutting, 50% coagulation)—power 10 to 15
  Setting 3: coagulation (90% coagulation, 10% cutting)—power 8 to 10
- Sterile technique
- Patient placement at the discretion of the practitioner, with most preferring to place the patient in the supine position

## Procedural Steps

1. Place the patient in a supine position with the grounding plate of the radiofrequency unit underneath the patient's back (if radiofrequency is being used).
2. Set up the surgical microscope or loupes.
3. Instill topical anesthetic (proparacaine, tetracaine) into both eyes to minimize reflex lacrimation, the blink reflex, and keep the patient comfortable during the procedure.
4. Use an alcohol prep pad to clean around the lesion and skin where the anesthetic will be injected.
5. Use a 30-gauge needle with bevel up to inject anesthesia (0.5%, 1%, or 2% lidocaine with 1:100,000 or 1:200,000 epinephrine) subcutaneously at a 10° to 15° angle around the chalazion (Figure 11-5). A bolus should be seen where the anesthesia was injected. Continue to inject as the needle is withdrawn. If additional anesthesia is needed, the patient will feel less pain if the needle is inserted in an area that was already anesthetized.
6. A gauze pad or cotton-tipped applicator can be used to massage the anesthesia into the area.
7. Use a 10% povidone–iodine (Betadine) swab stick to clean the lesion surface, ocular adnexal area, and eyelashes to maintain asepsis. Povidone–iodine should remain on the skin for 1 to 3 minutes.
8. Use a piece of gauze to remove any excess povidone–iodine if needed, with caution not to wipe uncleaned skin onto clean skin.
9. Apply two to three drops of ophthalmic 5% povidone–iodine into the eye being treated. Let sit for 30 to 60 seconds before rinsing the eye with sterile saline[26] (Figure 11-6).
10. Use the forceps to test the area to ensure it is anesthetized (Figure 11-7). If not, inject more anesthesia.
11. Use a correctly sized chalazion clamp and insert it around the lesion, with the open side toward the inner eyelid. The clamp should be the smallest clamp possible while still fitting around the chalazion (Figures 11-8 and 11-9).

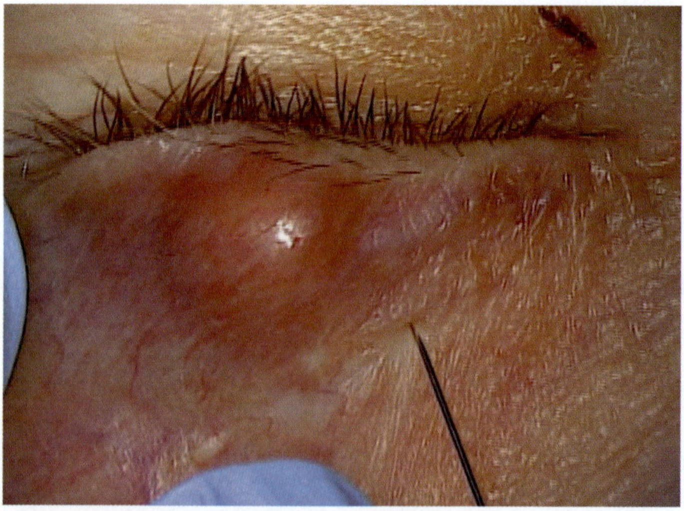

**FIGURE 11-5** Injection of lidocaine 1% with epinephrine to provide proper anesthesia for the patient.

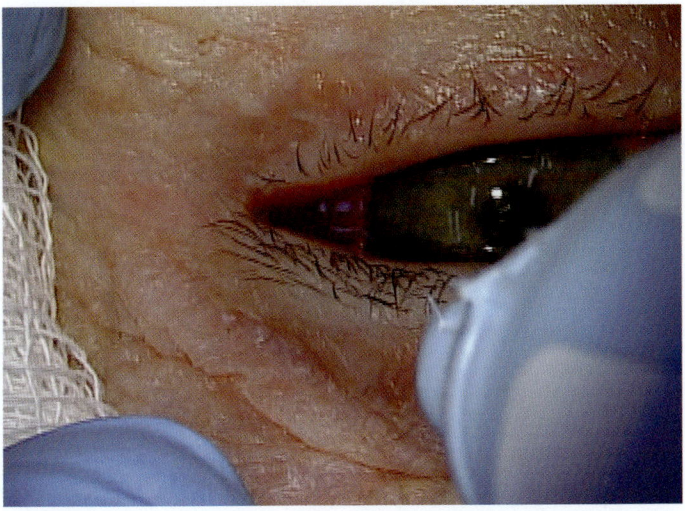

**FIGURE 11-6** Instillation of 5% ophthalmic povidone–iodine to assist in asepsis.

12. Slightly tighten the clamp, evert the eyelid, and fasten the clamp tightly (Figure 11-10).
13. Use the forceps to test the exposed side of the chalazion (palpebral conjunctiva) to ensure it is anesthetized.
14. If inadequate anesthesia is present on the palpebral conjunctiva, which commonly occurs, apply a few Weck-Cel sponges soaked in 4% topical lidocaine directly on the chalazion. Hold each sponge on the lesion for approximately 30 to 60 seconds.
15. Use the forceps to test the chalazion to ensure it is anesthetized. The patient is asked if they feel any pain or pinching. Pressure sensation is expected. Always ensure the lesion is fully anesthetized before performing the procedure.

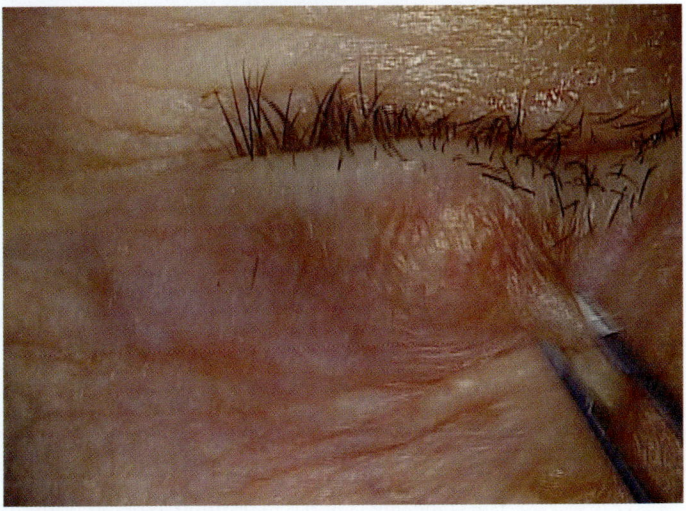

**FIGURE 11-7** Using forceps to test for adequate anesthesia.

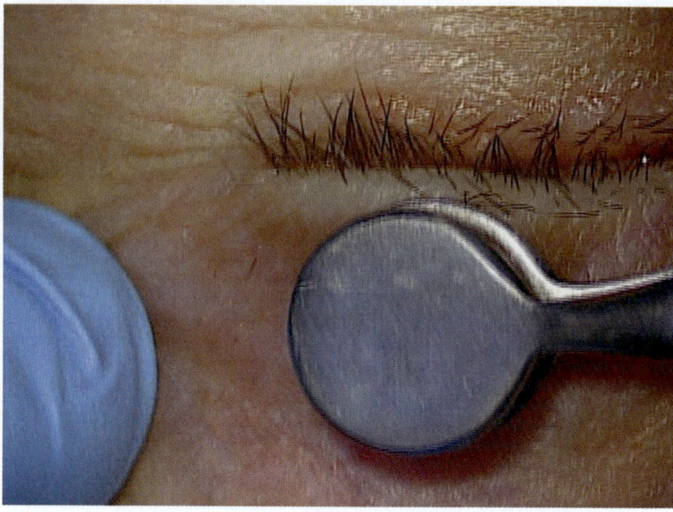

**FIGURE 11-8** Selecting the appropriate chalazion clamp size. The smallest clamp possible that will still fit around the chalazion is the desired clamp size.

16. Using a blade scalpel, make a vertical incision into the chalazion. The incision should not be closer than 2 to 3 mm from the eyelid margin.[27] Alternatively, a circular trephine blade can also be used to incise through the palpebral conjunctiva and into the chalazion (Figures 11-11 and 11-12).
17. The vertical incision may also be made with a radiofrequency unit using a fine wire electrode. Ensure the radiofrequency smoke evacuator is used to absorb the vapors. Caution should be taken not to incise too deep with the radiofrequency device as minimal to no tactile feedback is felt with that device. For that reason, it is recommended to incise with a blade scalpel.

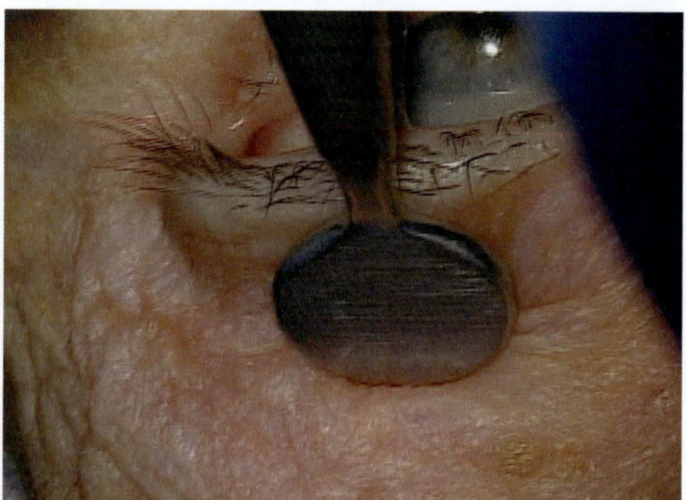

**FIGURE 11-9** The chalazion clamp is in position, is being tightened on the eyelid, and is about ready to evert the eyelid.

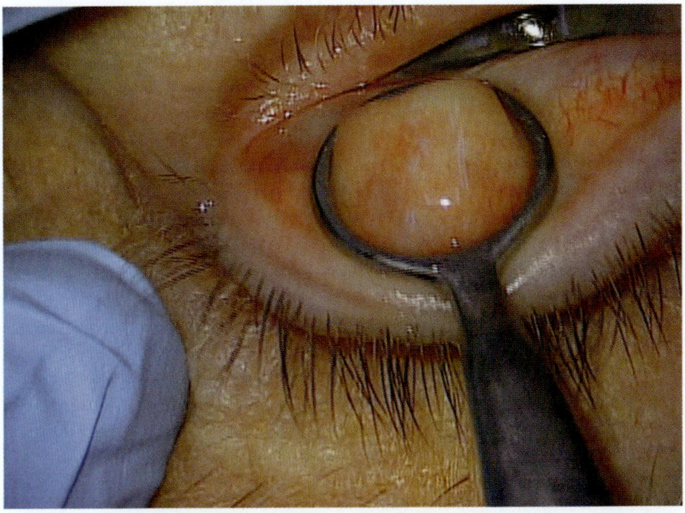

**FIGURE 11-10** Proper eversion of the eyelid with the chalazion clamp. Notice the fitting size of the chalazion clamp that isolates the chalazion very well.

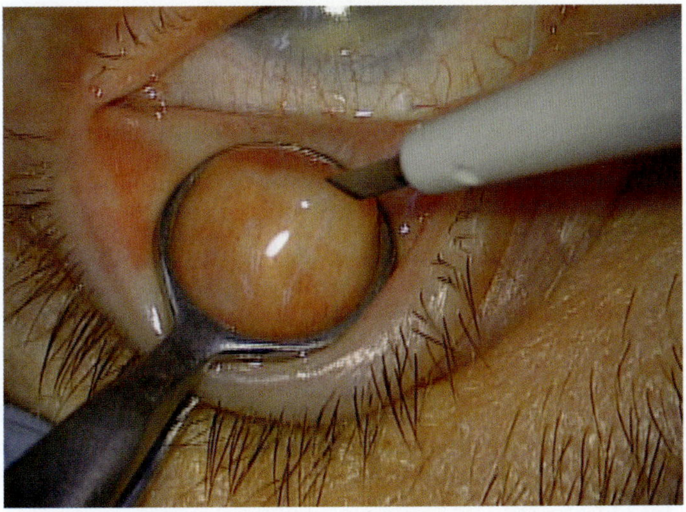

**FIGURE 11-11** Getting ready to use a small scalpel blade to vertically incise into the chalazion. Orient the sharp edge of the blade away from the globe if possible.

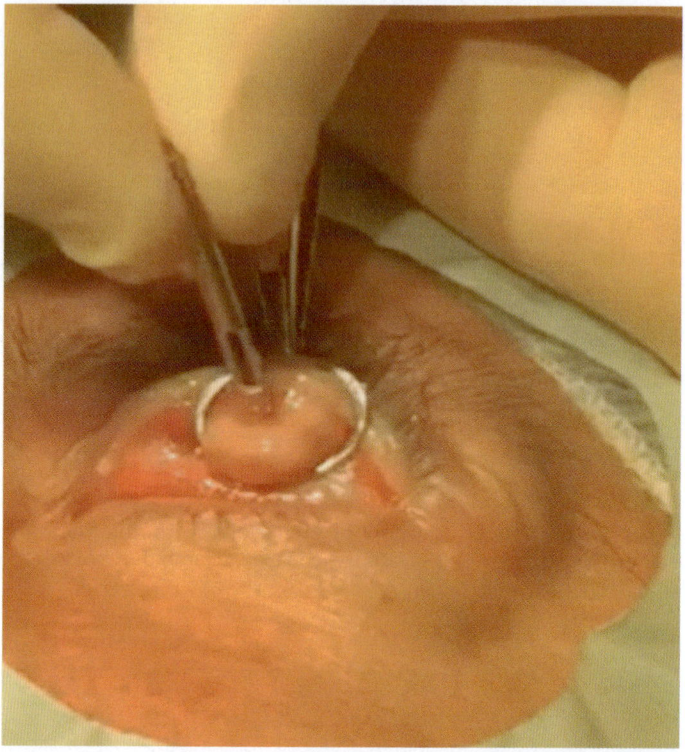

FIGURE 11-12 Alternatively, a trephine blade can also be used to make a circular incision through the palpebral conjunctiva into the chalazion.

18. Upon opening of the capsule, the chalazion contents may begin to express out of the lesion. Use a cotton-tipped applicator to remove this content (Figures 11-13 and 11-14).
19. Use a curette to remove the remainder of the chalazion contents (Figure 11-15). A cotton-tipped applicator can also be used to apply lateral pressure to aid in this removal.
20. Once the chalazion is drained, use the curette to traumatize the capsule (Figure 11-16). This helps avoid recurrence.
21. A horizontal incision parallel to the eyelid margin to make a cross-shaped incision may also be needed depending on the size of the chalazion and surgeon preference[23,24] (Figures 11-17 and 11-18). Westcott scissors may be needed to excise the fibrotic tarsal plate[24,27] (Figures 11-19 to 11-21).
22. An optional injection of 0.1 to 0.2 mL of steroid (triamcinolone acetonide suspension) may be given to aid resolution.[6]
23. Remove the chalazion clamp. No sutures or patches are needed.
24. There may be bleeding at the conclusion of the procedure once the clamp is removed as it was aiding in hemostasis. Rinse the eye with sterile saline and hold direct pressure with gauze to the closed eye to provide hemostasis (Figure 11-22). This may take 5 to 10 minutes.
25. Apply ophthalmic tobramycin 0.3%/dexamethasone 0.1% ointment to the eye.
26. Measure blood pressure and pulse.

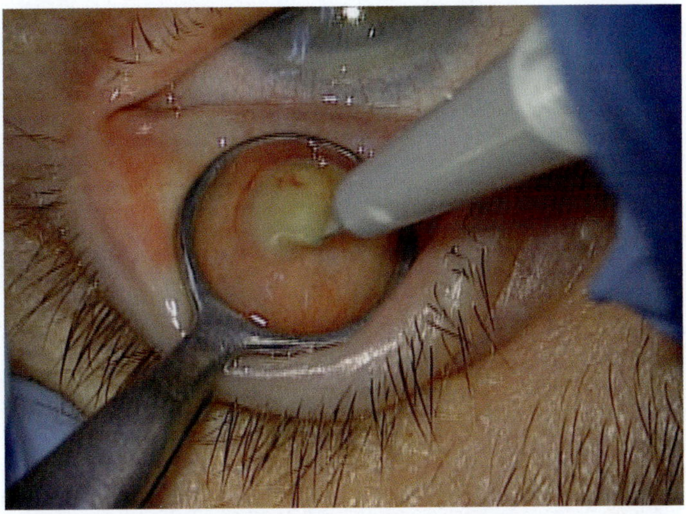

**FIGURE 11-13** Scalpel blade being used to make a vertical incision (parallel to the meibomian glands) through the palpebral conjunctiva and into the meibomian glands. Notice the cheesy material coming out.

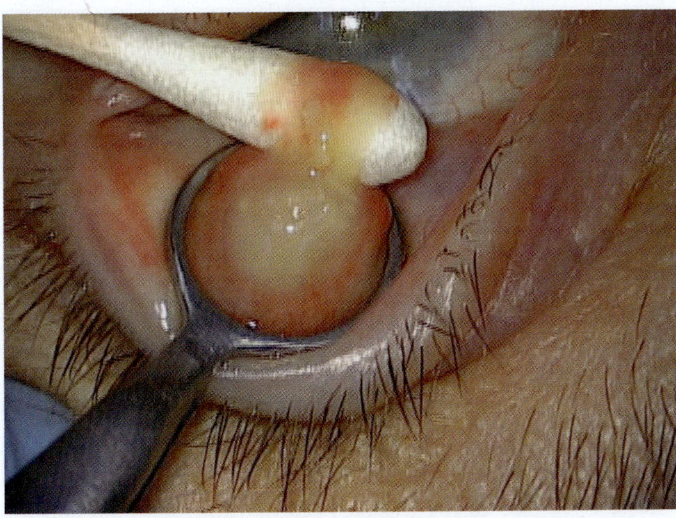

**FIGURE 11-14** Using a cotton tip applicator to soak up and remove some of the cheesy material. Weck-Cel sponges or other instruments can also be used to facilitate drainage of the chalazion.

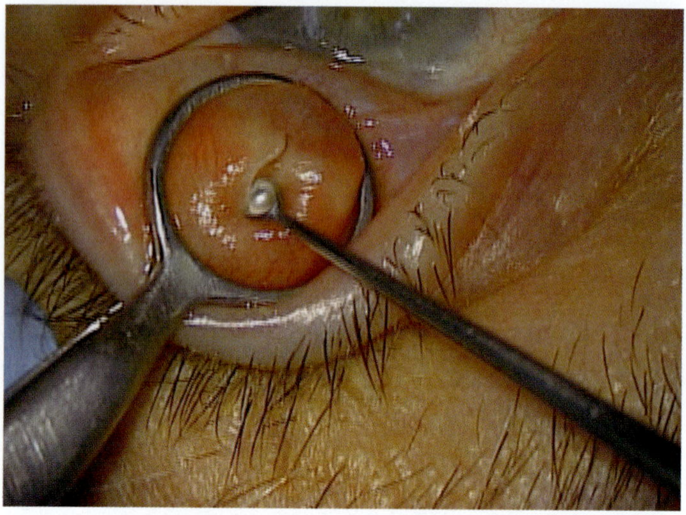

**FIGURE 11-15** The curette is used to facilitate scooping out inflammatory, cheesy material inside the chalazion. Move the curette in all directions to ensure the removal of as much content as possible.

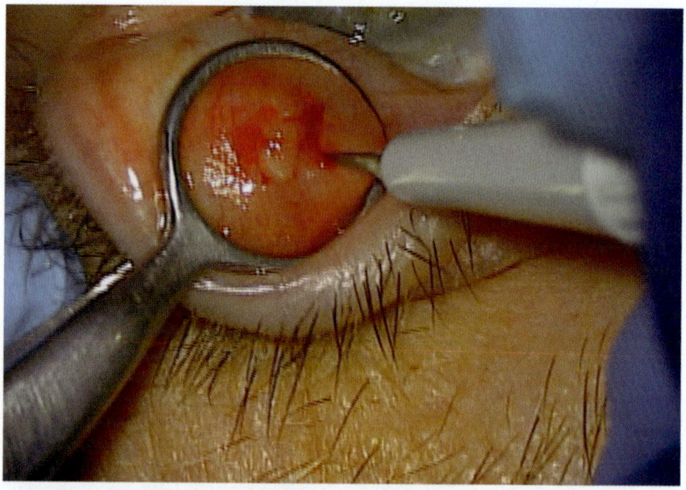

**FIGURE 11-16** Due to the chronic nature of this chalazion and the thick capsule, a horizontal incision was added to the initial vertical incision to form an "x" incision that helps with excising fibrotic capsule.

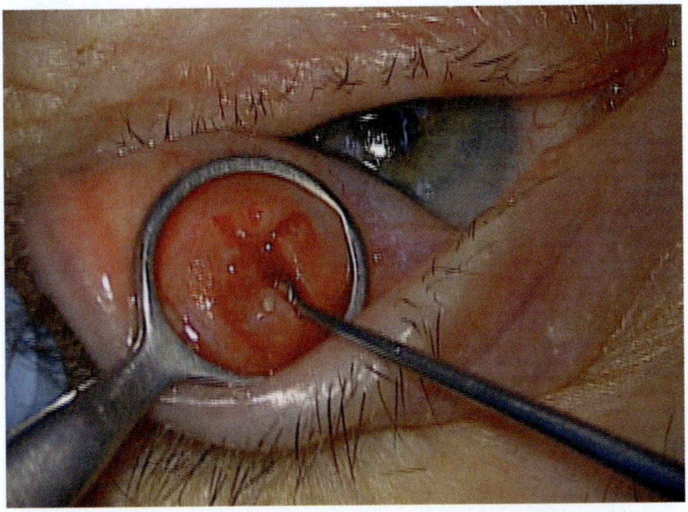

FIGURE 11-17 Following the horizontal incision, the curette was reintroduced to scoop out more material within the chalazion.

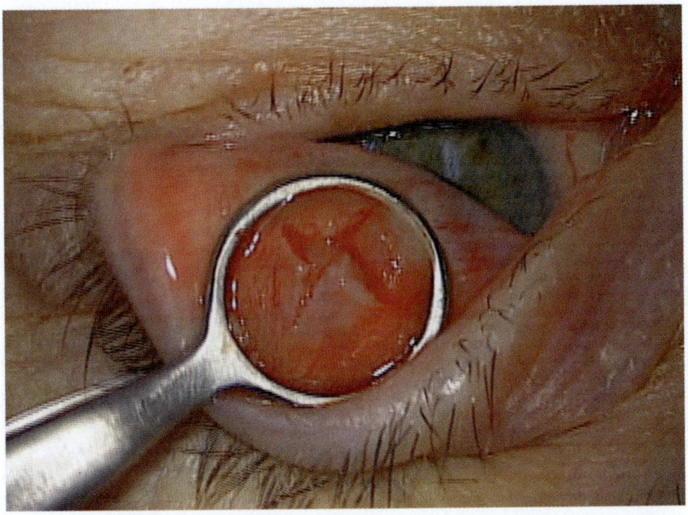

FIGURE 11-18 Classic "x" shaped incision. Notice the four flaps that are now ready to be excised.

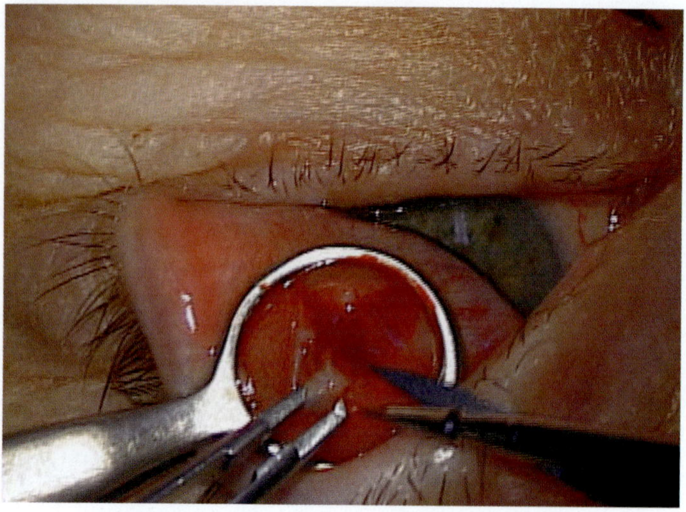

**FIGURE 11-19** Grabbing one of the flaps with a toothed forceps and getting ready to snip a portion of the anterior capsule.

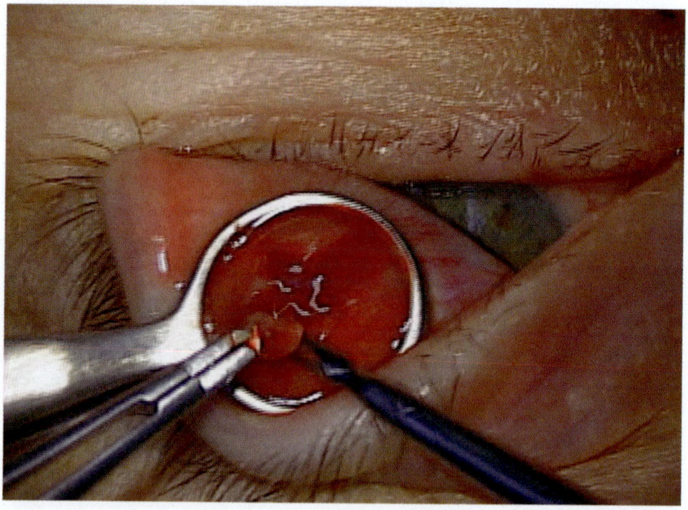

**FIGURE 11-20** Using forceps and small Westcott scissors to excise the four anterior flaps of the chalazion.

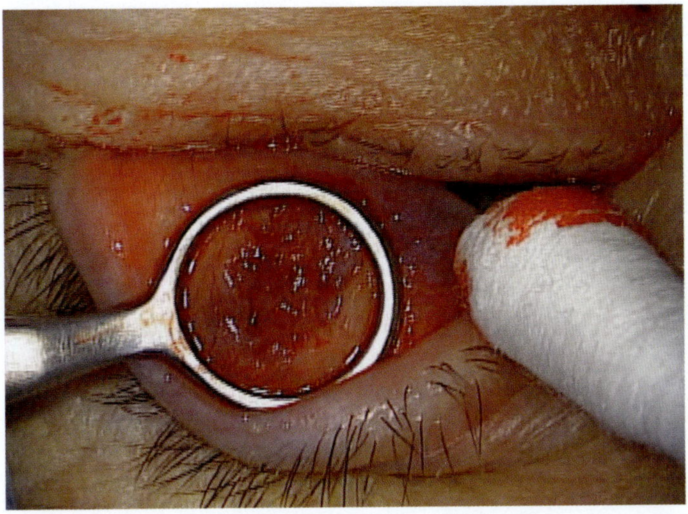

**FIGURE 11-21** At the completion of the chalazion I&C, notice the complete removal of the chalazion. The patient will be left with a conjunctival defect that will heal in the coming weeks.

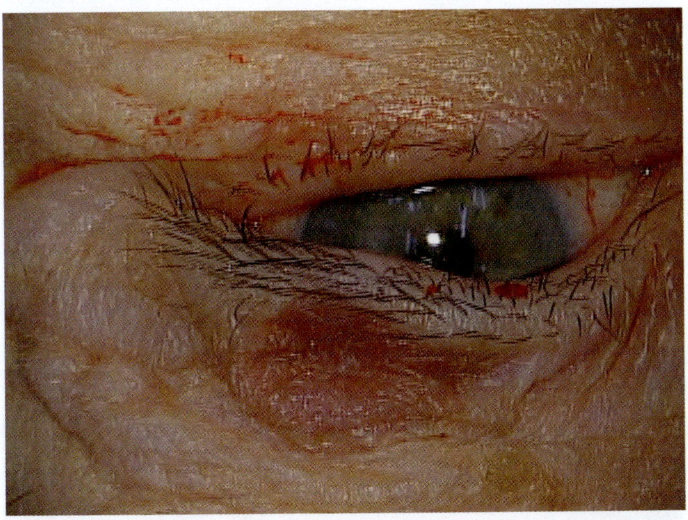

**FIGURE 11-22** The eyelid is now returned to its normal orientation, and the clamp is removed. Notice no bump remaining in the eyelid. Saline and gauze are used to clean up any residual blood on the eyelids or around the eyes.

# POSTOPERATIVE CARE/COMANAGEMENT (FOLLOW-UP SCHEDULE)

## Key Postoperative Considerations

- Documentation and operative report
- Blood pressure measurement
- Pulse measurement
- Ophthalmic antibiotic/steroid ointment (e.g., tobramycin 0.3%/dexamethasone 0.1%)
- Follow-up in 1 to 4 weeks

An operative report should be completed after every procedure that describes the steps taken to perform the procedure. Blood pressure and pulse are measured at the conclusion of the procedure due to the injection of epinephrine. An antibiotic/steroid combination ointment or antibiotic ointment is used three times a day for 7 days to prevent infection and control inflammation.[2,24] A 1- to 4-week follow-up appointment is typically scheduled to assess healing and chalazion resolution[8] (Figures 11-23 and 11-24). All patients should be educated to return to the clinic sooner if signs and symptoms of infection arise.

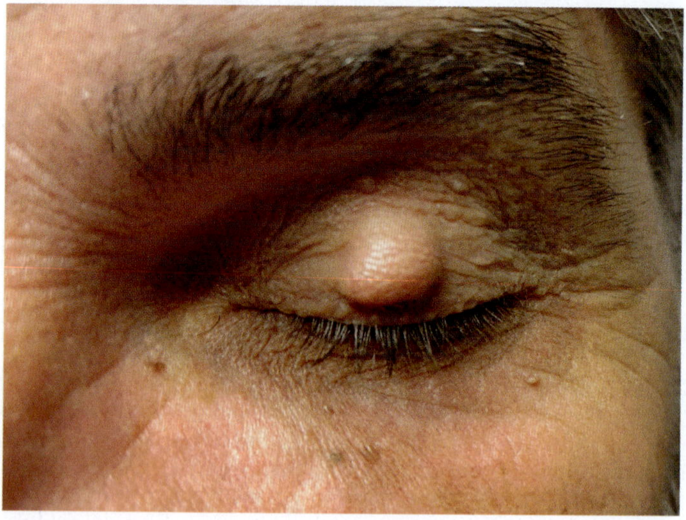

**FIGURE 11-23** Preoperative appearance of a patient prior to a chalazion I&C.

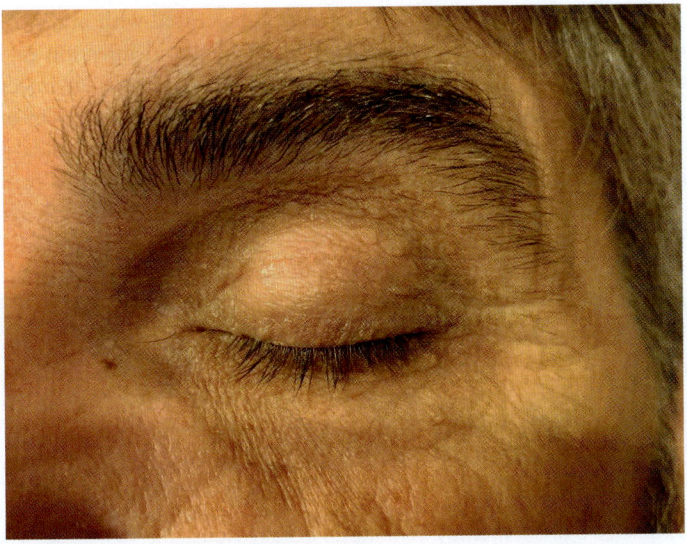

**FIGURE 11-24** One-month postoperative appearance of this same patient showing complete resolution of the chalazion, the desired result.

## POTENTIAL COMPLICATIONS AND THEIR TREATMENT

### Key Potential Complications to Look for

- Recurrence
- Redness
- Bruising
- Pain
- Infection
- Scarring of the tarsal plate
- Loss of eyelashes
- Eyelid notching
- Retinal vascular occlusion

Redness and mild pain are temporary during the postoperative phase and will self-resolve once completely healed. Bruising may occur from the injection of anesthesia and typically resolves within a week. Eyelash loss may occur if the radiofrequency device is used close to the eyelid margin and causes injury of the eyelash follicle. These eyelash bulbs are 2 mm from the eyelid margin; thus, caution should be taken to avoid this area.[27] Eyelid notching results from excessive excision of the tarsus close to the eyelid margin, which again should be performed 2 to 3 mm away from the eyelid margin.[27] Infection can be treated with oral antibiotics. Recurrence or a nonresolving chalazion may be retreated with steroid injection or I&C. Caution should be taken if malignancy is a suspicion. In rare cases, intravascular injections may lead to retrograde infiltration, which could lead to a central retinal artery or vein occlusion.[8] Two case reports have outlined individual patients who had a retinal and choroidal vascular occlusion after periocular injection of corticosteroid.[20,21] This can be avoided by injecting with low pressure to minimize retrograde arterial flow or by aspirating the needle and syringe to ensure it is not in a blood vessel.[6]

## VIDEOS OF PROCEDURES

**Video 11-2**—Chalazion I&C. In this video, a lower eyelid chalazion that had been present for approximately 4 to 6 weeks was drained via I&C. Not seen on the video was the area being prepped with an alcohol swab and 10% povidone–iodine (Betadine), as well as approximately 0.5 to 0.6 mL of lidocaine 1% with epinephrine being injected around the chalazion to provide the proper amount of local anesthesia. In the video, a large chalazion clamp is used to isolate the chalazion and flip the eyelid, and a feather blade is used to make a vertical incision through the palpebral conjunctiva, taking care to stay at least 2 to 3 mm away from the lid margin. Notice the immediate "cheesy material" that drains from the chalazion. The curette was then introduced to scoop out as much material as possible as well to traumatize the capsule. Because this chalazion was relatively new and only present for a matter of weeks, only the vertical incision was required. Once the chalazion was completely drained, the clamp was removed, the eye was rinsed with sterile saline, and gauze was held on the eye for a minute or two to help achieve hemostasis. The chalazion was completely removed, and it did not return. The patient was extremely satisfied. (Video courtesy of Nate Lighthizer.)

**Video 11-3**—Chalazion incision and curettage. In this video, a left upper eyelid chalazion that had been present for approximately 10 months was removed via I&C. The area was prepped with an alcohol swab and 5% povidone–iodine (Betadine). Approximately 0.7 to 0.8 mL of lidocaine 0.5% with epinephrine was injected around the chalazion to provide proper anesthesia. Notice multiple injections are done to ensure that enough anesthetic was injected to surround the chalazion. A perfect-fitting chalazion clamp was selected and placed around the chalazion to isolate the chalazion and flip the eyelid. A vertical incision was made with a feather blade, making sure to stay 2 to 3 mm away from the lid margin. Notice the immediate drainage of "cheesy" inflammatory material from the chalazion. A curette was introduced to help drain the contents of the chalazion. Due to the chronic nature of the chalazion (10 months), the walls of the capsule were thick and fibrotic, and therefore a horizontal incision was added to the vertical incision to form the classic "x-shaped" incision. The curette was again used, along with surgical spear sponges (Weck-Cel sponges), to scoop out as much chalazion contents as possible while at the same time traumatizing the capsule. A Westcott scissors along with 0.12 mm toothed forceps were used to excise portions of the thickened capsule (the four flaps of the "x-shaped" incision). Once the chalazion was completely drained, the clamp was removed, the eye was rinsed with sterile saline, and gauze was held on the eye for a minute or two to help achieve hemostasis. The chalazion was completely removed with no recurrence, and the patient was very happy. (Video courtesy of Nate Lighthizer.)

**Video 11-4**—Chalazion incision and curettage. In this video, a left upper eyelid chalazion that had been present for approximately 13 months was removed via I&C. The area was prepped with an alcohol swab and 10% povidone–iodine (Betadine). Approximately 0.7 to 0.8 mL of Lidocaine 0.5% with epinephrine was injected around the chalazion to provide proper anesthesia. Notice multiple injections are done to ensure that enough anesthetic was injected to surround the chalazion. Also, notice a blood vessel was nicked during the initial injection, which caused an almost immediate bruise of the eyelid. A chalazion clamp was selected and placed around the chalazion to isolate the chalazion and flip the eyelid. A vertical incision was made with a feather blade, making sure to stay 2 to 3 mm away from the lid margin. Notice the immediate drainage and forceful squirting out of "cheesy" inflammatory material from the chalazion. A cotton-tipped applicator was used to help soak up the liquid inflammatory material. A curette was introduced to help drain the contents of the chalazion. After the curette was introduced, a metallic foreign body emerged out of the chalazion through the incision! It was scooped up with the curette and placed aside. The patient could not recall getting any foreign body in the eye when his chalazion started. Due to the chronic nature of the chalazion (13 months), the walls of the capsule were thick and fibrotic, and therefore a horizontal incision was added to the vertical incision to form the classic "x-shaped" incision. A Westcott scissors along with 0.12-mm toothed forceps were used to excise portions of the thickened capsule (the four flaps of the "x-shaped" incision). Once the chalazion was completely drained and as much thickened capsule as possible excised, the clamp was removed, the eye rinsed with sterile saline, and gauze held on the eye for a minute or two to help achieve hemostasis. The chalazion was completely removed with no recurrence, and the patient was thrilled. See Figures 11.23 and 11.24 for preoperative and 1-month postoperative photos, respectively. (Video courtesy of Nate Lighthizer & Komal Patel.)

**Video 11-5**—Chalazion incision and drainage. (Video courtesy of Leonid Skorin Jr and Kynndyl Giannonatti.)

**Video 11-6**—Kissing chalazia incision and drainage. (Video courtesy of Leonid Skorin Jr and Andrew Krein.)

**Video 11-7**—Chalazion incision and drainage. (Video courtesy of Leonid Skorin Jr and Andrew Mackner.)

## EFFICACY

One prospective randomized treatment study found the resolution rate after triamcinolone acetonide injection and I&C to be 84% and 87%, respectively.[10] Pain scores were lower in the steroid injection group, but overall satisfaction scores were equal between both steroid injection and I&C.[10] Another prospective randomized clinical trial studied the outcomes of triamcinolone injection and I&C for primary chalazion. They found complete resolution in 79% of I&C patients and 81% of steroid injection patients.[28] Another group found a success rate of 79% after one I&C and 89% after a second I&C.[29]

A group of researchers studied the advantage of injecting subtarsal steroid after I&C. They found that steroid injection administered simultaneously with an I&C led to decreased rates of chalazion recurrence.[17] In the 25 patients who received steroid injection with I&C, all patients showed resolution within 1 week and no recurrence during the 6-month follow-up period. In the 25 patients who underwent I&C only, 14 patients showed a quicker resolution than the group who received I&C plus steroid, but 11 ended up having a chalazion recur in the same eyelid.[17] This lends support that steroid injection with I&C may be strongly considered if there are no contraindications to steroid use.

## CODING/BILLING

- **CPT code: 11900**—Inject into the skin lesion
- **CPT code: J3301**—Injection, triamcinolone acetonide, not otherwise specified, 10 mg, 40 mg
- **CPT code: 67800**—Chalazion excision, single

- **CPT code: 67801**—Chalazion excision, multiple, same lid
- **CPT code: 67805**—Chalazion excision, multiple, different lids
- **CPT codes: 11900, 67800, 67801, and 67805** have a 10-day postoperative global period.

Common ICD-10 codes that support this procedure include the following:

- **H00.11** (chalazion right upper eyelid)
- **H00.12** (chalazion right lower eyelid)
- **H00.13** (chalazion right eye, unspecified eyelid)
- **H00.14** (chalazion left upper eyelid)
- **H00.15** (chalazion left lower eyelid)
- **H00.16** (chalazion left eye, unspecified eyelid)
- **H00.19** (chalazion unspecified eye, unspecified eyelid)

## REFERENCES


1. Penne RB. *Oculoplastics*. 2nd ed. Lippincott Williams & Wilkins Health; 2012.
2. Bowling B, Kanski JJ. *Kanski's Clinical Ophthalmology: A Systematic Approach*. 8th ed. Elsevier; 2016.
3. Yanoff M, Fine BS. *Ocular Pathology: A Text and Atlas*. 2nd ed. Harper & Row; 1982.
4. Pe'er J. Pathology of eyelid tumors. *Indian J Ophthalmol.* 2016;64:177-190.
5. Nema HV, Nema N, eds. *Ocular Tumors*. Springer Singapore; 2021.
6. Bobby SK, Don K, eds. *Video Atlas of Oculofacial Plastic and Reconstructive Surgery*. 2nd ed. Elsevier; 2017.
7. Sun M, Huang S, Huilgol S, Silva D. Eyelid lesions in general practice. *Aust J Gen Pract.* 2019;48:509-514.
8. Ehler JP; Wills Eye Hospital, eds. *The Wills Eye Manual: Office and Emergency Room Diagnosis and Treatment of Eye Disease*. 5th ed. Lippincott Williams & Wilkins; 2008.
9. Lee JWY, Yau GSK, Wong MYY, Yuen CYF. A comparison of intralesional triamcinolone acetonide injection for primary chalazion in children and adults. *Sci World J.* 2014:1-4.
10. Goawalla A, Lee V. A prospective randomized treatment study comparing three treatment options for chalazia: triamcinolone acetonide injections, incision and curettage and treatment with hot compresses. *Clin Exp Ophthalmol.* 2007;35:706-712.
11. Krout C, Peter LA. Tetracyclines: history and current formulation review from a dermatology perspective. *Practical Dermatology*. 2015. https://practicaldermatology.com/articles/2015-feb/tetracyclines-history-and-current-formulation-review-from-a-dermatology-perspective#:~:text=Tetracyclines%20are%20essentially%20absorbed%20completely,in%20the%20urine%20and%20feces
12. Lighthizer N, ed. *The Ophthalmic Laser Handbook*. Wolters Kluwer; 2022.
13. Caravaca A, Alió del Barrio JL, Martínez Hergueta MC, Amesty MA. Intense pulsed light combined with meibomian gland expression for chalazion management. *Arch Soc Esp Oftalmol (Engl Ed)*. 2022;97:490-496.
14. Naik V, B Vasu S. Comparison of intralesional injection of triamcinolone—40 mg/ml and Triamcinolone—10 mg/ml in treatment of chalazion. *IP Int J Ocul Oncol Oculoplasty.* 2021;6:243-247.
15. Ho SY, Lai JSM. Subcutaneous steroid injection as treatment for chalazion: prospective case series. *Hong Kong Med J.* 2002;8:18-20.
16. Park J, Chang M. Eyelid fat atrophy and depigmentation after an intralesional injection of triamcinolone acetonide to treat chalazion. *J Craniofac Surg.* 2017;28:e198-e199.
17. Qurban Q, Kamil Z, Mahmood K. Added advantage of injecting subtarsal steroid injection after incision and curettage of multiple chalazion. *J Ayub Med Coll Abbottabad.* 2021;33:437-440.
18. Carnahan MC, Goldstein DA. Ocular complications of topical, peri-ocular, and systemic corticosteroids. *Curr Opin Ophthalmol.* 2000;11:478-483.
19. Hoşal BM, Zilelioğlu G. Ocular complication of intralesional corticosteroid injection of a chalazion. *Eur J Ophthalmol.* 2003;13:798-799.
20. Thomas EL, Laborde RP. Retinal and choroidal vascular occlusion following intralesional corticosteroid injection of a chalazion. *Ophthalmology.* 1986;93:405-407.

21. Yağci A, Palamar M, Eğrilmez S, Şahbazov C, Özbek SS. Anterior segment ischemia and retinochoroidal vascular occlusion after intralesional steroid injection. *Ophthalmic Plast Reconstruct Surg.* 2008;24:55-57.
22. Aycinena ARP, Achiron A, Paul M, Burgansky-Eliash Z. Incision and curettage versus steroid injection for the treatment of chalazia: a meta-analysis. *Ophthalmic Plast Reconstr Surg.* 2016;32:220-224.
23. Unal M. Chalazion treatment. *Orbit.* 2008;27:397-398.
24. Fowler GC, ed. *Pfenninger & Fowler's Procedures for Primary Care.* 4th ed. Elsevier; 2020.
25. Robinson JK, ed. *Surgery of the Skin: Procedural Dermatology.* 3rd ed. Saunders Elsevier; 2015.
26. Ferguson AW, Scott JA, McGavigan J, et al. Comparison of 5% povidone-iodine solution against 1% povidone-iodine solution in preoperative cataract surgery antisepsis: a prospective randomised double blind study. *Br J Ophthalmol.* 2003;87:163-167.
27. Dutton JJ. *Atlas of Oculoplastic and Orbital Surgery.* 2nd ed. Wolters Kluwer; 2019.
28. Ben Simon GJ, Rosen N, Rosner M, Spierer A. Intralesional triamcinolone acetonide injection versus incision and curettage for primary chalazia: a prospective, randomized study. *Am J Ophthalmol.* 2011;151:714-718.e1.
29. Ahmad S, Baig MA, Khan MA, Khan I-H, Janjua TA. Intralesional corticosteroid injection vs surgical treatment of chalazia in pigmented patients. *J Coll Physicians Surg Pak.* 2006;16:42-44.

## SUPPLEMENTAL READING

See McGee SR, Stonecipher K. Intense pulsed light therapy. In: Freisberg L, Lighthizer N, Skorin L, Stonecipher K, Zimmerman AB, eds. *The Ophthalmic Laser Handbook.* Wolters Kluwer; 2022: 371-391 for a detailed description on intense pulsed light therapy.

# 12 Lid-Everting Sutures for Entropion

**Brandon Runyon**

## BACKGROUND

Lid-everting sutures for entropion repair are a simple, noninvasive procedure that can be performed in the office or even bedside in a nursing home or hospital with minimal equipment. The utilization of lid-everting sutures for entropion repair was first described in 1971 by Marvin Quickert, MD, and has also been called "Quickert suture" repair of entropion.[1] Three sutures are placed in the lower lid, plicating the lower lid retractors. The sutures pull on the anterior lid causing eversion of the entropic lid.[2] Subsequent inflammation and fibrosis occur along the suture track, which are critical to the success of the procedure.[3] Sutures are then removed within the first 1 to 2 weeks following the procedure or left to dissolve on their own based on provider preference and patient healing.

Although surgery techniques for entropion repair have evolved over time to be more successful in correcting entropion and preventing recurrence, this procedure still remains a simple yet valuable tool in any clinician's armamentarium for the management of involutional entropion. It can be particularly useful for patients who would prefer less invasive options, are medically fragile, or unable to access an oculoplastic specialist.

## INDICATIONS

**Key Indications**

- Involutional entropion
- Spastic entropion

The primary indication for an entropion repair by suture is an involutional entropion, which may also be known as a "senile entropion." Involutional entropion is the most common form of entropion encountered by clinicians. Horizontal lid laxity is the primary factor in the development of involutional entropion resulting from medial and canthal tendon laxity in conjunction with age-related tarsal thinning.[4]

A second indication in which lid-everting sutures may be rarely used is spastic (intermittent) entropion. As the name implies, it is thought that inflammation, infection, or prior ocular surgery may cause an intermittent spasm of the orbicularis oculi muscle, resulting in a temporary inward rolling of the lower eyelid. Clinically, these patients may present with no issues in the office if the entropion is very infrequent. They may also present with frequent—but not constant—inward rolling of the lower eyelid. This event often is intermittent yet can still be frustrating for the patient, causing discomfort, irritation, and tearing. Because the etiology is primarily muscular, these patients often respond well to botulinum toxin (Botox) injections to relax these spasms temporarily.[5] See Chapter 23—Neurotoxin. However, for more frequent spasms or recalcitrant cases, lid-everting sutures may be a minimally invasive treatment option.

## CONTRAINDICATIONS

### Key Contraindications

- Cicatricial entropion
- Congenital entropion
- Allergy to chromic gut or Vicryl suture materials (rare)

Absolute contraindications to entropion repair by suture include any form of cicatricial entropion or congenital entropion due to etiologies that do not involve lower eyelid retractor dehiscence. In cases of cicatricial entropion, the inferior fornix is often shortened due to scar tissue formation whereas the lower eyelid retractors are usually intact and attached to the inferior tarsal plate. Cicatricial entropion usually occurs in chronic inflammatory conditions such as Stevens–Johnson syndrome (SJS), ocular cicatricial pemphigoid (OCP), and trachoma.

There is not a universally agreed upon surgical approach to repair congenital entropion as the etiology is not well understood. It has been postulated that perhaps there is overactivity of the orbicularis oculi in combination with disinsertion of the inferior lid retractor muscles.[4] Congenital entropion is often encountered secondary to epiblepharon in the Asian pediatric population.[6] However, persistent congenital entropion is encountered less frequently as the condition often improves and spontaneously resolves with facial bone growth during normal aging into adolescence, negating the need for surgical intervention in most cases.[7]

Other less frequent causes of congenital entropion include congenital facial nerve paralysis resulting in the absence of oppositional force to inferior tarsus muscle retraction by the orbicularis oculi.[8] Because of the neurogenic etiology, entropion repair by suture is contraindicated.

Finally, this procedure should not be utilized in patients with known hypersensitivity to the selected suture materials (usually chromic gut or Vicryl). In the event of lidocaine allergy, alternative agents may be used for local anesthesia such as chloroprocaine injection or diphenhydramine injection.

## INFORMED CONSENT CONSIDERATIONS

### Key Informed Consent Adverse Events Listed

- Infection
- Bleeding and bruising
- Scarring
- Pain or discomfort at the surgical site(s)
- Anaphylactic reaction to medications
- Foreign body sensation
- Tearing
- Blurred vision
- Undercorrection of entropion
- Overcorrection of entropion (i.e., "ectropion")
- Recurrence

The informed consent should describe the procedure in plain language, such as the following: "Your provider will instill eye drops and inject medication(s) to numb the eye and eyelid prior to the procedure. Multiple sutures will then be placed in the eyelid to help rotate the eyelid outward and prevent the eyelid and eyelashes from rubbing against the eye. This will reduce the risk of chronic eye irritation, chronic tearing, chronic discharge, and more serious eye conditions including corneal ulcers and corneal perforations."

Potential alternative treatments, such as eye drops, monitoring, Botox injection, or invasive surgery, should be listed. Risks and complications inherent to any procedure of the skin include but are not limited to infection, bleeding, bruising, and pain or discomfort at the surgical site(s). Due to the placement of sutures on the palpebral side of the conjunctiva, there may be resulting foreign body sensation, tearing, and blurred vision. Complications more specific to this procedure include undercorrection of entropion, overcorrection of entropion (i.e., "ectropion"), and recurrence of entropion.

## PREOPERATIVE CARE

### Key Preoperative Considerations

- Slit-lamp examination of anterior segment to confirm entropion diagnosis
- Careful examination of inferior conjunctival fornix to exclude findings consistent with cicatricial entropion such as symblepharon, shortened fornices, and so on
- Preoperative drops: topical anesthetic (e.g., proparacaine)
- Preoperative meds: lidocaine 1% with epinephrine

- Suggested materials:
  - Mayo stand with a sterile drape
  - Surgical skin marker
  - Sterile gloves
  - Sterile gauze
  - Sterile cotton-tipped applicators
  - Sterile saline
  - 3-cc syringe with 27G or 30G 1/2″ to 1″ needle
  - Antibiotic ointment
  - 5-0 double-armed chromic gut suture with reverse cutting needle *or* 5-0 double-armed Vicryl sutures with reverse cutting needle
  - 1 × 2 ophthalmic tissue forceps
  - Ophthalmic needle drivers
  - Westcott or Vannas micro-scissors
  - McPherson tying forceps (optional; knots may be tied by hand if desired)

Slit-lamp examination should confirm the diagnosis of involutional entropion and specifically exclude cicatricial and congenital etiologies. Careful examination of the inferior fornix should exclude the presence of symblepharon, shortened fornices, and other findings consistent with cicatricial entropion as this will require further workup and differing treatment approaches.

Clinical findings diagnostic of involutional entropion include an inward-turned lower eyelid with the lower lid margin and/or lower eyelashes in contact with the globe. The incorrect lid position and frictional force against the globe often lead to chronic tearing, foreign body sensation, conjunctivitis, and corneal scarring. Corneal ulceration or perforation is also possible in more severe cases.

A few additional tests can be used to properly diagnose involutional entropion. The first is direct observation of the lower lid movement in downgaze. Normally, while in downgaze, the lower eyelid should retract; however, due to weak or disinserted lower lid retractors in involutional entropion, the retraction may be reduced or completely absent.[9]

Second, the horizontal lid laxity test (also known as the "snap back test") is a direct measure of canthal tendon laxity and is simple to perform and easy to interpret for all clinicians. The test involves pulling the lower eyelid downward and releasing the lid. The clinician then observes the ability of the lid to return to the normal position in the absence of blinking. A normal result is the immediate return ("snap back") of the lower eyelid to its normal lid position. An abnormal result is subjectively graded on the basis of delayed return or complete absence of return of the lid to the normal lid position.[4,9]

Third, a careful slit-lamp examination of the inferior fornix is done to directly observe lower lid retractor dehiscence. Some clinicians have described lid retractor dehiscence appearing as a "delicate white line between the tarsus and the fornix," though this may be hard to appreciate for all clinicians. Although this is certainly a definitive feature of senile ectropion, the absence of this clinical feature alone does not exclude involutional entropion as a diagnosis.[9] Clinicians still need to assess for other clinical history and findings that may point toward spastic, cicatricial, or congenital etiologies.

Congenital entropion can usually be excluded by the age of the patient and/or the duration of symptoms. However, Asian descent and/or the presence of epiblepharon in an adult patient may also suggest a congenital etiology that might warrant an alternative surgical approach.

An array of surgical procedures may be utilized in the correction of senile entropion, ranging from simple procedures such as lid-everting sutures to more technical procedures such as lateral tarsal strip, suture canthopexy, or lower lid retractor reinsertion. Lid-everting sutures are often utilized with the lateral tarsal strip procedure to reduce recurrence rates.[10]

# PROCEDURE

## Key Procedural Points

- Subcutaneous and subconjunctival lidocaine 1% with epinephrine for procedural anesthesia
- Skin is marked in three target locations with a surgical skin marker:
  - Center of the lower lid
  - 4 to 5 mm lateral to the punctum
  - 4 to 5 mm medial to the lateral canthus
- Three 5-0 double-armed chromic gut sutures are placed through the inferior fornix, emerging approximately 2 to 3 mm below the lash line. (Note: Double-armed sutures have a needle on both ends of the suture.)
- Each arm of the suture should enter and emerge approximately 2 to 3 mm apart in the lower lid near the marked locations.
- The desired lid position is slightly ectropic at the conclusion of the procedure.
- Antibiotic ophthalmic ointment is applied to the fornix and exposed sutures.

In preparation for the procedure, a mayo stand should be draped with a sterile cover with all instrumentation readily available. A drop of topical anesthetic such as proparacaine is instilled in the eye. The external skin should be cleaned and prepped using an alcohol prep pad or betadine swab. Next, a subcutaneous injection of lidocaine 1% with epinephrine is injected into the external lid for anesthesia (Figure 12-1). The medication can be spread across the lid using gentle pressure with sterile gauze or a sterile cotton-tipped applicator. A sterile eye drape is then placed (Figure 12-2).

Following the application of the drape, skin markings should be placed on the external lid to aid in suture placement. The first mark should be made in the center of the lower lid approximately 2 to 3 mm below the inferior lash line (Figure 12-3). The second and third marks

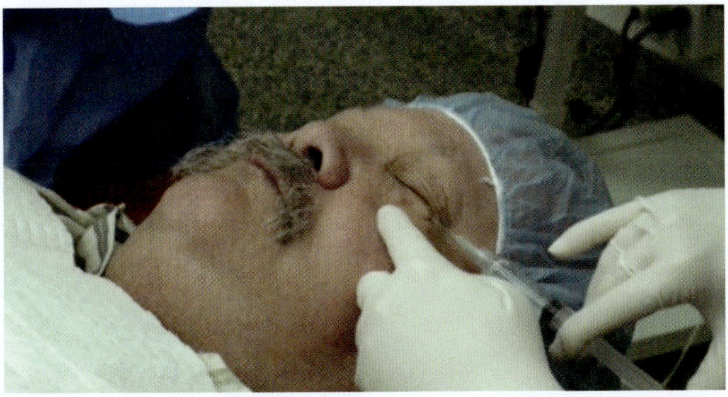

**FIGURE 12-1** Subcutaneous injection of lidocaine 1% with epinephrine into external eyelid prior to inserting sutures. (Photo courtesy of Nate Lighthizer, OD.)

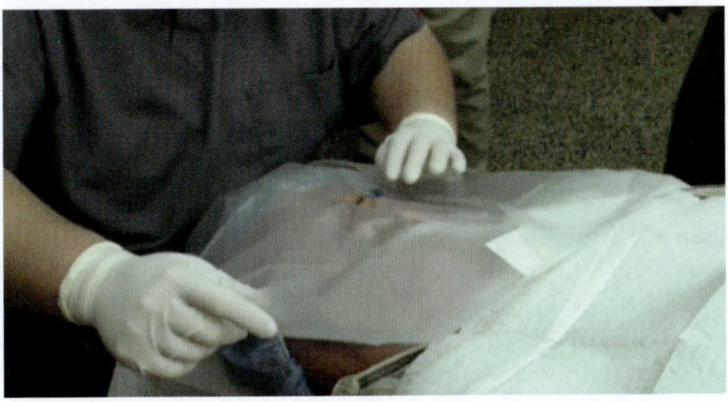

**FIGURE 12-2** Sterile ophthalmic drape placement. (Photo courtesy of Nate Lighthizer, OD.)

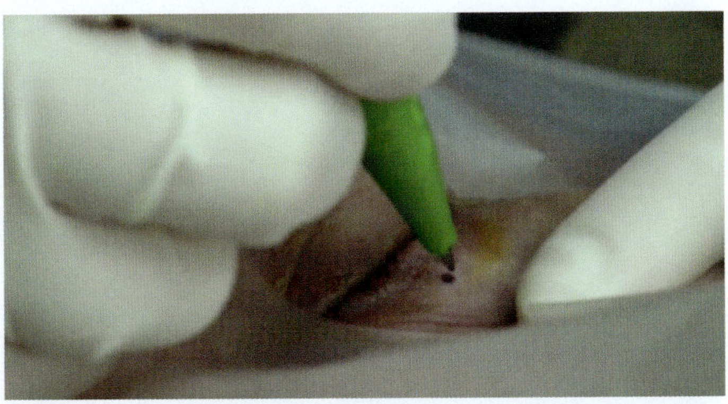

**FIGURE 12-3** Using a surgical skin marker to dot the external skin to provide a target for the reverse cutting needle as it is driven through the palpebral conjunctiva and eyelid skin. (Photo courtesy of Nate Lighthizer, OD.)

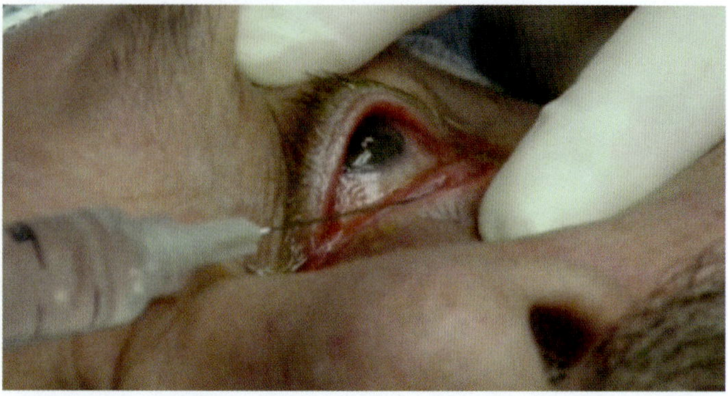

**FIGURE 12-4** Subconjunctival injection of lidocaine 1% with epinephrine injected into the posterior aspect of the eyelid. (Photo courtesy of Nate Lighthizer, OD.)

should be made 4 to 5 mm lateral to the punctum and 4 to 5 mm medial to the lateral canthus, respectively (see Figures 12-5 and 12-6 for examples of placement).

An injection of subconjunctival lidocaine 1% with epinephrine is then placed under the palpebral conjunctiva for additional patient comfort (Figure 12-4). Complete anesthesia of the palpebral conjunctiva and external skin of the eyelid should be confirmed before proceeding further.

Beginning near the central lower lid marking, the first arm of the 5-0 chromic gut suture should be passed through the palpebral conjunctiva in the inferior fornix to the external lid (Figures 12-5 and 12-6). An ophthalmic needle driver is then used to pull the needle through the skin of the eyelid (Figure 12-7). Moving 2 to 3 mm adjacent to the first pass of the suture, pass the second arm of the 5-0 chromic gut suture through the lid in the same manner, entering and emerging 2 to 3 mm adjacent to the first arm of the suture on the external lid (Figures 12-8 and 12-9).

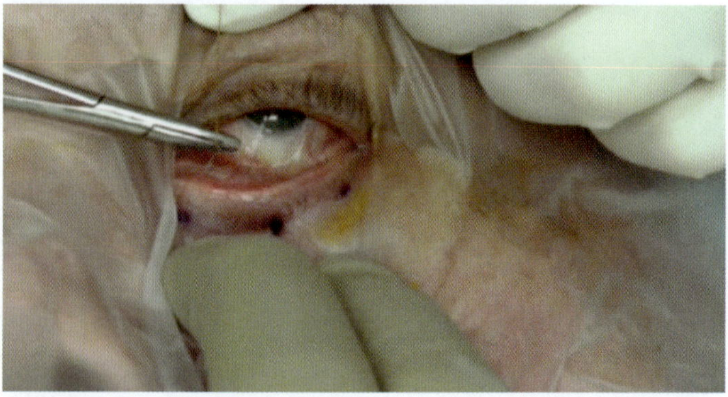

**FIGURE 12-5** Using a needle driver to place the first pass of double-armed suture through the palpebral conjunctiva. (Photo courtesy of Nate Lighthizer, OD.)

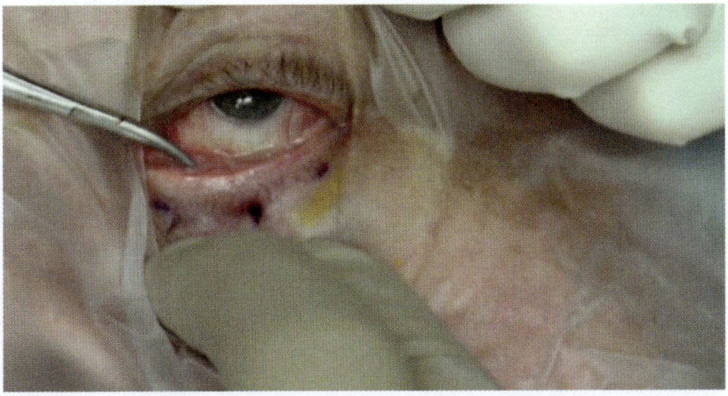

**FIGURE 12-6** Passing the double-armed suture through the posterior lid to the anterior lid with needle drivers. (Photo courtesy of Nate Lighthizer, OD.)

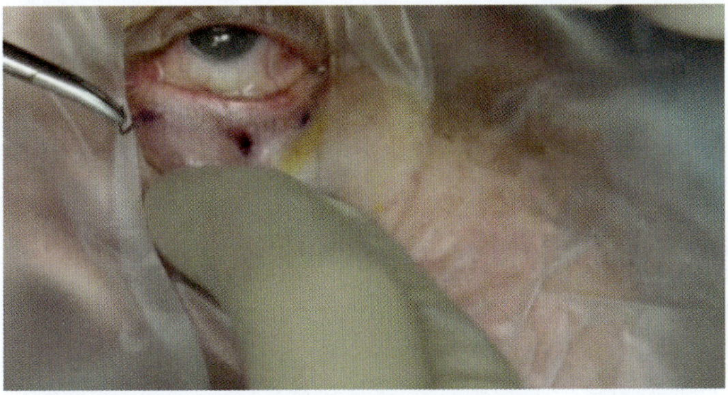

**FIGURE 12-7** Pulling the needle through the skin with needle drivers. (Photo courtesy of Nate Lighthizer, OD.)

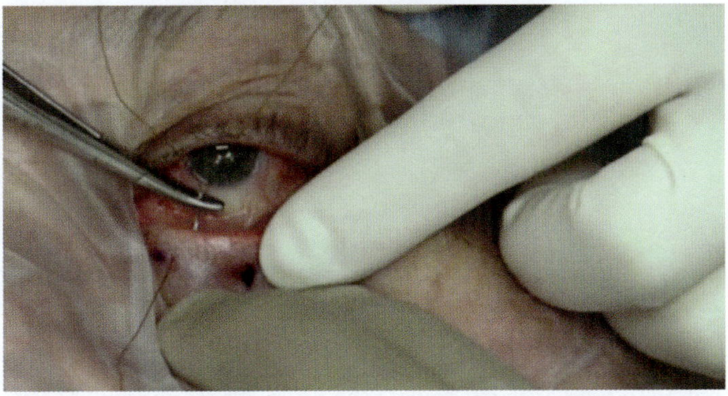

**FIGURE 12-8** Passing the needle of the second arm (on the opposite end of the suture) through the eyelid. Placement should be roughly 2 to 3 mm from where the first needle was passed through. (Photo courtesy of Nate Lighthizer, OD.)

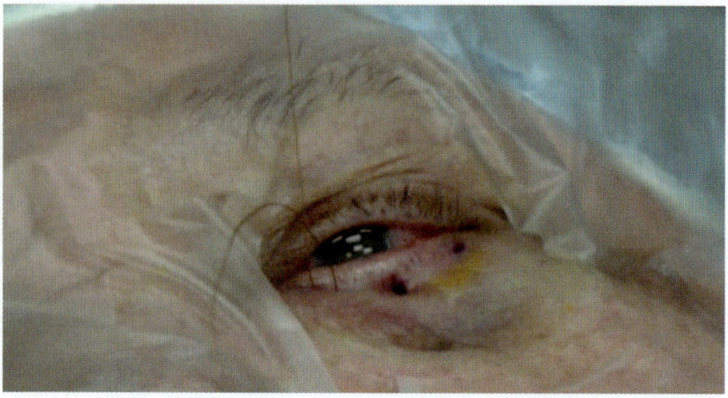

**FIGURE 12-9** The needles have now passed through the posterior lid to the anterior lid. (Photo courtesy of Nate Lighthizer, OD.)

A surgeon's knot should then be tied with enough tension to evert the lid to a slightly ectropic position (Figure 12-10). The tails of the surgeon's knot are then cut short with Vannas or Westcott scissors (Figure 12-11).

This process should be repeated at the medial and lateral target locations. It is critical to avoid the punctum at the medial suture location. The desired endpoint is a slightly ectropic lower lid immediately following the procedure (Figure 12-12). Antibiotic ophthalmic ointment should be placed in the conjunctival fornix and along the exposed sutures at the conclusion of the procedure. An additional example of the preoperative and postoperative appearances is demonstrated in Figures 12-13 and 12-14.

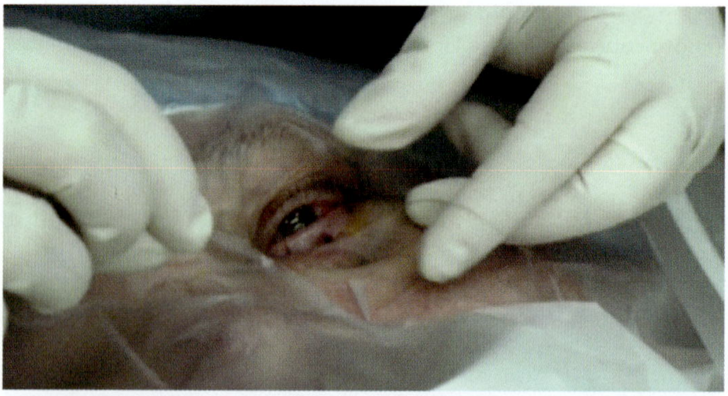

**FIGURE 12-10** A surgeon's knot is being tied to tightly secure the suture in place. The knot should indent or dimple the skin, but should not be so tight as to strangulate the tissue. (Photo courtesy of Nate Lighthizer, OD.)

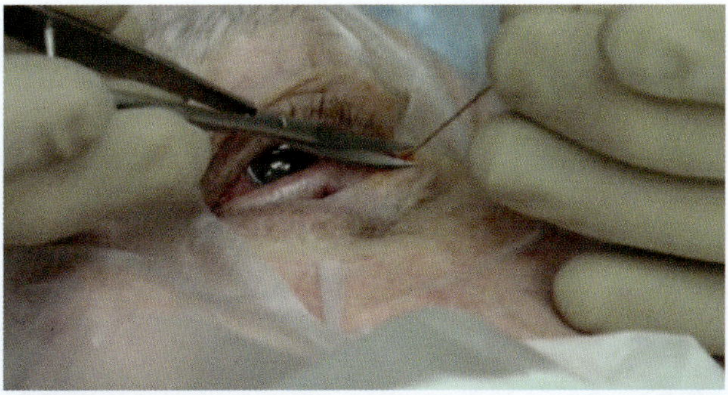

FIGURE 12-11 After tying the knot, the excess suture material is trimmed with Westcott or Vannas micro-scissors. (Photo courtesy of Nate Lighthizer, OD.)

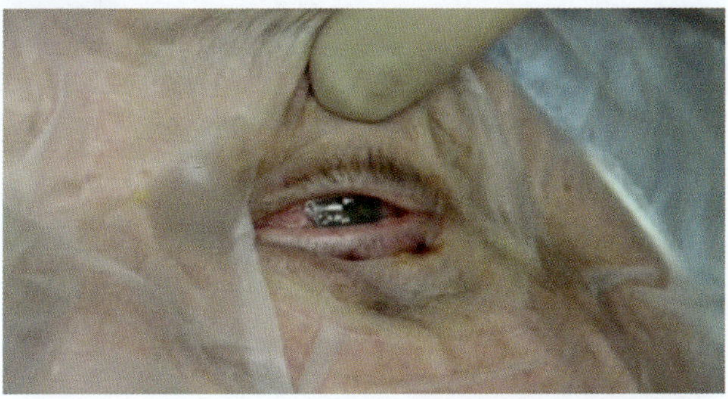

FIGURE 12-12 Completion of the three (3) lid-everting sutures laterally, centrally, and medially. The medial suture is not visible due to the angle of the photo. The endpoint of the procedure is a lid position that is slightly everted (mild ectropion) of the eyelid. (Photo courtesy of Nate Lighthizer, OD.)

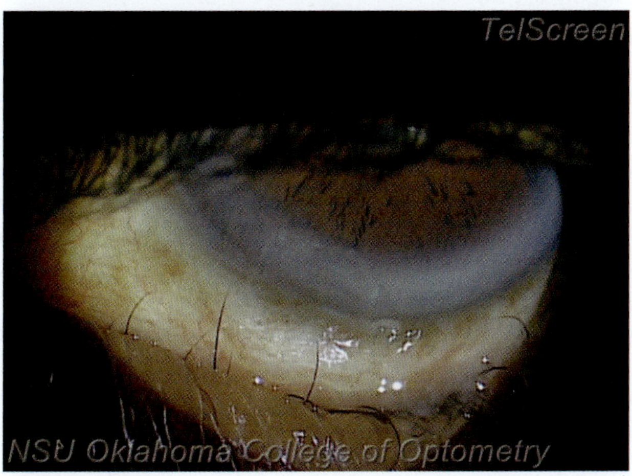


FIGURE 12-13 Preoperative photo of a patient with involutional entropion. (Photo courtesy of Nate Lighthizer, OD.)

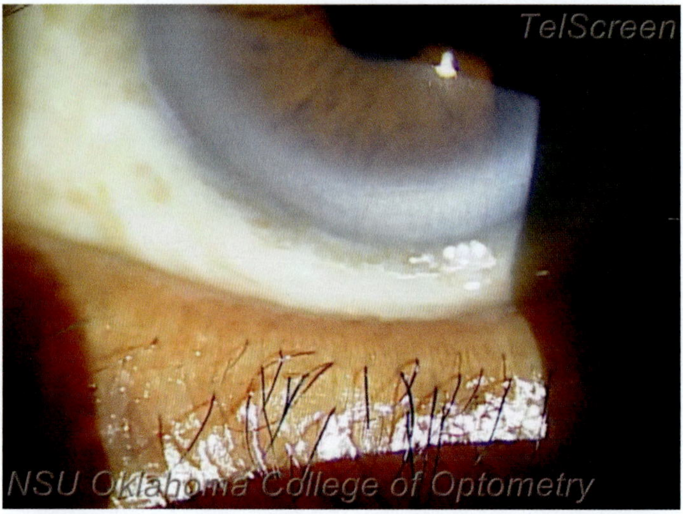


**FIGURE 12-14** Three-week postoperative photo of lid-everting sutures showing a corrected entropion. (Photo courtesy of Nate Lighthizer, OD.)

# POSTOPERATIVE CARE/COMANAGEMENT (FOLLOW-UP SCHEDULE)

## Key Postoperative Considerations

- Postoperative instructions:
  - Antibiotic ointment BID–TID × 1 week
  - Avoid rubbing eyelid.
  - Avoid water exposure (i.e., swimming) and dirty environments.
- 7 to 14 days postprocedure: infection check, suture removal

Immediately after completing the procedure, antibiotic ointment should be instilled into the postoperative eye. The patient should be instructed not to rub the eye or eyelids, to avoid dirty environments and getting water on the eye and eyelids, and to apply antibiotic ointment to the eye two to three times per day.

Antibiotic ointment two to three times a day for 1 week should be prescribed for the postoperative eye. A combination antibiotic steroid ointment may also be used; however, this may limit the wanted inflammatory and fibrotic reaction of the tissue to the suture material, so it is not recommended.

The procedure note should be recorded as performed including the medications used as well as the type, size, quantity, and location of sutures used. Importantly, a notation of the final eyelid position at the conclusion of the procedure should be documented, such as "The eyelid was everted successfully with lids and lashes no longer in contact with the globe at the conclusion of the procedure." Additionally, the provider should note the patient's tolerance of the procedure as well as their disposition upon discharge with a statement such as "The patient tolerated the procedure well and left in no apparent distress" should be added to the chart.

The patient should be given instructions not to rub the eyelid, as well as to avoid water on the face (i.e., swimming, showering, washing face, etc.) and dirty environments. A follow-up visit for 1 week is scheduled with instructions to the patient to return if any increased pain or decreased vision is noted. The patient should be specifically educated to expect some mild swelling that should improve over the following week.

At the 7- to 14-day follow-up, the doctor should evaluate the patient for signs of postoperative infection and remove the sutures. The lid position should be well apposed to the globe with perhaps a slight ectropion at this visit. Chromic gut and Vicryl sutures will retain tensile strength for approximately 2 to 4 weeks depending on the manufacturer, suture material, and patient healing. They may be left to dissolve in place if desired to prolong the wanted inflammation and fibrosis along the suture track. Leaving sutures to dissolve on their own is an option if follow-up may be challenging (such as for a bedfast patient with dementia). For patients that chronically rub their eyes, consider a clear eye shield until sutures are removed.

# POTENTIAL COMPLICATIONS AND THEIR MANAGEMENT

### Key Potential Complications to Look For

- Bleeding
- Anaphylactic reaction to medications
- Infection
- Undercorrection of entropion
- Overcorrection of entropion (i.e., ectropion)
- Recurrence of entropion

In the initial publication of this procedure by Quickert and Rathbun, the procedure was described as having "no known complications" in the 12 patients in the case series.[1] Another case series of 90 lid-everting suture procedures performed by ophthalmic nurses reported zero complications and concluded that the procedure "could be safely performed by ophthalmic nurses, with success rate comparable to the same technique performed by ophthalmologists."[11]

Because the procedure utilizes only sutures and does not require incisions or penetrate the orbital septum, a true postoperative complication of any kind should be exceedingly rare. Most of the potential complications are managed following other types of eyelid procedures, thus providing clinicians with a basis for managing them. A few potential complications will be discussed subsequently.

Mild bleeding is expected immediately postoperatively. This should in theory be minimal as the procedure does not require incisions. However, in patients taking blood thinners, there may be prolonged or excessive bleeding. Should excessive bleeding occur, this usually can be treated by applying 10 to 15 minutes of continuous firm pressure on the eye with sterile gauze (in office) or tissues (if at home). A cold pack may be considered in addition to the gauze. In office, pharmacologic agents such as topical 2.5% phenylephrine or a few drops of 1% lidocaine with epinephrine 1:100,000 instilled into the lower conjunctival sac or externally on the lid may also be helpful. A cotton tip applicator soaked in the medications may also be used for focal bleeds.

The most serious immediate intraoperative or postoperative concern is anaphylaxis. This should be managed by utilizing the appropriate epinephrine auto-injector pen as soon as anaphylaxis is suspected. Emergency services should be contacted immediately to transport the patient to the emergency room for ongoing medical monitoring outside of the office.

A postoperative infection might present within 3 to 7 days of the procedure as conjunctivitis or cellulitis. These should be managed with broad-spectrum topical and/or oral antibiotics and monitored closely as per usual treatment protocols. Special consideration can be given to cultures if treatment response is less than expected.

The most common complications of lid-everting sutures for entropion would include undercorrection, overcorrection, and recurrent entropion. These issues will most likely be identified after any swelling has resolved. Should undercorrection (i.e., early postoperative entropion) be present more than 1 month after the procedure, a second procedure with lid-everting sutures may be attempted or the patient may be referred to an oculoplastic surgeon for consideration of other procedures of the lids such as a lateral tarsal strip tarsorrhaphy.

For overcorrection resulting in ectropion, the management depends largely upon patient symptoms. In milder cases of ectropion, the patient may be largely asymptomatic. If mild symptoms exist, lubricant drops, gels, and ointments may be utilized for dry eye and foreign body sensation. Rarely should this procedure result in moderate to severe cases of postoperative ectropion. If these were to occur, referral for evaluation and management by an oculoplastic surgeon is likely indicated.

Finally, in the case of patients who had a successful initial procedure but later develop a recurrent entropion, the lid-everting suture procedure may be attempted a second time. Little data have been published on repeat procedures as the patient demographic requiring this procedure often skews toward older adults with an increasing yearly mortality rate. One study suggested a 30% mortality rate in the 4-year follow-up period.[2]

## VIDEOS OF PROCEDURES

**Video 12-1**—Step-by-step video of lid-everting suture procedure as performed by Rich Castillo, OD, DO. (Video courtesy of Rich Castillo, OD, DO.)

**Video 12-2**—In this video, three lid-everting sutures are placed for involutional entropion. Not shown is the lower eyelid being prepped with an alcohol swab and a 10% povidone–iodine swab stick (Betadine). Proper anesthesia is achieved with a subcutaneous and subconjunctival injection of lidocaine 2% with epinephrine. A sterile drape is placed, and the lower eyelid is "dotted" with three dots with a skin marker showing the points where the sutures are intended to be placed. The dots serve as an aiming point for where to pass the needles through the skin. Three double-armed (needle on both ends of the suture) 5-0 chromic gut (dissolvable) lid-everting sutures are placed (one medially, one centrally, and one laterally). Notice the needles are placed deep within the fornix on the palpebral conjunctival side, with the needles passed through the eyelid aiming to come out approximately 2 to 3 mm below the lash line (at the point of the dots). This is done for the needle on both ends of each suture. After the two needles are passed through the eyelid, the needles are then cut off, and the suture is tied with a surgeon's knot. This is repeated for each of the three lid-everting sutures. Notice at the conclusion of the procedure, a slight ectropion is seen, which is the immediate postoperative clinical endpoint. (Video courtesy of Nate Lighthizer, OD, and Michelle Welch, OD.)

## EFFICACY

The lid-everting suture procedure has been shown to be minimally complicated to perform and highly efficacious. Although only a few small studies on procedure outcomes and efficacy have been published to date, the documented recurrence rates have ranged from 0% to approximately 20%.

The initial series of 12 procedures published by Quickert and Rathbun reported no recurrences after 5 years of follow-up.[1] In another study of 62 eyelids with 48 months of follow-up, recurrence occurred in only 9 (15%) eyelids. Recurrence was not correlated to age, sex, lower lid excursion, or magnitude of horizontal lid laxity. Interestingly, all nine treatment failures occurred in primary entropion patients whereas there were no treatment failures in patients with recurrent entropion.[2]

A retrospective study of success rates of lid-everting sutures for entropion repair analyzed 90 procedures performed by nonphysician ophthalmic nurses in the United Kingdom over a period of 60 months. The entropion recurrence rate was reported to be 21.1%. A second lid-everting suture procedure was performed on 11 patients, and the recurrence rate was reported as 20%. The range of time to recurrence was reported to be between 6 weeks and 3 years, with 15 months as the mean time to recurrence.[11]

Other more invasive and complicated surgical options do exist for entropion and would likely be performed by an oculoplastic surgeon. However, this suture-based procedure may be an excellent first-line treatment for many patients.

## CODING/BILLING

For an entropion repair utilizing lid-everting sutures, CPT code 67921 is used: "Repair of Entropion, suture." This code has a 90-day postoperative global period. The E2 (left lower lid) or E4 (right lower lid) modifiers may need to be utilized depending on the insurance carrier.

If both eyes are done in the same session, use modifier −50 after the CPT code.

Common ICD-10 codes that support this procedure include:

- **H40.032**—Senile (involutional) entropion, right lower eyelid
- **H40.035**—Senile (involutional) entropion, right lower eyelid
- **H40.042**—Spastic entropion, right lower eyelid
- **H40.045**—Spastic entropion, left lower eyelid

# REFERENCES

1. Quickert MH, Rathbun E. Suture repair of entropion. *Arch Ophthalmol.* 1971;85(3):304-305. doi:10.1001/archopht.1971.00990050306012
2. Wright M, Bell D, Scott C, Leatherbarrow B. Everting suture correction of lower lid involutional entropion. *Br J Ophthalmol.* 1999;83:1060-1063.
3. Seiff SR, Kim M, Howes EL Jr. Histopathological evaluation of rotational sutures for involutional entropion. *Br J Ophthalmol.* 1989;73:628-632.
4. Guthrie AJ, Kadakia P, Rosenberg J. Eyelid malposition repair: a review of the literature and current techniques. *Semin Plast Surg.* 2019;33(2)92-102. doi:10.1055/s-0039-1685473
5. Steel DH, Hoh HB, Harrad RA, Collins CR. Botulinum toxin for the temporary treatment of involutional lower lid entropion: a clinical and morphological study. *Eye (Lond).* 1997;(11):472-475.
6. Carter SR, Seiff SR, Grant PE, Vigneron DB. The Asian lower eyelid: a comparative anatomic study using high-resolution magnetic resolution imaging. *Ophthalmic Plast Reconstr Surg.* 1998;14(4):227-234. doi:10.1136/bjo.73.2.126
7. Noda S, Hayasaka S, Setogawa T. Epiblepharon with inverted eyelashes in Japanese children. I. Incidence and symptoms. *Br J Ophthalmol.* 1989;73(2):126-127. doi:10.1136/bjo.73.2.126
8. Pasco NY, Kikkawa DO, Korn BS, Punja KG, Jones MC. Facial nerve paralysis: an unrecognized cause of lower eyelid entropion in the pediatric population. *Ophthalmic Plast Reconstr Surg.* 2007;23(2):126-129. doi:10.1097/IOP.0b013e318031d807
9. Faria-E-Sousa SJ, de Paula Gomes Vieira M, Silva JV. Uncovering intermittent entropion. *Clin Ophthalmol.* 2013;7:385-388. doi:10.2147/OPTH.S40572
10. Serin D, Buttanri IB, Karslioglu S, Sevim MS, Buttanri B, Akbaba M. The efficacy of the combined procedure in involutional entropion surgery: a comparative study. *Korean J Ophthalmol.* 2013;27(6):405-408.
11. Mohammed B, Ford R. Success rate of nurse-led everting sutures for lower lid entropion. *Eye (Lond).* 2017;31:732-735.

# 13 Entropion Repair

**Rachna Murthy • Jonathan Roos**

Entropion is an abnormal positioning of the eyelid margin where the eyelid turns inward toward the eye, resulting in the eyelashes pointing toward the cornea and the conjunctiva (Figure 13-1). The hallmark symptom of entropion is a feeling of intense pain or irritation on the eye caused by the eyelashes rubbing against the cornea and conjunctiva. Other symptoms can include watering of the eye, blurred vision, and redness.

This condition can be caused by age (involutional entropion) or damage to the eyelid structure, although congenital entropion can also occur. Entropion can also occur as a result of trauma or burns, certain infections of the conjunctiva such as trachoma, and cicatricial diseases of the conjunctiva such as ocular cicatricial pemphigoid (cicatricial entropion). Entropion is most common in older individuals but can affect people of any age and can be particularly bothersome. When the eye is irritated because of dryness or inflammation, excessive rubbing of the eye can contribute to laxity of the eyelid with excessive blinking and squeezing that results in spasm of the orbicularis oculi muscle (spastic entropion). Epiblepharon is commonly seen

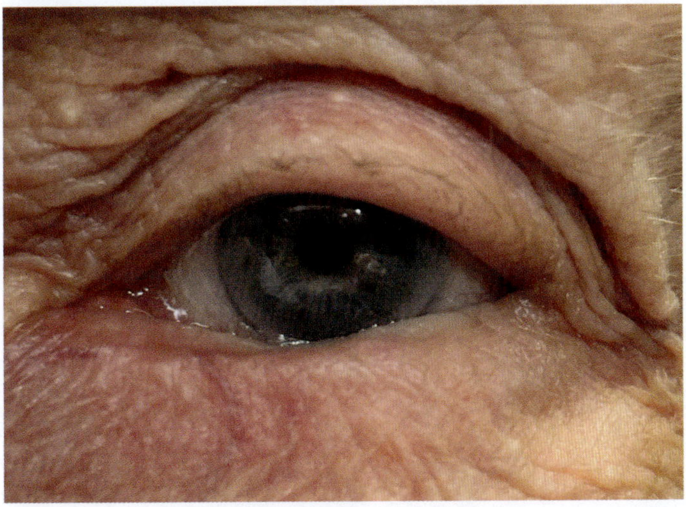

**FIGURE 13-1** Entropion. Note preseptal orbicularis oculi muscle has moved upward and overrides the pretarsal muscle. (Image courtesy of Leonid Skorin Jr, DO, OD, MS.)

in Asian patients and occurs when a fold of skin overrides the eyelid margin, pushing the lashes vertically toward the ocular surface. This is different to an entropion when the eyelid margin is rolled inward. In this chapter, we will explore the clinical features, diagnosis, and treatment of involutional entropion.

## CLINICAL FEATURES

Initially symptoms may be intermittent but become progressively more constant with time.

- Foreign body sensation
- Redness of the eye
- Irritation and soreness
- Excessive tearing
- Mucoid discharge (Figure 13-2)

Blurred vision and light sensitivity, rapidly worsening pain and redness can be symptoms and signs of corneal damage, and this warrants prompt treatment.

### Etiology of Involutional Entropion

Involutional changes in the orbicularis oculi muscle, lower eyelid retractors, tarsal plate, and horizontal lid contribute to the formation of involutional entropion. All these aspects need to be assessed and addressed for optimal treatment.

The orbital septum is a thin sheet of fibrous tissue, attached firmly to the orbital rim and loosely to the retractors. The lower eyelid retractors, responsible for the downward movement

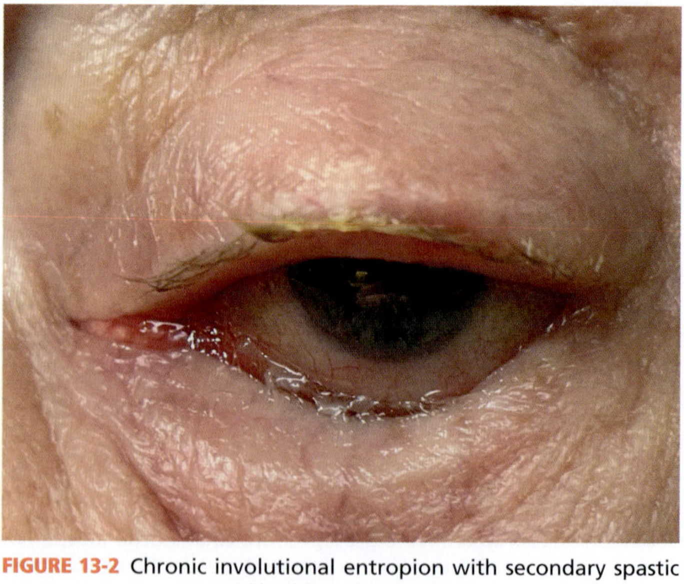

**FIGURE 13-2** Chronic involutional entropion with secondary spastic component. Note mucoid buildup along the inferior eyelid-lash line. (Image courtesy of Leonid Skorin Jr, DO, OD, MS.)

of the eyelid on downgaze, consist of a sheet of fibrous tissue extending from the inferior rectus muscle sheath, passing forward to enclose the inferior oblique muscle, and blending into the inferior suspensory ligament of Lockwood. Anteriorly, the retractors attach to the inferior border of the tarsal plate. The inferior suspensory ligament of the fornix is part of the fibrous tissue of the retractors (Figures 13-3 and 13-4). The lateral canthal tendon arises from Whitnall's tubercle, 2 mm posterior to the lateral orbital rim. The medial canthal tendon inserts into the lacrimal crest. The tendons support the eyelids. Involutional changes in the bony orbit can result in laxity of the tendons and contribute to horizontal laxity of the eyelid.

1. Orbicularis oculi muscle
   Involutional changes in the orbicularis oculi muscle allow the preseptal orbicularis to move upward and override the pretarsal muscle (Figure 13-1). Treatment involves prevention of overriding by creating a scar tissue barrier between the preseptal and pretarsal portions by transverse lid split, transverse sutures, or radiofrequency. As a temporizing measure, neuromodulation with botulinum toxin can be given to the preseptal orbicularis oculi muscle to reduce this overriding, which is often further contributed to by ocular surface irritation by eyelashes rubbing on the cornea.
2. Lower eyelid retractors
   Laxity of the lower eyelid retractors allows the lower border of the tarsal plate to rotate outward. Treatment to the lower eyelid retractors to strengthen by plication or eversion with sutures helps to address this.
3. Tarsal plate
   The tarsal plate loses its stiffness and bends, allowing the upper border to invert. Treatment is to transfer the vector pull of the lower lid retractors to evert the eyelid margin into a normal anatomic position with everting sutures.

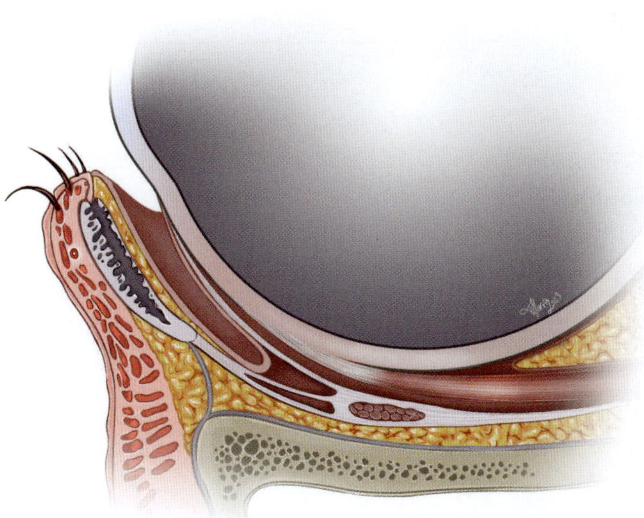

**FIGURE 13-3** Diagram showing a cross section of the lower eyelid demonstrating the lower eyelid retractors in normal state.

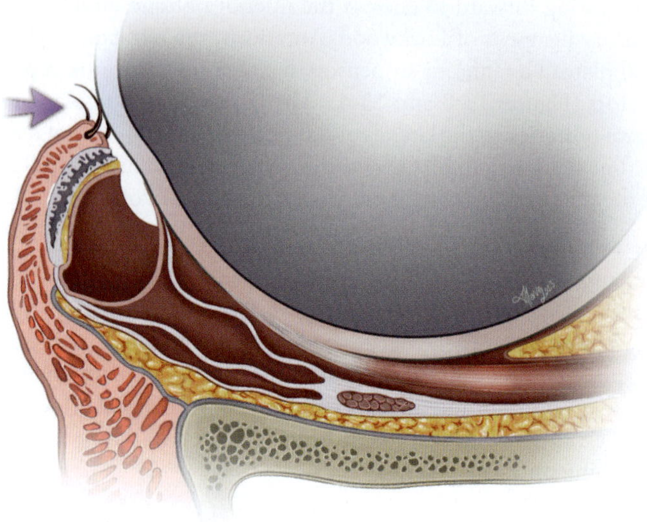

**FIGURE 13-4** Diagram showing a cross section of the lower eyelid demonstrating the lower eyelid retractors in entropion.

4. Horizontal lid laxity
Involutional changes to the canthal tendons, tarsal plate, and orbicularis oculi muscle result in laxity of the eyelid. Treatment involves assessing the position of laxity and shortening the eyelid horizontally.

# INDICATIONS

**Key Indications**

- Functional entropion
- Cosmetic entropion

Entropion can risk ocular surface irritation and corneal erosion because of the lashes rubbing against the ocular surface.

# CONTRAINDICATIONS

**Key Contraindications**

- Cicatricial disease of the conjunctiva
- Active symblepharon

Underlying cicatricial disease of the conjunctiva should be excluded with slit lamp examination. Active symblepharon suggestive of cicatricial disease would warrant treatment avoiding a conjunctival incision, which can lead to more scarring.

## INFORMED CONSENT CONSIDERATIONS

**Key Informed Consent Adverse Events Listed**

Informed consent should include the benefits and risks of surgery and any other alternatives.

**What are the benefits of surgery?**

- Improve comfort
- Prevent ocular surface disease
- Cosmetic improvement

**What are the alternatives to surgery?**

- There are no good alternatives to surgery. Other treatment modalities are either unpredictable or offer only temporary relief. Options are:
  - Ocular lubricants
  - Bandage contact lenses
  - Everting the eyelid with tape
  - Everting sutures or radiofrequency scar formation
  - Botulinum toxin to preseptal orbicularis oculi muscle

Topical lubricants can temporarily relieve symptoms of corneal irritation from the eyelashes rubbing the cornea.

**What are the risks of anesthesia?**

We usually perform entropion repair under local anesthesia without sedation as day case outpatient surgery.

- Local anesthetic may cause bruising, bleeding, and swelling
- May need additional anesthesia

The following is a sample of the consent Drs. Roos and Murthy use.

**What are the risks and possible complications of surgery?**

- *Infection:* might present as increased swelling and redness of the skin. There might also be yellow discharge from the wound. Infection is treated with antibiotics. You will be provided with a novel patent pending hypochlorous spray, Purifeyes, that we have developed. This will help to reduce postoperative infection and scar.
- *Bleeding:* may present as fresh blood oozing from the site of surgery or a lump appearing near the wound after the operation. Simple pressure on a skin wound is usually enough to control minor bleeding and is not of concern. In rare cases, a deeper hematoma may require review.
- *Loss of vision:* Total loss of vision in an eye because of this type of surgery is extremely rare. A blood hematoma collecting in the orbit, behind the eye, may compress the nerve of vision and threaten eyesight. It is extremely rare for this to occur. It presents as pain, loss of vision,

and a bulging forward of the eyeball and is an emergency. The eye prescription may change following surgery and new postoperative refraction may be required.

- *Scar:* Whenever the skin is incised a scar may form. Every attempt is made to minimize and hide scars but rarely they can be visible. The eyelid margin if involved in the repair may be left with a small indentation of notch, which should usually improve over time.
- *Further surgery:* Occasionally entropion may recur, and further surgery is required. The eyelid margin wound may dehisce and need to be resutured.
- *Dry eye:* Ocular surface disease can be worsened by entropion and surgery should help mitigate this.
- *Loss of sensation:* After surgery, there may be numbness of some of the skin around the incision. This is usually temporary returning gradually over months.
- *Inflammation:* Swelling and bruising of the skin or conjunctiva after surgery can occur but in varying degrees. A big improvement will be noticed after 2 weeks, with most resolved 3 months later. Rarely inflammation may cause small lumps to form called granulomas. Most resolve spontaneously but some require further treatment or surgery.
- *Secondary ectropion:* Overcorrection of the entropion can occur, resulting in out turning of the eyelid or an ectropion, this may require further surgery to repair this.

## PREOPERATIVE ASSESSMENT

**Key Preoperative Considerations**

- Full medical and ocular history including documentation of the duration and symptoms
- Clinical photographs
- Full ocular examination and eyelid evaluation

A full ocular examination is essential, including visual acuity, unaided and corrected, slit lamp ocular examination, assessment of the tear film, ocular surface for corneal staining, and conjunctiva for signs of cicatricial changes, such as symblepharon, or cicatricial disease.

Examination of the lower eyelid should also involve assessment of eyelid laxity with a snap test, canthal tendon laxity, and lower eyelid retractors, and septal deficiency (shallowing of the inferior conjunctival fornix). The eyelid excursion on upgaze and downgaze is a good way of examining for disinsertion of the lower eyelid retractors. If the retractors are still attached, the eyelid will move down with downgaze. This will inform whether the eyelid or tendon will require a tightening procedure and whether the retractors need reattaching to the inferior border of the tarsal plate.

### Preoperative Regimen

- Confirm the clinical findings.
- Confirm the treatment goals.

- Obtain full informed consent as earlier described.
- Ask if there are any unanswered questions.

We routinely prescribe benzodiazepine, diazepam 5 mg, 1 hour prior to the procedure.

The patient is positioned supine on the operating table and monitoring leads connected for pulse oximetry and cardiac telemetry. We use selective bipolar cautery and cold steel surgical instruments for surgery, which in our experience allows quicker postoperative recovery when compared with the use of radiofrequency, and does not necessitate a corneal shield.

## PROCEDURE

*Topical anesthesia*: A drop of proxymetacaine (proparacaine 0.5%) followed by tetracaine 0.5% is applied per eye for topical anesthesia of the cornea, conjunctiva, and inner surface of the eyelids.

*Local anesthesia infiltration*: We use bupivacaine 0.5% (Marcaine) with 1:200,000 epinephrine mixing 5 mL with 4 mL lidocaine 2% (Lignocaine) with adrenaline 1:80,000 and 1 mL dexamethasone 3 mg/mL.

### Surgical Technique

Several surgical methods have been described to treat entropion. The Hotz procedure involves excising skin and orbicularis oculi muscle in a crescent shape, followed by suturing the skin.[1] This procedure is suitable for epiblepharon, without lid laxity or retractor dehiscence.

Capsulopalpebral fascia repair involves a subciliary incision below the eyelashes, peeling the skin and orbicularis oculi muscle down to access the lower eyelid retractors, and attaching the lower eyelid retractors to the inferior border of the tarsal plate (Figures 13-5 and 13-6).[2] This addresses retractor dehiscence.

Lower eyelid everting sutures aim to plicate the lower eyelid retractor to the inferior tarsus without a skin incision (Figure 13-7). This method is quick but can be temporary if any horizontal lid laxity is present.

When there is horizontal lid laxity, this is addressed either by a wedge excision or by a lateral canthal tightening procedure, such as a lateral tarsal strip (Figure 13-8).

In the Wies procedure, a full-thickness transverse skin incision is made 4 mm inferior to the lashes, in the horizontal direction of the eyelid margin, and a suture passed through the skin from the posterior lamella of the proximal eyelid, that is, through the conjunctiva and lower lid retractors 2 mm below the incision into the orbicularis oculi muscle anterior to the tarsal plate in the upper wound edge, and the sutures emerged from the skin 2 mm inferior to the lashes.

Transverse blepharotomy and everting sutures have been used to prevent overriding. The sutures create scarring and adhesions between inferior retractors and the tarsal plate as they dissolve and prevent further inward rotation and recurrence.[3]

The procedure of choice is determined by the cause, pathology, and degree of entropion as well as what the patient can tolerate.[4] Procedures that address only one or two of the etiologic factors have been reported to have higher recurrence rates.[3]

We use a combined procedure of horizontal lid shortening and retractor plication. If there is no lateral canthal tendon laxity, we prefer to perform a full-thickness wedge excision of

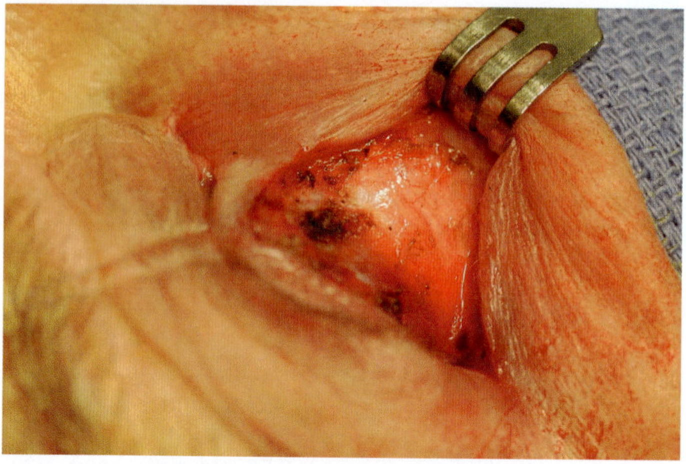

FIGURE 13-5 A traction suture is reflecting superior aspect of incised lower eyelid upward (left side of image). Subciliary incision can be seen to have been performed 2 to 3 mm below lash line. Orbicularis oculi muscle layer has been dissected to expose the orbital septum. Rake instrument used to reflect inferior aspect of incised lower eyelid, further exposing orbital septum (right side of image). (Image courtesy of Leonid Skorin Jr, DO, OD, MS.)

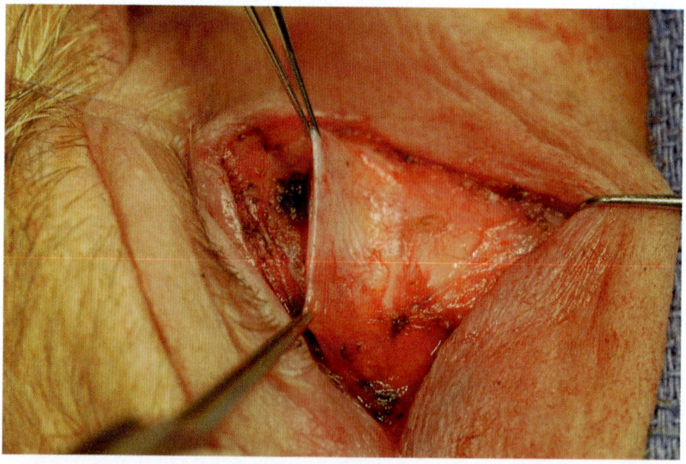

FIGURE 13-6 Lower lid retractors tented superiorly with two-toothed forceps. The leading edge of the retractors will be secured with dissolvable suture to the base of the tarsal plate. Note muscle hook instrument on the right side of the image being used to expose the orbital septum. A traction suture is seen reflecting the superior aspect of incised lower eyelid upward (left side of image). (Image courtesy of Leonid Skorin Jr, DO, OD, MS.)

the eyelid lateral to the corneal limbus. If there is lateral canthal laxity, a lateral tarsal strip procedure is performed. This involves exposing the lateral orbital rim periosteum and lateral canthal tendon. An approximately 1-cm-long skin incision is made from the lateral canthus to the orbital rim. A lateral canthotomy and inferior cantholysis to the lower limb of the lateral canthal tendon releases the lateral tendon that will be fashioned into a strip (Figure 13-8). Orbicularis fibers over the lateral orbital rim are dissected, and the lateral rim identified. We do not fashion a periosteal strip but fashion a tarsal strip that is sutured to the periosteum of the lateral orbital rim. Blunt-pointed scissors are used to spread anterior to the retractor layer, and the conjunctiva-retractor layer cut at the level of the inferior border of the tarsal plate transversely from the lateral canthal region to the required length of the strip. The lower lid is pulled laterally under moderate tension to assess the amount of horizontal shortening required. A tarsal strip is prepared by excising the superior mucocutaneous junctional tissue and the anterior lamella and debriding the conjunctival epithelium. A double-armed 5-0 Vicryl suture is passed through the tarsal strip and sutured to the periosteum of the internal aspect of the lateral orbital rim. The new canthal angle is formed and orbicularis over the rim and the skin closed with 6-0 Vicryl sutures.

Alternatively, if there is horizontal eyelid laxity, without lateral canthal tendon laxity, a full-thickness wedge excision of the eyelid is performed at the site of maximal laxity (Figure 13-9A–C) and the wedge closed by using 6-0 Vicryl buried sutures to oppose the cut edges of the tarsal plate and close the gray line and lash line at the lid margin (Figure 13-9D).

The retractors are plicated by making a horizontal skin incision as described earlier.

The retractor layer is dissected posteriorly from the conjunctiva and then shortened using three 6-0 Vicryl sutures passed in the following order: preseptal orbicularis, retractor layer and the conjunctiva in the lower wound edge, inferior border of the tarsal plate, and pretarsal orbicularis. The sutures are tied to achieve a slight ectropion of the eyelid (Figure 13-9E and F).

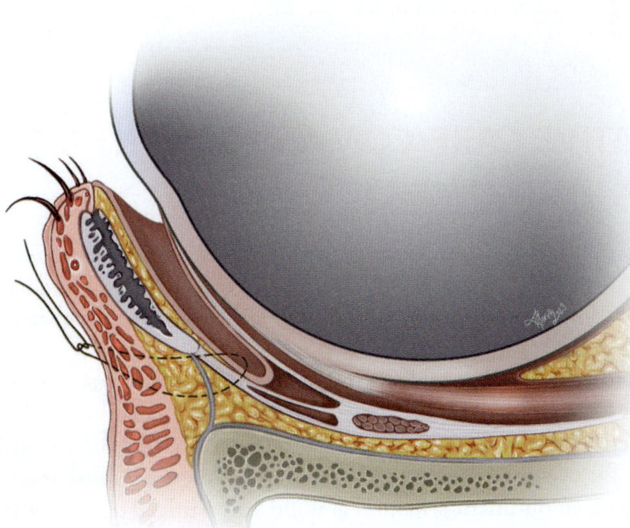

**FIGURE 13-7** Lower eyelid everting suture placement.

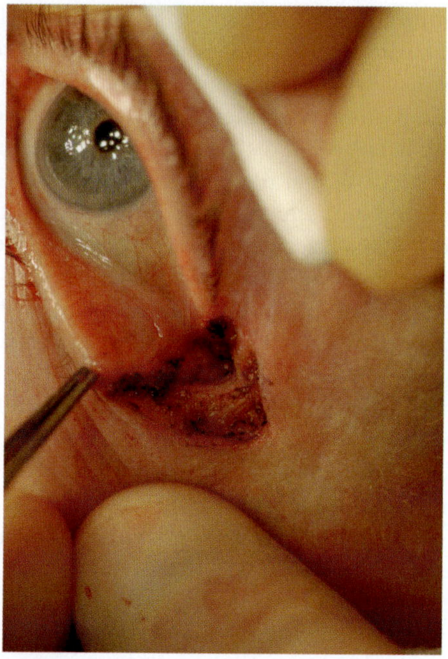

**FIGURE 13-8** Lateral canthal strengthening (tightening). Full thickness, 1 cm in length, horizontal lateral canthal incision is performed with a No. 15 surgical blade down to the periosteum. Tarsal strip not yet completed in this image. (Image courtesy of Leonid Skorin Jr, DO, OD, MS.)

## POSTOPERATIVE CARE/COMANAGEMENT (FOLLOW-UP SCHEDULE)

The natural history of healing includes ingrowth of blood vessels and extracellular matrix that last 5 to 6 weeks. At this time, incision lines become tight, firm, and red, and this can cause some patients frustration. Following this period, incision lines soften and fade, for around 4 to 5 months.

Usually, antimicrobial antibiotic tablets are not required and we have moved to the use of hypochlorous spray. (Purifeyes is a pH balanced ocular and periocular hypochlorous spray with antimicrobial properties, and anti-inflammatory properties, that is convenient for patients to use postoperatively for eyelid hygiene.) For lubrication of the eyes when there is tightness of the eyelids postsurgery, an ointment is helpful at night and artificial tears by day for a few days, which are less likely to blur vision.

Following is an example of the patient information we give to our patients.

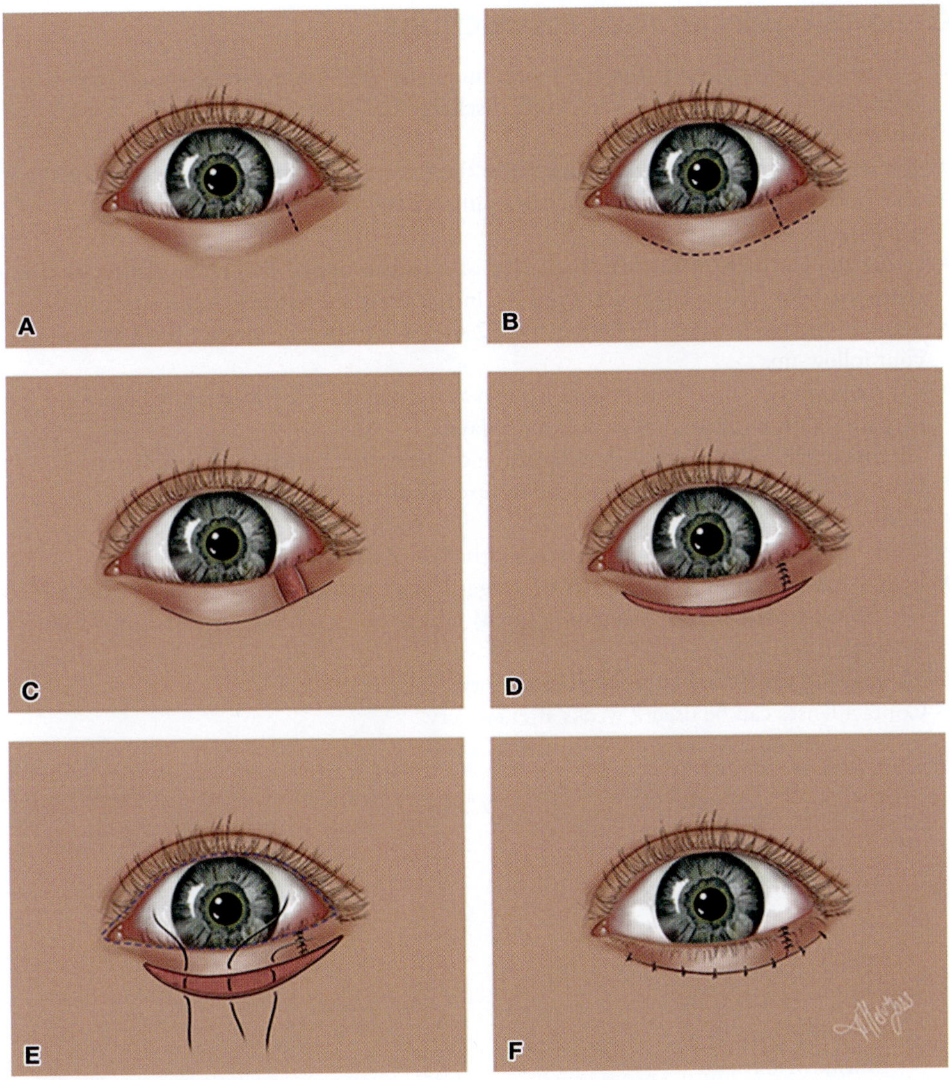


**FIGURE 13-9** Left lower eyelid entropion repair. **A,** Full-thickness vertical eyelid incision into lower eyelid lateral to the corneal limbus. **B,** Horizontal eyelid incision in skin and orbicularis oculi muscle. **C,** Excision of lateral wedge of lower eyelid. **D,** Closure of eyelid margin and vertical incision. **E,** Plication of lower eyelid retractors to tarsal plate. **F,** Skin closure.

## Postoperative Instructions

If any swelling, bruising, discomfort, or pain worsens or a discharge (pus) appears around suture line, contact your surgeons/clinic immediately.

We will give you a prescription for an oral antibiotic that you can take should any symptoms appear though we think this is most unlikely.

## General Postoperative Instructions

- A firm eye pad is put on after the procedure for at least 1 hour. This should stay on until instructed. It is usually removed before discharge but may remain until the next morning when you can remove it yourself.
- You will be given teardrops or ointment for the eye—usually three times per day for 1 week.
- You will be given a broad-spectrum eye ointment for any external wound before you are discharged.
- Apply the ointment with clean fingertips or a cotton-tipped bud along the incision lines twice a day for 2 weeks, running from the inside along the stitches to the outer end.
- Your absorbable stitches will fall out after 2 to 3 weeks, but we remove these as required at your follow-up.
- Cool compresses should commence as soon as the pad is removed or immediately if there is no pad: 5 minutes, five times a day, for 5 days.
- Cleanse the lids with cotton wool dipped in cooled boiled water or sterile saline for 10 days.
- Do walk but avoid any form of strenuous exercise for 10 days.
- Reading and watching television is fine.
- Please try not to bend over very much for the first 2 days after surgery.
- If you have pain within 2 hours of surgery, start taking the painkiller prescribed (or two 500 mg paracetamol [acetaminophen] tablets every 6 hours) for 48 hours following surgery.
- Eye makeup can be used 1 week after surgery.
- Contact lenses can be used 2 weeks after surgery.

# POTENTIAL COMPLICATIONS AND THEIR TREATMENT

### Key Potential Complications

- Allergy
- Bruising
- Hematoma
- Blurred vision
- Vision loss
- Infection
- Asymmetry
- Scar
- Dry eyes
- Wound dehiscence
- Lower eyelid secondary ectropion
- Corneal abrasion

Common patient worries include bruising and blurring of vision with tightness and swelling of the eyelids immediately postoperatively and with the ointment used.

Overcorrection can result in secondary ectropion, which may need return to the operating room.

If the procedure involves a lid margin incision, there may rarely be wound dehiscence requiring return to the operating room.

Lateral canthal tightening can result in chemosis of the conjunctiva, dehiscence or rounding of the canthus, or a suture granuloma.

With good consent and communication, patient expectations can be met and reassurance given.

Complications are fortunately rare and can be on the whole avoided with good preoperative modulation and good surgical technique.

## VIDEO OF PROCEDURE

**Video 13-1**—Entropion repair. Reattachment of lower eyelid retractors and lateral canthal strengthening procedure. (Video courtesy of Leonid Skorin Jr and Stephanie Norberg.)

# EFFICACY

There are no good alternatives to surgery. Conservative nonsurgical treatment modalities are either unpredictable or offer only temporary relief. The longest lasting nonsurgical modality is botulinum toxin injections. These may deliver from 3 to 4 months of relief. These injections can be repeated as necessary. For poor surgical candidates, botulinum toxin injection therapy is the most practical and effective nonsurgical treatment approach.

The surgical procedure of choice is determined by the cause, pathology, and degree of entropion as well as what the patient can tolerate.[4] Surgical procedures that address only one or two of the etiologic factors have been reported to have higher recurrence rates.[3] Particularly for elderly patients, and those with complex medical issues, minimally invasive entropion management, such as the placement of everting or "temporizing" sutures, should be considered before more extensive surgical intervention.

# CODING/BILLING

- CPT code: 67921—Repair of entropion; suture
- CPT code: 67922—Repair of entropion; thermocauterization
- CPT code: 67923—Repair of entropion; excision tarsal wedge
- CPT code: 67924—Repair of entropion; extensive (e.g., tarsal strip or capsulopalpebral fascia)
- CPT code: 67961—For repair of cicatricial entropion requiring scar excision or skin graft up to one-fourth of lid margin
- CPT code: 67966—For repair of cicatricial entropion requiring scar excision or skin graft over one-fourth of lid margin

Common International Classification of Diseases (ICD)-10 codes that support entropion repair include the following:

- H02.001 to H02.009—Unspecified entropion
- H02.011 to H02.019—Cicatricial entropion of eyelid
- H02.021 to H02.029—Mechanical entropion of eyelid
- H02.031 to H02.039—Senile entropion of eyelid
- H02.041 to H02.049—Spastic entropion of eyelid

Eyelid modifiers can be used as such: E1 for upper left eyelid, E2 for lower left eyelid, E3 for upper right eyelid, and E4 for lower right eyelid.

## REFERENCES

1. Ding J, Chen F, Zhai W, et al. Orbicularis oculi muscle transposition for repairing involutional lower eyelid entropion. *Graefes Arch Clin Exp Ophthalmol.* 2014;252(8):1315-1318. doi:10.1007/s00417-014-2694-3
2. Kreis AJ, Shafi F, Madge SN. Transconjunctival entropion repair—the backdoor approach. *Orbit.* 2013;32(5): 271-274. doi:10.3109/01676830.2013.815230
3. Scheepers MA, Singh R, Ng J, et al. A randomized controlled trial comparing everting sutures with everting sutures and a lateral tarsal strip for involutional entropion. *Ophthalmology.* 2010;117(2):352-355. doi:10.1016/j.ophtha.2009.06.056
4. Serin D, Buttanri IB, Karslioglu S, et al. The efficacy of the combined procedure in involutional entropion surgery: a comparative study. *Korean J Ophthalmol.* 2013;27(6):405-408. doi:10.3341/kjo.2013.27.6.405

# 14 Ectropion Repair

**Leonid Skorin, Jr • Zurriat Syed**

Ectropion is the outward rotation or sagging of the eyelid (Figure 14-1).[1] This malposition leaves the inner lining of the lower eyelid exposed and at risk for irritation and infection. Because the inferior cornea may also be exposed, the patient will experience foreign-body sensation and will potentially exhibit superficial punctate keratopathy, corneal erosion, and even corneal ulceration in severe cases. Patients usually present with either severe dry eyes or tearing.[2] Ectropion has a higher incidence of presenting in the lower eyelids and is rarely found in the upper eyelids. The likelihood of this condition increases with age.[3]

Common risk factors that increase the likelihood of ectropion development include age, floppy eyelid syndrome (Figure 14-2), long-term eye drop use, prior eyelid operation, and ocular trauma.[1,4] Less common risk factors include inflammation, infection, cancer, and certain hereditary conditions such as Down syndrome. Most studies indicate that ectropion prevalence is equal between men and women; however, certain studies have found a higher prevalence in men aged 80 years or older than women of similar ages.[5] Skin cancer history and sun sensitivity are factors that correlate with higher ectropion occurrence. Individuals who smoke or have a history of hypertension, diabetes, or stroke are also predisposed to ectropion development.[5]

Malposition of the eyelid can cause irritation, pain, excess tearing without proper drainage, dry eyes, and other symptoms associated with corneal exposure. The inability to close the eyes fully due to ectropion leads to chronically dry eyes, which can inversely lead to epiphora or watery eyes. This can thicken the conjunctiva, causing worsening of symptoms (Figure 14-3). Clinically, ectropion can be seen on physical and slit-lamp examination of the eyes. The normal excursion of the lid margin is 6 mm or less, and the greater the amount of excursion correlates with ectropion severity.

Treatment can be lubrication and keeping the eyes moist with artificial tears or ophthalmic bland ointment in mild cases.[2] Taping is also beneficial in reducing ectropion, but it is only a temporary measure (Figure 14-4). For more advanced ectropion cases, surgical treatment is recommended. Specific treatments depend on the underlying etiology of the ectropion. Left untreated, ectropion can result in corneal ulcers, corneal and conjunctival abrasions, and ocular infections. If severe, it can cause blindness and impaired visual acuity.

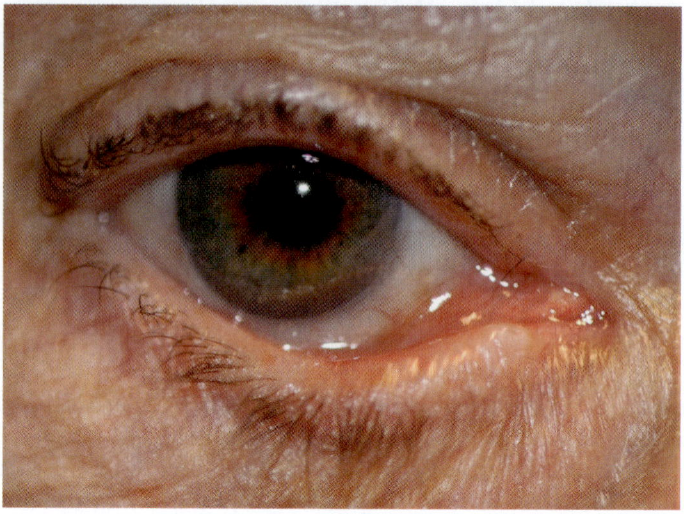

FIGURE 14-1 Lower eyelid ectropion with punctal eversion.

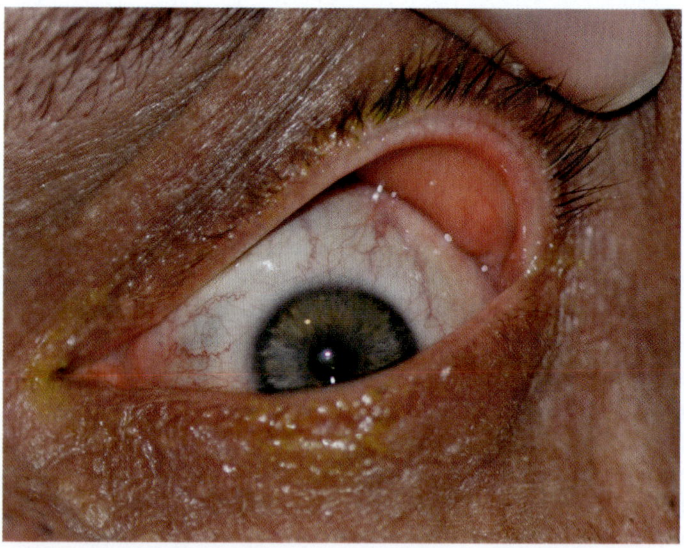

FIGURE 14-2 Floppy eyelid syndrome. Note easy manual eversion of the upper eyelid. The upper eyelid can sometimes even evert spontaneously. Floppy eyelid syndrome is strongly associated with obstructive sleep apnea.

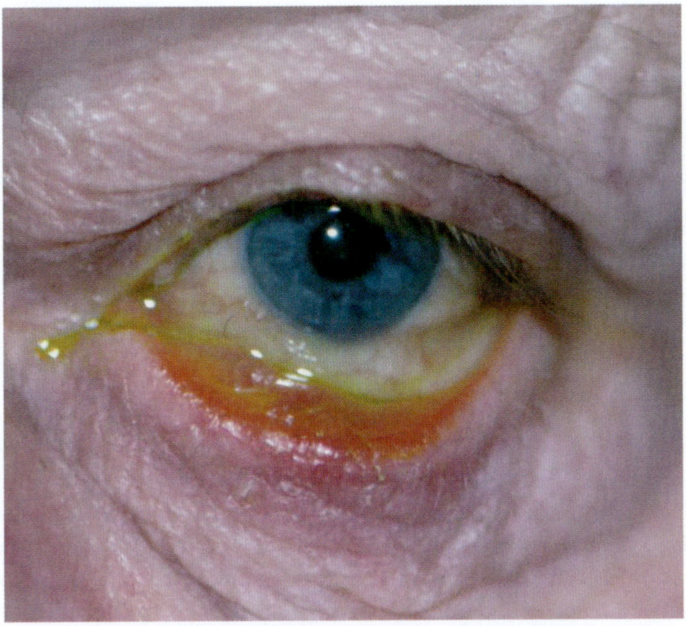

**FIGURE 14-3** Chronic ectropion of lower eyelid. Note the thickening of conjunctival tissue and redness from chronic exposure and inflammation. (Image courtesy of Gladstone GJ. Ectropion. In: Onofrey BE, Skorin L, Holdeman NR, eds. *Ocular Therapeutics Handbook: A Clinical Manual*. 4th ed. Wolters Kluwer; 2020:649-652.)

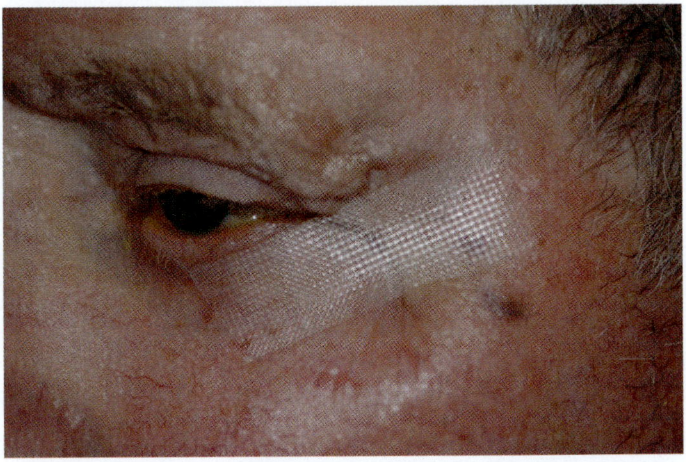

**FIGURE 14-4** Taping of ectropic lower eyelid temporally. This is only a temporary measure.

# INDICATIONS

**Key Indications**

- Punctal eversion
- Lateral canthal laxity
- Medial canthal laxity
- Overall eyelid laxity
- Excessive dry eyes or tearing

Ectropion can be classified as either congenital or acquired. Congenital causes include primary and secondary ectropion. Primary ectropion occurs in the absence of any other condition whereas secondary ectropion occurs in the presence of another pathologic condition. Congenital ectropion is rare and often found with coexisting health conditions, particularly Down syndrome and blepharophimosis syndrome.[5] This type of ectropion more commonly appears on the lower eyelids. It is caused by an eyelid skin deficiency. The eyelid is a bilamellar structure. In congenital ectropion, the anterior lamella is shorter toward the lateral portion of the lower eyelid. This can also be in conjunction with laxity of the lateral canthal tendon.

Acquired causes include cicatricial, mechanical, involutional, and paralytic etiologies (Table 14-1).[2] Of these, the highest prevalence is involutional ectropion (Figure 14-5). Involutional ectropion occurs gradually, increasing with age and presents with vertical eyelid instability and progressive horizontal eyelid laxity. Evaluation of the amount of punctal

**TABLE 14-1 TYPES OF ACQUIRED ECTROPION**

| TYPE | INVOLUTIONAL | PARALYTIC | CICATRICIAL | MECHANICAL |
|---|---|---|---|---|
| Epidemiology | Older age; M = F | Any age; M = F | Any age; M = F | Older patients; M = F |
| Etiology | Older age | Palsy, stroke, tumor, surgery | Trauma, surgery, scarring, dermatitis | Mass (e.g., dermatochalasis, edema, chalazion, eyelid tumor) pushes the eyelid out. |
| Examination | Eyelid sagging inferiorly and away from globe; look for the amount of horizontal laxity, corneal exposure, punctal stenosis. | Check for Bell phenomenon, corneal sensation, etiology of facial palsy. | External scarring or possible skin changes | Asymptomatic or corneal irritation and redness |
| Special considerations | Tarsal ectropion—repair with horizontal strengthening and reattachment of retractors. | Corneal sensation will determine the severity. | Rule out skin carcinoma. | Determine the degree of involutional changes and etiology of mass. |

**TABLE 14-1 TYPES OF ACQUIRED ECTROPION (*continued*)**

| TYPE | INVOLUTIONAL | PARALYTIC | CICATRICIAL | MECHANICAL |
|---|---|---|---|---|
| Treatment | Lubricate if mild; treat with horizontal shortening and punctoplasty for long-term benefit. | Depends on the duration of paralysis—if resolution is expected, use lubrication, temporary tarsorrhaphy, or gold weight in the upper eyelid; partial permanent tarsorrhaphy is used for cases in which resolution is less likely. | Treat underlying skin condition; lysis of any deep scar tissue with horizontal strengthening; if severe, may need a full-thickness skin graft | Excision of mass and correction of involutional factors of the eyelid |
| Prognosis | Excellent; 5%–10% recurrence rate after surgery | Variable; tends to recur over time if paralysis is permanent | Trauma cases do well; chronic cases have a poorer prognosis. | Good if the mass is eliminated |

From Skorin L, Lange R. Ectropion: classification, diagnosis, and management. *Consultant*. 2018;58(6):e180. https://www.consultant360.com/articles/ectropion-classification-diagnosis-and-management

stenosis secondary to chronic punctal eversion, corneal exposure, and horizontal lid laxity should be performed. If the eyelid has fully rotated outward from the eye in an involutional ectropion, it can be called a tarsal ectropion. In tarsal ectropion, the eyelid turns outward by being hinged at the inferior tarsal border.[1] Treatment for all types of involutional ectropion

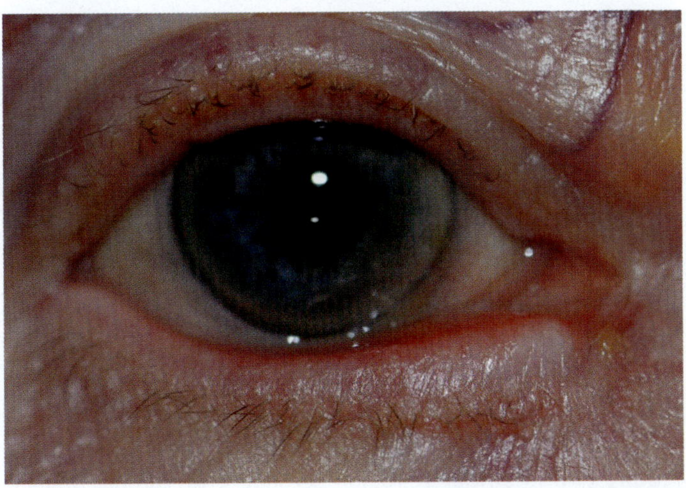

**FIGURE 14-5** Involutional ectropion of lower eyelid with significant punctal eversion.

includes lubrication for mild cases. Surgical treatment for more severe cases includes horizontal eyelid shortening and punctoplasty. Specific surgical treatment for tarsal ectropion is horizontal eyelid strengthening and reattaching detached retractors. The prognosis with involutional ectropion is excellent.

Trauma to the face or conjunctiva can cause cicatricial ectropion. Lower eyelid blepharoplasty or eyelid reconstruction after tumor removal can cause vertical skin deficiency.[1] Scarring, dermatitis, infection, history of skin diseases such as herpes zoster and rosacea, and inflammation can also result in cicatricial changes to the eyelid (Figure 14-6).[1] Exclusion of skin cell carcinoma is necessary with cicatricial ectropion. In cicatricial ectropion, the anterior lamellae of the eyelid contract and pull the eyelid downward. It can cause tears to spill over the eyelid margin instead of draining to the puncta (Figure 14-7). Treatment involves management of underlying conditions, horizontal strengthening with deep scar tissue lysis, and if foreshortening of the skin is present, a full-thickness graft is usually necessary. Chronic cicatricial ectropion has a poorer prognosis, unlike traumatic cicatricial cases that have an overall better prognosis.

Mechanical ectropion involves the presence of a physical anatomical factor causing the eyelid to move downward (Figure 14-8). This is the rarest of the ectropion types. It can result from eyelid tumors as seen with neurofibromatosis, chalazion, swelling, orbital fat, and dermatochalasis. Older age is often associated with mechanical ectropion. It can also be asymptomatic until it becomes quite advanced. Treatment involves excision and resolving any secondary involutional components. If the mass can be eliminated, the prognosis is good.

Facial nerve paralysis is associated with paralytic or neurogenic ectropion (Figure 14-9).[6] Tumors, postoperative complications injuring the facial cranial nerve, and stroke can cause this type of ectropion. It can occur at any age. Evaluation for Bell's palsy versus stroke should be initiated. Treatment is based on how long the paralysis lasts. If a quick resolution of symptoms

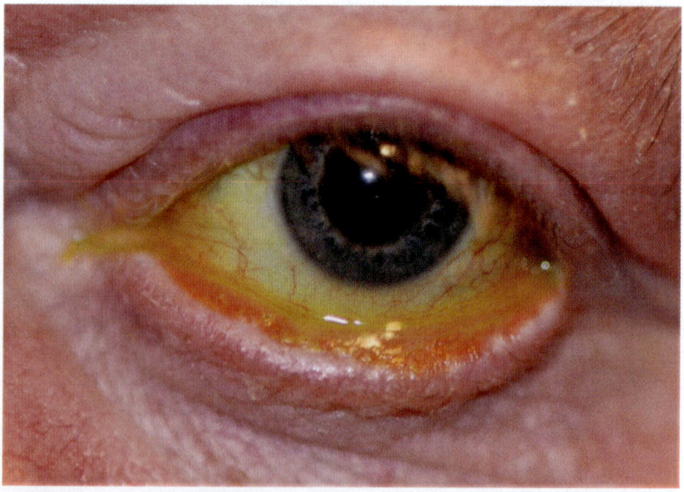

**FIGURE 14-6** Cicatricial ectropion secondary to chronic dermatitis. Note the thickening of conjunctival tissue and signs of chronic inflammation.

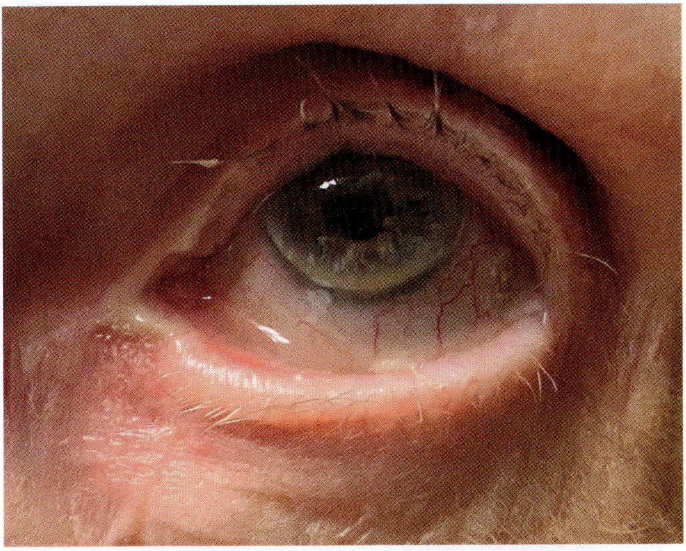

**FIGURE 14-7** Cicatricial ectropion from chronic involutional ectropion with punctal ectropion and punctal stenosis. (Image courtesy of Nate Lighthizer, OD.)

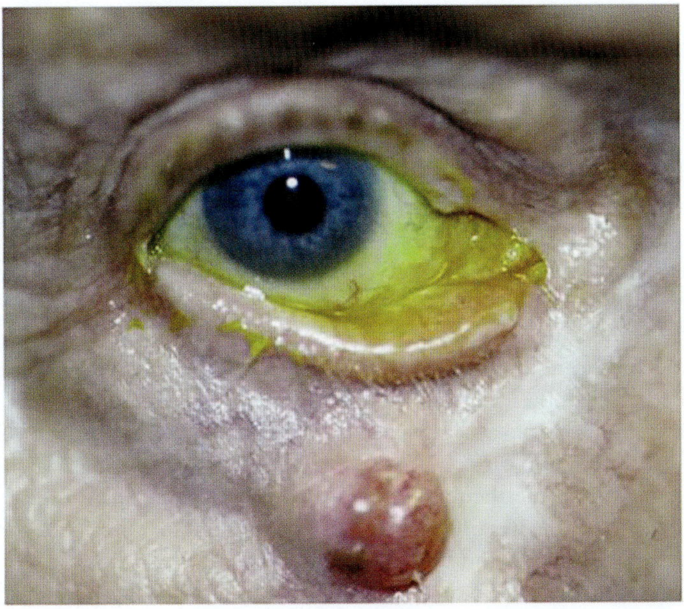

**FIGURE 14-8** Mechanical ectropion caused by basal cell carcinoma that is physically pulling the lower eyelid downward and away from the globe.

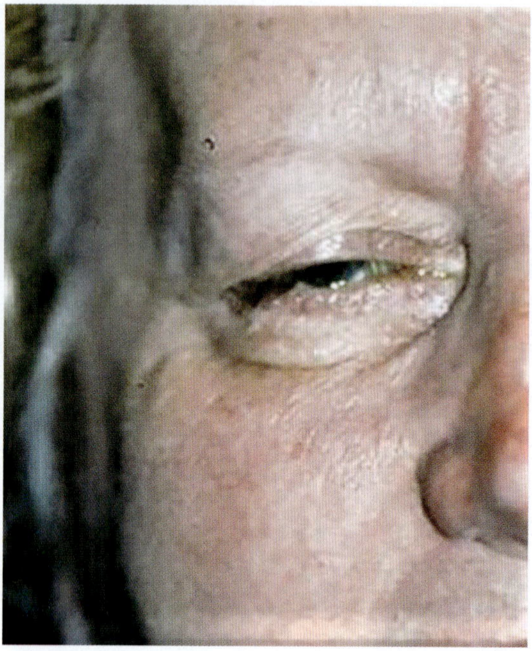

**FIGURE 14-9** Paralytic ectropion in a patient with Bell's palsy. The patient is trying to close her right eye and smile. Note the lids do not close completely, there is mild paralytic ectropion, there is a flattening of the nasolabial fold, and there is no wrinkling of the forehead (frontalis) muscle.

is expected, then lubrication, gold weight placement in the upper eyelids, or temporary tarsorrhaphy may be sufficient treatment. If no resolution is anticipated or symptoms do not improve, partial permanent tarsorrhaphy is the preferred treatment (Figure 14-10). Prognosis depends on several factors including whether normal corneal sensation is present or absent. If paralysis is irreversible, then ectropion will recur.

There are several diagnostic measures for ectropion. Punctal eversion is seen clinically on eye examination and if present, it suggests the presence of medial ectropion (see Figures 14-1 and 14-5). The use of fluorescein stain in the eye will show any compromise of the corneal surface and other signs of dryness. If dryness is present, then artificial tears or bland ointment is suggested. Tear production can be measured as well with the Schirmer/Basal secretion test.[2] Instill topical ophthalmic anesthetic and then place the Schirmer strips over the lower lateral lid margin.[2,7] This test measures the basal component of total tear production.[2,7] Less than 10 mm of test strip wetness in 5 minutes is abnormal.[2,7]

Measuring eyelid laxity can be done with the distraction test. By pulling the lower eyelid away from the globe of the eye, the distance between the globe and the eyelid margin can be measured (Figure 14-11). If the amount is greater than 10 mm, then significant eyelid laxity

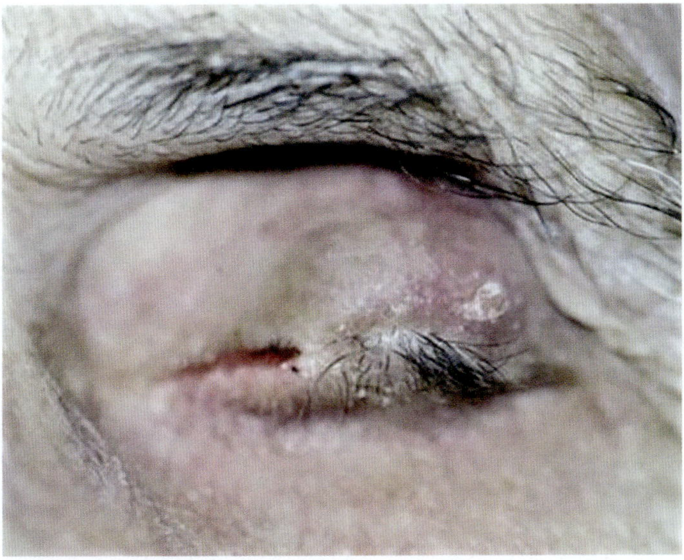

**FIGURE 14-10** Partial permanent tarsorrhaphy.

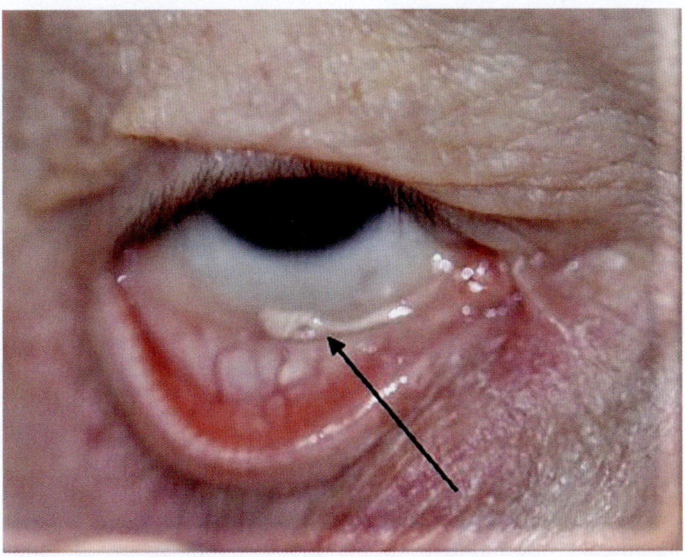

**FIGURE 14-11** The distraction test is performed to evaluate ectropion. Note the white band of mucus in the lower cul-de-sac (arrow). (From Skorin L, Lange R. Ectropion: classification, diagnosis, and management. *Consultant*. 2018;58(6):e180. https://www.consultant360.com/articles/ectropion-classification-diagnosis-and-management)

is present. Another method to assess eyelid laxity is the snap-back test. The patient must not blink during this test. The eyelid is pulled downward and released. The time it takes for the lower eyelid to return to baseline (reapproximate to the globe) after release will determine laxity (Figure 14-12). If it takes more than 2 to 5 seconds for the eyelid to return to normal positioning, laxity is present. If the lid only returns after the patient blinks, this should also be noted.[2]

Medial canthal laxity can be measured by grasping the medial eyelid and pulling it laterally away from the medial canthus (Figure 14-13). The amount of displacement at the medial canthus is measured and directly correlates with medial lid laxity. Normally, the punctum should only move 0 or 1 mm laterally.[2] The greater the amount of displacement, the more laxity is present.[2] Lateral canthal laxity can be evaluated by pulling the lateral eyelid medially away from the lateral canthus and measuring displacement at the lateral canthal corner (Figure 14-14). The greater the displacement, the more laxity is present.[2] A displacement of 10 mm is not uncommon when significant laxity is present. The snap-back and laxity tests are graded measurements where Grade 0 is normal and Grade IV is severe (Table 14-2).

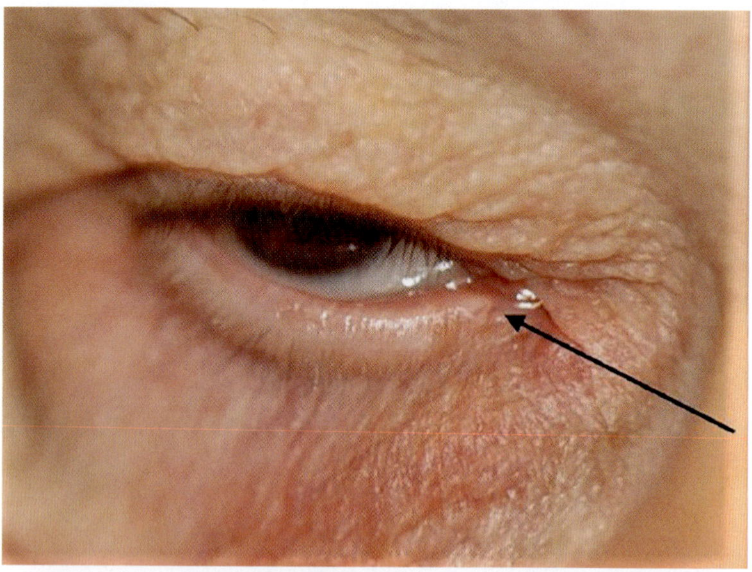

**FIGURE 14-12** The eyelid position 1 second after release during the snap-back test. Note the punctal eversion (arrow) and the medial eyelid margin not apposed to the globe. (From Skorin L, Lange R. Ectropion: classification, diagnosis, and management. *Consultant*. 2018; 58(6):e180. https://www.consultant360.com/articles/ectropion-classification-diagnosis-and-management)

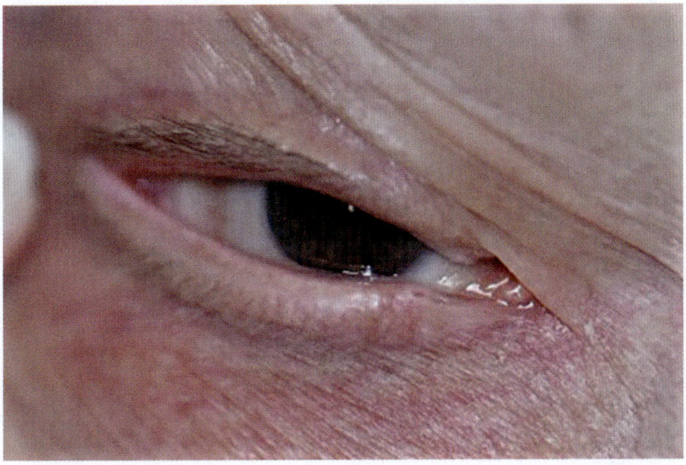

**FIGURE 14-13** The medial canthal laxity test is performed to evaluate ectropion. (From Skorin L, Lange R. Ectropion: classification, diagnosis, and management. *Consultant*. 2018;58(6):e180. https://www.consultant360.com/articles/ectropion-classification-diagnosis-and-management)

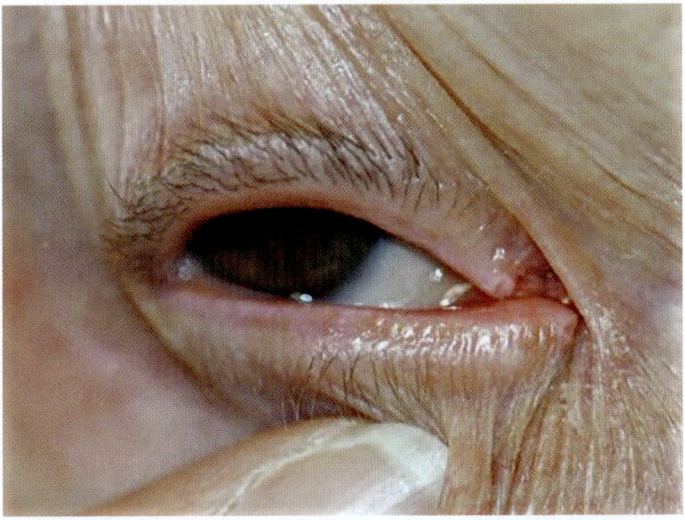

**FIGURE 14-14** The lateral canthal laxity test is performed to evaluate ectropion. (From Skorin L, Lange R. Ectropion: classification, diagnosis, and management. *Consultant*. 2018;58(6):e180. https://www.consultant360.com/articles/ectropion-classification-diagnosis-and-management)

**TABLE 14-2 TESTS FOR ASSESSMENT OF EYELID LAXITY**

| TEST | GRADE 0 (NORMAL) | GRADE I | GRADE II | GRADE III | GRADE IV (SEVERE LAXITY) |
| --- | --- | --- | --- | --- | --- |
| Snap-back test | Returns to position immediately | ~2–3 sec to return to position | ~4–5 sec to return to position | >5 sec to return to position | Never returns to position, may continue to hang down |
| Medical canthal laxity test | 0–1 mm displacement | ~2 mm displacement | ~3 mm displacement | >3 mm displacement | Does not return to baseline |
| Lateral canthal laxity test | 0–2 mm displacement | 2–4 mm displacement | 4–6 mm displacement | >6 mm displacement | Does not return to baseline, even with blink |

From Skorin L, Lange R. Ectropion: classification, diagnosis, and management. *Consultant*. 2018;58(6):e180. https://www.consultant360.com/articles/ectropion-classification-diagnosis-and-management

# CONTRAINDICATIONS

**Key Contraindications**

- Unstable medical condition
- Infection
- Inflammation
- Unable to discontinue blood thinners (relative contraindication)

If a patient does not consent or cannot undergo this surgical procedure, it should not be performed. Patients should be counseled on the procedure and any risks or potential adverse effects. Expected results and goals of the procedure should be discussed prior to the procedure. General risks in any surgical operation include infection. Risks specific to ectropion including ectropion recurrence, corneal ulcer, infection, and blindness should be discussed with the patient beforehand. They should complete and sign a consent form prior to the procedure.

Any underlying health condition should be treated before any surgical intervention. Because certain ectropion types are associated with connective tissue or dermatologic disorders such as cicatricial ectropion, management of the patients' health conditions should be a priority. If uncontrolled infection or inflammation is present, surgical intervention should be avoided as the risk of complications is increased.

# PREOPERATIVE PREPARATION

## Necessary Instrumentation

1. Ophthalmic topical anesthetic (e.g., tetracaine 0.5%, proparacaine 0.5%)
2. Lidocaine 1% or 2% with 1:100,000 epinephrine

3. Povidone–iodine 10% swabs for cleaning eyelids and surrounding areas
4. Povidone–iodine 5% ophthalmic topical
5. Sterile fenestrated surgical drape
6. Plastic corneal shield
7. 10-mL syringe for anesthetic
8. 25 gauge × 1 1/2″ needle
9. 4 × 4 surgical gauze pads
10. Cotton-tipped applicators
11. No. 15 surgical blade
12. Bowman dilating probes
13. Vannas and Westcott scissors
14. 0.5-mm toothed forceps
15. 6-0 silk suture, 5-0 Vicryl or chromic suture, double-armed 5-0 or 6-0 Vicryl suture
16. Millimeter ruler and surgical marking pen
17. Topical ophthalmic antibiotic ointment

A standard oculoplastic tray will include most of the instrumentation required.[4]

# PROCEDURE

## Medial Spindle Procedure

1. Patient should be supine with eyelids and head stabilized.
2. Administer topical and local anesthetic.
3. Placement of corneal shield.
4. Perform elliptical tarsoconjunctival excision incorporating the lower eyelid retractors.
5. Place double-armed 5-0 or 6-0 absorbable suture through the lower eyelid retractors.
6. Sutures are tied on the eyelid skin surface to invert the punctum.
7. Remove the corneal shield.
8. Administer topical ophthalmic antibiotic ointment.

The medial spindle procedure can also be referred to as medial conjunctivoplasty or medial palpebral conjunctival excision. When the patient has a medial ectropion, the medial spindle procedure can turn back the medial portion of the eyelid to the globe. At the start of the procedure, topical and local anesthetic is administered. After corneal shield placement, the eyelid margin is everted. An elliptical excision using Vannas scissors of tarsoconjunctival tissue with capture of the lower eyelid retractors is performed a few millimeters temporally from the punctum (Figure 14-15). Cautery is applied as necessary. A double-armed 5-0 or 6-0 Vicryl absorbable suture is passed through the lower eyelid retractors and reapproximates the excision site on the conjunctival side (Figure 14-16). Then these needles are redirected anteriorly and passed through the full thickness of the eyelid to the skin surface where they are secured (Figure 14-17). Tying these sutures inverts the punctum and eyelid margin. Remove plastic corneal shield. Apply topical ophthalmic antibiotic ointment.

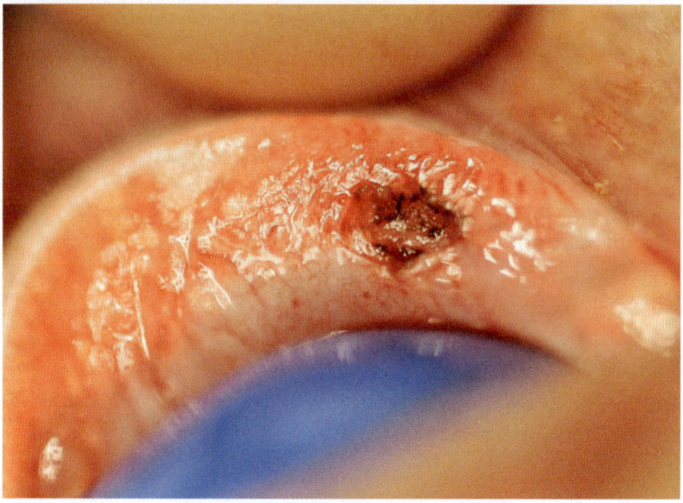

**FIGURE 14-15** Medial spindle procedure. The inferior eyelid has been everted to expose the palpebral conjunctiva. Elliptical excision of tarsoconjunctival tissue has been performed. The black streaks and spots on the surface are char from cautery. Note that the excision has been performed a few millimeters lateral to the punctum. The blue-colored object is a plastic corneal shield used to protect the globe during the surgery.

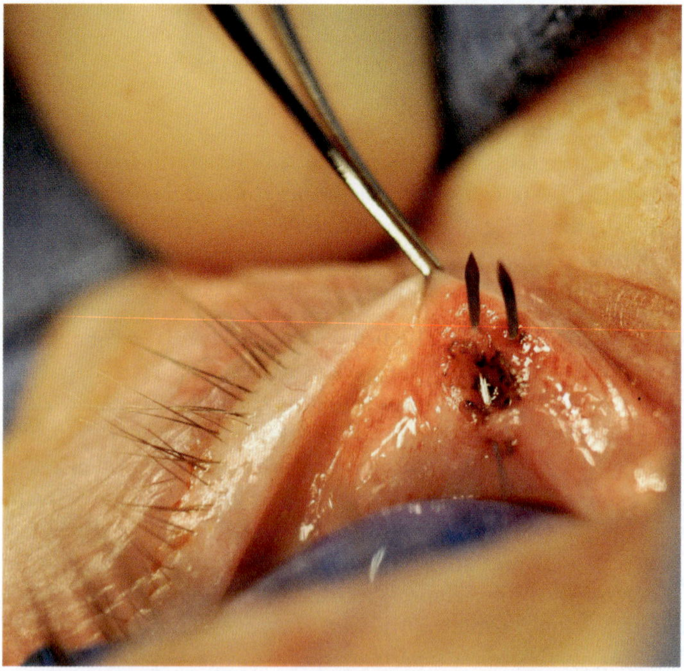

**FIGURE 14-16** Medial spindle procedure. Double-armed 5-0 or 6-0 Vicryl absorbable suture is passed through the lower eyelid retractors and reapproximates the excision site on the conjunctival side.

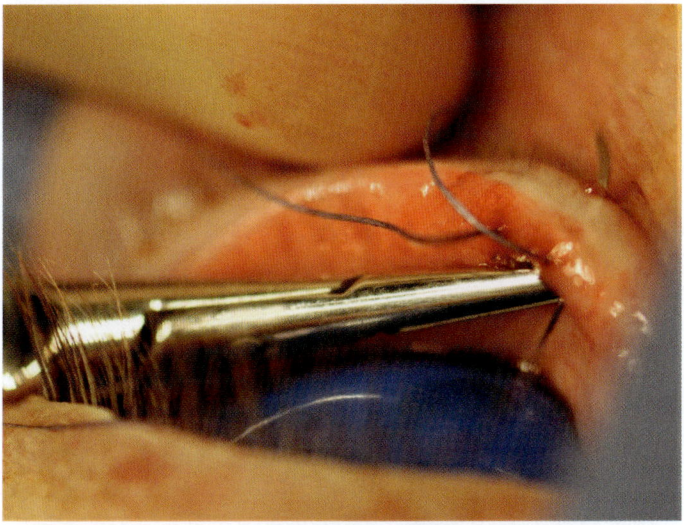

FIGURE 14-17 Medial spindle procedure. Each needle of the double-armed Vicryl suture is redirected anteriorly and passed through the full thickness of the eyelid to the skin surface where they are secured.

## Lateral Canthal Strengthening

1. Patient should be supine with eyelids and head stabilized.
2. Administer topical and local anesthetic to include the lateral lower eyelid, lateral canthus, and lateral orbital rim regions.
3. Perform a lateral canthotomy.
4. Incise the lateral canthal tendon (cantholysis).
5. Measure lateral lower eyelid for excision and excise excess lateral lid tissue.
6. Perform a tarsal strip of the lateral-most lower eyelid margin epithelium.
7. Reattach tarsal strip/lateral aspect of eyelid to the periosteum with a suture at the level of the lateral orbital tubercle.
8. Reform angle of lateral canthus and close with a nondissolvable suture.
9. Remove the plastic corneal shield.
10. Apply topical ophthalmic antibiotic ointment.

The lateral canthal strengthening procedure is performed for ectropion repair routinely but can be performed as an acute medical operation for correction of orbital compartment syndrome. It can also be performed in retrobulbar hemorrhage with high intraocular pressure (IOP).

With lateral canthal strengthening procedure, the first step is a lateral canthotomy. This is when the upper and lower eyelids are separated at the lateral canthus. Using a millimeter ruler and surgical marking pen, 1 cm is measured horizontally from the lateral canthus. At the start of the procedure, topical and local anesthetic is administered. The plastic corneal shield is positioned to protect the cornea and globe. A full-thickness, 1 cm in length, horizontal incision is performed with a No. 15 surgical blade down to the periosteum (Figure 14-18). Cautery is applied as necessary (Figure 14-19). Incision with Westcott scissors of the canthal tendon

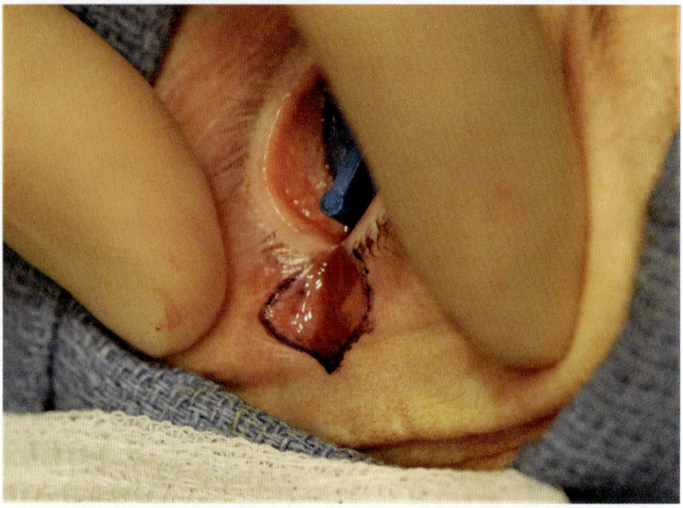

FIGURE 14-18 Lateral canthal strengthening. Full-thickness, 1 cm in length, horizontal lateral canthal incision is performed with a No. 15 surgical blade down to the periosteum. Note the blue-colored plastic corneal shield used to protect the globe during the surgery.

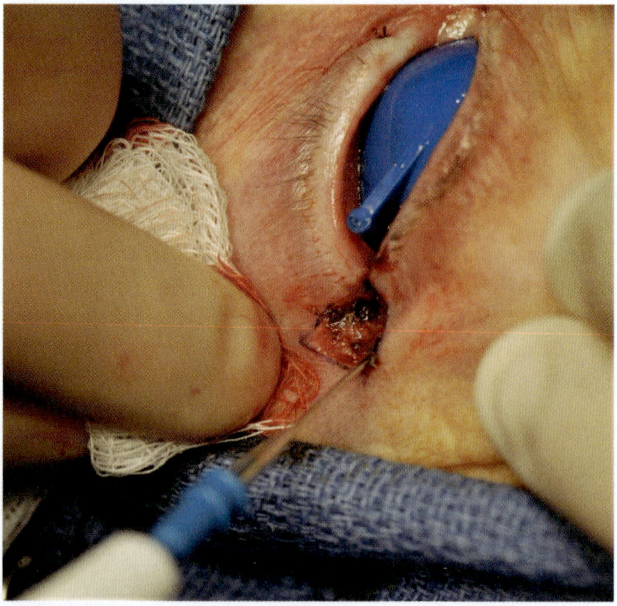

FIGURE 14-19 Cautery is applied at the lateral canthal incision site.

separates the lower eyelid away from the globe. The excess lateral lower eyelid is measured for excision. In order to achieve accurate measurement, the lower eyelid is held tightly against the inferior globe. The excess lid tissue is marked with the surgical marking pen and then excised using Westcott scissors. A tarsal strip is fashioned by excising the lateral-most eyelid margin epithelium with Westcott scissors. This prevents epithelial cyst formation. The lateral aspect of the lower eyelid is attached by a 5-0 chromic or Vicryl suture at the lateral orbital rim to the periosteum at the level of the lateral orbital tubercle (Figure 14-20). The lateral canthal angle is reformed with an interrupted 6-0 silk suture (Figure 14-21). This repositions the lower eyelid tightly against the globe and thus correcting the ectropion. Remove the plastic corneal shield. Apply topical ophthalmic antibiotic ointment.

## Repair of Cicatricial Ectropion with Autologous Graft

1. Patient should be supine with eyelids and head stabilized.
2. Administer topical and local anesthetic.
3. Placement of corneal shield.
4. Set traction sutures in the lash line and tent lower lid superiorly.
5. Perform subciliary incision with No. 15 surgical blade.
6. Dissect and free posterior lamella with Westcott scissors.

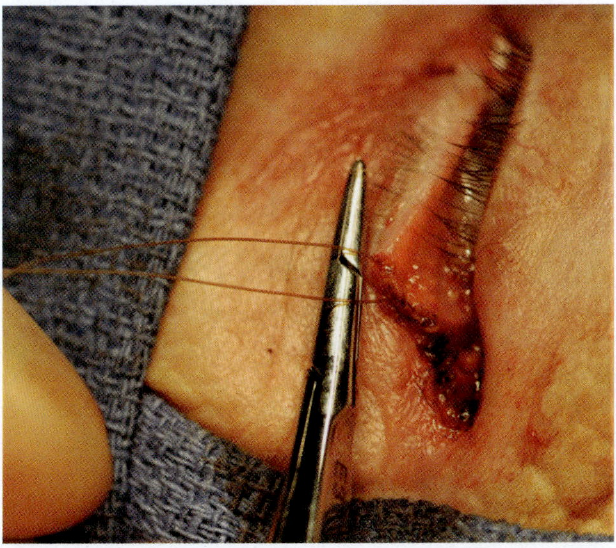

**FIGURE 14-20** The excess lid tissue has been excised using Westcott scissors. A tarsal strip is fashioned by excising the lateral-most eyelid margin epithelium with Westcott scissors. The lateral aspect of the lower eyelid is attached by a 5-0 chromic suture that is passed through the tarsal plate (shown here in the image). This suture is then attached at the lateral orbital rim to the periosteum at the level of the lateral orbital tubercle.

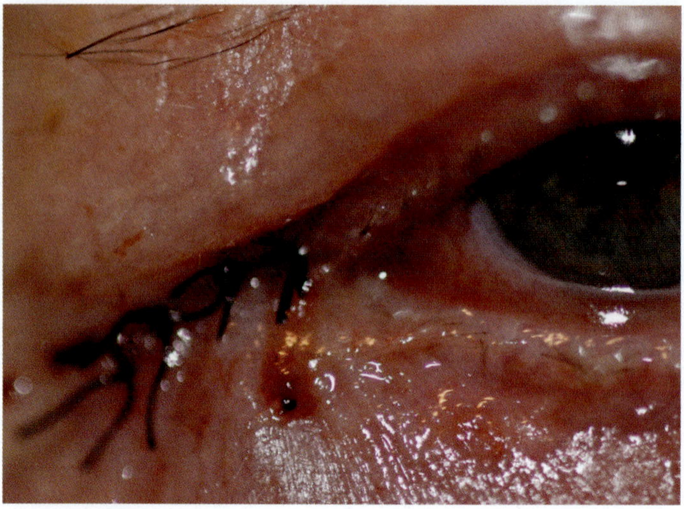

**FIGURE 14-21** The lateral canthal angle is reformed with an interrupted 6-0 silk suture.

7. Perform lateral canthal strengthening procedure.
8. Create graft template from residual wound site.
9. The template is used to measure the tissue needed to be removed from the donor site.
10. The autologous graft is removed, and the donor site is closed.
11. The autologous graft is sutured with interrupted 6-0 silk suture to the wound (recipient) site.
12. Remove the corneal shield.
13. Xeroform dressing and ophthalmic antibiotic ointment are applied.
14. Pressure patch and/or frost sutures are placed.

At the start of the procedure, topical and local anesthetic is administered. After corneal shield positioning, traction sutures are set in the lash line and the lower eyelid is tented upward. A subciliary incision with a No. 15 surgical blade is performed approximately 2 mm below the eyelash margin. It is extended horizontally along the entire length of the lower lid, stopping before reaching the puncta. Dissection of the underlying scar tissue with Westcott scissors should free the posterior lamella to its original anatomical location (Figure 14-22). Cautery is applied as necessary. A lateral canthal strengthening procedure, as described earlier is now performed.

After the area for the graft is measured with calipers from the residual wound site, a template is created. Either Telfa or the stiffer cardboard from the suture packaging can be used to create a template of the required donor tissue.[8] Either the upper eyelid skin, especially if the patient has significant dermatochalasis, or postauricular area can serve as autologous donor tissue sites (Figure 14-23). The supraclavicular and infraclavicular areas can also be used to harvest tissue for an autologous graft. The donor skin graft should be slightly larger (because of shrinkage) than the defect and should be excised as thinly as possible.[8] Once the autologous graft is obtained, the donor site incision is closed. The graft is then attached with interrupted

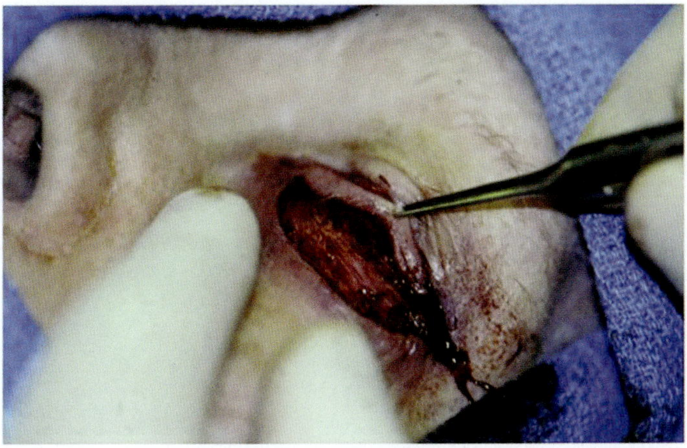

**FIGURE 14-22** A subciliary incision with a No. 15 surgical blade is performed approximately 2 mm below the eyelash margin. It is extended horizontally along the entire length of the lower lid, stopping before reaching the puncta. Dissection of the underlying scar tissue with Westcott scissors should free the posterior lamella to its original anatomical location.

6-0 silk sutures to the residual wound (Figure 14-24). Small drainage holes are made in the graft to prevent hematomas from forming underneath the graft, which would lead to graft rejection.[8] A Xeroform dressing is applied to hold the graft securely against the recipient site (Figure 14-25).[8] Either a pressure patch and/or frost sutures can be placed after the corneal shield is removed and ophthalmic antibiotic ointment is applied (Figure 14-26).

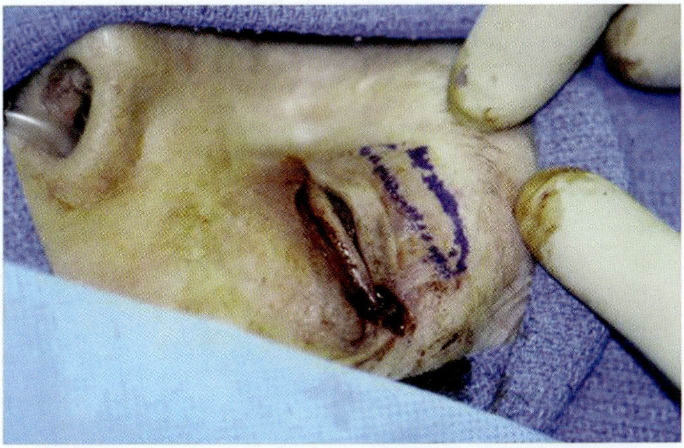

**FIGURE 14-23** The upper eyelid skin, especially if the patient has significant dermatochalasis as in this case, will serve as an autologous donor tissue site. The upper eyelid has been marked using a surgical marking pen.

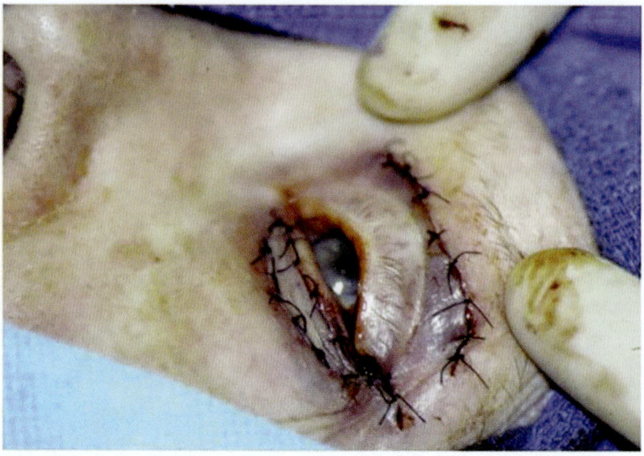

**FIGURE 14-24** Once the autologous graft is obtained, the donor site incision is closed with interrupted 6-0 silk sutures (in this case the upper eyelid). The graft is then attached with interrupted 6-0 silk sutures to the residual wound (recipient site) located on the lower eyelid.

If during the clinical evaluation of the patient, it is found that the eyelid can be repositioned manually back to the globe and there is no medial ectropion noted, then the lateral canthal strengthening procedure is all that would be necessary to correct the eyelid laxity. If there is persistent medial ectropion during the clinical evaluation, then a combined lateral canthal strengthening procedure with the medial spindle procedure will need to be done to eliminate the eyelid laxity. In this situation, the medial spindle procedure is always performed as the first surgical intervention, before the lateral canthal strengthening procedure. If there is only a medial ectropion present, then only the medial spindle procedure will need to be done. This is rare because in most cases of medial ectropion there is usually an accompanying eyelid laxity

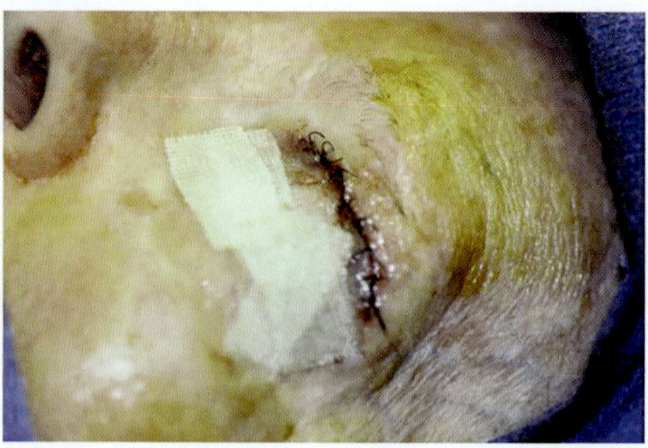

**FIGURE 14-25** Xeroform dressing is applied to hold the graft securely against the recipient site. Note the placement of frost sutures used to suture together the upper and lower eyelids.

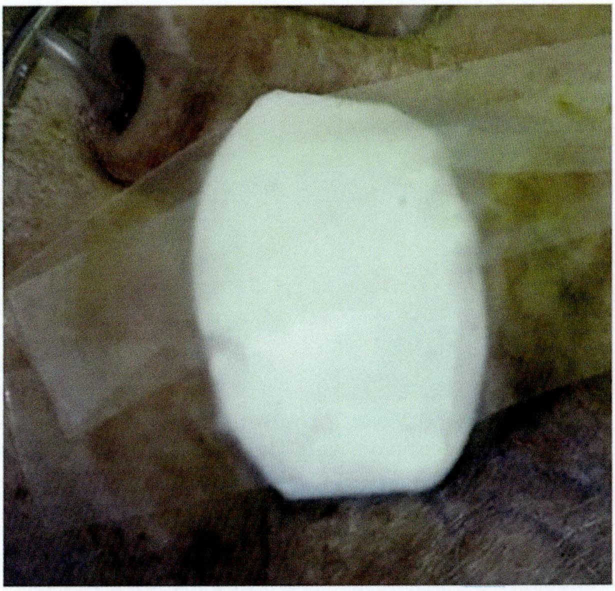

**FIGURE 14-26** A pressure patch is placed after the corneal shield is removed and ophthalmic antibiotic ointment is applied.

requiring the tightening of the eyelid laxity with a lateral canthal strengthening procedure. Repair of cicatricial ectropion with an autologous graft always needs to have a concurrent lateral canthal strengthening procedure performed. This surgery usually corrects any accompanying medial ectropion.

## POSTOPERATIVE CARE/COMANAGEMENT (FOLLOW-UP SCHEDULE)

### Key Postoperative Considerations

- Over-the-counter pain medications as necessary
- Topical ophthalmic antibiotic ointment twice a day (BID) until all sutures are removed
- Lateral canthal sutures removed in 1 week
- Medial spindle sutures removed in 2 weeks
- Autologous graft placement information as follows.

It is recommended that patients use over-the-counter pain medications. Eyelids should also be covered with ice packs. This will reduce any pain, swelling, and bruising. Patients should be prescribed ophthalmic antibiotic ointment BID to hydrate sutures, promote healing, and reduce the risk of infection. After 1 week postoperatively, the lateral canthal sutures are removed. The medial spindle sutures are removed 2 weeks following the procedure at which time the ophthalmic antibiotic ointment can be discontinued (Figures 14-27 to 14-29).

For those cases involving autologous graft placement, the pressure patch, frost sutures, and Xeroform dressing are removed approximately 5 days following surgery.[8] Traction sutures, lateral canthal sutures, and graft sutures can be removed in 7 to 10 days.[8]

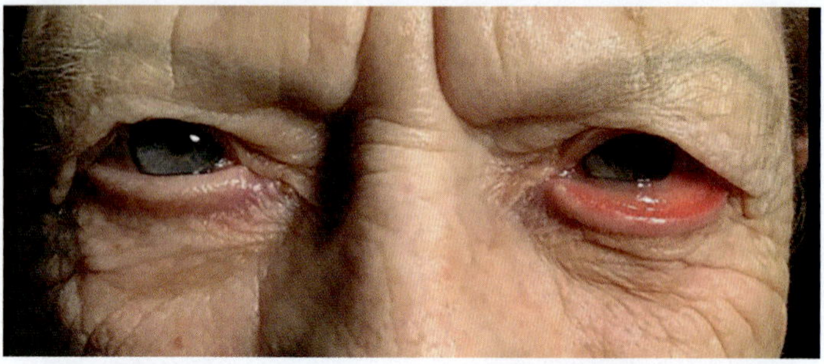

**FIGURE 14-27** Bilateral lower eyelid ectropion. Right lower eyelid with involutional ectropion. Left lower eyelid with involutional ectropion and secondary cicatricial component. The patient was instructed to apply a combination dexamethasone–neomycin–polymyxin B ophthalmic ointment to the left lower eyelid and massage the lid upward BID. After 6 weeks, the left lower eyelid was repositioning itself against the globe. The patient was scheduled for combination medial spindle procedure and lateral canthal strengthening for both lower eyelids.

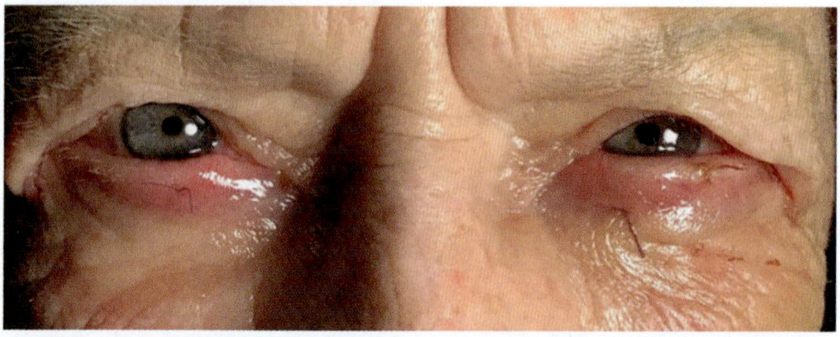

**FIGURE 14-28** One-week postoperative medial spindle procedure and lateral canthal strengthening, both lower eyelids. Note that the lateral canthal sutures have been removed at this visit, but the medial spindle sutures remain.

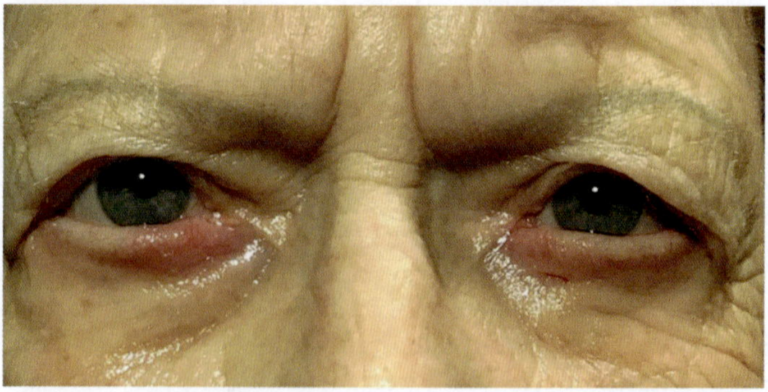

**FIGURE 14-29** Two weeks postoperative. The medial spindle sutures have been removed at this visit.

## POTENTIAL COMPLICATIONS AND THEIR TREATMENT

**Key Complications**

- Infection
- Bleeding/hematoma
- Pain
- Ectropion recurrence
- Graft failure
- Granuloma formation/scarring
- Corneal damage
- Epiphora

Complications of any eyelid surgery including ectropion include infection, bleeding, and pain.[4] Infection is to be treated aggressively and often cultures are taken to treat with more specific antibiotics. Monitoring of patients is done in the clinic and is dependent on which symptoms present. Conservative management of pain is suggested. Scarring, corneal damage, and corneal injury can occur after ectropion repair. Canthal dystopia and suture erosion can also occur.[9] The cornea is dry because of increased exposure in ectropion and postoperatively, surgery can aggravate dry eyes, which exacerbates the risk of corneal injury. This can be managed with topical ophthalmic eye drops, antibiotic ointment, and in severe cases, with surgery.

Ectropion recurrence is an adverse effect of ectropion surgical intervention. Cases of very severe or recurrent ectropion can warrant extensive surgical intervention. This could include a combination of tarsal strip and pentagonal wedge resection or temporalis muscle transfer procedures.[3]

## VIDEO OF PROCEDURE

**Video 14-1**—Ectropion repair. Three-snip procedure, medial spindle, and lateral canthal strengthening procedure. (Video courtesy of Leonid Skorin, Jr)

## EFFICACY

Lateral canthal strengthening is a gold standard in ectropion repair with reliable patient outcomes. The resolution of epiphora after the lateral canthal strengthening procedure is a favorable effect and promotes eye health postoperatively.[10] For severe lid laxity and involutional ectropion, lateral canthal strengthening remains the superior surgical choice of treatment.[11] The aesthetic result of the procedure is favorable, and the postoperative recovery period is relatively short.[12]

Cicatricial repair is recommended with full-thickness autologous graft. Studies have shown that this approach causes less ectropion recurrence and increased graft success.[13] A common complication with cicatricial repair is graft failure and contracture of the graft. When this happens, the graft is removed and replaced. Full-thickness autologous grafting along with a lateral block excision shows great success in repeat ectropion repair and virtually no cases of graft failure.[13]

## CODING/BILLING AND MODIFIERS

- **CPT code: 67924**—Ectropion repair
- **CPT code: 67914**—Ectropion repair with suture
- **CPT code: 67915**—Ectropion repair with thermocauterization
- **CPT code: 67916**—Ectropion repair with excision tarsal wedge
- **CPT code: 67917**—Ectropion repair with a tarsal strip operation

Common ICD-10 codes that support this procedure include the following:

- **H02.100 to H02.109**—Unspecified ectropion
- **H02.110 to H02.119**—Cicatricial ectropion of eyelid
- **H02.120 to H02.129**—Mechanical ectropion of eyelid
- **H02.130 to H02.139**—Senile ectropion of eyelid
- **H02.140 to H02.149**—Spastic ectropion of eyelid
- **H02.150 to H02.159**—Paralytic ectropion of eyelid

Eyelid modifiers can be used as such: E1 for upper left eyelid, E2 for lower left eyelid, E3 for upper right eyelid, and E4 for lower right eyelid.

## REFERENCES

1. Gladstone GJ. Ectropion. In: Onofrey BE, Skorin L, Holdeman NR, eds. *Ocular Therapeutics Handbook: A Clinical Manual.* 4th ed. Wolters Kluwer; 2020:649-652.
2. Skorin L, Lange R. Ectropion: classification, diagnosis, and management. *Consultant360.* 2018;58(6): e180. https://www.consultant360.com/articles/ectropion-classification-diagnosis-and-management
3. Gladstone GJ, Nesi FA, Nesi-Eloff F, Castillo F. Ectropion. In: *Oculoplastic Surgery Atlas: Eyelid and Lacrimal Disorders.* Springer; 2019:30-36.
4. Bergstrom R, Czyz CN. Ectropion lower eyelid reconstruction. In: *StatPearls [Internet].* StatPearls Publishing; 2022. Updated October 7, 2022.
5. Mitchell P, Hinchcliffe P, Wang JJ, et al. Prevalence and associations with ectropion in an older population: the Blue Mountains Eye Study. *Clin Exp Ophthalmol.* 2001;29(3):108-110. doi:10.1046/j.1442-9071.2001.00412.x
6. Bedran EG, Pereira MV, Bernardes TF. Ectropion. *Semin Ophthalmol.* 2010;25(3):59-65. doi:10.3109/08820538.2010.488570
7. Mick AB. Lacrimal tests and procedures. In: Onofrey BE, Skorin L, Holdeman NR, eds. *Ocular Therapeutics Handbook: A Clinical Manual.* 4th ed. Wolters Kluwer; 2020:320-323.
8. Marx DP, Yen MY. Management of ectropion and floppy eyelids. In: Yen MY, ed. *Surgery of the Eyelids, Lacrimal System and Orbit.* 2nd ed. Oxford University Press; 2012:91-101.
9. McKelvie J, Papchenko T, Carroll S, Ng SG. Cicatricial ectropion surgery: a prospective study of long-term symptom control, patient satisfaction and anatomical success. *Clin Exp Ophthalmol.* 2018;46(9):1002-1007. doi:10.1111/ceo.13338
10. Vick VL, Holds JB, Hartstein ME, Massry GG. Tarsal strip procedure for the correction of tearing. *Ophthalmic Plast Reconstr Surg.* 2004;20(1):37-39. doi:10.1097/01.IOP.0000103005.81708.FD
11. Georgescu D. Surgical preferences for lateral canthoplasty and canthopexy. *Curr Opin Ophthalmol.* 2014;25(5):449-454. doi:10.1097/ICU.0000000000000094
12. Kam, K., Cole, C., Bunce, C. et al. The lateral tarsal strip in ectropion surgery: is it effective when performed in isolation? *Eye (Lond).* 2012;26:827-832. doi:10.1038/eye.2012.34
13. Mol I, Paridaens D. Efficacy of lateral eyelid-block excision with canthoplasty and full-thickness skin grafting in lower eyelid cicatricial ectropion. *Acta Ophthalmologica.* 2018;97(4):e657-e661. doi:10.1111/aos.13958

# 15 Blepharoplasty

**Rachna Murthy • Jonathan Roos**

The eyelids and eyebrows frame and protect the eyes and are an area of focus when we interact with others. With age, skin loses collagen, hydration, elasticity, and support. The eyelid skin, being less than a millimeter in thickness, is the thinnest in the body and often shows the earliest signs of aging.[1] The eyelid contains no subcutaneous fat. With every blink, there is movement of the orbicularis and levator muscles. This continuous muscle movement under the increasingly less supple skin can result in sagging and loss of plumpness, called dermatochalasis. This can go on to hang loosely over the eyelids and cover the eyelashes. This is known as hooding. With age, hooding can appear worse in the outer part of the eyelid owing to the additional effect of lateral eyebrow ptosis. With more extensive hooding, dermatochalasis can result in a heavy sensation in the upper eyelids or a mechanical secondary ptosis. This can impact the visual field and visual acuity adversely as well as result in eyelash entropion.

With loosening of the skin, there may also be weakening of the orbital septum, a thin sheet of connective tissue in the eyelid under the orbicularis muscle. This can result in herniation of the orbital fat, although this is seen mostly in the lower eyelid owing to gravity. Sometimes, the lacrimal gland also can be found to have prolapsed out from its normal location in the superolateral orbit, and in the inner aspect the medial fat may also be seen as a bulge.

With aging, there are anatomical shifts in all layers of the face, and changes occur in all layers, including in the bone. Bony resorption with age affects the orbital rim, which results posteriorly in enlargement of the orbit and superomedially in collapse of the medial brow and forehead fat pads. In the inferior lid, the orbital rim becomes more visible topographically as resorption occurs and with downward descent of the malar (cheek) fat pads, baring the rim.[2] This appearance of the rim is often described as the "tear trough."

## CAUCASIAN UPPER EYELID

The upper eyelid skin and orbicularis are divided into three contiguous portions: a pretarsal and preseptal forming the palpebral portion and an orbital portion. The orbital portion surrounds the orbital rim and is responsible for forced eyelid closure. The pretarsal portion arises from the lateral canthal tendon and inserts medially by two heads. The superficial head forms the superficial part of the medial canthal tendon, and the deep head inserts onto the posterior lacrimal crest, forming the posterior limb of the medial canthal tendon. With contraction of the pretarsal portion, the eyelid closes, and the lacrimal puncta are pulled medially into the tear lake. The preseptal muscle similarly inserts by a superficial and deep head. The deep head inserts into the lacrimal fascia on the lateral side of the lacrimal sac. With contraction of the preseptal muscle, the lacrimal fascial is pulled laterally, creating a vacuum in the lacrimal sac that draws in the tears, which are pipetted into the lacrimal puncta by the pretarsal portion. Normal orbicularis muscle is very efficient in eyelid closure, and debulking this muscle does not compromise eyelid closure.

The orbital septum is a tough sheet of fibrous tissue that is firmly attached to the orbital rim and fuses with the levator aponeurosis in the upper eyelid. It divides the eyelid from the orbit and holds the orbital fat pads back.

In the upper eyelid, the preaponeurotic fat lies immediately behind the orbital septum and is divided into a medial and central compartment. The lacrimal gland lies laterally. This is an important consideration if excising fat for a blepharoplasty, not to mistake fat and lacrimal gland which is pinker in appearance (Figure 15-1). Blood vessels run through the fibrous septa in the fat pads connecting to the posterior ciliary circulation. Traction on the fat pads should be avoided because this can result in rupture of the septa and deep orbital vessels.

The levator muscle arises from the lesser wing of the sphenoid bone and extends forward, splitting into the levator aponeurosis and the Müller's muscle. The nerve supply is from the superior division of the third cranial nerve, which runs through the superior rectus muscle.

In Caucasians, aponeurosis inserts between the orbicularis oculi to form the skin crease. As the preseptal skin is not anchored to underlying structures, a fold of skin often overhangs the pretarsal skin and obscures the crease. The preaponeurotic fat pad lies behind the orbital septum and above the levator aponeurosis. This serves as an invaluable aid in its identification during surgery.

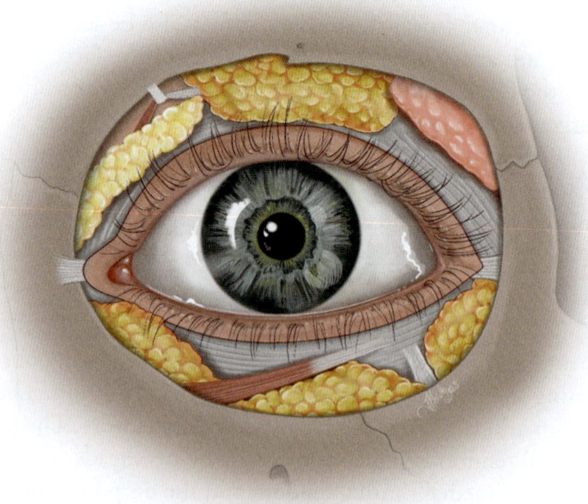

**FIGURE 15-1** Diagram demonstrating the eyelid fat pads on the left side. The lacrimal gland is pinker hued, and the medial upper fat pad is usually paler than the central fat pad.

The Müller's muscle is a thin strip of smooth muscle that extends from the striated levator muscle to the tarsal plate. In Caucasians, the tarsal plate height ranges from 9 to 10.5 mm. The aponeurosis lies anterior and conjunctiva posterior. Its innervation is from the sympathetic nervous system. Denervation causes the ptosis of Horner's syndrome.

## ASIAN UPPER EYELID

Approximately 50% of Asians will have some form of skin crease. The tarsal plate is within 6.5 to 7.5 mm in height, and the upper border corresponds to where a natural upper lid crease would sit. This is an important consideration in Asian skin crease forming blepharoplasty. In those without a crease, it has been postulated that the orbital septum fuses to the anterior surface of the tarsus, with a lower positioning of the preaponeurotic fat pad. Upper eyelid fat consists of pretarsal, preseptal, postseptal (preaponeurotic) and subbrow. In Caucasians, the preseptal and subbrow fat is contiguous, as in Asians without a crease, and often this is contiguous with pretarsal fat also.[3]

## LOWER EYELID

The orbital septum is a thin sheet of fibrous tissue, attached firmly to the orbital rim and loosely to the retractors. The lower eyelid retractors, responsible for the downward movement of the eyelid on downgaze, consist of a sheet of fibrous tissue extending from the inferior rectus muscle sheath, passing forward to enclose the inferior oblique muscle and blending into the inferior suspensory ligament of Lockwood. Anteriorly, the retractors attach to the inferior border of the tarsal plate (Figure 15-2). Laxity of the retractors contributes to involutional entropion and has implication in transconjunctival blepharoplasty postoperative care to avoid iatrogenic entropion. The inferior suspensory ligament of the fornix is part of the fibrous tissue of the

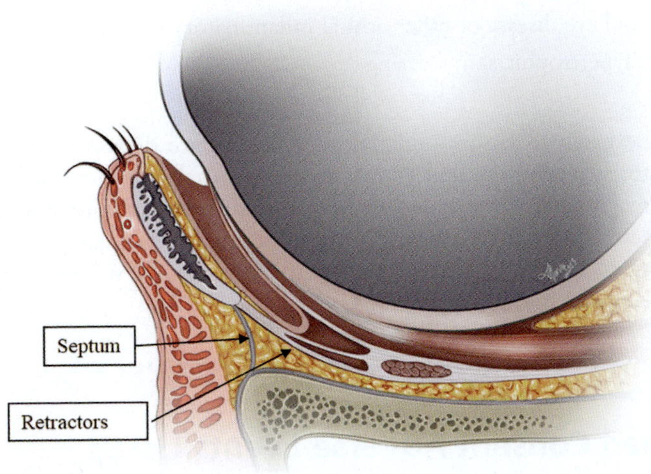


FIGURE 15-2 Cross section of the lower eyelid demonstrating the position of the lower eyelid retractors, which are posterior to the orbital septum.

retractors. Laxity of this results in shallowing of the fornix and allows orbital fat to bulge into the fornix, the "fornix fat sign." Laxity of the orbital septum allows orbital fat to bulge forward above the orbital rim, producing the appearance of "eyebags." The lateral canthal tendon arises from Whitnall's tubercle, 2 mm posterior to the lateral orbital rim. The medial canthal tendon inserts into the lacrimal crest. The tendons support the eyelids. Involutional changes in the bony orbit can result in laxity of the tendons and contribute to horizontal laxity of the eyelid.

## INDICATIONS

### Key Indications

Upper Eyelid:

- Cosmetic improvement
- To improve visual field defect secondary to hooding from excess skin
- To improve secondary lash entropion
- To obtain a full-thickness skin graft

Lower Eyelid:

- Cosmetic improvement

## CONTRAINDICATIONS

### Key Contraindications

- Ocular surface disease
- Brow ptosis causing the appearance of dermatochalasis
- Active thyroid eye disease or other orbital inflammatory disease
- History of hypertrophic skin scarring

Care should be taken to ensure underlying ocular surface disease is diagnosed and optimized. Brow ptosis causing the appearance of dermatochalasis should be excluded, and a brow procedure may be felt to be more suitable or considered in conjunction with upper lid blepharoplasty. Active thyroid eye disease and other orbital inflammatory disease should be stable prior to surgery. History of hypertrophic skin scarring would warrant consideration of a transconjunctival approach to lower eyelid blepharoplasty.

## INFORMED CONSENT CONSIDERATIONS

### Key Informed Consent Adverse Events Listed

Informed consent should include the benefits and risks of surgery and any other alternatives.

**What are the benefits of surgery?**

- Cosmetic improvement
- Improve upper lid hooding
- Improve lower lid laxity
- To appear less tired
- To reduce heavy sensation

**What are the alternatives to surgery?**

- There are no good alternatives to surgery. Other treatment modalities are either unpredictable or offer only temporary relief.
- There is always an option of not doing anything.

**What are the risks of anesthesia?**
We usually perform blepharoplasty under local anesthesia without sedation as day case outpatient surgery, although many surgeons prefer deep sedation (twilight sleep) or general anesthesia, particularly when combined with midface lift. Local anesthesia affords the patient quick surgical recovery and the surgeon the ability to assess the eyelid position on opening and closing and ocular surface protection.

- Local anesthetic may cause bruising, bleeding, and swelling.
- May need to administer additional anesthesia.

The following is a sample of the consent Drs. Roos and Murthy use.

**What are the risks and possible complications of surgery?**

- *Infection*: might present as increased swelling and redness of the skin. There might also be yellow discharge from the wound. Infection is treated with antibiotics. You will be provided with a novel patent-pending hypochlorous spray, Purifeyes, which we have developed. This will help to reduce postoperative infection and scar.
- *Bleeding*: may present as fresh blood oozing from the site of surgery or a lump appearing near the wound after the operation. Simple pressure on a skin wound is usually enough to control minor bleeding and is not of concern. In rare cases, a deeper hematoma may require review.
- *Loss of vision*: Total loss of vision in an eye caused by this type of surgery is extremely rare. A blood hematoma collecting in the orbit, behind the eye, may compress the nerve of vision and threaten eyesight. It is extremely rare for this to occur. It presents as pain, loss of vision, and a bulging forward of the eyeball and is an emergency. The eye prescription may change if there is significant hooding that is affecting the vision. A new postoperative refraction may be required.
- *Scar*: Whenever the skin is incised, a scar may form. Every attempt is made to minimize and hide scars, but rarely they can be visible.
- *Further surgery*: We will take great care to excise the correct amount of skin for your eyelid and brow position. It is possible, but in our hands most unlikely, for too much or too little to be excised. Underexcision may be addressed by further surgery to excise more.

Overexcision is even less likely but could cause eyelid retraction, ectropion, exposure of the eye, corneal ulceration, and loss of vision and may require further surgery to correct this.

- *Dry eye*: If you have a preexisting dry eye problem or weakness of the eyelids, these symptoms may be worsened by blepharoplasty surgery. However, we are trained, as ophthalmologists, in how to avoid this.
- *Skin puckering*: If deep sutures are placed, for instance, in the eyebrow area for brow pexy, there is a risk of puckering of the skin above them or discomfort. This is usually temporary but may necessitate further surgery to remove the suture if persistent.
- *Loss of sensation*: After surgery, there may be numbness of some of the skin around the incision. This is usually temporary, returning gradually over months. Extremely rarely, it is permanent and may involve larger areas like the forehead.
- *Inflammation*: Swelling and bruising of the skin or conjunctiva after surgery can occur but in varying degrees. A big improvement will be noticed after 2 weeks, with most resolved 3 months later. Rarely, inflammation may cause small lumps, called granulomas, to form. Most resolve spontaneously, but some require further treatment or surgery.
- *Altered appearance*: One of the goals of surgery may be to positively improve appearance. Some people may be unhappy with their appearance after surgery owing to asymmetry of facial features; hollowed appearance; eyelid contour or position changes.

## PREOPERATIVE ASSESSMENT

### Key Preoperative Considerations

- Full medical, aesthetic, and ocular history, including documentation of the patient's concern and goals from treatment
- Clinical photographs
- Full ocular examination and eyelid evaluation

A blepharoplasty consultation involves a full medical, aesthetic, and ocular history, including documentation of the patient's concern and goals from treatment. Preparation for surgery to the periocular area should be holistic and include ocular examination, dynamic facial examination and skin assessment, as well as assessment of the periocular area and eyelid and brow subunits. Clinical photographs with standardized lighting are essential.

When considering an upper eyelid blepharoplasty, a full ocular examination is essential, including visual acuity, unaided and corrected; slit-lamp ocular examination; assessment of the tear film; visual field testing; and ocular motility examination. Examination of the periocular area should include the eyelid margin, lash position, lid position, skin crease, tarsal plate show, brow position, and levator function. Any underlying eyelid ptosis should be identified at preassessment. This can be unmasked by blepharoplasty and should be preempted and addressed with a combined procedure. Brow ptosis, as a cause of secondary dermatochalasis, should be excluded and a discussion had with the patient regarding the brow contribution and a brow procedure. Lacrimal gland position and prolapse should be assessed and, if present, repositioning discussed as part of the procedure.

Examination of the lower eyelid should involve assessment of eyelid laxity and skin laxity with a snap test, canthal tendon laxity, fat pad prolapse, and retractor and septal deficiency (shallowing of the inferior conjunctival fornix). This will inform whether an anterior skin approach or posterior (transconjunctival approach) is suitable. Both approaches can also be combined. If there is horizontal lid laxity or canthal tendon laxity, the eyelid or tendon will require a tightening procedure.

Once the patient has confirmed they wish to proceed with surgery, it is good clinical practice to allow at least a 2-week cooling-off period to allow the patient time to confirm they wish to proceed for cosmesis.

## PREOPERATIVE REGIMEN

- Confirm the clinical findings.
- Confirm the treatment goals.
- Obtain full informed consent as earlier.
- Ask if there are any unanswered questions.

Perform preoperative and prelocal anesthesia marking to clearly mark skin incisions (if skin approach), amount of skin to be excised, and position of prolapsed fat pads with the patient sitting up and eyes closed.

We routinely prescribe the benzodiazepine, diazepam 5 mg, 1 hour prior to the procedure.

The patient is positioned supine on the operating table and monitoring leads are connected for pulse oximetry and cardiac telemetry. We use selective bipolar cautery and cold steel surgical instruments for surgery, which, in our experience, allows quicker postoperative recovery when compared with the use of $CO_2$ laser blepharoplasty or radiofrequency and does not necessitate a corneal shield.

## PROCEDURE

Topical anesthesia and marking:

A drop of proxymetacaine (proparacaine 0.5%) followed by tetracaine 0.5% is applied per eye for topical anesthesia of the cornea, conjunctiva, and inner surface of the eyelids.

The eyelids are marked with a fine surgical marker pen, with the patient sitting up. The inferior incision line is placed in the upper lid skin crease at the superior tarsal border, about 10 mm from the lash line in Caucasians. The superior line is determined by grasping the excess skin with fine nontoothed forceps, such as Moorfield's forceps, taking care to allow complete lid closure while pinching the skin.

Local anesthesia infiltration:

We use bupivacaine 0.5% (Marcaine) with 1:200,000 epinephrine mixing 5 mL with 4 mL lidocaine 2% (Lignocaine) with adrenaline 1:80,000 and 1 mL dexamethasone 3 mg/mL.

- *Upper lid blepharoplasty*

To remove skin and orbicularis muscle, use a No.15 surgical blade for the incision and Spring scissors for the excision. Alternatively, a radiofrequency device or a $CO_2$ laser can be used, although we prefer the cold steel approach, as explained previously. Skin and orbicularis muscle can then be excised in a single layer[4] or as two separate flaps,[5] making the muscular flap a little bit smaller in order to leave some muscle fibers concentric to the skin. Bipolar cautery is used to seal any localized bleeding points. A 5-0 Vicryl suture can be placed superolaterally at the border of two-thirds and lateral third of the orbicularis incision, in order to anchor some fibers of the orbicularis muscle from the upper and lower edge of the wound to the periosteum of the orbital rim (see Video 15-1). The expected effect is to give support to the lateral eyebrow, reducing lateral skin hooding (internal brow support). The retro-orbicularis oculi fat (ROOF) differs from the orbital fat in that it is located anteriorly to the orbital septum and posteriorly to the orbicularis muscle extending toward the eyebrow.[6] Careful but not excessive sculpting or excision will help to achieve a good aesthetic result. The medial fat pad, if excessive, can be sculpted carefully. The medial orbital septum is opened with sharp straight scissors, and gentle retropulsion on the globe allows the fat to prolapse out. The appearance of this orbital fat is paler and less yellow than the ROOF or preaponeurosis fat (Figure 15-1). The surplus is clamped with fine curved mosquito forceps, cut, and cauterized. The clamp is gently released, avoiding traction on the vessels, which risks orbital hemorrhage (Figure 15-3). We prefer to close the skin with 6-0 Vicryl interrupted sutures, although a 6-0 nylon running suture can be used (Figure 15-4).

- *Lower lid blepharoplasty*

A lower lid blepharoplasty can be performed either through a transcutaneous or transconjunctival approach.[7]

The transcutaneous approach is helpful when one wishes to excise skin.[8] Care should be taken to avoid excessive skin removal because this can lead to rounded appearance to the eye, lagophthalmos, or cicatricial ectropion. The skin is classically marked 1.5 to 2 mm below the lashes, starting medially from the lower punctum level and continuing laterally into the "crow's feet" lateral skin creases. A small incision with a scalpel is performed, and then the

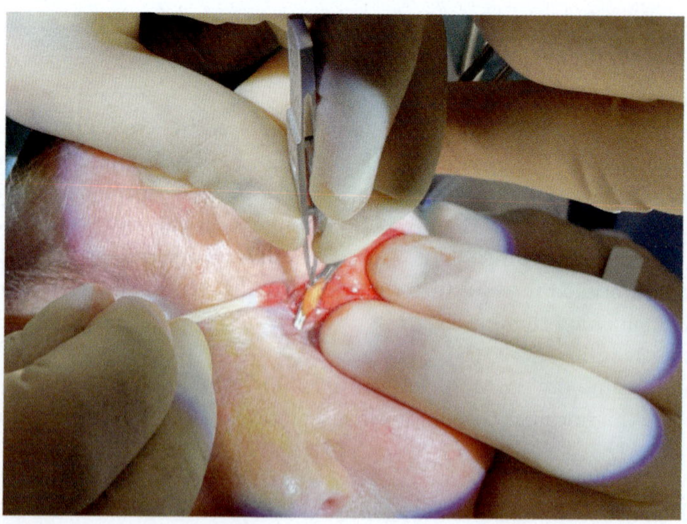

**FIGURE 15-3** Photograph on table of medial fat upper fat pad.

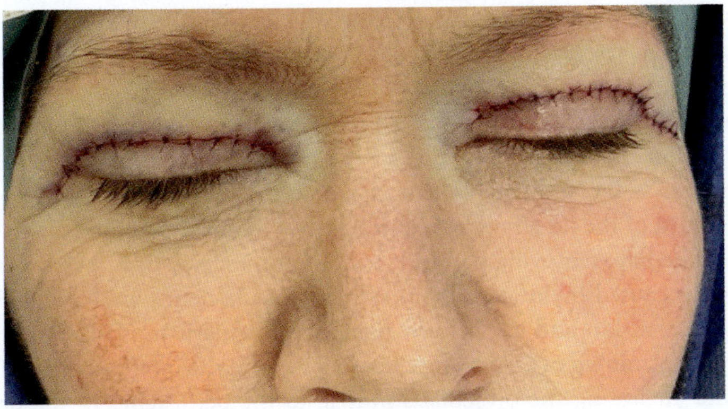

**FIGURE 15-4** Photograph on table following wound closure with 6-0 Vicryl interrupted sutures.

suborbicularis plane is identified and undermined with blunt scissors passing medially. This skin–muscle flap is cut with scissors, freeing it as far as the line of the inferior punctum. Just as with the upper lid blepharoplasty, skin and muscle can be undermined and excised separately in order to preserve more muscle and ensure good lid closure. The exposed septum is then incised, and the surplus fat cauterized and removed. The skin–muscle flap is finally laid and gently stretched upward and laterally while opening the mouth, in order to determine the amount of excess skin to be taken away. Six-0 Vicryl interrupted or a 6-0 nylon suture is used to close the skin. A lower lid strengthening procedure such as a strip or pexy can be placed if there is lid laxity or risk of lid laxity detected during the preoperative examination.

In contrast, the transconjunctival approach is thought to have a reduced risk of complications such as round eye or ectropion because the middle lamella is not disturbed.[9] It can also be less time-consuming, not requiring closure. However, the approach can be challenging with a tight eyelid, requiring surgery through a small opening.[10] This procedure is often appropriate for young patients with tight skin who do not require any skin excision. The procedure is performed by placing a Desmarres retractor in the lower lid, and the conjunctiva is then incised halfway between the tarsal border and the fornix. The capsulopalpebral fascia is opened and the fat exposed. The conjunctival incision is extended to almost the total length of the eyelid, toward the orbital rim, medial to lateral. Alternatively, two incisions can be performed, leaving a small central bridge that covers the inferior rectus muscle and avoids a rare complication when retractors fail to reattach spontaneously. The herniated fat is resected: a gentle retropulsion on the globe simulates gravity and can help in calculating the amount of fat to be removed. Alternatively, instead of resecting, the fat can be redistributed and draped to fill the tear trough deformity.

Occasionally, a transconjunctival blepharoplasty can be combined with a skin pinch technique to trim excess skin.[11] Although requiring two separate incisions, the advantage is that the middle lamella is untouched. The skin is pinched with forceps or hemostat in order to determine the amount that could be resected without risk of eyelid malposition.[12] Skin excision should be performed in a linear shape, not parallel to the inferior eyelid border at 5 mm from it.[13] Some surgeons prefer to follow the skin tension lines, where the skin fold forms. As the pinch does not incise the orbicularis muscle, the scar is usually not visible. Alternatively, chemical or laser skin resurfacing can be used together with transconjunctival blepharoplasty to treat skin excess.

An alternative to the skin pinch is a mixed transcutaneous and transconjunctival approach. This is a transconjunctival blepharoplasty for the medial and central fat pad, associated with temporal skin–muscle flap and lateral fat pad excision. The creation of a skin–muscle flap in the lateral one-third of the lid allows one to reach the lateral fat pad more easily and to stretch up and laterally the flap, removing part of it to correct skin excess.

Malar festoons caused by inflammatory exudate, insufficient lymphatic drainage near the orbital rim, or excess skin and a weak low-hanging orbicularis muscle, should be addressed. Extending the undermining of a skin-muscular flap beyond the inferior orbital rim and redraping the flap and anchoring the orbicularis muscle to the periosteum of the orbital rim may minimize their appearance. If festoons originate from lymphedema, direct resection may be required to correct this deformity. Although a scar is less disfiguring than a festoon, informed consent must be sought because some patients may otherwise be disappointed with the postoperative result.

## POSTOPERATIVE CARE/COMANAGEMENT (FOLLOW-UP SCHEDULE)

The natural history of healing includes ingrowth of blood vessels and extracellular matrix that last 5 to 6 weeks. At this time, incision lines become tight, firm, and red, and this can cause some patient frustration. Following this period, incision lines soften and fade for around 4 to 5 months.

Usually, antimicrobial antibiotic tablets are not required, and we have moved to the use of Hypochlorous spray (Purifeyes is a pH-balanced ocular and periocular hypochlorous spray with antimicrobial properties, and anti-inflammatory properties, that is convenient for patients to use postoperatively for eyelid hygiene). For lubrication of the eyes when there is tightness of the eyelids post surgery, an ointment is helpful at night and artificial tears by day for a few days, which are less likely to blur vision.

The following is an example of the information we give to our patients.

### Postoperative Instructions

If any swelling, bruising, discomfort, or pain worsens or a discharge (pus) appears around the suture line, contact your surgeons/clinic immediately.

We will give you a prescription for an oral antibiotic that you can take should any symptoms appear, although we think this is most unlikely.

### General Postoperative Instructions

- A firm eye pad is put on after the procedure for at least 1 hour. This should stay on until instructed. It is usually removed before discharge but may remain until the next morning when you can remove it yourself.

- You will be given teardrops or ointment for the eye—usually used three times per day for 1 week.
- You will be given a broad-spectrum ophthalmic antibiotic ointment for any external wound before you are discharged.

Apply the prescribed ophthalmic ointment with clean fingertips or a cotton-tipped bud along the incision lines twice a day for 2 weeks, running from the inside along the stitches to the outer end.

- Your absorbable stitches will fall out after 2 to 3 weeks, but we remove these as required at your follow-up.
- Cool compresses should commence as soon as the pad is removed or immediately if there is no pad. 5 minutes, five times a day, for 5 days.
- Cleanse the lids with cotton wool dipped in cooled boiled water or sterile saline for 10 days.
- Do walk but avoid any form of strenuous exercise for 10 days.
- Reading and watching television is fine.
- Please try not to bend over very much for the first 2 days after surgery.
- If you have pain within 2 hours of surgery, start taking the painkiller prescribed (or two 500-mg acetaminophen tablets every 6 hours) for 48 hours following surgery.
- Eye makeup can be used 1 week after surgery.
- Contact lenses can be used 2 weeks after surgery.

## POTENTIAL COMPLICATIONS AND THEIR TREATMENT

### Key Potential Complications

- Allergy
- Bruising
- Hematoma
- Blurred vision
- Vision loss
- Infection
- Asymmetry
- Scar
- Too little/too much skin removal
- Too little/too much fat removal
- Feminizing male lids
- Exaggerated sulcus/tarsal show
- Dry eyes
- Lower eyelid retraction
- Lower eyelid lash entropion/orbicularis roll
- Corneal abrasion

Common patient worries include initial appearance change when the eyelids are tight, puffy, and may be bruised. Blurring of vision is also a concern while the blink is incomplete with tightness and swelling of the eyelids immediately postoperatively and with the ointment used.

With good consent and communication, patient expectations can be met and reassurance given.

Complications are, fortunately, rare and can, on the whole, be avoided with good preoperative modulation and good surgical technique.

## VIDEOS OF PROCEDURES

**Video 15-1**—Internal suture brow support with 5-0 Vicryl closing orbicularis oculi fibers from inferior wound to superior wound with a pass through the superolateral orbital rim periosteum at the junction of the medial two-thirds and lateral third of the incision. (Video courtesy of Rachna Murthy and Jonathan Roos.)

**Video 15-2**—Blepharoplasty of upper eyelid. (Video courtesy of Leonid Skorin, Jr. and Taylor Lauermann.)

# EFFICACY

According to a 2019 survey of 28 studies, an upper blepharoplasty is accompanied by a great variety of beneficial functional outcomes, including an increased visual field and improvement in headache-related quality of life and vision-related quality of life[14] (Figure 15-5).

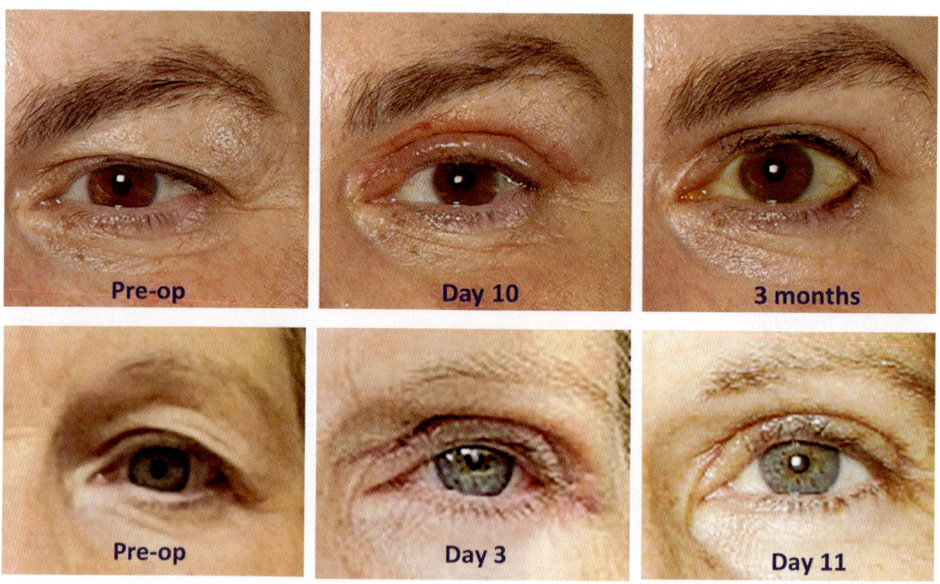


**FIGURE 15-5** Two patients demonstrating preoperative appearance of upper eyelid dermatochalasis and postoperative recovery following upper eyelid blepharoplasty with brow supporting sutures.

## CODING/BILLING

- **CPT code: 15820**—Blepharoplasty, lower lid
- **CPT code: 15821**—Blepharoplasty, lower lid: with extensive herniated fat pad
- **CPT code:15822**—Blepharoplasty, upper lid
- **CPT code:15823**—Blepharoplasty, upper lid; with excessive skin weighting down

Common ICD-10 codes that support blepharoplasty include the following:

- **H02.831** (dermatochalasis of right upper eyelid)
- **H02.832** (dermatochalasis of right lower eyelid)
- **H02.833** (dermatochalasis of right eye, unspecified eyelid)
- **H02.834** (dermatochalasis of left upper eyelid)
- **H02.835** (dermatochalasis of left lower eyelid)
- **H02.836** (dermatochalasis of left eye, unspecified eyelid)
- **H02.839** (dermatochalasis of unspecified eye, unspecified eyelid)

## REFERENCES


1. Chopra K, Calva D, Sosin M, et al. A comprehensive examination of topographic thickness of skin in the human face. *Aesthet Surg J.* 2015;35(8):1007-1013. doi:10.1093/asj/sjv079
2. Kim J, Park SW, Choi J, et al. Ageing of the bony orbit is a major cause of age-related intraorbital fat herniation. *J Plast Reconstr Aesthet Surg.* 2018;71(5):658-664. doi:10.1016/j.bjps.2017.11.029
3. Seiff S, Seiff B. Anatomy of the Asian eyelid. *Facial Plast Surg Clin North Am.* 2007;15:309-314, v. doi:10.1016/j.fsc.2007.04.010
4. Bosniak S. Upper lids: anatomy and surgical techniques. In: Bosniak S, ed. *Cosmetic Blepharoplasty.* Raven Press; 1990:37-58.
5. Carroll R, Manhanti R. En bloc resection in upper eyelid blepharoplasty. *Ophthalmic Plast Reconstr Surg.* 1992;8(1):47-49.
6. May J, Fears J, Zingarelli P. Retro-orbicularis oculus fat (ROOF) resection in aesthetic blepharoplasty: a 6-years study in 63 patients. *Plast Reconstr Surg.* 1990;86(4):682-689.
7. Bosniak S. Lower lids: anatomy and surgical techniques. In: Bosniak S, ed. *Cosmetic Blepharoplasty.* Raven Press; 1990:59-80.
8. Bourguet J. Orbital fat herniation: our surgical treatment. *Bull Acad Natl Med.* 1924;92:1270-1271.
9. Baylis HI, Long JA, Groth MJ. Transconjunctival lower eyelid blepharoplasty. Technique and complications. *Ophthalmology.* 1989;96(7):1027-1032.
10. Schwarz F, Randall P. Conjunctival incision for herniated orbital fat. *Ophthalmic Surg.* 1980;11:276-279.
11. Parkes ML, Bassiloios JI. Experience with the pinch technique in blepharoplasty. *Laryngoscope.* 1976;88:364-366.
12. Rosenfield LK. The pinch blepharoplasty revisited. *Plast Reconstr Surg.* 2005;115(5):1405-1412.
13. Kim EM, Bucky LP. Power of the pinch: pinch lower lid blepharoplasty. *Ann Plast Surg.* 2008;60(5):532-537.
14. Hollander MHJ, Contini M, Pott JW, et al. Functional outcomes of upper eyelid blepharoplasty: a systematic review. *J Plast Reconstr Aesthet Surg.* 2019;72(2):294-309. doi:10.1016/j.bjps.2018.11.010

# 16 Ptosis Repair

**Karina Richani • Thai Do**

Blepharoptosis, or ptosis, is a unilateral or bilateral drooping of the upper eyelid caused by dysfunction of the upper eyelid retractor(s). This can result in functional impairment of daily activities (e.g., driving, reading, or near work) and cosmetic dissatisfaction. The two upper eyelid retractors are the levator palpebrae superioris and Müller's muscle.

The levator palpebrae superioris is the major retractor muscle.[1] It is a skeletal muscle that originates from the orbital apex, above the annulus of Zinn, and is innervated by the superior branch of the oculomotor nerve. As it travels anteriorly, the muscular segment gradually transitions to the aponeurotic segment at the level of Whitnall's ligament.[2,3] The levator aponeurosis has multiple insertion points: anteriorly, into the subcutaneous fibers of the skin to form the eyelid crease; inferiorly, on the anterior surface of the tarsal plate for mechanical eyelid elevation; and posteriorly, to the Müller's muscle.[2,3]

The Müller's muscle is a sympathetically innervated smooth muscle that originates from the undersurface of the levator aponeurosis and inserts on the superior tarsal border.[2,3] This muscle provides approximately 2 mm of upper eyelid lift.

Aponeurotic ptosis is the most common form and accounts for approximately 60% of cases.[1,3] This degenerative process is caused by dehiscence of the aponeurotic fibers from the tarsal plate and fatty degeneration of the levator muscle.[4,5] Risk factors leading to aponeurotic ptosis are eyelid trauma, postsurgical changes, and contact lens wear.[3] Patients with aponeurotic ptosis often present with high or absent lid crease, thin upper eyelid skin, and good levator function. Other categories of ptosis include myogenic, neurogenic, traumatic, and mechanical. The following etiologies are several "cannot-miss" diagnoses that should be ruled out with every ptosis evaluation.

## "CANNOT-MISS" DIAGNOSES

### Myasthenia Gravis

Myasthenia gravis (MG) is an autoimmune disease characterized by muscle fatigue and weakness. Auto-antibodies directed against acetylcholine (ACh) receptor sites at the postsynaptic neuromuscular junction cause blockage and degradation of the signal receptors.[3,6] With sustained muscle activation, the amount of ACh released from the presynaptic terminal saturates the reduced number of postsynaptic receptors, resulting in muscle fatigue. Ptosis and diplopia may be the only manifestation of MG. The sleep test and ice-pack test are safe in-office evaluations for MG.[7]

Laboratory workup includes ACh receptor (binding, blocking, modulating) and Muscle-Specific Kinase (MuSk) receptor auto-antibodies.[8] Approximately 10% of MG patients have no auto-antibodies[8] and should receive single fiber electromyography (EMG) if there is a high clinical suspicion. Confirmed MG patients should receive a computed tomography (CT) of the chest to rule out thymoma.

Surgical intervention to address the ptosis should only be considered when MG is medically controlled.

## Third Nerve Palsy[3,9]

Disruption of the oculomotor nerve tract can result in ptosis, motility (adduction, elevation, and depression) deficits, and pupillary dilation. Ptosis associated with third nerve palsy is severe, with poor levator function. Acute presentation of a pupil-involving third nerve palsy may be a neurosurgical emergency, and urgent CT angiography or magnetic resonance angiography is required to rule out a compressive lesion.

The degree to which third-nerve-palsy-associated ptosis recovers is highly variable and depends on the underlying etiology. Once diagnosed and treated, patients should be monitored for at least 3 months for improvement. Significant ocular misalignment may require strabismus surgery before lid elevation. Patients with persistent poor levator function may require a frontalis sling for adequate lid elevation.

## Horner's Syndrome[3,9]

Horner's syndrome results from a disruption of the sympathetic pathway that supplies the head and neck. The differential diagnosis for the cause of Horner's syndrome is broad and includes intracranial infarction, Pancoast tumor, vascular dissection, cavernous sinus thrombosis, and demyelinating diseases. The classic triad of Horner's syndrome is mild ptosis, pupillary miosis, and facial anhidrosis. Loss of sympathetic innervation to the Müller's muscle causes subtle upper eyelid ptosis (≤2 mm). A careful pupillary examination should be performed in light and dark conditions on every patient with unilateral ptosis. In-office evaluation with topical apraclonidine 0.5% or cocaine 10% solution may help diagnose Horner's syndrome.

Patients with newly diagnosed Horner's syndrome require neuroimaging of the head and neck to evaluate the sympathetic tract. Patients with Horner's syndrome are excellent candidates for Müller's muscle conjunctival resection (MMCR) ptosis procedure, which directly addresses the affected retractor muscle.[10]

# INDICATIONS

**Key Indications**

- Visual impairment resulting from eyelid position with or without excess skin weighing down the eyelids
- Cosmetically displeasing owing to lid positioning, lid crease deformity, deep superior sulcus, or lid asymmetry

The most common indication for ptosis repair is visual impairment caused by superior visual field constriction. Clinical findings that may support the need for functional ptosis repair include decreased margin corneal light reflex distance 1 (MRD1), improvement of visual field with lid elevation, and subjective interference with activities of daily living. Cosmetic deformity (high eyelid crease, deep superior sulcus) and lid position asymmetry are other indications for cosmetic ptosis repair.

## CONTRAINDICATIONS

### Key Absolute Contraindications

- Poor levator function (≤4 mm)
- Significant lagophthalmos

**Key Relative Contraindications**

- Severe dry eyes
- Superior trabeculectomy
- Bell's palsy
- Corneal hypoesthesia
- Unrealistic expectation

Patients with poor levator function are unlikely to have improvement with external levator advancement or MMCR. These patients require a frontalis sling or frontalis muscle flap, which couples the upper eyelid with the frontalis muscle. Elevation of the upper eyelid in patients with preexisting lagophthalmos will exacerbate and worsen their ocular surface disease. Depending on the severity, this may result in a vision-threatening complication and ultimately lead to a poor outcome.

The most common ocular complaint following ptosis surgery is worsening dry eye symptoms. Patients with known ocular surface disease can have successful surgical outcomes with appropriate preoperative counseling and treatment. Ocular surface and dry eye symptoms and the ocular surface itself should be optimized with artificial tears, lubricating gel or ointment, topical anti-inflammatory medications (steroids, cyclosporine, or lifitegrast), and/or punctal plugs. Patients should be aware that a diminished blinking reflex is expected, and recovery may take up to 3 months to return to baseline.

Patients with superior trabeculectomy blebs, decreased corneal sensation, or decreased blinking from Bell's palsy may not be ideal candidates for internal ptosis repair. Disruption of the palpebral conjunctiva and tear film and potential suture exposure may lead to corneal abrasion, bleb irritation/inflammation, and corneal ulceration.

# PREOPERATIVE PREPARATION

**Key Preoperative Considerations**

- Obtain a detailed history to help identify ptosis etiology.
- A complete ophthalmic examination should be performed.
- Photographic and visual field documentation is important in demonstrating medical necessity.

## History

A careful and detailed history is critical to identifying the ptosis etiology and recognizing cannot-miss diagnoses. The history should include the time of onset, progression over time, visual complaints and effect on daily activities, and possible associated symptoms, including double vision, generalized weakness, fluctuation in eyelid position, and difficulty swallowing or talking. Questions regarding general health and systemic illnesses should be asked to identify potential anesthesia risks. A review of the medication list may help identify general health conditions that may have been overlooked. Any use of aspirin or other blood thinners should be covered. Questions regarding previous surgeries, trauma, and reactions to anesthesia are helpful for preoperative planning. Old photographs of the patient may help determine the type and onset of the ptosis.

## Physical Examination

A complete ophthalmic examination should be performed. Visual acuity, intraocular pressure, and confrontation visual field may identify concurrent intraocular pathology, which would not improve with eyelid surgery. Pupil size and light reactivity should be measured. Anisocoria should be evaluated in light and dark conditions. Extraocular motility is crucial to rule out cranial nerve palsy, MG, and other myogenic or neurogenic causes.

Eyelid measurements are the objective information necessary to determine the appropriate surgical approach. The two primary measurements are MRD1 and levator function. The MRD1 is the distance between the upper lid margin and the corneal light reflex from a handheld penlight in primary gaze. The normal MRD1 is 3 to 4.5 mm. The levator function is the amount of upper eyelid excursion from the maximal downgaze to the maximal upgaze. The normal levator function is 12 to 18 mm. Frontalis recruitment affects the levator function and should be negated by applying firm pressure on the ipsilateral frontalis muscle while evaluating the levator function. Levator function can be categorized as poor ($\leq$4 mm), fair (5–9 mm), or good ($\geq$10 mm). Patients with poor levator function are not candidates for external levator advancement or MMCR.

In unilateral ptosis, the nonptotic eye should be evaluated with the suppression of Hering's reflex. To perform this maneuver, first measure the MRD1 of the nonptotic eyelid in the neutral position. Repeat the measurement with elevation of the ptotic eyelid. If the MRD1 decreases, this indicates that the Hering's reflex is affecting the position of the nonptotic eyelid and that the eyelid position is expected to drop with unilateral ptosis surgery. If there is a significant decrease, bilateral surgery should be considered.

The vertical skin distance and eyelid crease height should also be measured. Excess upper eyelid skin may cause lateral hooding and contribute to a superior visual field defect. Dehiscence of the levator aponeurosis may increase the lid crease height and contribute to crease asymmetry. These concurrent issues may be addressed simultaneously via the external approach.

Facial and orbital asymmetry may affect the eyelid position. Exophthalmometry helps assess for globe position and orbital asymmetry. Full-face photographs are also helpful for documenting preexisting asymmetry and for patient counseling.

Dry eye disease should be assessed with tear breakup time, Schirmer's test, and/or tear osmolarity. The orbicularis muscle tone and Bell's phenomenon should also be checked. Slit-lamp examination can reveal underlying dry eye disease or ocular surface conditions.

### Photography[11]

Photographic documentation is important in demonstrating medical necessity for insurance purposes. Furthermore, photographs may help a surgeon explain and discuss eyelid asymmetry and surgical approach. A comparison between the preoperative and postoperative photographs may be helpful to allow patients to see improvements in eyelid position following surgery and help provide information in medicolegal disputes. The preoperative and postoperative photographs should, ideally, be taken with the same type of camera, lens, and lighting conditions. The background should be nondistracting, and heavy use of makeup should be discouraged.

Most insurers require photographs in the primary upright position, full face, and side view with the brow in a neutral position. The photographs should demonstrate the upper eyelid margin within 2 mm of the corneal light reflex. Additional shots at 45°, downgaze, or with Hering's reflex suppressed may also be beneficial.

### Visual Fields

Visual field testing may be performed in several different ways, including tangent screen visual field testing, Goldmann perimetry, or programmable automated perimetry. In general, visual fields must demonstrate a minimum of 12° or 30% loss of the upper field of vision owing to the position of the upper eyelid to demonstrate functional needs for surgical correction.[11]

## INFORMED CONSENT CONSIDERATIONS

#### Key Informed Consent Adverse Events Listed

- Pain
- Bleeding
- Infection

- Undercorrection
- Overcorrection
- Scarring
- Possibility of repeat surgery
- Exacerbation of dry eye symptoms
- Ocular injury
- Vision loss

Informed consent is an essential step in achieving optimal surgical outcomes. This is a step to discuss surgical goals as well as potential risks and complications associated with surgery. The risks associated with ptosis surgery include pain, bleeding, infection, undercorrection, overcorrection, eyelid asymmetry, exposure keratopathy or worsening dry eye, vision loss, and the need for repeat surgery.

In most cases, patients with ptosis seek surgery for improvement in vision and cosmetic outcomes. The patient must be aware that their central visual acuity and visual clarity will not change following ptosis surgery. Their peripheral visual field is expected to improve.

Subtle eyelid asymmetry (≤1 mm) may be challenging to address perfectly. Observation or medical treatment with topical oxymetazoline should be considered in these cases. Facial or orbital asymmetry may contribute to eyelid asymmetry and can be challenging to correct with eyelid surgery alone.

Patients with uncontrolled dry eye, ocular surface disease, poor blinking, or lid closure should be informed of potential postoperative increase in dryness.

Several factors that can improve patient satisfaction with ptosis surgery include honest, open communication between surgeon and patient; realistic expectations of what will occur before, during, and after surgery; and a clear understanding of the goals involved in ptosis surgery.

## INSTRUMENTATION

### External Levator Advancement (Figure 16-1)

- Local: 50–50 mixture of 2% lidocaine with epinephrine and 0.5% bupivacaine with epinephrine
- 30 gauge × ½ inch needle
- Fine tip surgical marking pen
- Serrated, nontoothed forceps
- Blunt tip Westcott scissors
- 0.5 toothed forceps × 2
- Castroviejo needle holder
- No. 15 Bard Parker blade
- High-temperature cautery or Bovie monopolar with needle tip

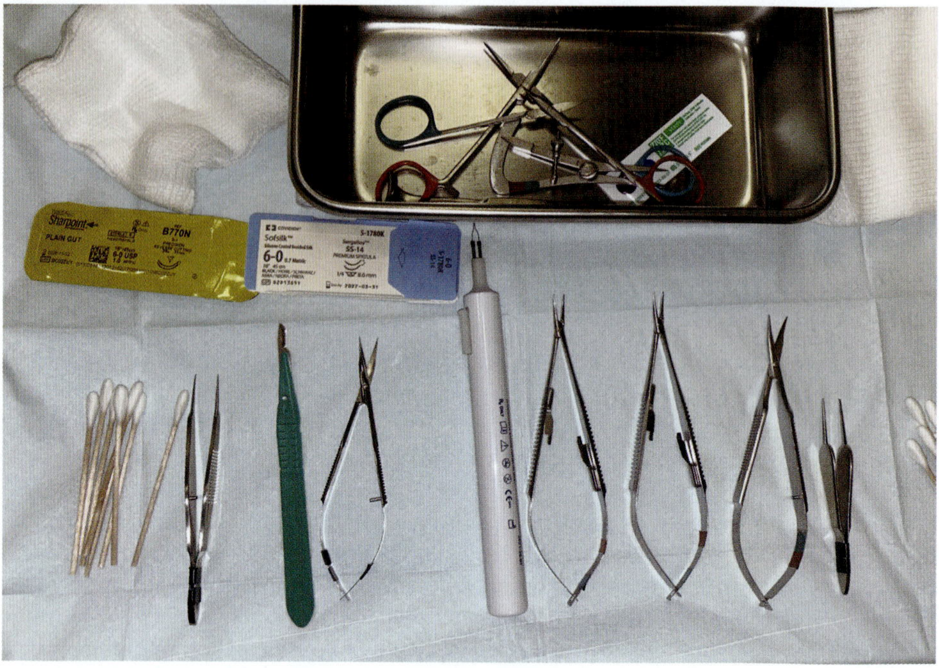


**FIGURE 16-1** Instrumentations for external levator advancement.

- Double-arm 6-0 silk suture (C1, taper needle, double arm, 3/8c, 18″)
- Double-armed 6-0 fast absorbing plain gut suture (PC-1 needle, 3/8c, conventional cutting, 13 mm, 18″)
- 4 × 4 gauze
- Cotton tip applicators

## Müller's Muscle Conjunctival Resection (Figure 16-2)

- Local: 50-50 mixture of 2% lidocaine with epinephrine and 0.5% bupivacaine with epinephrine
- 30 gauge × ½ inch needle
- Desmarres retractors
- Castroviejo calipers
- Putterman Conjunctiva-Müller's resection clamp
- Blunt tip Westcott scissors
- 0.5 toothed forceps × 2
- Castroviejo needle holder
- No. 15 Bard Parker blade
- High-temperature cautery or Bovie monopolar with a needle tip
- Single-armed 4-0 silk suture (reverse cutting, 3/8c, 13 mm, 18″)

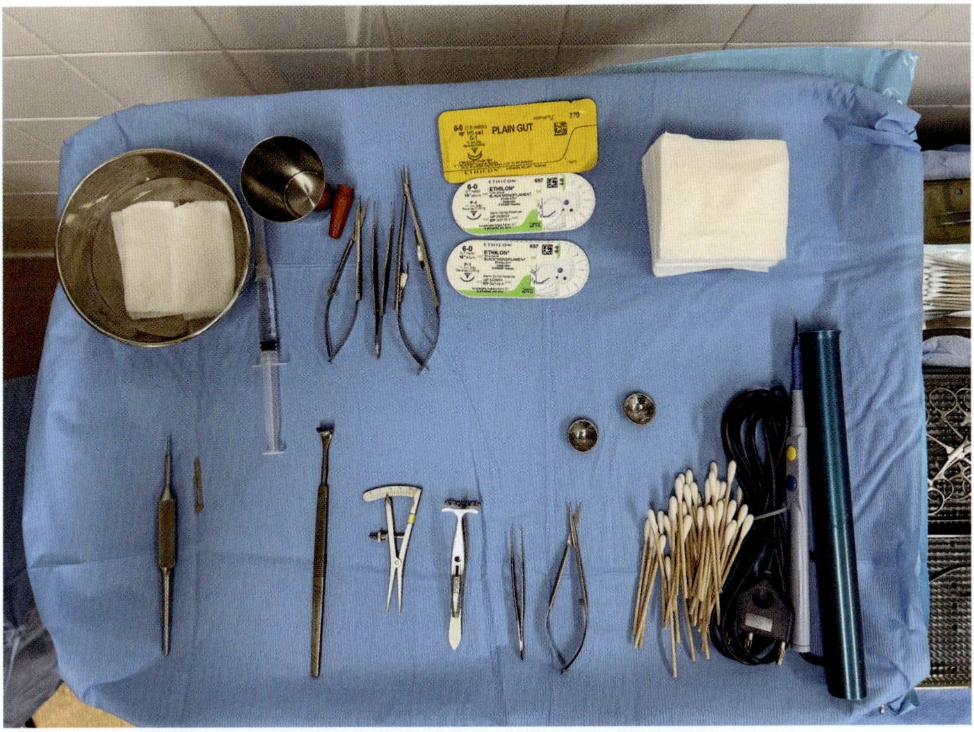

FIGURE 16-2 Instrumentations for Müller's muscle conjunctival resection.

- Double-armed 6-0 fast absorbing plain gut suture (PC-1 needle, 3/8c, conventional cutting, 13 mm, 18″)
- 4 × 4 gauze
- Cotton tip applicators

# PROCEDURE

## External Levator Advancement

### *Step 1: Lid Crease Marking*

Topical anesthetic drops are instilled onto the surface of both eyes. The eyelid skin is wiped with an alcohol wipe to remove residual oil and debris. The supratarsal lid crease is marked with a marking pen. This can be identified by asking the patient to open their eyes to a neutral opening position. If the lid crease is poorly defined, greater than 10 mm, or if there is significant asymmetry, the lid crease should be marked at a new position (Figure 16-3).

For most non-Asian patients, the lid crease is between 7 and 10 mm. For Asian patients, the crease is between 4 and 7 mm. Once the crease is marked, a skin flap can be drawn, leaving behind 20 mm of upper eyelid skin for adequate eyelid closure. A skin pinch test with nontooth

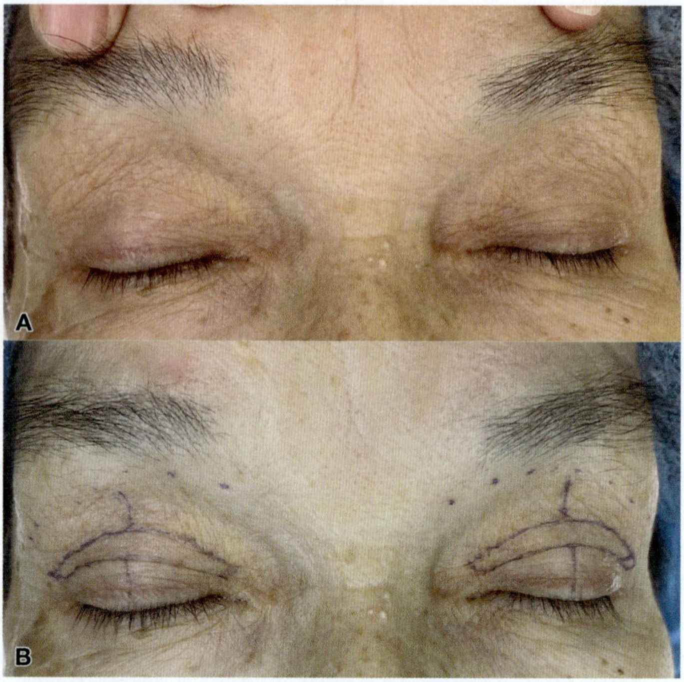

**FIGURE 16-3** **A,** The lid crease of both upper eyelids is poorly defined. **B,** The upper eyelid blepharoplasty incision is marked at 10 mm.

forceps can confirm that lagophthalmos will not result from the skin excision. If eversion of the eyelashes is noted with the skin pinch, remeasure or decrease the amount of skin taken.

### *Step 2: Local Anesthesia*

Local anesthesia can be injected just below the skin to prevent any anesthetic effect on the levator or Müller's muscles.

The closed eyelids are scrubbed and prepped in the usual fashion for oculoplastic surgery, typically with 5% povidone–iodine (Betadine) prep.

### *Step 3: Skin Incision*

The skin is held taut to prevent buckling, and the incision is then performed with a No. 15 blade or a monopolar cautery with a needle tip along the marked lines. A skin flap is elevated and excised with Wescott scissors or monopolar cautery. The orbicularis muscle should be preserved, particularly in patients with poor eyelid closure or Bell's phenomenon.

### *Step 4: Tarsal Plate Dissection*

Dissection is then carried out inferiorly over the surface of the tarsus. This can be done by tenting the skin edges overlying the tarsal plate with forceps, then using Westcott scissors or a high-temperature cautery to cut through the orbicularis muscle over the anterior surface of the tarsal plate. Fibrous attachment of the levator aponeurosis over the anterior surface of the tarsal plate should be cleared to reveal a clean tarsal plate (Figure 16-4).

### Step 5: Isolating the Levator Aponeurosis

Superiorly, the edge of the levator aponeurosis is identified and isolated. The levator aponeurosis has a white, fibrous appearance. In patients with significant dehiscence, the levator aponeurosis is not directly visible on the superior tarsal border. The preaponeurotic fat pads and the peripheral arcades are helpful landmarks to identify the levator aponeurosis. Once identified, an assistant can retract the levator inferiorly, and the preaponeurotic fat pads can be retracted superiorly. This should expose the septal attachment, which can then be separated (Figure 16-5) with a high-temperature cautery or Westcott scissors.

The surgeon can palpate the superior orbital rim while applying inferior traction on the levator aponeurosis to verify that the levator aponeurosis is sufficiently freed. Because the septum is firmly attached at the arcus marginalis, the surgeon will feel this traction if the septum is pulled inferiorly. Septal attachments should be released until no traction is felt.

### Step 6: Levator Advancement

A 6-0 double-arm silk suture can be used to pass through the tarsus in a partial thickness fashion for approximately 5 mm in length near the superior tarsal border (Figure 16-6).

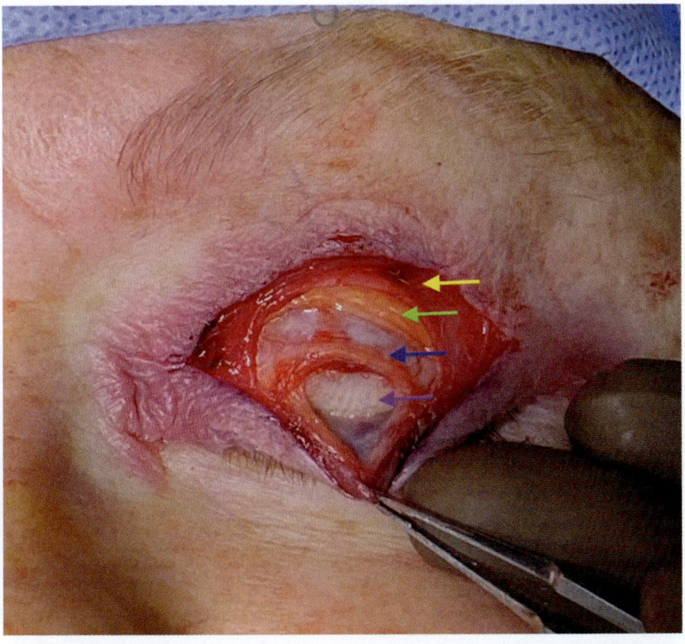

**FIGURE 16-4** Upper eyelid structures. Purple arrow: tarsus with the superior peripheral arcade. Blue arrow: levator aponeurosis. Green arrow: preaponeurotic fat. Yellow arrow: orbicularis oculi.

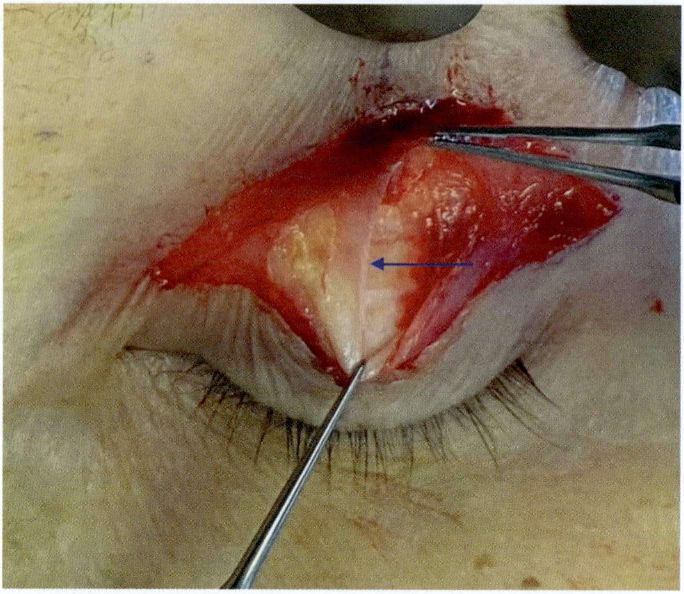

**FIGURE 16-5** The septum is a thin, fibrous layer between the levator aponeurosis and the preaponeurotic fat pads. With the levator and preaponeurotic fat retracted in opposite direction, the septal bands (blue arrow) become visible and can be released by Westcott scissors or a high-temperature cautery.

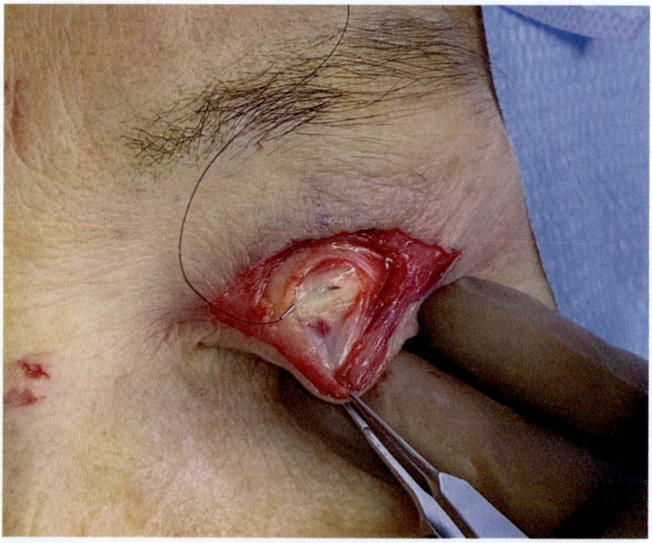

**FIGURE 16-6** Partial thickness pass through the center of the tarsus.

Note that the tarsus lateralizes with age and does not match up perfectly with the height of the eyelid. Therefore, the tarsal pass should be centered at the midpupil line and not at the peak of the tarsus. The eyelid should be everted to ensure that the pass is partial thickness. Each arm of the suture is then passed superiorly through the levator aponeurosis in a horizontal mattress fashion. For each 3 mm of levator aponeurosis advancement, one can expect approximately 1 mm of eyelid lift. Once both arms of the suture are passed, the eyelid should be everted again to ensure that the pass is not full thickness through the Müller's muscle and conjunctiva. The suture can be tied in a temporary fashion with a single interrupted square knot. The same procedure can be repeated on the opposite side for bilateral surgery. The patient is then asked to open their eyes, and the sutures can be adjusted until the ideal lid height, contour, and symmetry are achieved. Then the sutures are tied off completely and cut over the knot. Be careful not to apply additional tension on the temporary sutures, which may overtighten and alter the lid height.

### *Step 7: Skin Closure*

The skin is then closed with a running 6-0 plain gut, nylon, or Prolene suture. Eyelid crease reformation sutures can be placed by attaching the deeper levator aponeurosis to the skin closure.

## Before and after Images of External Levator Advancement (Figures 16-7 to 16-11)

### *Müller's Muscle Conjunctival Resection*

Ptosis repair by resection of the conjunctiva and Müller's muscle was first described by Putterman and Urist in 1975.[12] Different methods have been used to determine the amount of Conjunctival-Müller's resection, and most are based on the desired ptosis correction and the response to the phenylephrine test. If there is a significant increase in the eyelid height with the phenylephrine test, the patient may be a candidate for MMCR (Figure 16-12).

The phenylephrine test is performed preoperatively to determine the amount of tissue resection, which can vary between 6.5 mm and 9.5 mm.[13-16] A drop of phenylephrine 10% is instilled in the eye, and the result is monitored 3 to 10 minutes later.[17] If the eyelid achieves the desired height after the phenylephrine test, a resection of 8.0 mm can be performed. If the lid responds to the phenylephrine but not to the desired height, a larger resection can be performed up to 9.5 mm. If the eyelid height is higher than intended, the resection amount can be decreased to 6.5 mm. Typically, the MMCR procedure is avoided in patients with ocular surface disease, glaucoma filtration surgery, and conjunctival disease such as ocular cicatricial pemphigoid.

## Procedure

The patient is placed in a supine position. If concomitant blepharoplasty is planned, then the upper lid blepharoplasty incision is also marked. A corneal protective shield is placed in the eye.

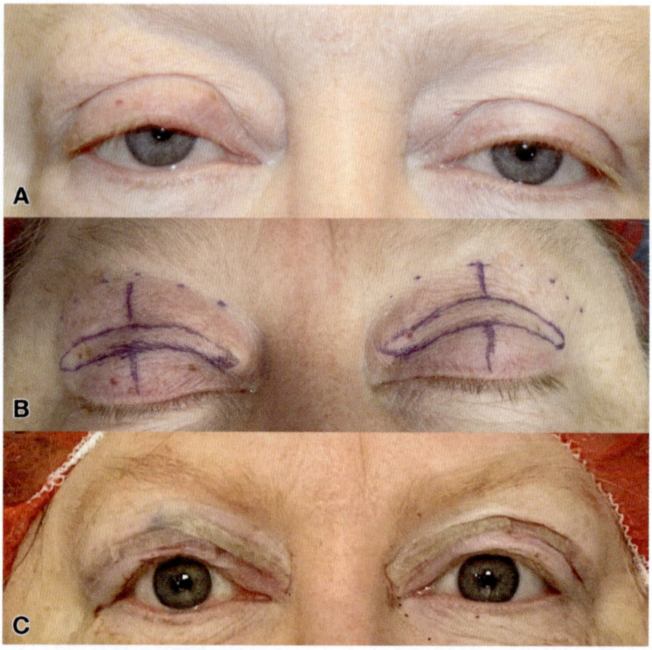

**FIGURE 16-7** **A,** Preoperative photograph. **B,** Bilateral upper lid blepharoplasty marking. **C,** Improved eyelid position following bilateral external levator advancement.

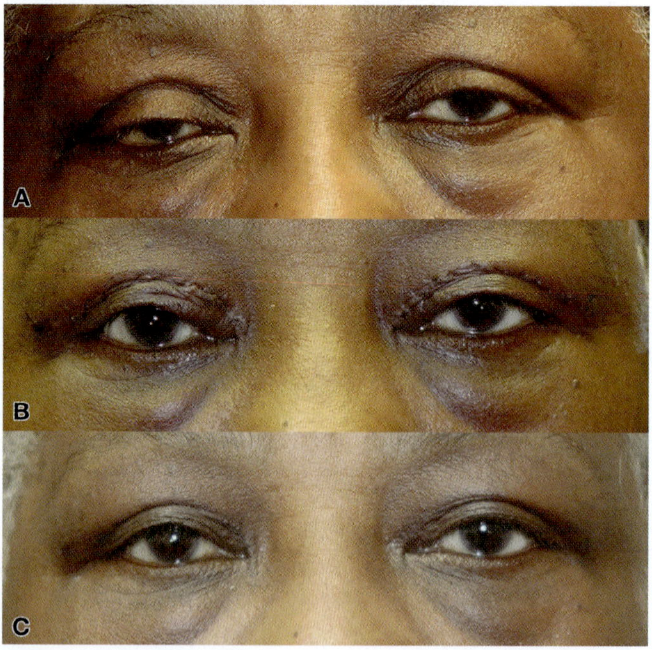

**FIGURE 16-8** **A,** Preoperative photograph. **B,** 1 Week postlevator advancement. **C,** 2 Months postlevator advancement.

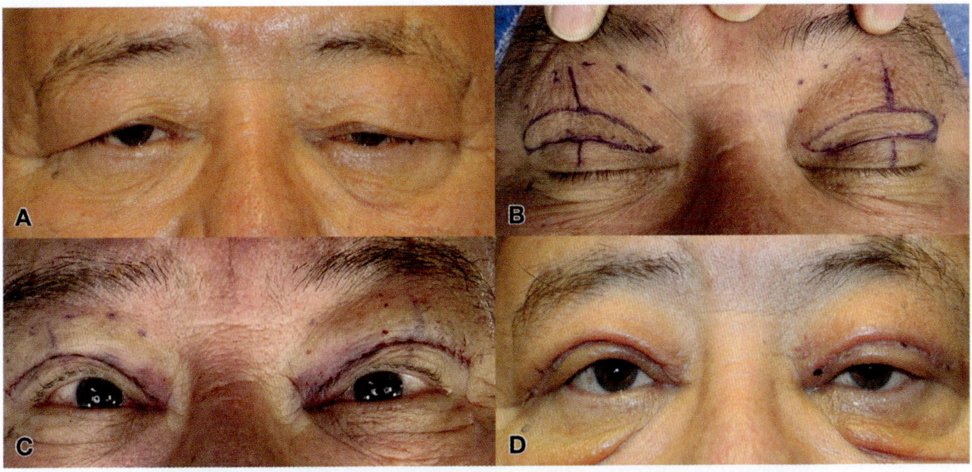

**FIGURE 16-9** **A,** Preoperative photograph. **B,** Bilateral upper eyelid blepharoplasty marking. **C,** Improved eyelid position immediately following levator advancement. **D,** Mild upper eyelid asymmetry at 1 week caused by postoperative edema.

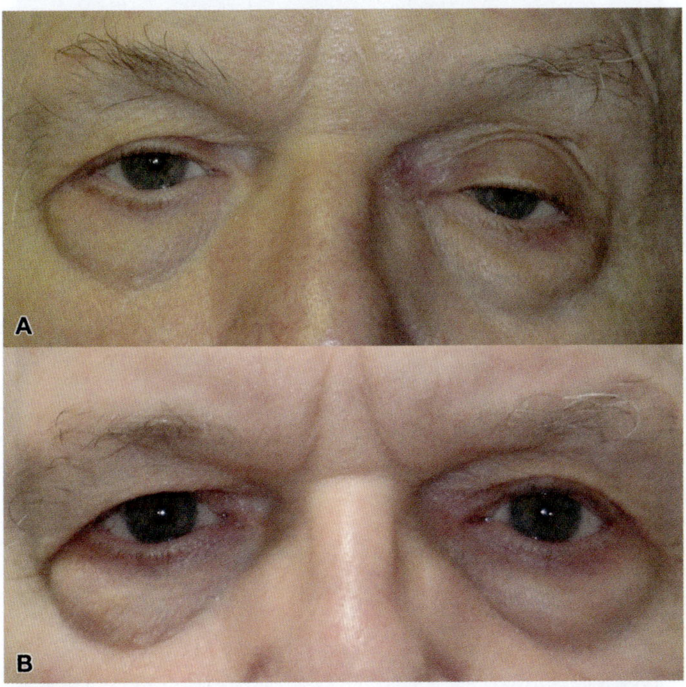

**FIGURE 16-10** **A,** Preoperative photograph. **B,** 6 Weeks postlevator advancement.

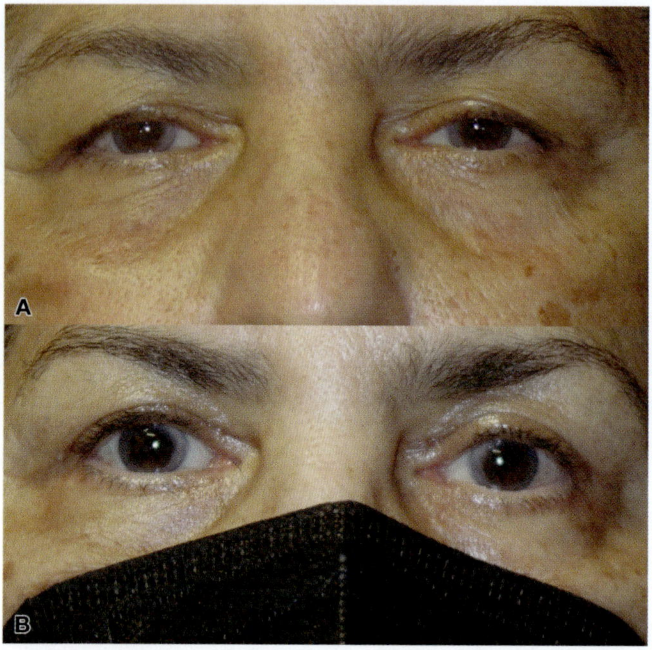


**FIGURE 16-11** **A,** Preoperative photograph. **B,** 2 Months post-levator advancement.

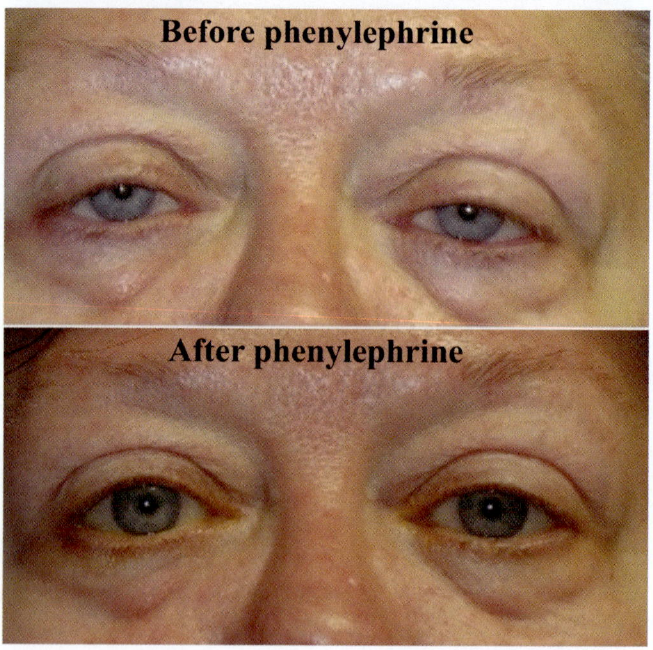


**FIGURE 16-12** Improved eyelid position following application of 10% phenylephrine.

### Step 1: Local Anesthesia

Topical anesthetic drops are placed in the eye. Then, the local anesthetic is administered to the upper lid skin and conjunctiva. The face and lids are prepped and draped in the usual sterile fashion for oculoplastic surgery, typically with 5% povidone–iodine (Betadine) prep. A drop of 5% ophthalmic povidone–iodine can also be instilled in the eye.

### Step 2: Eyelid Eversion and Marking Planned Resection

If blepharoplasty is planned, it is performed before ptosis repair, as described previously in the levator advancement section.

Attention is directed to the upper eyelid ptosis. A 6-0 silk traction suture is passed through the central upper lid margin, and the lid is everted over a Desmarres retractor (Figure 16-13). The conjunctiva and Müller's muscle are grasped and loosened from the levator aponeurosis (Figure 16-14), and the predetermined amount of resection is marked (e.g., 8 mm) from the superior border of the tarsus using calipers and a marking pen or Bovie/high-temperature cautery (Figure 16-15).

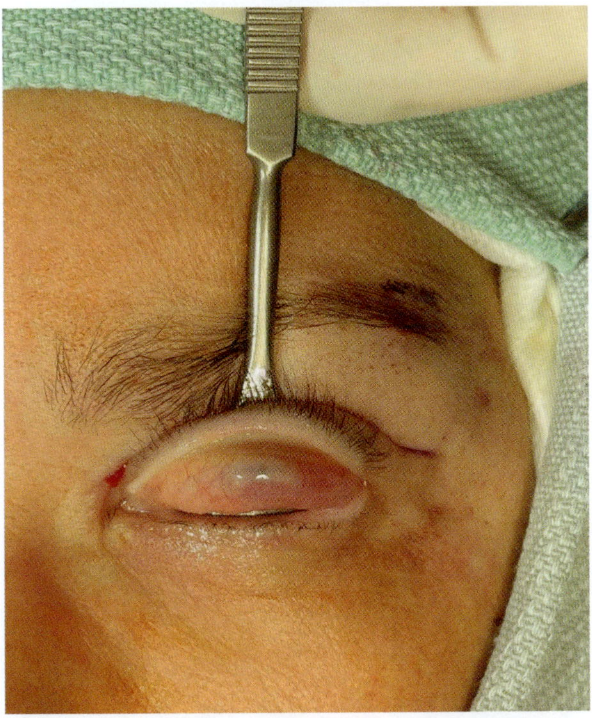

**FIGURE 16-13** Left upper eyelid everted over a Desmarres retractor.

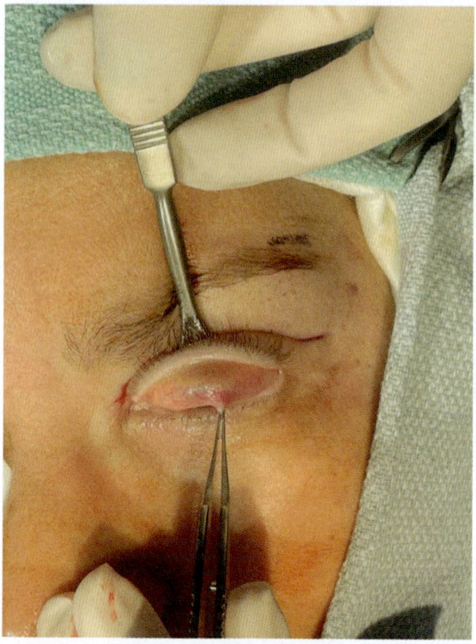

**FIGURE 16-14** Forceps are used to grasp and loosen the conjunctiva and Müller's muscle from the levator aponeurosis.

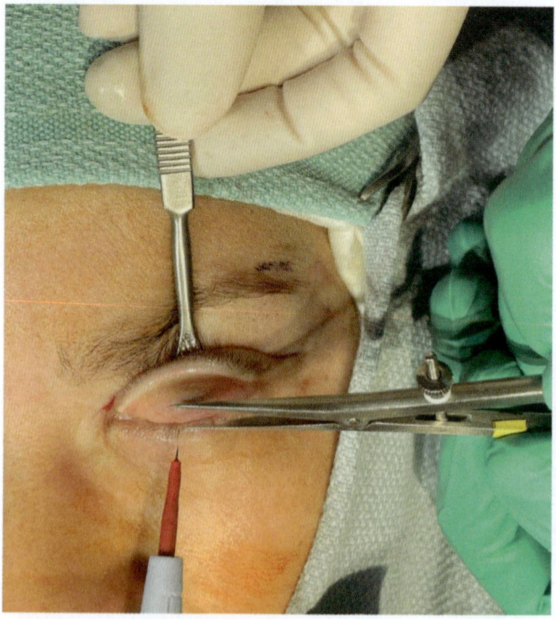

**FIGURE 16-15** Caliper and monopolar cautery were used to mark the predetermined resection amount from the superior border of the tarsus.

### Step 3: Müller's Muscle and Conjunctival Resection

A Putterman Conjunctiva-Müller's resection clamp is placed between the marked area and the superior border of the tarsus and closed tightly. The tissue is tested to confirm that the septum is not incorporated into the clamp. A 6-0 plain gut suture that is tied on the skin at the eyelid crease nasally is passed through the skin and conjunctiva and then passed through the clamped tissue in a running mattress fashion just below the clamp. The tissue is carefully excised using a No. 15 Bard Parker blade cutting against the border of the muscle clamp, maintaining metal-on-metal contact between the blade and the clamp in order to avoid cutting the suture (Figure 16-16).

### Step 4: Closure

The 6-0 plain gut suture is then passed full thickness back through the eyelid exiting the lid crease laterally and tied down, avoiding the septum. Alternatively, a double-armed 6-0 plain gut suture can be used for the procedure, and each arm of the suture is externalized and tied at the level of the lid crease medially and laterally.

If a blepharoplasty incision is performed, then it is closed with the preferred suture in a running or interrupted fashion. The silk retraction suture is removed from the upper lid.

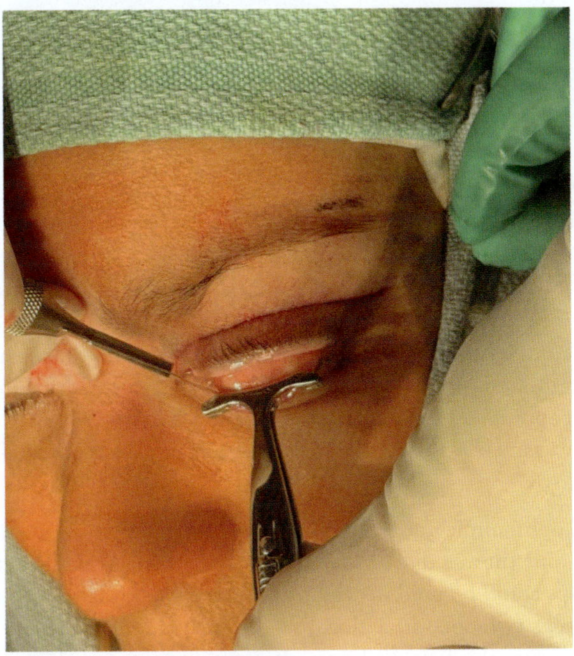

**FIGURE 16-16** Excision of the conjunctival-Müller's muscle against the Putterman clamp.

## Before and after Images of MMCR (Figure 16-17)

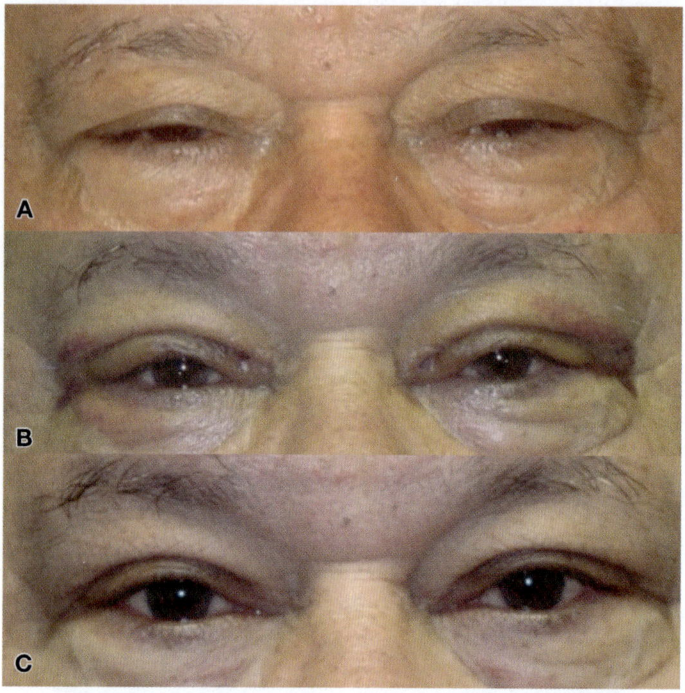


**FIGURE 16-17 A,** Preoperative photograph. **B,** 1 Week post-MMCR. **C,** 6 Weeks post-MMCR.

# POSTOPERATIVE CARE (FOLLOW-UP SCHEDULE)

Immediately after completing the procedure and removing the drapes and eye shields, the face and eyelids should be washed with saline solution and patted dry. Ophthalmic antibiotic ointment should be applied on the incisions and on the eye (if MMCR was performed). Cold compresses/ cold packs are placed over the incisions. The wound is checked for active bleeding.

- Incision care:
  - Apply topical ophthalmic antibiotic ointment or steroid/antibiotic ointment to incision site(s) two to four times a day. If the patient underwent MMCR without skin excision, antibiotic drops could be used instead. Alternatively, petrolatum jelly may be used.
  - Apply cold packs (wrapped in a cloth) to the eyelids for 10-minute periods every hour while awake during the first 48 hours after surgery. Then reduce to three times a day until follow-up visit.
  - Avoid rubbing the eyes or direct makeup to the incision site(s) for 2 weeks.
  - Eye shadow or false eyelashes should not be applied.

    - Avoid excessive sun exposure during the first 30 days after the procedure.
- Medications:
    - Blood thinner can be resumed the day after surgery in most cases.[18]
    - Oral acetaminophen for pain management
    - Artificial tears (Systane, Refresh, etc.) can be used as needed for comfort.
- Activities:
    - Recommend sleeping with the head elevated on two to three pillows or in an upright position.
    - Use eye shields at bedtime.
    - Avoid bending over or lifting heavy things (over 8 lbs.) for 1 week.
    - No swimming, gym, or strenuous athletic activity for 1 week
    - Not to wear contact lenses for 2 weeks.
    - Always inform the patient about contacting the office/on-call doctor if experiencing signs and symptoms of sight-threatening complications such as pain, proptosis, decreased vision, and uncontrolled bleeding.

At the postoperative week one visit, the physician should inspect the incision to ensure there are no signs of infection or wound dehiscence, to check the eyelid contour, and for the presence of lagophthalmos. The sutures should be removed if nonabsorbable sutures were used for skin closure. Absorbable suture remnants can also be removed after 7 days because they can cause local inflammation and granuloma formation. The lid position should be assessed but not fixated on because the eyelid position will continue to fluctuate as edema and muscle contusion resolve with time. The corneal surface and tear film should be evaluated at this time. If there is a concern for worsening ocular surface disease, topical artificial tears and lubricating ointment should be started. As the orbicularis tone restores to the preoperative level, dry eye symptoms should improve with time.

A second postoperative visit is usually scheduled 6 to 8 weeks after surgery to assess the incision, the eyelid contour, and position and determine the presence of lagophthalmos. Postoperative photographs should be taken at this visit for comparison.

# POTENTIAL COMPLICATIONS AND THEIR TREATMENT

### Key Short-term Complications

- Corneal abrasion
- Ecchymosis
- Infection
- Hemorrhage
- Loss of vision
- Suture granuloma
- Wound dehiscence

**Key Long-term Complications**

- Overcorrection
- Undercorrection
- Dry eyes
- Lagophthalmos
- Recurrence of ptosis
- Hypertrophic scar
- Lid asymmetry

Most patients are expected to have some degree of postoperative edema and ecchymosis. This is expected to resolve after 1 to 2 weeks but can be longer for patients on anticoagulation or antiplatelet therapy. Postoperative soft tissue infection typically occurs four to seven days after the procedure. An infected incision appears erythematous, may be tender and warm to touch, and may have mucopurulent discharge. Patients with suspected eyelid infection should be started on oral antibiotics, such as cephalexin or trimethoprim–sulfamethoxazole, for 7 days and monitored for improvement. Significant hemorrhage with upper eyelid surgery is rare but can occur with ptosis surgery. Because the septum is violated during external ptosis repair, retrobulbar hemorrhage may occur. Patients who are on anticoagulation or who have fat debulking are at a higher risk of significant postoperative bleeding. If there is a concern for a retrobulbar hemorrhage, the skin suture should be removed. A lateral canthotomy and inferior cantholysis may be indicated.

## Corneal Abrasion

Corneal abrasion can occur after internal ptosis correction, particularly if the sutures were placed below the superior tarsal border. In this case, ophthalmic antibiotic ointment or drops can be used three to four times a day until the corneal defect heals.

## Overcorrection

Overcorrection is an expected complication of this procedure. Mild asymmetry (≤2 mm) is expected in the immediate recovery phase. This is caused by eyelid edema, muscle contusion or edema, and weakened orbicularis muscle tone. Mild overcorrection is managed with lubrication and observation. If needed, lid stretching exercises can be started 2 weeks after surgery by instructing the patient to hold the lashes down toward the anterior cheek and then look far up and down repeatedly. If performed correctly, this stretches the tissues to drop the lid height. Be cautious with using this technique, because it can undo the surgical procedure.

Moderate to severe overcorrection may require a secondary procedure to correct the eyelid position. Unless there is significant exposure keratopathy, wait at least 3 months to allow the eyelid height to stabilize. Cutting or replacing the tarsal-levator suture may be required.

## Undercorrection

Postoperative edema and ecchymosis can mechanically push down the lid position. Early cold compresses to the incision site(s) can accelerate the recovery phase. Patients with decreased levator function preoperatively (e.g., severe congenital ptosis or myogenic ptosis) have a higher likelihood of undercorrection. Intraoperative observation and documentation of the levator muscle may help determine why an eyelid may be undercorrected. A levator muscle with high fibrotic and fatty infiltration may have a myogenic component and is more likely to be undercorrected than pure levator dehiscence. Wait at least 3 months to allow postoperative edema and ecchymosis to be entirely resolved prior to reoperation. In rare cases, the tarsal-levator suture may slip, causing a recurrence of the ptosis. Early intervention to reinsert the levator muscle may be indicated in these cases.

## Dry Eyes and Exposure Keratopathy

Patients with a known history of dry eye syndrome or poor lid closure are at higher risk for worsening dry eye and exposure keratopathy following ptosis repair. Aggressive lubrication with preservative-free artificial tears and lubricating ointment at bedtime is recommended for exposure keratopathy. Over time, the orbicularis muscle tone should return to normal, and lid closure should improve. Punctal plugs may be helpful in some cases.

## Hypertrophic Scar, Suture Cyst, or Granuloma

Scar gel, steroid ointment, and massage are usually recommended to smoothen incisional scars. Surgical revision may be required for persistent hypertrophic scar, suture cyst, or granuloma.

## VIDEOS OF PROCEDURES

**Video 16-1**—Tarsal and levator dissection. The dissection was performed through a blepharoplasty incision. A No. 15 blade was used to incise the skin along the marking. Westcott scissors were used to elevate and excise the skin flap. Care was taken to preserve the orbicularis oculi muscle. Pinpoint hemostasis was achieved with a high-temperature cautery. The left ring finger was used to stabilize the tarsal plate. The high-temperature cautery was used to dissect and expose the anterior surface of the tarsus. Superiorly, the levator aponeurosis can be identified by its fibrosis appearance. Inferior retraction of the aponeurosis revealed the surrounding septal attachment, which can be released with a high-temperature cautery. Once the levator is completely freed, it can be advanced to complete the external ptosis repair.

**Video 16-2**—Unilateral levator advancement. First, a No. 15 blade was used to incise the skin along the marked supratarsal lid crease. Pinpoint hemostasis was achieved with a high-temperature cautery. Dissection was carried out inferiorly using a high-temperature cautery to expose the anterior surface of the tarsus. With the patient looking inferiorly, the levator aponeurosis was identified and grasped. A high-temperature cautery was used to separate the levator aponeurosis from the surrounding septal attachments. Once the levator was completely freed and mobilized, a double-armed 6-0 silk suture was used to place a 5-mm partial thickness bite through the center of the tarsus. The eyelid was everted to evaluate for suture exposure. The eyelid contour was assessed by pulling on both ends of the suture. Then, each arm of the suture was passed superiorly through the levator aponeurosis. The eyelid was everted over a cotton tip applicator to make sure there was no suture exposure in the superior fornix. The suture was tied in a temporary fashion. The patient was asked to open her eyes, and the suture was adjusted until the ideal lid height, contour, and symmetry were achieved. Afterward, the suture was tied off completely and cut over the knot. The skin incision was closed with a running 6-0 plain gut suture.

**Video 16-3**—Bilateral levator advancement. First, a No. 15 blade was used to incise the skin along the marked upper lid blepharoplasty incision. A skin flap was elevated and excised with Westcott scissors. Hemostasis was achieved with a high-temperature cautery. An inferior dissection was carried out using a high-temperature cautery to expose the anterior surface of the tarsus. Superiorly, the levator aponeurosis was identified. With the assistant retracting the levator inferiorly, a high-temperature cautery was used to separate the levator aponeurosis from the preaponeurotic fat pads and septal attachments. Afterward, a double-armed 6-0 silk suture was used to place a partial thickness bite through the center of the tarsus. The lid was everted to evaluate for suture exposure. The eyelid contour was assessed by pulling on both ends of the suture. Afterward, each arm of the suture was advanced superiorly through the levator aponeurosis. The suture was tied in a temporary fashion. Attention was turned to the right upper lid, where the same procedure was performed up to this point. The upper lids were everted to evaluate for suture exposure in the superior fornices. The patient was asked to open the eyes, and the sutures were adjusted until the ideal lid height, contour, and symmetry were achieved. Afterward, the suture was tied off completely and cut over the knot. The skin incisions were closed with a running 6-0 plain gut suture. Erythromycin ophthalmic ointment was applied to the incisions at the conclusion of the case.

**Video 16-4**—MMCR. After the eyelid has been anesthetized and the face prepped and draped, a 6-0 plain gut suture is secured to the eyelid at the level of the eyelid crease medially. Then the suture is passed through the skin and exits through the conjunctiva side. A Desmarres retractor was used to evert the eyelid. The desired amount of resection is measured using a caliper and marked with a monopolar cautery from the superior tarsal border. A Putterman clamp is used to clamp the tissues to be excised. The suture is run in a horizontal mattress fashion across the length of the planned resection. An assistant can hold the clamp while the surgeon reloads the needle. A No. 15 Bard Parker blade is used to excise the conjunctiva-Müller's muscle against the border of the clamp. The suture is externalized and secured at the level of the eyelid crease, laterally.

**Video 16-5**—MMCR with blepharoplasty. After the face has been prepped and draped, and the incision of the skin and the excision of the skin flap is performed, a 6-0 plain gut suture is tied at the medial edge of the incision. The suture is then passed full thickness from the skin incision through the conjunctiva. A Desmarres retractor is used to evert the eyelid. Forceps are used to grasp the conjunctiva and Müller's muscle. A Bovie cautery and calipers are used to measure the desired resection. A Putterman clamp is used to grasp the tissues to be excised. The previously placed 6-0 plain gut is passed in a running horizontal mattress fashion 1 mm below the clamp across the length of the desired resection. An assistant holds the clamp while the surgeon loads the needle. A No. 15 Bard Parker blade is used to excise the conjunctiva-Müller's muscle. The blade is beveled up against the clamp to prevent cutting the suture. The 6-0 plain gut is then externalized and secured at the eyelid crease laterally.

## EFFICACY

External levator advancement and MMCR are effective procedures to correct upper eyelid ptosis. The success rate of external levator advancement ranges between 74% and 95%,[19-21] and for MMCR 80% to 100%.[20,22,23] Multiple factors contribute to these surgical outcomes, including the surgeon's comfort with surgical technique, underlying ptosis etiology, suture type, and associated complications.

External levator advancement is technically more challenging and has a higher learning curve. The procedure requires a detailed understanding of the upper eyelid anatomy to dissect and isolate the levator palpebrae superioris muscle. The lid height, symmetry, and contour are affected by multiple factors: incision design, crease height, placement of tarsal pass, amount of levator advancement, and degree of suture tension. Conversely, MMCR can be performed without the patient's cooperation, and the amount of tissue resection can be determined preoperatively based on the phenylephrine test. In several studies, MMCR has been shown to have better postoperative symmetry and lower reoperation rate compared with external levator advancement.[20,21]

For an optimal outcome, surgeons should select the technique best suited for each patient's needs. Several considerations that would favor external levator advancement include fair to good levator function, poor response to phenylephrine test, and crease asymmetry that require lid crease reformation. MMCR is ideal for patients that respond to phenylephrine test, have good levator function, and have symmetric eyelid crease.

## CODING/BILLING AND MODIFIERS

- **CPT code: 67904**—"Repair of blepharoptosis; (tarso) levator resection or advancement, external approach." This code specifies an external approach through a skin incision to reach the levator muscle and does not differentiate between levator resection and advancement.
- **CPT code: 67908**—"Repair of blepharoptosis; conjunctivo-tarso-Müller's muscle-levator resection."
- Modifier 50 is used for CPT 67904 and 67908 when performed bilaterally. These codes have a 90-day postoperative global period.
- The CPT codes 67904 and 67908 are bundled with 15822 ("Blepharoplasty, upper eyelid") and 15823 ("Blepharoplasty, upper eyelid; with excessive skin weighing down the lid"). The only appropriate time to unbundle ptosis from blepharoplasty surgery with the modifier −59 is when functional ptosis is performed on one side and functional blepharoplasty is performed on the other side at the same time.

Common ICD-10 codes that support this procedure include:

- **H02.401** (unspecified ptosis of right eyelid)
- **H02.402** (unspecified ptosis of left eyelid)
- **H02.403** (unspecified ptosis of bilateral eyelids)
- **H02.411** (mechanical ptosis of right eyelid)
- **H02.412** (mechanical ptosis of left eyelid)
- **H02.413** (mechanical ptosis of bilateral eyelids)
- **H02.421** (myogenic ptosis of right eyelid)
- **H02.422** (myogenic ptosis of left eyelid)
- **H02.423** (myogenic ptosis of bilateral eyelids)
- **H02.431** (paralytic ptosis of right eyelid)
- **H02.432** (paralytic ptosis of left eyelid)
- **H02.433** (paralytic ptosis of bilateral eyelids)

# REFERENCES


1. Bacharach J, Lee WW, Harrison AR, et al. A review of acquired blepharoptosis: prevalence, diagnosis, and current treatment options. *Eye (Lond).* 2021;35(9):2468-2481.
2. Ng SK, Chan W, Marcet MM, et al. Levator palpebrae superioris: an anatomical update. *Orbit.* 2013;32(1):76-84.
3. Siddens JD, Kim JM, Gladstone GJ. Acquired ptosis: classification and evaluation. In: Servat JJ, Black EH, Nesi FA, et al, eds. *Smith and Nesi's Ophthalmic Plastic and Reconstructive Surgery.* 4th ed. Springer; 2021:295-306.
4. Beard C. Ptosis surgery: past, present, and future. *Ophthalmic Plast Reconstr Surg.* 1985;1(1):69-72.
5. Shore JW, McCord CD Jr. Anatomic changes in involutional blepharoptosis. *Am J Ophthalmol.* 1984;98(1):21-27.
6. Dresser L, Wlodarski R, Rezania K, et al. Myasthenia gravis: epidemiology, pathophysiology and clinical manifestations. *J Clin Med.* 2021;10(11):2235.
7. Kubis KC, Danesh-Meyer HV, Savino PJ, et al. The ice test versus the rest test in myasthenia gravis. *Ophthalmology.* 2000;107(11):1995-1998.
8. Lazaridis K, Tzartos SJ. Autoantibody specificities in myasthenia gravis; implications for improved diagnostics and therapeutics. *Front Immunol.* 2020;11:212.
9. Koka K, Patel BC. Ptosis correction. In: *StatPearls [Internet].* StatPearls Publishing; 2022.
10. Glatt HJ, Putterman AM, Fett DR. Muller's muscle-conjunctival resection procedure in the treatment of ptosis in Horner's syndrome. *Ophthalmic Surg.* 1990;21(2):93-96.
11. Edelstein JP, Mazow ML, Slonim CB. Coding assistant: oculofacial. *American Academy of Ophthalmology* 2022:4-7.
12. Putterman AM, Urist MJ. Muller muscle-conjunctiva resection. Technique for treatment of blepharoptosis. *Arch Ophthalmol.* 1975;93(8):619-623.
13. Putterman AM, Fett DR. Muller's muscle in the treatment of upper eyelid ptosis: a ten-year study. *Ophthalmic Surg.* 1986;17(6):354-360.
14. Weinstein GS, Buerger GF Jr. Modification of the Muller's muscle-conjunctival resection operation for blepharoptosis. *Am J Ophthalmol.* 1982;93(5):647-651.
15. Dresner SC. Further modifications of the Muller's muscle-conjunctival resection procedure for blepharoptosis. *Ophthalmic Plast Reconstr Surg.* 1991;7(2):114-122.
16. Perry JD, Kadakia A, Foster JA. A new algorithm for ptosis repair using conjunctival Mullerectomy with or without tarsectomy. *Ophthalmic Plast Reconstr Surg.* 2002;18(6):426-429.
17. Ramesh S, Mancini R. Dynamic analysis of Muller's muscle response to phenylephrine. *Ophthalmic Plast Reconstr Surg.* 2016;32(1):46-48.
18. Kim C, Pfeiffer ML, Chang JR, et al. Perioperative considerations for antithrombotic therapy in oculofacial surgery: a review of current evidence and practice guidelines. *Ophthalmic Plast Reconstr Surg.* 2022;38(3):226-233.
19. Berlin AJ, Vestal KP. Levator aponeurosis surgery. A retrospective review. *Ophthalmology.* 1989;96(7):1033-1036; discussion 1037.
20. Saonanon P, Sithanon S. External levator advancement versus Muller muscle-conjunctival resection for aponeurotic blepharoptosis: a randomized clinical trial. *Plast Reconstr Surg.* 2018;141(2):213e-219e.
21. Mangan MS, Cakir A, Imamoglu S. Cumulative sum analysis of the learning curve of ptosis surgery: external levator advancement versus Müller muscle-conjunctival resection. *Korean J Ophthalmol.* 2021;35(5):383-390.
22. Samimi DB, Erb MH, Lane CJ, et al. The modified Fasanella-Servat procedure: description and quantified analysis. *Ophthalmic Plast Reconstr Surg.* 2013;29(1):30-34.
23. Carruth BP, Meyer DR. Simplified Müller's muscle-conjunctival resection internal ptosis repair. *Ophthalmic Plast Reconstr Surg.* 2013;29(1):11-14.


# SUPPLEMENTAL READINGS


1. Dutton JJ. Posterior Muller's muscle-conjunctival resection. In: Dutton JJ, ed. *Atlas of Oculoplastic and Orbital Surgery.* Lippincott Williams & Wilkins; 2012:86-87.
2. Dutton JJ. External levator aponeurosis advancement. In: Dutton JJ, ed. *Atlas of Oculoplastic and Orbital Surgery.* Lippincott Williams & Wilkins, 2012:88-91.
3. Holds JB, Anderson RL. Blepharoptosis. In: David TT, ed. *Color Atlas of Oculoplastic Surgery.* Lippincott Williams & Wilkins; 2011:82-93.

4. Long JA. Ptosis. In: Long JA, ed. *Surgical Techniques in Ophthalmology Series: Oculoplastic Surgery.* Saunders Elsevier; 2009: 13-28.
5. Nerad JA. Evaluation and treatment of the patient with ptosis. In: Nerad JA, ed. *Techniques in Ophthalmic Plastic Surgery. A Personal Tutorial.* Saunders Elsevier; 2010:201-235.
6. Periocular malpositions and involutional changes. In: Korn BS, Burkat CN, Carter KD, Perry JD, Stabutr P, Steele EA, Vagefi MR, eds. *2019-2020 AAO Basic Clinical Science Course. Section 7: Oculofacial Plastic and Orbital Surgery.* American Academy of Ophthalmology; 2020:310-322.
7. Siddens JD, Kim JM, Gladstone GJ. Management of acquired ptosis. In: Servat JJ, Black EH, Nesi FA, Gladstone GJ, Calvano CJ, eds. *Smith and Nesi's Ophthalmic Plastic and Reconstructive Surgery.* 4th ed. Springer Nature; 2021:307-322.
8. Vrcek I, Hogan RN, Rossen J, Mancini R. Conjunctiva-sparing posterior ptosis surgery: a novel approach. *Ophthalmic Plast Reconstr Surg.* 2016;32(5):366-370.

# 17 Lid Debridement

Jacob Lang • Nicole Harris

Mechanical debridement of the lid margin and line of Marx (LOM) removes debris and keratin that can disrupt tear flow and migration as well as obstruct lipid expression from the meibomian glands. In a previous study, by Korb and Blackie, debridement on its own provided statistically significant symptom relief and improved meibomian gland function.[1,2] The LOM is described as the mucocutaneous junction (MCJ) posterior to the meibomian gland orifices where the cornified epidermis stops and is replaced by parakeratinized (pk) cells.[3] The LOM stains with lissamine green, rose bengal, and fluorescein. This continuous layer of pk cells is about 0.2 mm wide and extends across the upper and lower lids.[3] Debridement of the LOM is a quick and beneficial in-office procedure for many dry eye patients that requires minimal instruments and setup.

## INDICATIONS

### Key Indications

- Ocular surface disease related to meibomian gland dysfunction
- Sjogren's syndrome

The primary indication for lid debridement is ocular surface disease related to meibomian gland dysfunction. With meibomian gland dysfunction, the most common changes observed with the LOM are thickening and anterior displacement of the staining[3] (Figures 17-1 to 17-7). When comparing the medial, central, and lateral thirds of the LOM, it has been observed that the anterior shift occurs sooner in the medial and lateral sections than the middle section.[3]

Lid debridement has also been shown to be effective at improving some clinical signs and symptoms of patients with Sjogren's syndrome.[2] Although patients with Sjogren's have primarily aqueous deficient ocular surface disease, the meibomian glands also often have functional changes that can be seen by assessing the lid margin and LOM.

Excessive makeup or other lid debris along the waterline can easily be removed with a lid debrider under the slit lamp during the ocular exam or before other therapies are applied to the eyelid or ocular surface as well (Figure 17-8). Lid debridement may have even greater effects when combined with other treatments that use light, heat, and/or mechanical expression of the meibomian glands in conjunction with LOM debridement.[4]

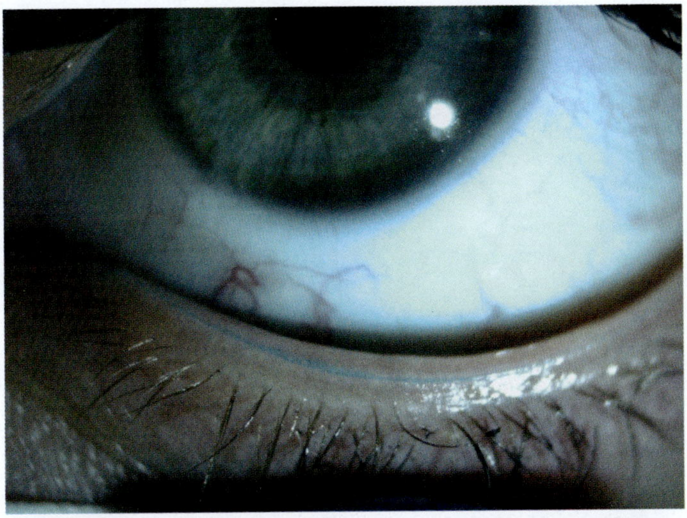

FIGURE 17-1 Lissamine staining of the line of Marx (LOM) in a patient with mild meibomian gland dysfunction (MGD). Note that the LOM is posterior to the meibomian gland (MG) orifices nasally and overlies the orifices temporally.

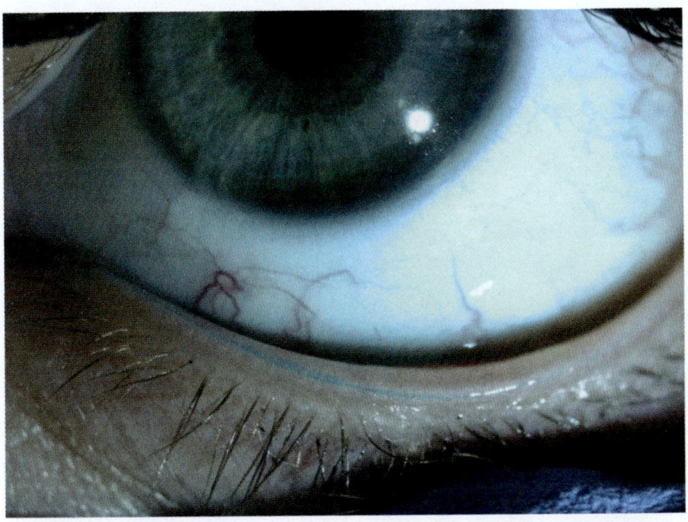

FIGURE 17-2 Lissamine staining of the line of Marx in a patient with mild MGD. Note that the LOM is posterior to the MG orifices nasally and overlies the orifices temporally.

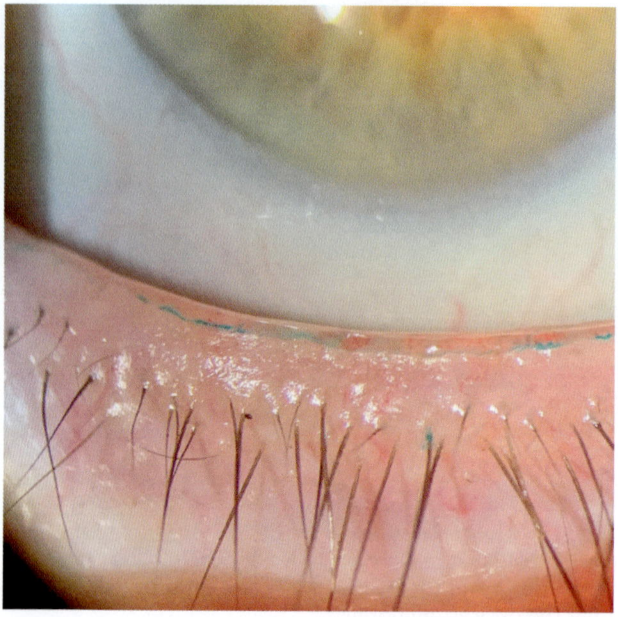

**FIGURE 17-3** Lissamine staining of the line of Marx (LOM) in moderate MGD. Note the anterior positioning of the LOM in reference to the MGs.

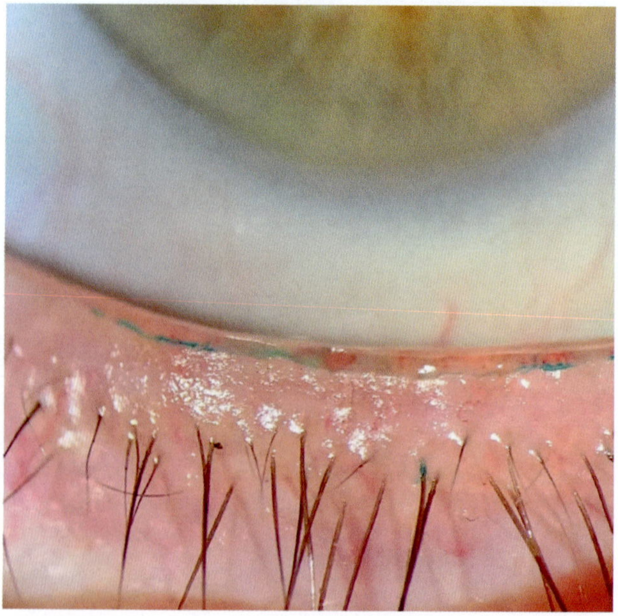

**FIGURE 17-4** Lissamine staining of the line of Marx (LOM) in moderate MGD demonstrating anterior migration of the LOM.

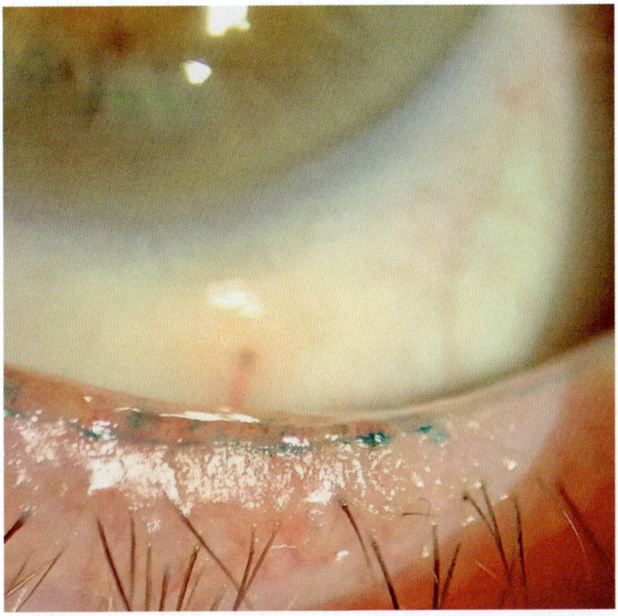

FIGURE 17-5 Lissamine staining of the line of Marx (LOM) in moderate MGD demonstrating anterior migration of the LOM and irregular uptake of lissamine across the LOM, consistent with increasing and irregular keratin and scale along the LOM.

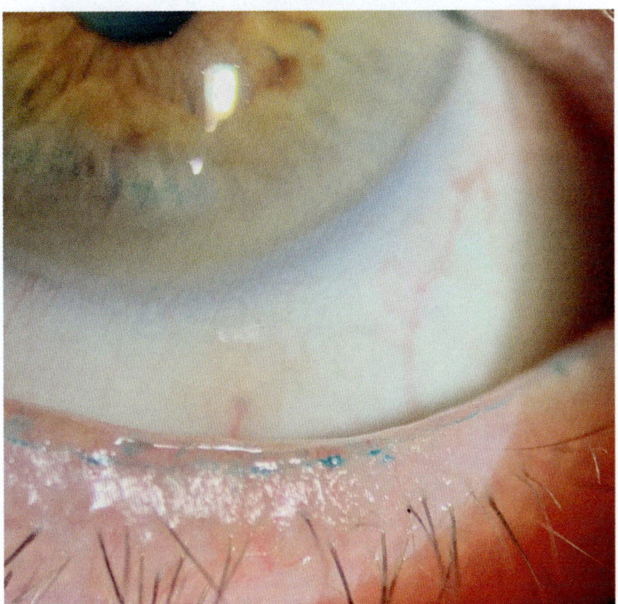

FIGURE 17-6 Lissamine staining of the line of Marx (LOM) in moderate MGD demonstrating anterior migration of the LOM.

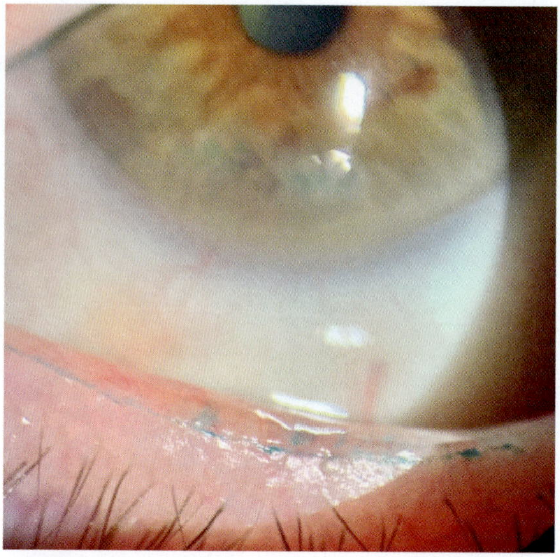

**FIGURE 17-7** Lissamine staining of the line of Marx (LOM) in moderate MGD demonstrating anterior migration of the LOM and irregular uptake of lissamine consistent with increasing and irregular keratin and scale along the LOM.

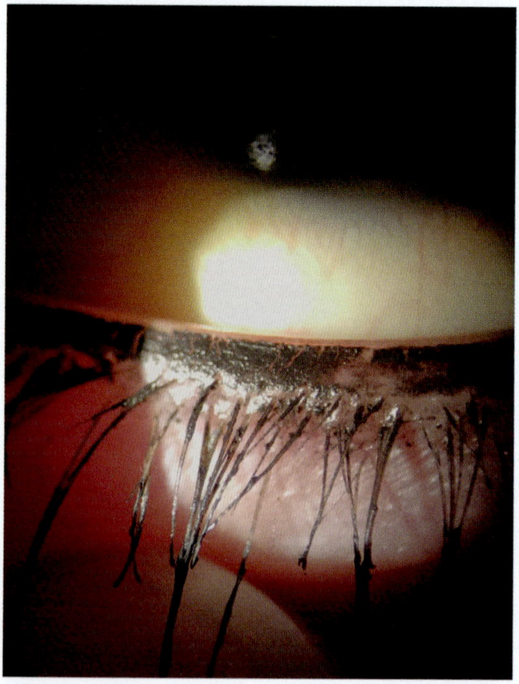

**FIGURE 17-8** Excessive makeup along the waterline may be best removed with a lid debrider under the slit lamp during the exam or before other therapies are applied to the eyelid or ocular surface.

## CONTRAINDICATIONS

### Key Contraindications

- Active ocular infection
- Recent eyelid trauma
- Ocular or eyelid anomalies

This procedure should not be performed if there is active ocular infection or recent ocular trauma involving the lid margins. It should also be avoided in patients with other ocular or eyelid anomalies, pathologies, or findings that may increase the risk of complications.

## PREOPERATIVE PREPARATION

### Key Preoperative Considerations

- The patient's symptoms should be evaluated and documented.
- The patient's ocular surface and meibomian gland function should be evaluated and documented.
- The patient's LOM should be evaluated and documented.
- Evaluation of symptoms can be done using the Standard Patient Evaluation of Eye Dryness (SPEED) questionnaire or similar surveys that quantify the patient's dry eye symptomatology.
- For standardized, repeatable evaluation of meibomian gland function, a meibomian gland evaluator (Johnson and Johnson Vision) can be used. Practitioners may also utilize a cotton-tipped applicator or even digital expression to evaluate the meibum consistency and force required to evacuate the meibum.
- Meibography can be used to document the structure and extent of meibomian gland disease and atrophy.
- After evaluating the eyelids, meibomian glands, and ocular surface, lissamine green dye is the preferred vital dye used to visualize the LOM and the dysplastic or keratinization at this ocular interface (see Figures 17-1–17-7). Rose bengal, and, to a lesser degree, fluorescein, can be used as well; however, we find lissamine significantly outperforms others. The location and thickness of the LOM should be evaluated.
- The main features of the LOM to note are:
    - Grade or measure the thickening in any area of the LOM by section (medial, lateral, central).
    - Grade or measure the height of the LOM (or height of the scale along the LOM) by section.
    - Grade or measure the placement of the LOM anterior to the meibomian gland orifices in any area of the LOM by section.

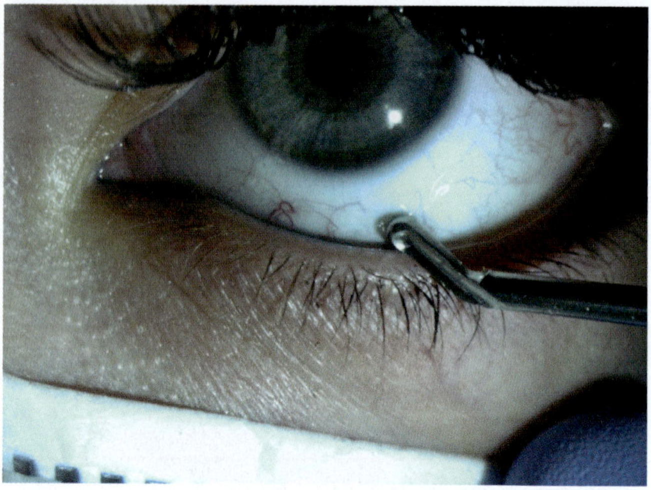

FIGURE 17-9 Epstein debrider (Medirix). Note the rounded terminal edge of this debrider, designed to avoid damaging the globe.

The preoperative preparation for this procedure is fairly straightforward. The patient will be seated at the slit lamp or procedure chair, and the following items are needed:

- Proparacaine hydrochloride 0.5% or other topical anesthetic may be used (optional).
- Lissamine green strips
- Debridement tool, which may include any of the following and/or others dependent on the provider's preference
- Epstein debrider (Medirix) (Figures 17-9 and 17-10)
- Karpecki debrider (Hilco Vision) (Figures 17-11 and 17-12)
- Stainless steel golf club spud (Hilco Vision) (Figures 17-13–17-15)

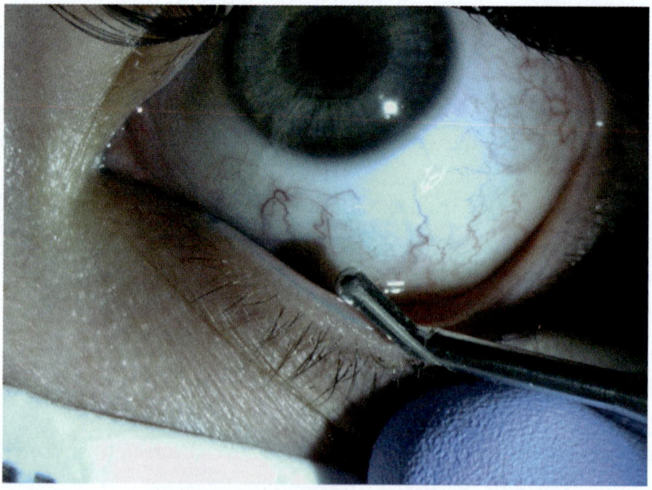

FIGURE 17-10 Epstein debrider (Medirix) positioned over the line of Marx with proper lid retraction.

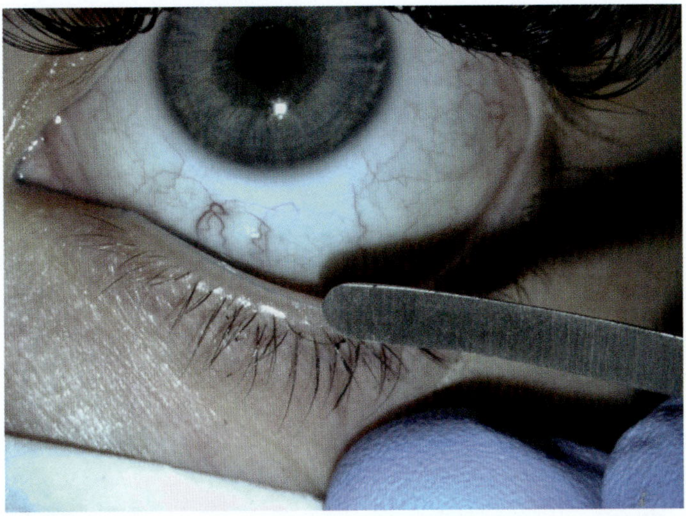

FIGURE 17-11 Karpecki debrider (Hilco Vision).

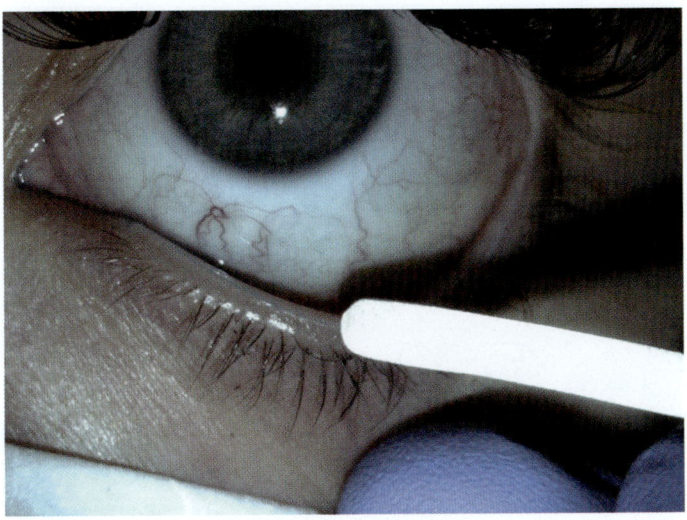

FIGURE 17-12 Karpecki debrider (Hilco Vision) positioned over the line of Marx with proper lid retraction.

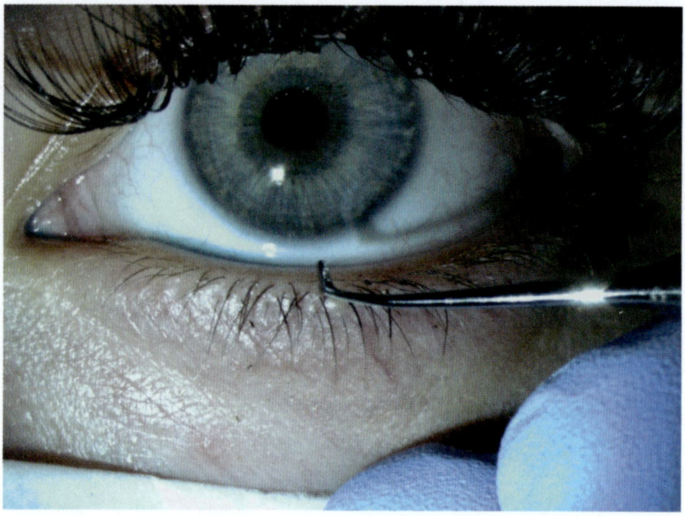

**FIGURE 17-13** Golf club spud (Hilco Vision).

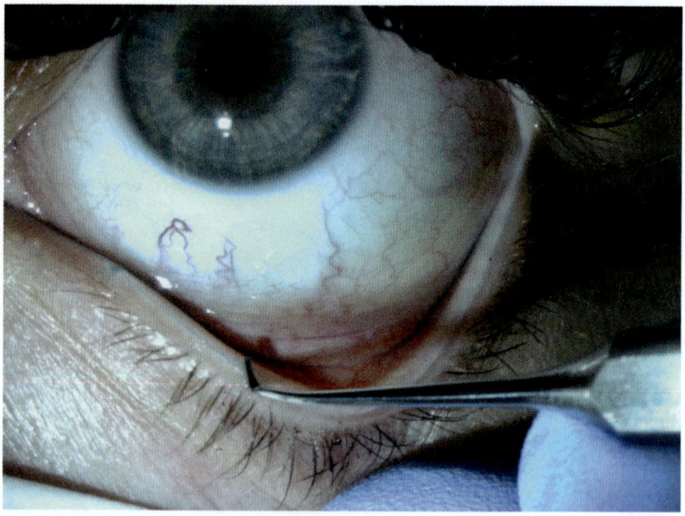

**FIGURE 17-14** Golf club spud (Hilco Vision) positioned over the line of Marx with proper lid retraction.

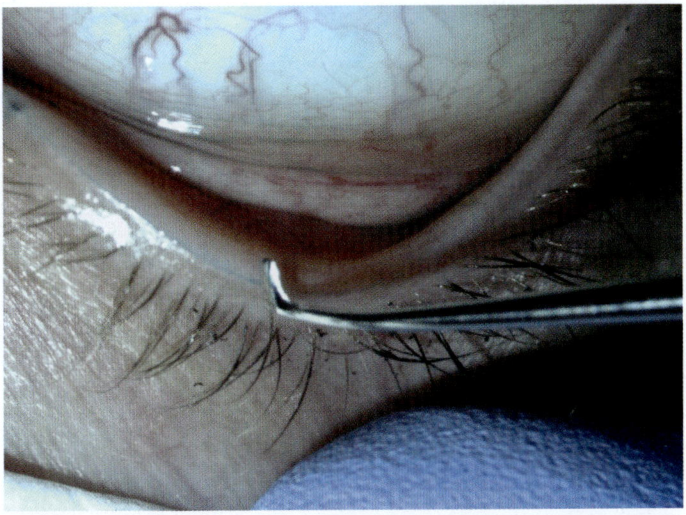

**FIGURE 17-15** Golf club spud (Hilco Vision) debriding the line of Marx (right side of lid complete, left side remains).

# PROCEDURE

## Key Procedural Points

- Consider topical anesthetic ophthalmic drops or gel.
- Optional placement of contact lens or shield to protect cornea
- Patient seated behind slit lamp
- Use 10× to 16× magnification and white light.
- Roll lid away from globe.
- Patient looks away from targeted lid.
- Gently sweep debridement tool laterally using mild pressure.
- Cover entire length of LOM.

No anesthetic is required; however, it is not contraindicated and should be left to the practitioner's discretion. Tetracaine gel may have more anesthetic effect on the lids than solution-based anesthetics and should be considered in sensitive patients. This procedure is not intended to remove any tissue that could not be removed with the gentle motion and mild pressure of the debriding utensil. The patient experiences minimal discomfort, and there should be no

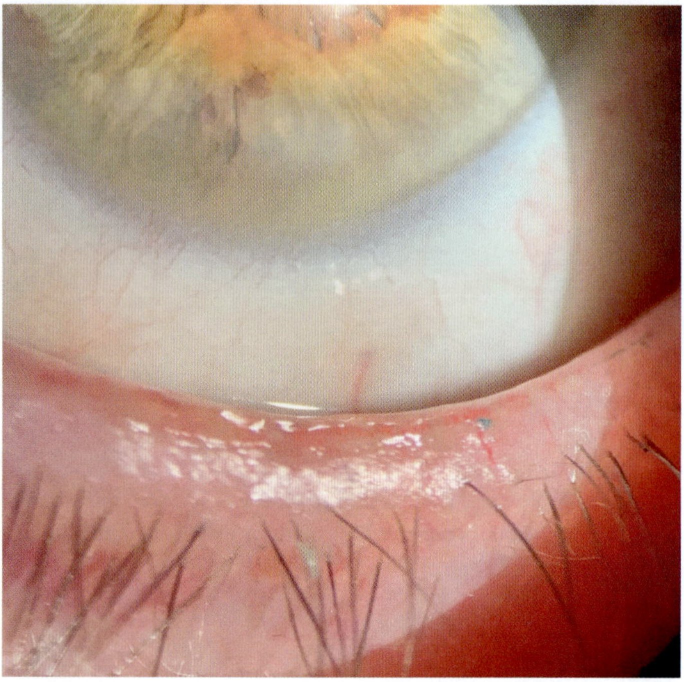

FIGURE 17-16 Lid margin post debridement, with lissamine stained tissue removed.

observable tissue damage after the procedure is completed. A soft contact lens, a scleral lens, or even laser corneal shields can easily be used as a safety lens to protect the cornea in the case of an erroneous slip of the debridement tool.

The goal of the procedure is to remove the accumulated lissamine green-stained debris from the LOM (Figures 17-16–17-21). With the patient comfortably seated at the slit lamp (10–16× magnification with white light), or in a procedure chair with adequate magnification such as loops, the lower lid should be gently rolled away from the globe to avoid accidental contact with the globe. The patient is directed to look away from the targeted lid (up for the lower lid, down for the upper lid). The debridement tool is placed onto the lid margin directly over the LOM. It is then gently swept laterally (nasal to temporal or vice versa) in small wiping motions with mild pressure across the entire length of the LOM (see Figure 17-15). The pressure applied with the debridement tool should be adapted to the specifics of the individual lid tissue morphology and resistance, to accomplish removal of the lissamine green-stained cells, scale, and debris.

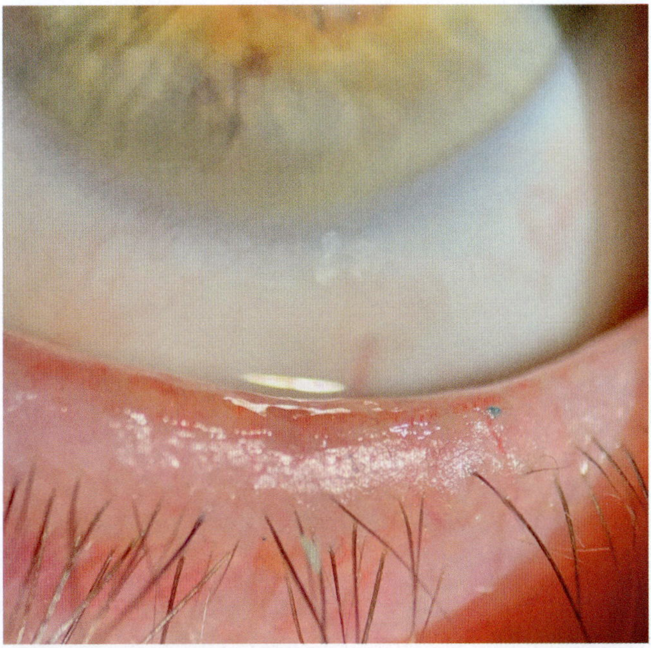

FIGURE 17-17 Lid margin post debridement, with lissamine stained tissue removed.

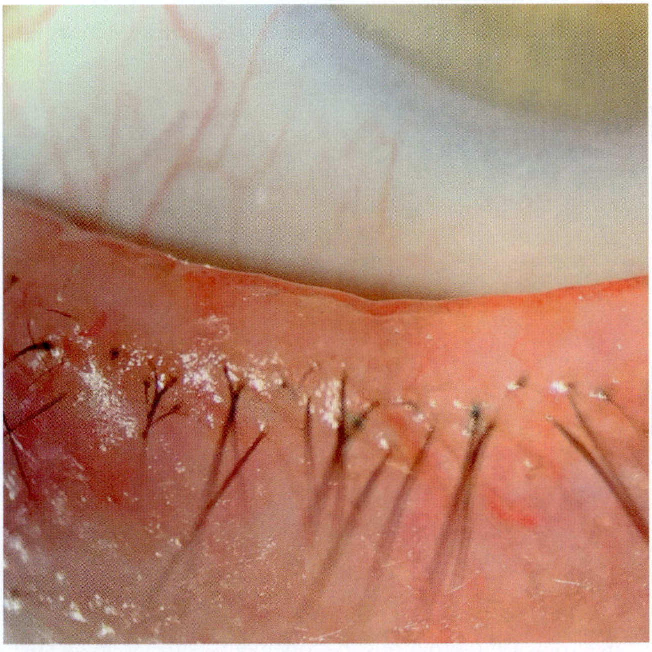

FIGURE 17-18 Lid margin post debridement, with lissamine stained tissue removed.

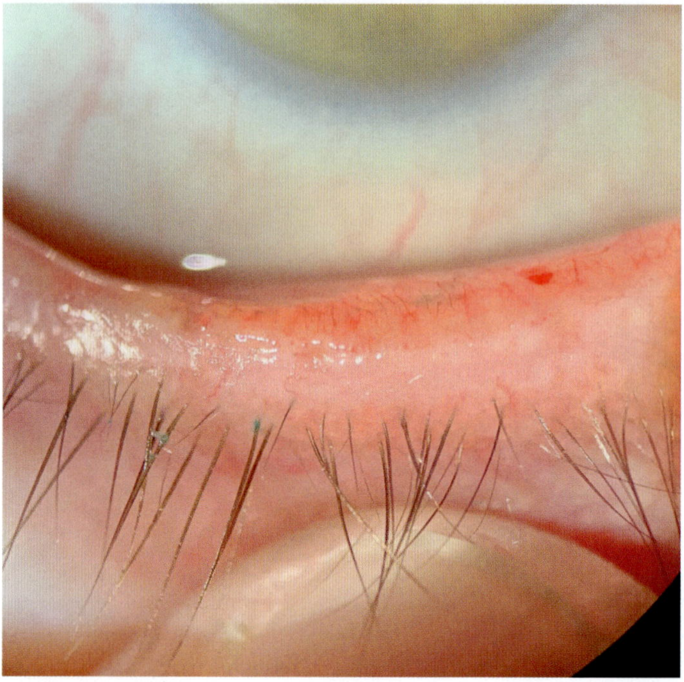

FIGURE 17-19 Lid margin post debridement, with lissamine stained tissue removed.

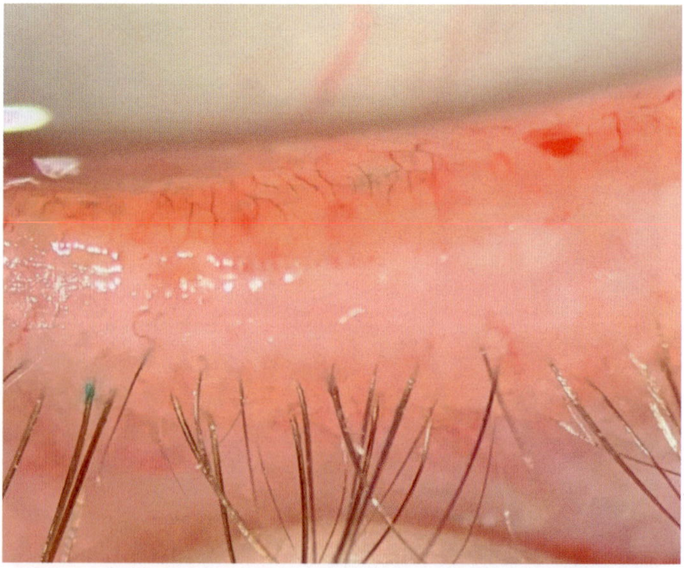

FIGURE 17-20 Lid margin post debridement, with lissamine stained tissue removed.

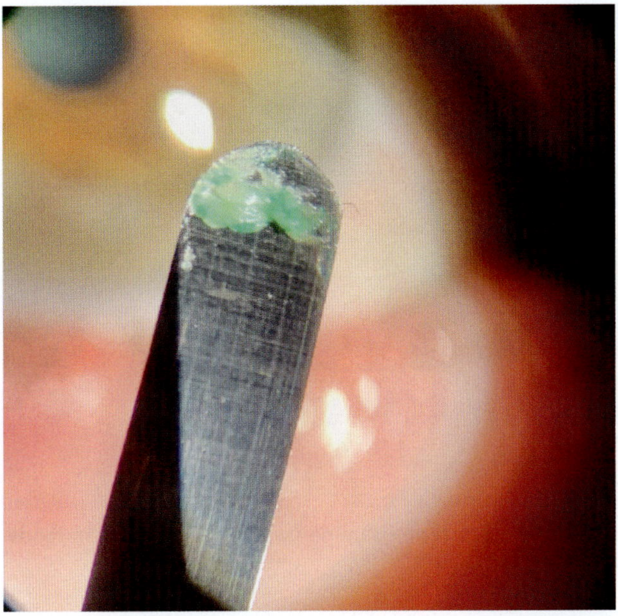

**FIGURE 17-21** Lissamine stained debris and keratinized tissue removed after debridement procedure.

# POSTOPERATIVE CARE (FOLLOW-UP SCHEDULE)

## Key Postoperative Considerations

- Follow up with the patient in 6 to 8 weeks.
- Reassess response to treatment and possible recurrence of lid margin disease.

This procedure is commonly done in conjunction with or alongside other therapies. These procedures' follow-up routine often eclipses that of LOM debridement alone; however, we generally recommend following up with the patient in 6 to 8 weeks to reassess the patient's response to the treatment and possible recurrence of lid margin disease, including dysplasia and keratin buildup along the LOM (Figure 17-22). It should be noted that improvement in symptoms and meibomian gland function was noted at 1 month during two case series clinical trials.[1,2]

# POTENTIAL COMPLICATIONS AND THEIR TREATMENT

## Key Potential Complications to Look for

- Excessive removal of tissue
- Focal tissue abrasion

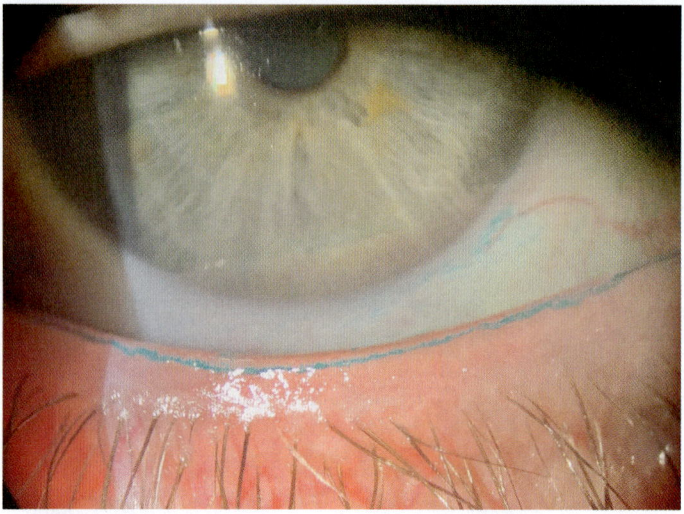

**FIGURE 17-22** Recurrent lissamine staining of the LOM in moderate MGD.

Possible complications center around excessive removal of tissue along the lid margin or loss of control to the utensil, which could lead to focal tissue abrasion. If this occurs, prophylactic antibiotic therapy should be utilized to minimize the risk of infection; however, this is not typically needed in standard outcomes because the epithelium should be left intact. Again, a soft contact lens, scleral lens, or ocular laser shields could be used to protect the globe in patients with fragile ocular surfaces or if the risk of slippage or unpredictable movement by the patient is expected.

## VIDEOS OF PROCEDURES

**Video 17-1**—Lissamine staining of the LOM. Note that the LOM is posterior to the meibomian gland orifices nasally and overlies the orifices temporally and is not displaced anterior in this patient.

**Video 17-2**—Lid debridement with an Epstein debrider. Note the lateral sweeps with this debrider and repeated sweeps across areas with increased pressure in areas where lissamine is persistent.

**Video 17-3**—Lid debridement with a Karpecki debrider. Note that the patient is directed to look up before the lower lid is debrided.

**Video 17-4**—Lid debridement with a golf club spud.

# EFFICACY

Dr. Marx first described the LOM in 1924.[1,5,6] Most of the recent research and publication surrounding the LOM and eyelid debridement was initiated and authored by Drs. Donald Korb, Caroline Blackie, and Erich Knop.[1-3,5,7,8] Several other publications have described this demarcation line in the settings of dry eye, blepharitis, and meibomian gland disease.[1-9] The process of mechanical debridement of the LOM was first described by Korb and Blackie in 2013.[1] In this publication, the authors describe a case series of 16 patients that underwent LOM debridement. The authors reported a statistically significant increase in the meibomian gland function 1 month post debridement for the test group, as opposed to no improvement in the control group. The number of functional meibomian glands also improved in the treatment group as opposed to the control group. Their results imply that there are benefits to LOM and keratinized lid margin debridement. The benefits were measured as decreased symptoms and increased the meibomian gland function 1 month after the procedure. A similar trial revealed similar results in a Sjogren's syndrome cohort with 14 subjects.[2] These authors concluded that lid debridement was effective in improving some clinical signs and symptoms in subjects with Sjogren's syndrome who exhibited severe dry eye and that it may play a helpful role in the management of Sjogren's syndrome-related dry eye.[2]

Other publications reference the LOM and, specifically, its anterior migration as a finding in ocular surface disease.[3,6,9] The location and thickness of this line is reported as a marker of disease state and could, theoretically, be used to track progression or improvement.[3,6,9]

## CODING/BILLING AND MODIFIERS

Currently, there is no CPT code for this procedure. It is typically considered part of the examination code and level determination.

## REFERENCES


1. Korb DR, Blackie CA. Debridement-scaling: a new procedure that increases Meibomian gland function and reduces dry eye symptoms. *Cornea.* 2013;32(12):1554-1557.
2. Ngo W, Caffery B, Srinivasan S, Jones LW. Effect of lid debridement-scaling in Sjogren syndrome dry eye. *Optom Vis Sci.* 2015;92(9):316-320.
3. Knop E, Knop N, Zhivov A, et al. The lid wiper and muco-cutaneous junction anatomy of the human eyelid margins: an in vivo confocal and histological study. *J Anat.* 2011;218(4):449-461. doi:10.1111/j.1469-7580.2011.01355.x
4. Moon SY, Han SA, Kwon HJ, et al. Effects of lid debris debridement combined with meibomian gland expression on the ocular surface MMP-9 levels and clinical outcomes in moderate and severe meibomian gland dysfunction. *BMC Ophthalmol.* 2021;21(1):175. doi:10.1186/s12886-021-01926-2
5. Korb DR. Marx's line publication 1924: critical in dry eye research 86 years later. *Optom Vis Sci.* 2010;87(10):716-717. doi:10.1097/OPX.0b013e3181f97a54
6. Doughty MJ. Morphological features of cells along Marx's line of the marginal conjunctiva of the human eyelid. *Clin Exp Optom.* 2013;96(1):76-84. doi:10.1111/j.1444-0938.2012.00763.x
7. Knop E, Korb DR, Blackie CA, Knop N. The lid margin is an underestimated structure for preservation of ocular surface health and development of dry eye disease. *Dev Ophthalmol.* 2010;45:108-122. doi: 10.1159/000315024
8. Korb DR, Blackie CA, McNally EN. Evidence suggesting that the keratinized portions of the upper and lower lid margins do not make complete contact during deliberate blinking. *Cornea.* 2013;32(4):491-495. doi:10.1097/ICO.0b013e31826a1e6f
9. Yamaguchi M, Kutsuna M, Uno T, et al. Marx line: fluorescein staining line on the inner lid as indicator of meibomian gland function. *Am J Ophthalmol.* 2006;141:669-675.

# 18 Maskin Intraductal Meibomian Gland Probing

Steven L. Maskin • Natalia A. Warren • Claire Toland

## BACKGROUND

Intraductal Meibomian gland probing (MGP) with Maskin probes and dilator, Maskin Small and Large Bore MicroTubes, and Maskin Expressor, is used in the diagnosis and treatment of the proximate cause of obstructive Meibomian gland dysfunction (MGD), periductal fibrosis, and fibrovascular tissue (Figure 18-1) that

1. contracts around the basement membrane and external wall of the duct, constricting and obstructing its lumen and
2. disrupts the normal differentiation of distal duct basal epithelium and basement membrane.[1]

Diagnostically, the procedure reveals the presence of occult fibrosis when the probe encounters fixed, firm, focal unyielding resistance (FFFUR) within the duct lumen. Therapeutically, the procedure confirms or establishes a patent outflow channel for the unobstructed flow of meibum through the central duct proximally to the lid margin.

When the probe releases fibrotic tissue in functioning glands, meibum sequestered behind the obstruction flows immediately, thereby equilibrating intraductal pressure and relieving lid tenderness and soreness. Immediately after MGP, pressure on acini is also released. Over time and with pressure normalized, glandular epithelial precursor cells are activated,[2] improving gland function and allowing dormant acini to resume the synthesis of meibum. Research has also shown the growth of gland tissue in areas of gland atrophy after MGP[3] (Figure 18-2). In addition, intraductal adjunct therapy is supported with MGP.

## INDICATIONS

**Key Indications**

- Can be utilized for diagnostic evaluation of fibrotic obstructions
- Ocular surface disease related to MGD
- Obstructive MGD secondary to fibrosis

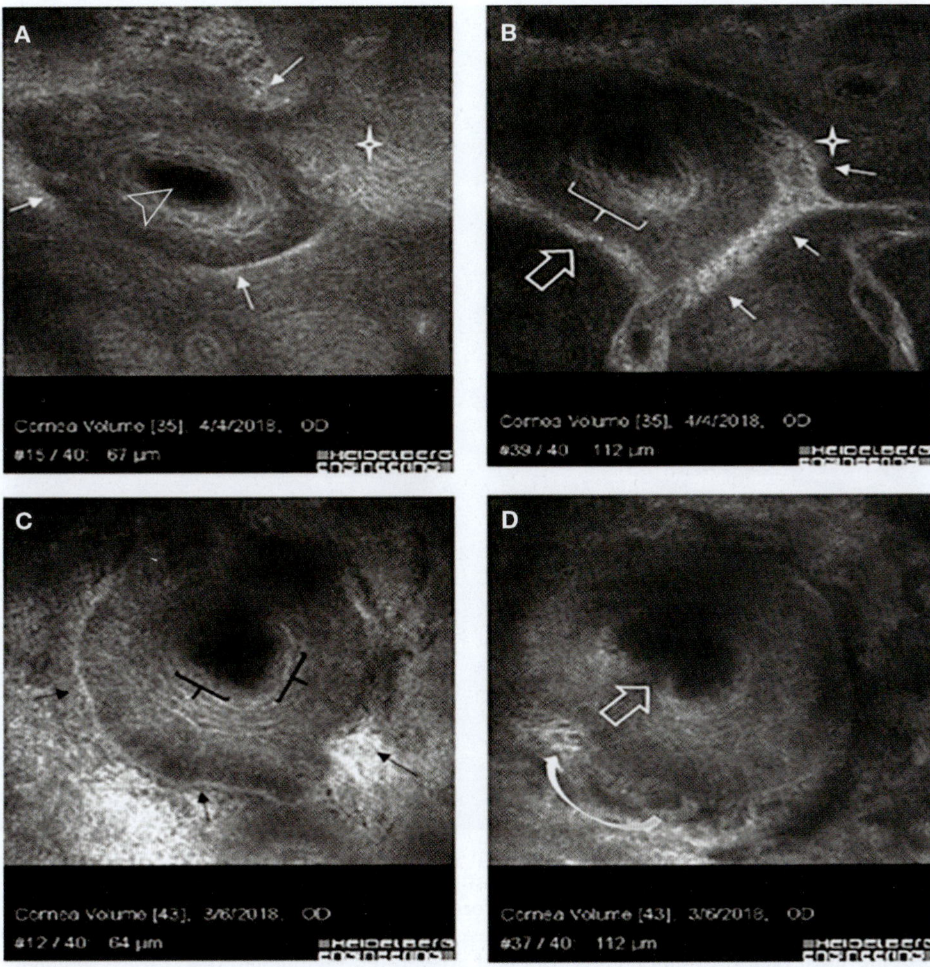


**FIGURE 18-1** Periductal fibrosis of two Meibomian gland distal ducts. **A and B,** Images of the same gland, where **B** is at a greater depth than **A**, (**A**) showing an oval-shaped patent lumen (open arrowhead) at a depth of 67 µm with apparent periductal fibrosis (arrows) and fibrotic sheets (star) that appears in (**B**) as a tight periductal fibrotic band (star and arrows) surrounding, constricting, and invading the external duct wall at 112 µm. **B** also shows an oval lumen with the flattest border (bracket), corresponding to the tightest area of fibrosis (open arrow). **C and D,** Images of the same gland, where **D** is at a greater depth than **C**, (**C**) showing scalloping and pinching of the external duct wall from apparent fibrosis (arrows), with flattening of oval lumen at corresponding meridians (brackets), which appears in (**D**) as an indentation of the external duct wall (arc) with corresponding lumen stricture (open arrow). (From Maskin SL, Alluri S. Expressible Meibomian glands have occult fixed obstructions: findings from Meibomian gland probing to restore intraductal integrity. *Cornea*. 2019;38(7):880.)

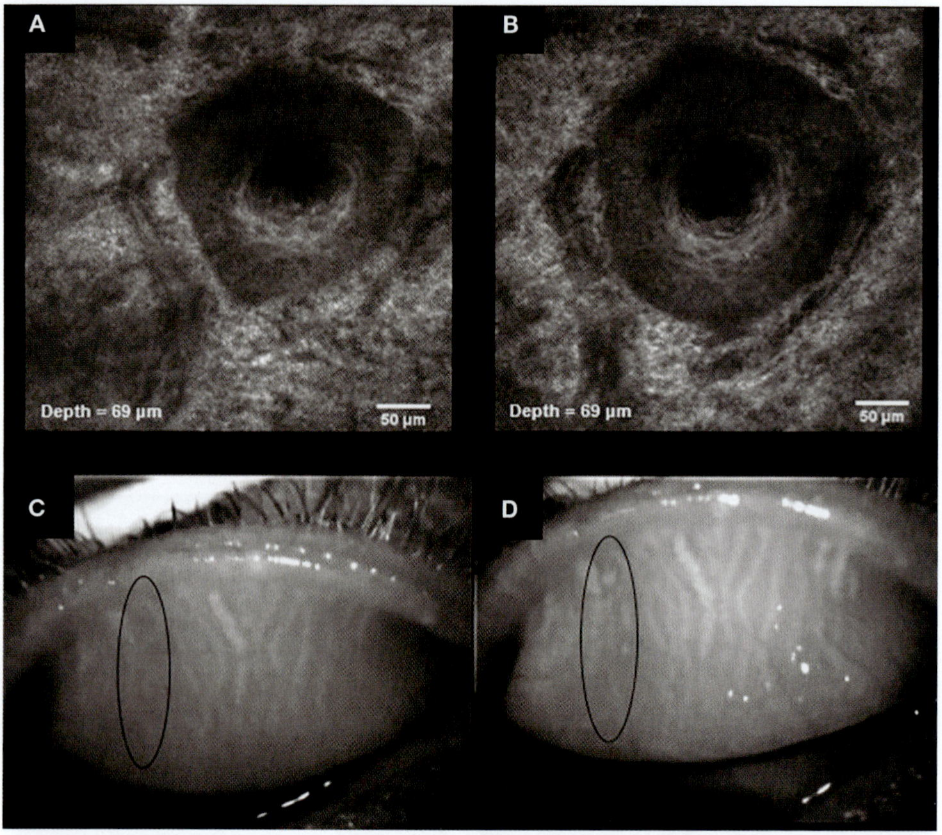


**FIGURE 18-2** Meibomian gland increased duct wall thickness and gland growth on confocal microscopy and infrared meibography suggesting stem cell activation. **A and B**, Confocal microscopy images of a Meibomian gland before probing (**A**) and after probing (**B**) with an increase in duct wall thickness of 38.3%. (Maskin SL, Toland C. Intraductal Meibomian gland probing (MGP) leads to more superficial and accelerated Meibomian gland (MG) basement membrane (BM) differentiation with increased ductal epithelial cell layers (ECL). Poster presented at: World Cornea Congress; 2022; Chicago, IL, manuscript in preparation). **C and D**, Infrared meibography images of an upper lid before probing (**C**) and after probing (**D**), showing growth of gland tissue of 21% ($p = 0.03$). Postprobing showed a statistically significant increase in glandular tissue and greater overall demarcation and density of acinar-ductular units (oval). (Maskin SL, Testa WR. Growth of Meibomian gland tissue after intraductal Meibomian gland probing in patients with obstructive Meibomian gland dysfunction. *Br J Ophthalmol*. 2018;102(1):59-68.) (Adapted from Maskin SL, Warren NA. *Your Dry Eye Mystery Solved: Reversing Meibomian Gland Dysfunction, Restoring Hope*. Yale University Press; 2022.)

## MGP for Diagnostic Evaluation

After a slit-lamp examination or after meibography indicating obstructive MGD, MGP confirms the presence of occult fibrotic obstructions. Using a 1-mm probe on lids with MGD, 67% of glands had fixed fibrotic obstructions, and with the longer, 2- or 4-mm, probes, 90% of glands had these obstructions.[1]

As obstructive MGD is known to develop and progress in asymptomatic patients even with expressible glands, probing individual glands helps stage the disease by revealing the presence and extent of occult fixed fibrotic *proximal* obstruction prior to the development of symptoms. It is also true that patients that have been probed are routinely "wowed" by the elimination of symptoms not recognized prior to probing. The slow progression of symptoms with this disease escapes awareness until probing reverses the proximate cause of these symptoms first appreciated during the postprobing period. These improvements in previously unnoticed symptoms were reported by patients in addition to the resolution of the presenting complaint.[4]

When the probe encounters resistance in the glands, it reveals the presence of obstruction as well as its status: extent and location. Resistance that is FFFUR suggests glands that are obstructed with periductal fibrotic tissue. Resistance that is "soft" or that yields easily, is nonfixed, and nonfocal, instead suggests a nonfibrotic alteration of ducts or their contents. No resistance may indicate a healthy gland or indicate dilation of the distal duct caused by loss of periglandular tissue support or poor external basement membrane differentiation with decreased rigidity of the duct wall allowing the duct to microdilate.[5]

Resistance may occur anywhere along the length of a gland and in more than one location. Resistance near the orifice suggests distal obstruction and may prevent gland expressibility, whereas deeper within the gland, beyond at least one course of acini, fixed resistance reveals proximal obstruction that allows expressibility of meibum from more distal acini. Resistance that creates a single audible "popping" sound when fibrosis is released suggests a single band of fibrosis. Resistance that creates a "gritty" sound when it is released suggests the presence of multiple bands of fibrosis.[1] The location of FFFUR at the 1-, 2-, 4-, or 6-mm distance may indicate a differential depth analysis, potentially revealing the underlying source of the pathology such as distal duct, orifice, lid margin, and tear film versus a more proximal conjunctival or periglandular/autoimmune source of inflammation.[6]

## MGP as a Therapeutic Intervention[6]

Indications with the following signs and symptoms of mild to severe obstructive MGD:

- Lid tenderness, lid soreness (on exam or as reported by the patient)
- Deficient meibum production and lipid tear deficiency with burning, stinging, and photophobia
- Nonexpressible glands
- Reduced number of expressible glands without signs of MGD (nonobvious MGD:NOMGD)

- Expressible glands with visible MGD: lid margin hyperemia, tarsal hyperemia, lid margin telangiectasia, thickening or irregularity, notches or grooves, orifice metaplasia, and anterior migration of mucocutaneous junction
- Early hordeolum or chalazion (patients may also benefit from therapeutic gland lavage)
- Transillumination or infrared meibography of lids showing gland irregularity: atrophic abnormalities, dilation, cystic acini, tortuous glands
- Previous diagnosis of ocular neuropathic pain

Patients with early and advanced MGD may be asymptomatic. Indications for asymptomatic patients:

- Nonexpressible glands
- Expressible glands with signs of MGD
- Reduced numbers of expressible glands without signs of MGD (NOMGD)
- Transillumination or infrared meibography of lids showing gland irregularity: atrophic abnormalities, dilation, cystic acini, tortuous glands

Patients with MGD and other ocular surface comorbidities that have not been adequately diagnosed and treated will need earlier repeat probing as the comorbidities create inflammation leading to recurrence of fixed periductal fibrosis. For patients in preop for cataract, refractive and other eye surgery, it is important to identify MGD and other comorbidities and begin their treatment prior to surgery, which has been shown to be a significant cofactor in exacerbation of MGD.[7] Ocular surface comorbidities frequently occurring may include (Figure 18-3):

- Aqueous tear deficiency (ATD)
- Blepharitis
- Allergies
- Other ocular surface disease such as conjunctivochalasis
- Side effects or irritation from scleral and other contact lenses

MGP is suitable and indicated for all patients with obvious and nonobvious MGD. After initial therapy with MGP, annual maintenance probing is performed to retain ductal integrity by helping prevent or release recurrent obstructions, maintain patency of the ductal outflow tracts, and help prevent subclinical progression of disease and possible initial or progressive gland atrophy. An analogy may be dentistry with periodic prophylactic tooth scaling and cleaning in the absence of cavities or gingival disease. Early repeat probing may be indicated if contributing factors or comorbidities are not concurrently and effectively treated.

## INDICATIONS: ADDITIONAL CONSIDERATIONS

### Indications for Selecting Glands for Treatment

Generally, when MGD is diagnosed, all glands in a lid are treated. However, some patients may need additional or repeat probing in only one lid or in a section of a lid, particularly in cases with new or persistent comorbidities that cause inflammation and exacerbate the development of periductal fibrosis.

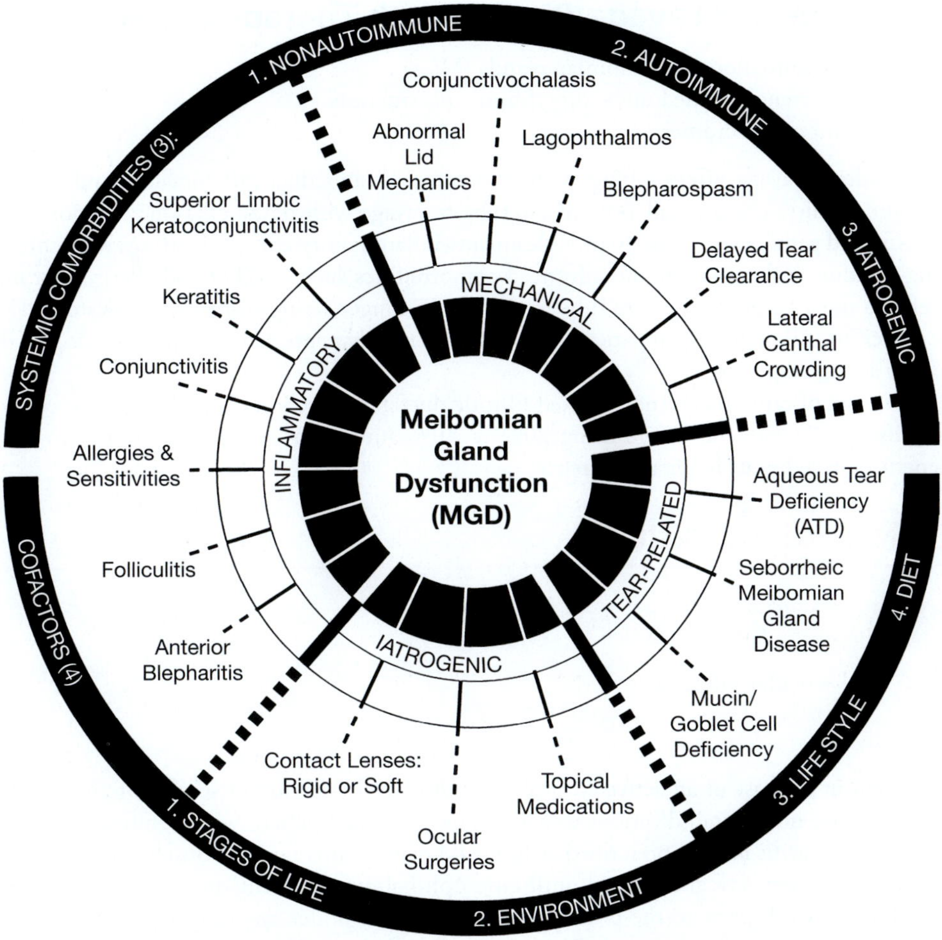


**FIGURE 18-3** If dry eye were a wheel, MGD would be its hub. Although each patient will experience a unique combination of comorbidities and react to cofactors differently, at the core of an interconnected hub and wheel we virtually always find MGD. (From Maskin SL, Warren NA. *Your Dry Eye Mystery Solved: Reversing Meibomian Gland Dysfunction, Restoring Hope*. Yale University Press; 2022.)

## Indications for Dilating Glands

Severe fixed obstruction: In some cases, severe periductal fibroses that prove difficult to release with routine probes may be encountered when probing glands. If the shortest and stiffest 1-mm probe is unable to release the dense fibrotic band, the dilator probe is typically able to do so. I have both routine and dilator probes available on hand when beginning the procedure in case they are needed.

Preparation for therapeutic intraductal lavage with corticosteroid: The dilator probe creates the larger lumen diameter able to accommodate the large bore tube required for this lavage with small particle suspension such as Celestone.

### Indications for Lavage/Rinsing with Therapeutic Agent

- Severe inflammation of Meibomian glands (MGs)
- Rapid recurrence of fixed unyielding fibrotic obstruction
- Significant comorbidities

Intraductal lavage, after probing, with corticosteroid can reduce inflammation and improve meibum quality. Use a Small Bore MicroTube to lavage with dexamethasone solution, after probing and gentle expression, to provide an anti-inflammatory effect. In settings with chronic long-standing inflammation and advanced comorbidities such as ATD and allergy, you may prefer to use a Large Bore MicroTube to deliver the longer acting suspension Celestone. (My ocular cicatricial pemphigoid patients, for example, readily appreciate the salutary effect of the longer acting suspension.)

For cases of rapid recurrence of fixed fibrotic ductal obstruction despite managing comorbid diseases, intraductal lavage using 20% to 50% autologous serum appears to provide a benefit in delaying its further recurrence.

## CONTRAINDICATIONS

**Key Contraindications**

- Active ocular infection

Except in the case of an active corneal or conjunctival infection or severe anterior blepharitis, there are no contraindications to MGP. The occasional patient with significant bacterial anterior blepharitis may be prescribed at-home lid hygiene therapy with Stone Crop Gel Wash cleanser twice per day and topical antibiotic ophthalmic ointment on lid margins at bedtime for one week prior to the procedure. For severe Demodex anterior blepharitis, clearing the lashes with topical compounded Ivermectin Ophthalmic Ointment has shown to be very successful.

## PREOPERATIVE PREPARATION

**Key Preoperative Considerations**

- Patient education is important leading up to procedure to minimize anxiety.
- The patient's symptoms should be evaluated and documented.
- The patient's ocular surface and function of MGs assessed
- Proper instrumentation is essential.
- Maskin Intraductal Meibomian Gland Probing Kit
- Determine if lavage will be performed.

Patient comfort to minimize anxiety:

- If necessary, reduce caffeine intake during the previous 1 to 2 weeks.
- Provide adequate anesthesia with two rounds of topical jojoba anesthetic ointment or supraorbital and infraorbital nerve block.
- Pretreat anterior blepharitis with antibiotic ophthalmic ointment to reduce lid sensitivity.
- Prescribe anxiolytics such as Valium or Xanax.

Patient sits at the slit lamp with staff gently supporting back of head.

- Instrumentation: Anesthetic
  - Topical tetracaine or proparacaine drop and bandage contact lens
  - Topical antibiotic ophthalmic ointment, cotton-tipped applicators, and latex-free gloves
  - Jojoba anesthetic ophthalmic ointment (JAO), 8% lidocaine in a petrolatum base ointment containing 25% jojoba (O'Brien Pharmacy in Mission, Kansas)
  - 2% Lidocaine with 1:100,000 epinephrine for nerve block, with betadine swab and alcohol wipe with sterile 4 × 4 and JBP 33-gauge needles (4 mm depth) with 3- or 5-mL syringe
- Maskin Intraductal Meibomian Gland Probing Kit
  - Maskin Meibomian gland intraductal probe: 1-, 2-, 4-, and 6-mm-long probe tips, 76 μm outer diameter, nonsharp (Figure 18-4)
  - Maskin Meibomian gland intraductal dilator probe, 150 μm outer diameter, 2 mm long, nonsharp (Figure 18-5)
  - Maskin Small Bore MicroTube, 110 μm outer diameter, 1 mm long, nonsharp (Figure 18-6)
  - Maskin Large Bore MicroTube, 150 μm outer diameter, 2 mm long, nonsharp (Figure 18-6)
- For intraductal lavage or rinse therapy (optional)
  - Dexamethasone solution (4 mg/mL)
  - Celestone small particle corticosteroid suspension (6 mg/mL)
  - Autologous serum 20% or 50% in 0.9% sterile preservative-free saline
- Individual vials of sterile, preservative-free, 0.9% saline solution
- Tissues (unscented with no emollients)
- Preservative-free lubricating drops

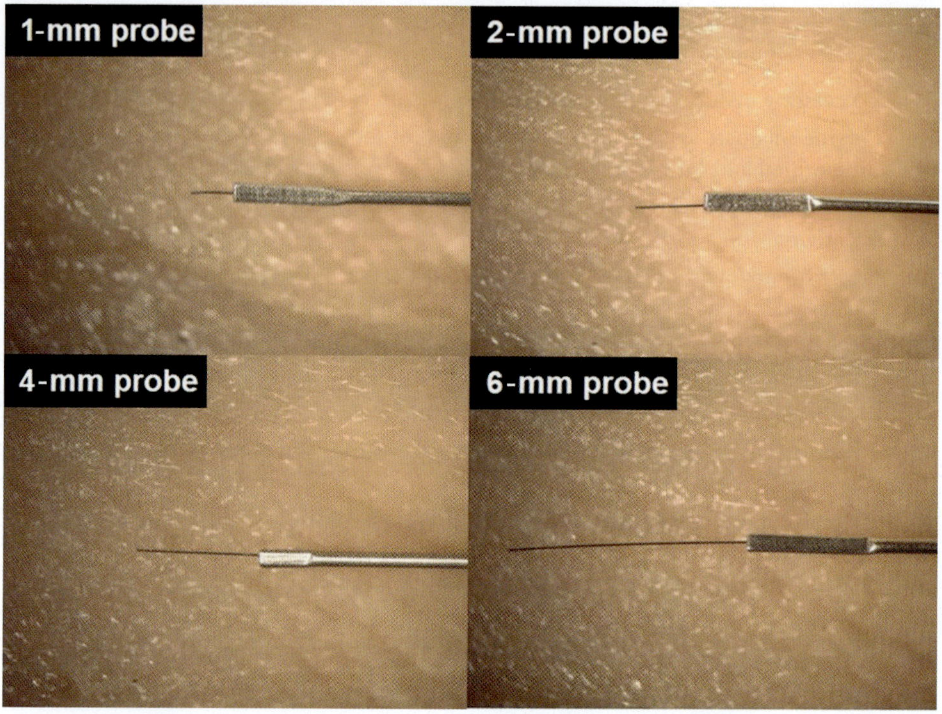


FIGURE 18-4 Maskin probes. Images of 1-, 2-, 4-, and 6-mm stainless steel Maskin probes (76 μm diameter), respectively. (Courtesy of Steven L. Maskin, MD.)

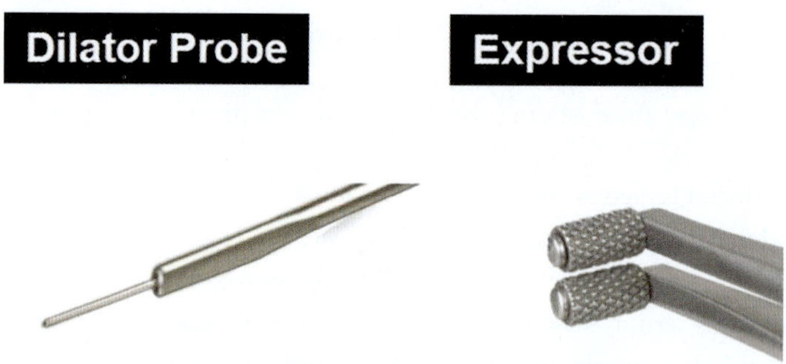


FIGURE 18-5 Maskin dilator probe and Maskin Meibum Expressor. Stainless steel Maskin dilator probe (150 μm) and stainless steel Maskin Meibum Expressor designed to gently express meibum from patent Meibomian gland ducts. (Courtesy of Steven L. Maskin, MD; obtained from mgdi.com)

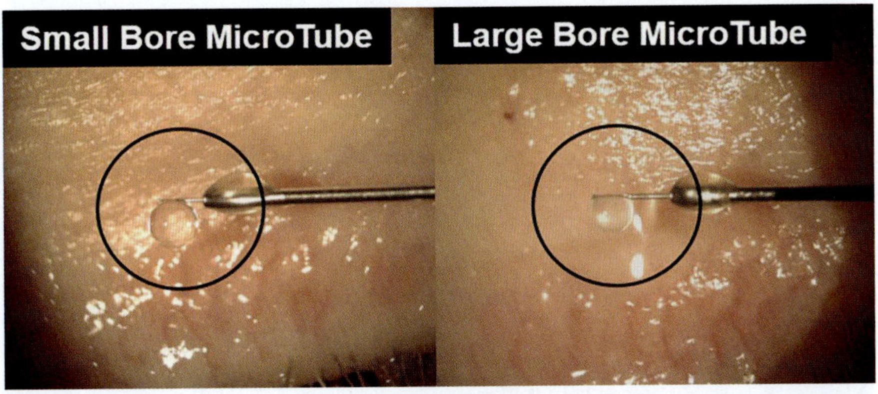


FIGURE 18-6 Maskin MicroTubes. Images of 1-mm Maskin Small Bore MicroTube (110 μm diameter) and Large Bore MicroTube (150 μm diameter), respectively. Small and Large Bore MicroTubes showing drops of dexamethasone solution (4 mg/mL) and Celestone (6 mg/mL) small particle suspension (encircled), respectively. (Courtesy of Steven L. Maskin, MD.)

# PROCEDURE

## Key Procedural Points

- Ensure proper application of anesthetic
- Gland Probing: diagnostic application and therapeutic application
- Dilation of orifice and expansion for therapeutic lavage
- Express to evacuate glands
- Intraductal lavage and rinse
- Irrigation of ocular surface and bandage contact lens removal

The six-step procedure involved in MGP, probing all glands in both lids of one eye, takes less than one hour, including the time for the topical anesthetic to take effect. Steps 3 through 5 are optional, depending on patient comorbidities (see Indications).

Step 1. Applying Anesthetic (Video 18-1, Figure 18-7)

- Place an anesthetic drop in the fornix of the eye.
- When numb, place a bandage contact lens on the eye.
- Swab lid margin and lash roots with topical ophthalmic antibiotic ointment on a sterile cotton-tipped applicator (CTA).
- Apply JAO with a sterile CTA to the lower lid margin. Patient is reclined in exam room chair, looking upward while the lower lid is everted and ointment placed along the entire lower lid margin. (Any stinging will dissipate in approximately 60 seconds.)
- Instruct patient to keep eyes closed for 10 minutes.

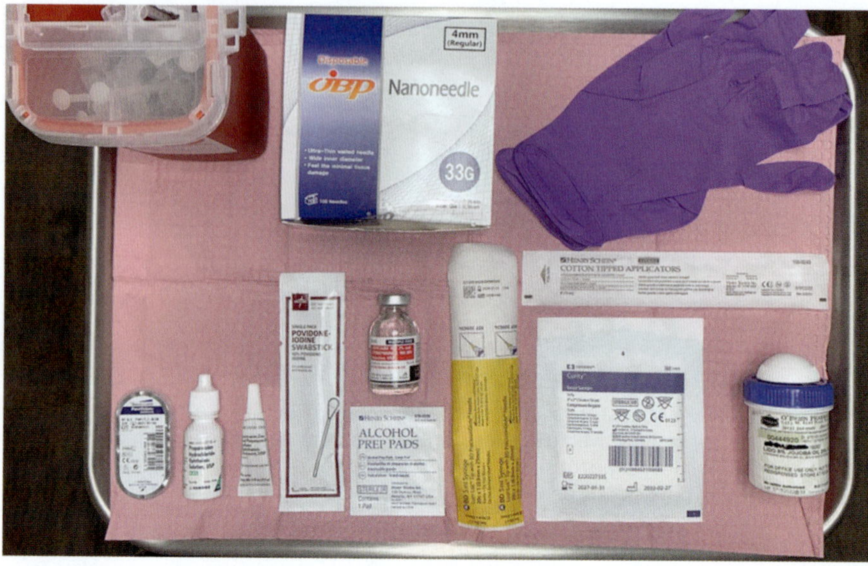


**FIGURE 18-7** Materials used for anesthesia protocol. From left to right, top row: sharps container, JBP nanoneedle 4-mm length and 33G, gloves; bottom row: bandage contact lens, proparacaine 0.5% solution, ophthalmic antibiotic ointment, povidone–iodine swab, Xylocaine 2% with epinephrine, alcohol wipe, 5-mL syringe, cotton-tipped applicator, 3″ × 3″ gauze sponge, jojoba anesthetic ophthalmic ointment (JAO). (Courtesy of Steven L. Maskin, MD.)

- For patients with chronic, long-term inflammation after 5 minutes:
  - Apply a second dose of JAO (Jojoba ointment appears to aid delivery of lidocaine to lid and MG tissues, eliminating the need for infiltrative anesthetic in most cases).
  - Five minutes later, apply a second anesthetic drop.
- For patients with chronic lid inflammation and sensitive lids, use a supraorbital and infraorbital nerve block before placing the jojoba anesthetic ointment. After the topical tetracaine and bandage contact lens is applied and lid margins cleaned with topical antibiotic ointment, the eyebrow over the superior orbital rim is wiped with povidone–iodine swab, followed 3 minutes later by a wipe with an alcohol pad for the upper lid nerve block and over the inferior orbital rim and cheek for the lower lid nerve block.
  - 2% Lidocaine with epinephrine (1:100,000) is then injected along the superior orbital notch, aiming superonasally through the JBP 33G/4-mm needle on a sterile 3-mL syringe, delivering 1.25 mL.
  - The same as mentioned earlier but aiming superonasally for the infraorbital nerve notch just below the inferior orbital rim in line with the pupil in primary gaze to anesthetize the lower lid.
  - The jojoba anesthetic ointment is then applied as earlier.

Step 2. Gland Probing (Video 18-2, Figure 18-8)

The operator wears clean latex-free gloves. The probing procedure begins with the 1-mm probe, the shortest and stiffest. The probe handle is placed within the sterile probing device

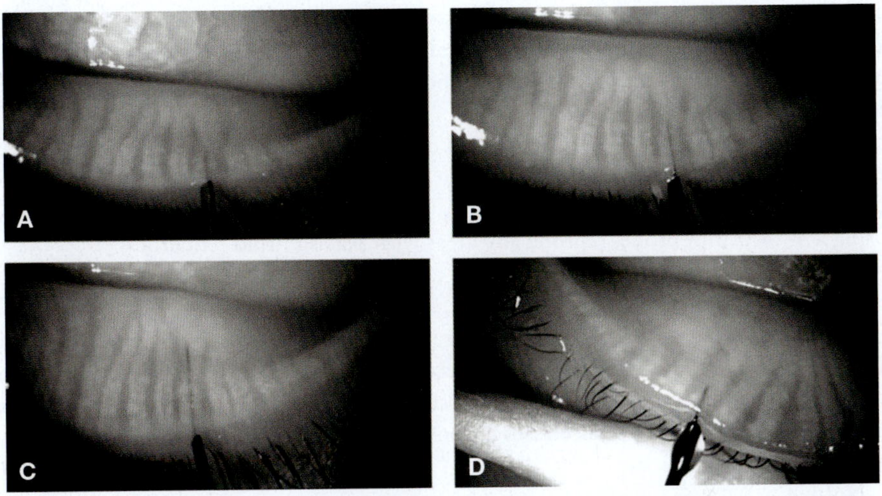


**FIGURE 18-8** Intraductal placement of probe and microtube. **A–C**, Presence and location of a 1-, 2-, and 4-mm probe (76 μm diameter), respectively, as well as (**D**) a 1-mm Maskin Small Bore MicroTube (110 μm diameter) within the central duct of a Meibomian gland. All images were obtained using the Mediworks S390L WDR FireFly Digital Slit Lamp from Eyefficient. (All images were obtained using the Mediworks S390L WDR FireFly Digital Slit Lamp from Eyefficient. Reproduced from Maskin SL, Alluri S. Meibography guided intraductal Meibomian gland probing using real-time infrared video feed. *Br J Ophthalmol*. 2020;104(12):1676-1682, with permission from BMJ Publishing Group Ltd.)

hub, which is then removed from its sterile pouch. The probe handle is designed ergonomically for comfort with a tapered handle. While a staff member supports the patient head within the slit lamp so the chin and forehead are against the respective supports, the probe tip is placed on the orifice, and a short dart-like motion is made with the wrist to advance the probe into the orifice. An adjustment in the probe angle may be made to find the correct entry angle, particularly with orifice dragging. The lid is held taut with a finger or thumb of the fellow hand or the tip of a CTA or a forceps for the lower lid. The hand holding the probe balances and steadies itself using facial structures, including the nose and cheek. Continue to use the 1-mm probe until all the glands have been probed or the probe gets fatigued and bends or breaks. For glands that show dense periductal fibrosis that the 1-mm probe is unable to release, use the dilator probe. The dilator probe is 150 μm in diameter and 2 mm long and successfully releases the denser fibroses. Return to using the 76-μm 1-mm long probe to complete the procedure.

When replacing the probe, simply twist off the probe hub from the handle, place the used probe into the biohazard container, and replace with a fresh probe.

Overview:

- Advance probe through orifice into gland with a quick motion.
- When the probe encounters resistance, apply additional mild force to release the constriction.
- Probe each gland in a lid, adjusting the angle of entry as necessary and replacing probe tip, if necessary, in case of a weak, bent, or broken probe tip.
- Once all glands in a lid are probed, check for residual tenderness by applying moderate pressure to the eyelid after probing. Apply moderate pressure along the entire span of the lid.

If the lid is still tender, this indicates persistent deeper obstruction and periductal fibroses, requiring a 2- and/or 4-mm probe. This test of persistent lid tenderness is useful if topical anesthetic is used without the nerve block because the nerve block can eliminate persistent lid tenderness.

- Using a 2-mm probe, reprobe the entire lid or any areas where patient reports persistent lid tenderness.
- Check for lid tenderness again.
- Using a 4- or 6-mm probe, reprobe any areas with persistent lid tenderness.

To record pre- and postprobing MG diagnostic expression results and probe findings:

- For MG diagnostic expression findings, use Meibomian gland classification form, MCF[8] (Figure 18-9), obtained at mgdi.com: Record the number of expressible glands, using mild to moderate pressure on lid just posterior to lid margin, preprobing and 1 week after probing. The functional classifications for each lid as a meibum-secreting unit are as follows[8]:
    - Normal
        - Five or more expressible glands
        - No tenderness (normal intraductal pressure)
    - PDO: Partial distal obstruction
        - Visible threadlike keratin may be noted within the orifice (orifice metaplasia).
        - Five or more expressible glands
        - No tenderness because obstruction is partial and does not cause elevated intraductal pressure
    - PDO-NF: Partial distal obstruction-nonfunctional
        - Visible threadlike keratin may be noted within the orifice (orifice metaplasia).
        - Four or fewer expressible glands
        - No tenderness because obstruction is partial and meibum is not being produced, as though the glands were dormant.
    - CPO: Complete proximal obstruction
        - Five or more expressible glands
        - Tenderness caused by increased intraductal pressure from blockage deeper within the gland
    - CPO-PA: Complete proximal obstruction-partial atrophy
        - Five or more expressible glands
        - Decreasing tenderness as meibum synthesis decreases behind the blockage
        - Truncated, short glands later visualized with infrared meibography and or transillumination
    - CDO: Complete distal obstruction
        - Four or fewer expressible glands
        - Tenderness caused by increased intraductal pressure from blockage deeper within the gland
    - CDO-NF: Complete distal obstruction-nonfunctional
        - Four or fewer expressible glands
        - Decreasing tenderness as gland deteriorates and meibum synthesis decreases behind blockage

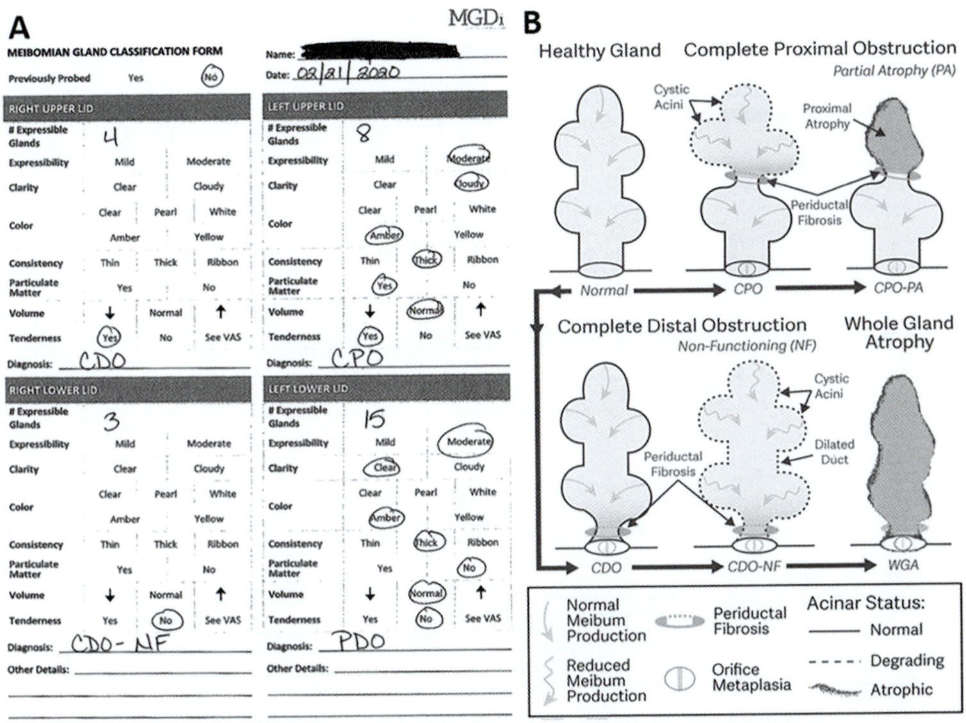


**FIGURE 18-9** **A,** Completed Meibomian gland Classification Form (MCF). This form is used to record the number of Meibomian glands per lid that are expressible, meibum quality, meibum volume, and lid tenderness. The number of expressible glands and lid tenderness findings provide a basis for each lid's diagnosis. **B,** Position of fixed fibrotic obstruction determines disease progression. Complete proximal obstruction (CPO), beyond the first acinus allows for the gland to still be expressible, yet leads to a gland's partial atrophy (CPO-PA). Complete distal obstruction (CDO), at the orifice or before the first acinus, leads to a nonfunctional gland (CDO-NF), which may lead to whole gland atrophy (WGA). Diagnostic classification of a lid is based on the predominant status of glands in that lid. (From Maskin SL, Warren NA. *Your Dry Eye Mystery Solved: Reversing Meibomian Gland Dysfunction, Restoring Hope*. Yale University Press; 2022.)

- For recording of in-depth probe findings:
  - Use the Probe Findings Form (Figure 18-10) obtained at mgdi.com
  - Number the glands, starting with #1. Always probe in the same direction (left eye, start temporally and move nasally. Right eye, start nasally and move temporally.)
  - Technician fills out the form in real time.
  - Tabulate findings, including Firm, Soft, or No Resistance. For Firm, specify Pop (FP) or Gritty (FG). Pop is a single focus of pressure release, whereas Gritty is multiple foci.

  There can be variation in the intensity level of tactile intraductal resistance, which is consistent with the audible volume generated by relief of the obstruction, at times heard across the room. The volume may correlate with severity of obstruction. The FP and FG produce sudden bursts of brief, not prolonged sounds. With FG, the multiple individual sounds may occur immediately after each other in rapid succession or after a

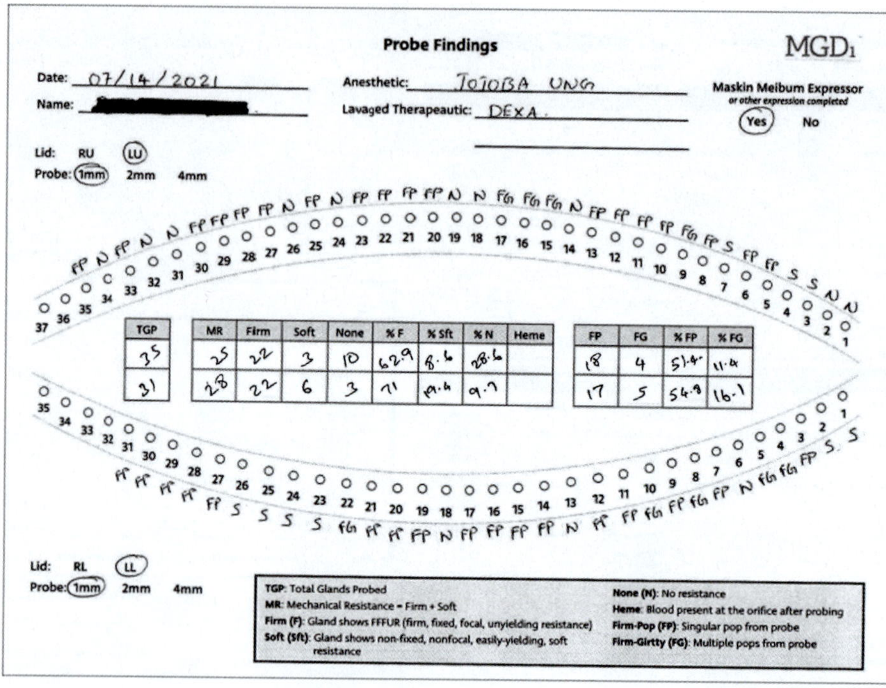

**Probe Findings** MGD1

Date: 07/14/2021
Name: [redacted]

Anesthetic: JOJOBA UNG
Lavaged Therapeautic: DEXA.

Maskin Meibum Expressor (or other expression completed): (Yes) No

Lid: RU (LU)
Probe: (1mm) 2mm 4mm

| TGP | MR | Firm | Soft | None | %F | %Sft | %N | Heme |
|---|---|---|---|---|---|---|---|---|
| 35 | 25 | 22 | 3 | 10 | 62.9 | 8.6 | 28.6 | |
| 31 | 28 | 22 | 6 | 3 | 71 | 19.4 | 9.7 | |

| FP | FG | %FP | %FG |
|---|---|---|---|
| 18 | 4 | 51.4 | 11.4 |
| 17 | 5 | 54.9 | 16.1 |

Lid: RL (LL)
Probe: (1mm) 2mm 4mm

TGP: Total Glands Probed
MR: Mechanical Resistance = Firm + Soft
Firm (F): Gland shows FFFUR (firm, fixed, focal, unyielding resistance)
Soft (Sft): Gland shows non-fixed, nonfocal, easily-yielding, soft resistance
None (N): No resistance
Heme: Blood present at the orifice after probing
Firm-Pop (FP): Singular pop from probe
Firm-Girtty (FG): Multiple pops from probe

**FIGURE 18-10** Completed Total Glands Probed (TGP) form. Probe findings form, for a single eye documenting findings from probing the upper and lower lids using a 1-mm probe. Probe findings include Firm Resistance that can be either a single pop (FP) or multiple pops, described as gritty (FG), or nonfixed resistance, described as soft (S). There may also be no resistance (N). (From Maskin SL, Warren NA. *Your Dry Eye Mystery Solved: Reversing Meibomian Gland Dysfunction, Restoring Hope*. Yale University Press; 2022.)

short delay if the probe advanced through an interim nonstrictured course of the duct lumen. Less commonly, a mild back pressure or "soft" resistance (SFT) may be noted, which is not fixed, not firm, and easily yielding. With SFT, the probe encounters mild resistance, akin to a drag on the to-and-fro movement of the probe but advances into the lumen without the application of significant additional mechanical pressure. When the probe passes through SFT resistance, an audible sound is not generated. SFT is not focal, in contrast to the FFFUR, which was characteristically focal or multifocal.

Infrequently, there may be a lack of resistance designated as no resistance "(NR)," where the probe enters the orifice and duct without any resistance or drag.[1]

Step 3: Dilating (Video 18-3)

- After probing, use the Maskin dilator probe to expand the orifice and the distal duct in preparation for therapeutic lavage with a small particle corticosteroid such as Celestone.
- Place the handle within the dilator device hub.
- Advance the dilator probe through the orifice into the gland as far as it will go.
- Repeat for all glands in a lid.

Step 4: Expressing (Video 18-4)

Mild expression to evacuate intraglandular stagnant material is safe after dilating ducts because duct patency is ensured after probing.

Cradle the lid between the rollers of the Maskin Meibum Expressor (Figure 18-5). Roll from the proximal tarsus deep part of the lid to the distal duct orifice and lid margin, directing meibum and other stagnant materials toward the orifices. Pass the rollers gently over the lid, ensuring that all glands have been expressed.

Step 5: Lavaging (Video 18-5)

Intraductal lavage of glands, with or without prior dilation or expression, reduces inflammation and recurrence of FFFUR.

- Draw up approximately 200 μL (0.2 mL) of the therapeutic agent into 1-mL syringe. Remove needle and replace with Maskin MicroTube.
- Insert tube tip into duct for full depth of tip.
- Apply slow, steady pressure to plunger for about 5 seconds (delivering approximately 2–6 μL).
- Repeat for each gland in a lid.
- Use Small Bore MicroTube for lavage with solution of dexamethasone (4 mg/mL) or autologous serum. Use dilator probe prior to lavage using Large Bore MicroTube to deliver small particle suspension such as Celestone (6 mg/mL).

Step 6: Irrigating

When all steps have been completed,

- Remove the bandage contact lens.
- Rinse copiously with sterile, preservative-free, 0.9% saline solution.
- Use sterile cotton swab to remove residual JAO from lid margins and lashes.

## POSTOPERATIVE CARE/COMANAGEMENT (FOLLOW-UP SCHEDULE)

### Key Postoperative Considerations

- Frequent lubrication postop can be helpful.
- Broad-spectrum ophthalmic antibiotic ointment
- Maintenance probing is necessary.

Patients may use preservative-free lubricating drops, 1 drop every hour per eye, if needed, until bedtime in case the eye is irritated from topical anesthetic ointment with 8% lidocaine. Also, the lubricating drops can be useful to lubricate for a few hours until the nerve block with decreased blink strength wears off. Eye closure for a few hours will also help.

Broad-spectrum ophthalmic antibiotic is applied to lid margins at bedtime for 5 nights. For eyes with more inflamed ocular surfaces, topical corticosteroid drops may be used 4× per day for 4 days.

Follow-up can be customized per patient, for example, the next day if patient needs closer follow-up owing to severe comorbidities, 3 months or more if doing well.

After initial probing, the procedure is repeated annually for maintenance. Annual probing ensures MGs remain unobstructed, synthesizing, and secreting good quality and quantities of meibum.

Early probing may be necessary in the presence of new or unresolved comorbidities.

## POTENTIAL COMPLICATIONS OR POST-PROCEDURE FINDINGS

### Key Potential Complications or Post-Procedure Findings to Look For

- Signs and symptoms of an infection
- Bruising

To reduce risk of infection, patients are instructed to avoid touching eyes and to wash hands before applying ointment to lid margin, best done with a sterile CTA. The incidence of gland infection is less than 1:100,000, and if occurs, would require systemic antibiotics.

A self-limiting hemorrhage is sometimes seen at the lid margin. This drop of blood is a good sign, indicating the release of vascularized periductal fibrosis. No therapy is required. With heavy vascularized periductal fibroses, mild bruising of the lid margin may be noted during examination with slit-lamp microscope, which resolves without treatment.

Author SLM Note: When I first began probing, twice the probe tips broke off partly within an orifice. I easily removed these with a forceps. On one other occasion, the probe remained inside the central duct, but without sequelae. As an aside, I have placed the probe next to an active MRI magnet on the patient table without showing any movement, suggesting the probes, being microscopic, are not sufficiently large to be deflected.

## VIDEOS OF PROCEDURES

**Video 18-1**—Anesthetic procedure. (Video courtesy of Steven L. Maskin, MD.)

**Video 18-2**—Probing the Meibomian gland. (Video courtesy of Steven L. Maskin, MD.)

**Video 18-3**—Dilating the Meibomian gland. (Video courtesy of Steven L. Maskin, MD.)

**Video 18-4**—Expressing the Meibomian gland. (Video courtesy of Steven L. Maskin, MD.)

**Video 18-5**—Lavaging the Meibomian gland. (Video courtesy of Steven L. Maskin, MD.)

# EFFICACY

The effect of MGP on patient symptoms of lid tenderness and excluding lid tenderness (symptoms such as burning, stinging, photophobia, increased blinking, and frequent eye closure) was studied using a visual analog scale (VAS) for up to 6 months post MGP[9] (Figure 18-11). This study showed an immediate and dramatic reduction of lid tenderness, which remained at 75% relief at 1 month, with further improvement to 79% at 3 months, and 90% at 6 months post MGP. Improvement of symptoms excluding lid tenderness was more gradual, with an immediate improvement of 36% and further improvement to 66% at 1 month, 78% at 3 months, and 80% at 6 months post MGP.

The percentage of lids showing reduced tenderness post MGP was further evaluated in patients with lid tenderness and a classification of CDO and CPO (Figure 18-12). Results

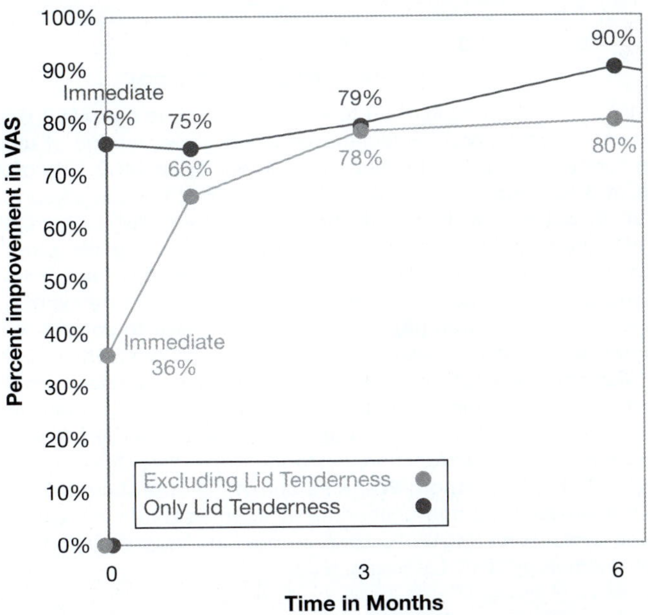


**FIGURE 18-11** The effect of MGP on visual analog scale for lid tenderness as well as excluding lid tenderness symptoms of MGD. Graph shows an immediate and dramatic reduction of lid tenderness, which remained at 75% relief at 1 month, with further improvement to 79% at 3 months, and 90% at 6 months post MGP. Improvement of symptoms excluding lid tenderness was more gradual with an immediate improvement of 36% and further improvement to 66% at 1 month, 78% at 3 months, and 80% at 6 months post MGP. (From Maskin SL, Kantor K. Intraductal Meibomian gland probing to restore functionality for obstructive meibomian gland dysfunction. In Poster presented at AAO 2011, Orlando.)

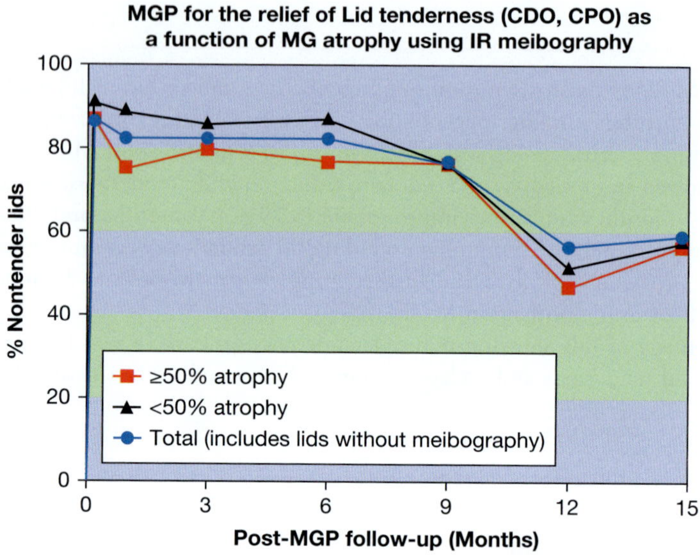


**FIGURE 18-12** Reduction of lid tenderness over time post MGP. Graph shows a dramatic and immediate reduction of percentage of tender lids for 86% of 144 treated lids within 1-week post MGP, 82% of 215 lids at 3 to 6 months post MGP, and 58% of 113 lids at 1-year post MGP in patients with classification of complete distal obstruction (CDO) and complete proximal obstruction (CPO). Complete proximal and distal obstruction refers to tender lids. CDO has four or fewer expressible glands per lid, whereas CPO has five or more expressible glands per lid. Infrared (IR) meibography was used to determine the degree of Meibomian gland atrophy. Although lids with less than 50% atrophy received better results than lids with greater than 50% atrophy at each time point, this finding did not reach significance. (From Maskin SL, Warren NA. *Your Dry Eye Mystery Solved: Reversing Meibomian Gland Dysfunction, Restoring Hope*. Yale University Press; 2022; Maskin SL, Hethorn WR. Meibomian gland probing (MGP) for lid tenderness (LT) & nonfunctioning Meibomian glands in Meibomian gland dysfunction (MGD). Poster presented at: American Academy of Ophthalmology 2015, Las Vegas, NV.)

showed a dramatic and immediate reduction of the percentage of tender lids for 86% of 144 lids within 1 week post MGP, 82% of 215 lids at 3 to 6 months post MGP, and 58% of 113 lids at 1 year post MGP. Infrared meibography was then used to determine the degree of MG atrophy in these lids that were studied. Although lids with less than 50% atrophy received better results than lids with greater than 50% atrophy at each time point, this finding did not reach significance.

The effect of MGP on gland expressibility was evaluated in patients with nonfunctional lids (≤4 expressible glands per lid)[10] (Figure 18-13). Results showed an increase of 412.86% in

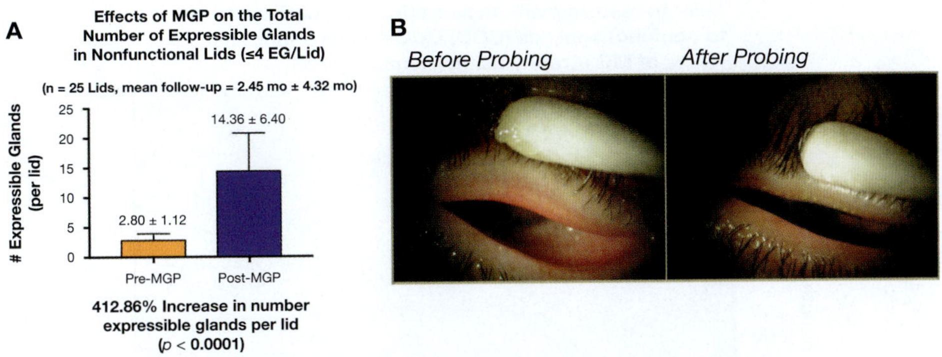


**FIGURE 18-13** Increase in number of expressible glands post MGP. **A,** The increase in number of expressible glands per lid after probing. **B,** Representative images showing the increase in gland expressibility post probing. (Adapted from Maskin SL. Meibomian gland probing (MGP): safely providing outflow patency with positive physical proof: concepts, literature review and results. AAO Instructional Course; 2018; Chicago, IL.)

the number of expressible glands per lid ($p < 0.0001$) at an average follow-up of 2.5 (±4.32) months post MGP.

The effect of MGP on restoring meibum-secreting lid functionality (MSLF; when lids show five or greater expressible glands) was also studied in patients with a classification of CDO and CDO-NF, which both have four or less expressible glands per lid (with CDO the lids are also tender)[9] (Figure 18-14). Results showed a restoration of MSLF in 94% of 64 lids at 1 week, 92% of 102 lids at 3 to 6 months, and 74% of 46 lids at 1 year post MGP. Infrared meibography was used to determine the degree of MG atrophy. Although lids with less than 50% atrophy received better results than lids with greater than 50% atrophy at each time point, this finding did not reach significance.

The efficacy of MGP has also been evaluated by other investigators and published in the peer-reviewed literature. From the published literature, there are five randomized control trials that are summarized as follows:

- Kheirkhah et al[11] compared posttreatment results at 1-month follow-up compared with baseline within three groups: (1) MGP with blephamide, (2) MGP with GenTeal, and (3) control: Sham MGP with GenTeal. They found statistical significance for improvement of symptoms only in the groups that received MGP. No statistically significant change was noted in patients that received Sham MGP plus GenTeal (see Table 18-1).
- Huang et al[12] compared three groups: (1) a series of treatments using intense pulse light therapy (IPL), (2) MGP alone, and (3) MGP with subsequent IPL. They found statistically significant improvement in signs and symptoms for all three groups compared with baseline (see Table 18-2). When compared between groups, they found that MGP with subsequent IPL had the greatest improvement. When comparing MGP alone to IPL alone, 100% of patients with MGP alone reported relief of symptoms compared

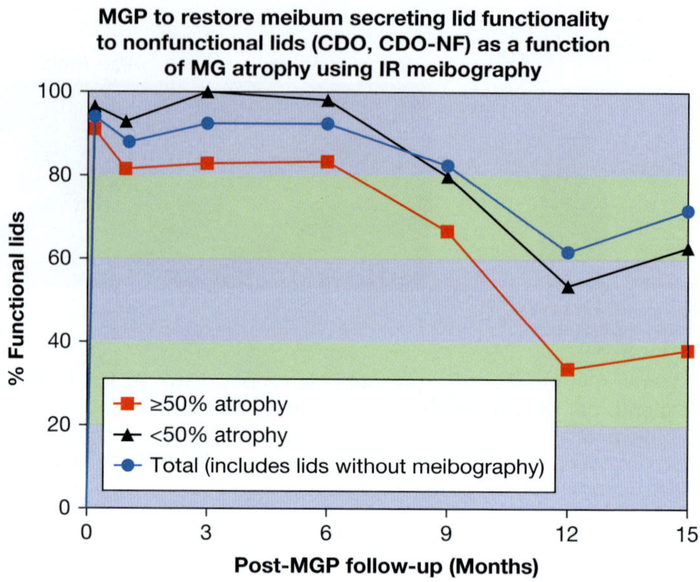


**FIGURE 18-14** Restoration of meibum-secreting lid functionality (MSLF) post MGP. Graph shows a restoration of MSLF (when lids show five or greater expressible glands) for 94% of 64 lids at 1 week, 92% of 102 lids at 3 to 6 months, and 74% of 46 lids at 1-year post MGP in patients with classification of complete distal obstruction (CDO) and complete distal obstruction-nonfunctional (CDO-NF). CDO and CDO-NF have four or fewer expressible glands per lid (with CDO, the lids are also tender). Infrared meibography was used to determine the degree of Meibomian gland atrophy. Although lids with less than 50% atrophy received better results than lids with greater than 50% atrophy at each time point, this finding did not reach significance. (From Maskin SL, Warren NA. *Your Dry Eye Mystery Solved: Reversing Meibomian Gland Dysfunction, Restoring Hope*. Yale University Press; 2022; Maskin SL, Hethorn WR. Meibomian gland probing (MGP) for lid tenderness (LT) & non functioning Meibomian glands in Meibomian gland dysfunction (MGD). Poster presented at: American Academy of Ophthalmology 2015, Las Vegas, NV.)

with 85.7% with IPL alone. Standard Patient Evaluation of Eye Dryness (SPEED) scores improved to less than or equal to 9 for 26.7% of MGP-alone compared with 14.3% of IPL-alone cases. The need for retreatment after 6 months was 20% of the MGP-alone group versus 35.7% in the IPL-alone group. Tear breakup time (TBUT) after treatment increased to greater than 5 seconds for 37% of MGP-alone eyes versus 18% of IPL-alone eyes. Patients that received MGP alone had significantly less lid tenderness than IPL alone after treatment ($p < 0.001$).

**TABLE 18-1 RANDOMIZED CONTROLLED TRIALS (RCT) SIGNIFICANT FINDINGS AND AUTHOR COMMENTS**

| TREATMENT GROUPS | SYMPTOMS (SUBJECTIVE)<br>KEY FINDING COMPARED WITH BASELINE | COMMENTS |
|---|---|---|
| 1) MGP + Blephamide | SANDE ($p = 0.002$)<br>OSDI ($p = 0.02$) | • "The MG probing was safe and no adverse events related to the study treatments were noted in any group." |
| 2) MGP + GenTeal | SANDE (0.01) | • "In conclusion, our study showed that MG probing can be an effective procedure to reduce patients' symptoms in patients with obstructive MGD, particularly if it is combined with an appropriate post-procedural regimen." |
| 3) Control: Sham MGP + GenTeal | No significance | |

MG, Meibomian gland; MGD, Meibomian gland dysfunction; MGP, Meibomian gland probing; OSDI, Ocular Surface Disease Index; SANDE, Symptom Assessment in Dry Eye.

From Kheirkhah A, Kobashi H, Girgis J, Jamali A, Ciolino JB, Hamrah P. A randomized, sham-controlled trial of intraductal meibomian gland probing with or without topical antibiotic/steroid for obstructive meibomian gland dysfunction. *Ocul Surf.* 2020;18(4):852-856.

- Incekalan et al[13] compared two groups: (1) MGP with conventional treatment and (2) control: conventional treatment alone. They found a statistically significant faster improvement of both signs and symptoms in the group receiving MGP when compared with the control group of conventional treatment alone (see Table 18-3).
- Ma and Lu[14] compared two groups: (1) MGP with topical steroid and (2) control: topical steroid only. They found statistically significant improvement in signs and symptoms in the group receiving MGP compared with the control group receiving topical steroid alone. In the group receiving MGP, 76% of patients reported relief in 1 day after MGP and before starting topical steroid (see Table 18-4).
- Dongju et al[15] compared three groups (1) MGP, (2) MGP with adjunctive intraductal steroid antibiotic lavage, and (3) control: conventional treatment only. They found statistically significant improvement in signs and symptoms in each of the groups receiving MGP compared with the control group of conventional treatment alone. The addition of intraductal steroid antibiotic lavage with MGP led to further improvement compared with MGP alone but did not reach statistical significance (see Table 18-5).

## CODING/BILLING AND MODIFIERS

There is no universally accepted Current Procedural Terminology (CPT) code for this procedure. Many doctors perform this procedure on a cash basis.

**TABLE 18-2** RANDOMIZED CONTROLLED TRIALS (RCT) SIGNIFICANT FINDINGS AND AUTHOR COMMENTS

| | SYMPTOMS (SUBJECTIVE) | | | | SIGNS (OBJECTIVE) | | |
|---|---|---|---|---|---|---|---|
| | KEY FINDING COMPARED WITH BASELINE | | | | KEY FINDING COMPARED WITH BASELINE | KEY FINDING COMPARED WITH IPL | |
| TREATMENT GROUPS | RELIEF OF SYMPTOMS | SPEED SCORE IMPROVEMENT ≤9 ($p = 0.02$) | NEED FOR RETREATMENT AFTER 6 MON | OTHER | INCREASED TBUT >5S ($p = 0.009$) | LID TENDERNESS | COMMENTS |
| 1) IPL | 85.7% of pts reported relief | 14.3% | 35.7% | 14.8% of pts reported worse symptoms | 18% | | "IPL, MGP, and combined MGP-IPL are all effective methods for refractory o-MGD patients; however, the combination of MGP-IPL method could maximize the therapeutic benefits which is especially helpful for patients who have severe Meibomian gland obstruction and obvious intraductal or eyelid margin inflammation, who want to gain the greatest amelioration in all clinical signs and subjective symptoms or still remain frustrated to either MGP or IPL treatments." |
| 2) MGP | 100% of pts reported relief | 26.7% | 20% | | 37% | $p < 0.001$ | |
| 3) MGP + IPL | | 64.3% | 0% | | 93% | | |

IPL, intense pulse light therapy; MGD, Meibomian gland dysfunction; MGP, Meibomian gland probing; SPEED, standard patient evaluation of eye dryness; TBUT, tear breakup time.

From Huang X, Qin Q, Wang L, et al. Clinical results of intraductal Meibomian gland probing combined with intense pulsed light in treating patients with refractory obstructive Meibomian gland dysfunction: a randomized controlled trial. *BMC Ophthalmol.* 2019;19(1):1-9.

**TABLE 18-3** RANDOMIZED CONTROLLED TRIALS (RCT) SIGNIFICANT FINDINGS AND AUTHOR COMMENTS

| TREATMENT GROUPS | SYMPTOMS (SUBJECTIVE) | SIGNS (OBJECTIVE) | COMMENTS |
|---|---|---|---|
| | KEY FINDING COMPARED WITH CONTROL | | |
| 1) MGP + Conventional Treatment<br>2) Control: Conventional Treatment Only | OSDI faster ($p = 0.0001$) | Sch1 faster ($p = 0.0001$)<br>BUT faster ($p = 0.0001$)<br>OS faster ($p = 0.0001$)<br>MQ faster ($p = 0.034$)<br>ME faster ($p = 0.0001$) | • "Considering that probing is a simple, reproducible and safe technique the data in the studies mentioned above can be regarded as satisfactory in terms of long-term effectiveness of probing."<br>• "In summary, our study plays an important role in revealing the rapid efficacy of probing in addition to conventional treatment versus conventional treatment alone. We demonstrate that intraductal meibomian gland probing is effective in accelerating the efficacy of conventional treatment."<br>• "Hereby, probing may become part of primary treatment as well as being an option in the patients resistant to conventional therapy in the future." |

BUT, breakup times; ME, meibum expressibility; MQ, meibum quality; OS, Oxford grading of ocular surface; OSDI, Ocular Surface Disease Index; Sch1, Schirmer 1 test.

From Incekalan TK, Harbiyeli II, Yagmur M, Erdem E. Effectiveness of intraductal meibomian gland probing in addition to the conventional treatment in patients with obstructive meibomian gland dysfunction. *Ocul Immunol Inflamm.* 2019;27(8):1345-1351. Reproduced by permission of Taylor and Francis Group, LLC, a division of Informa plc.

**TABLE 18-4** RANDOMIZED CONTROLLED TRIALS (RCT) SIGNIFICANT FINDINGS AND AUTHOR COMMENTS

| TREATMENT GROUPS | SYMPTOMS (SUBJECTIVE) | SIGNS (OBJECTIVE) | COMMENTS |
|---|---|---|---|
| 1) MGP + Topical Steroid | Key Finding Compared with Control<br><br>76% of pts reported relief in 1 day (19/25)[a] | <br><br>Immediate release of meibum (38/46) | "However, from our results, intraductal meibomian gland probing had significant efficacy regarding symptom relief and tear film stabilization. Probing helped release accumulated, abnormal meibum and helped increased [*sic*] the accessibility of the diseased Meibomian gland to topical corticosteroids to control inflammation. We propose that intraductal meibomian gland probing could be a valuable technique in the treatment of refractory O-MGD." |

(*continued*)

**TABLE 18-4 RANDOMIZED CONTROLLED TRIALS (RCT) SIGNIFICANT FINDINGS AND AUTHOR COMMENTS (*continued*)**

| TREATMENT GROUPS | SYMPTOMS (SUBJECTIVE) | SIGNS (OBJECTIVE) | COMMENTS |
|---|---|---|---|
| | Key Finding Compared with Control | | |
| | Various symptoms ($p < 0.001$) | LM Score ($p < 0.001$)<br>MG ($p < 0.001$)<br>TBUT ($p = 0.0293$) | |
| 2) Control: Topical Steroid Only | Key Finding Compared with Baseline | | |
| | 0% of pts reported relief in 1 day (0/24) | | |

[a]Before starting topical steroid.

LM Score, lid margin abnormalities; MG, meibum grade; TBUT, tear breakup time.

From Ma X, Yan L. Efficacy of intraductal meibomian gland probing on tear function in patients with obstructive meibomian gland dysfunction. *Cornea.* 2016;35(6):725-730.

**TABLE 18-5 RANDOMIZED CONTROLLED TRIALS (RCT) SIGNIFICANT FINDINGS AND AUTHOR COMMENTS**

| TREATMENT GROUPS | SYMPTOMS (SUBJECTIVE) | SIGNS (OBJECTIVE) | COMMENTS |
|---|---|---|---|
| | KEY FINDING COMPARED WITH CONTROL | | |
| 1) MGP | OSDI ($p < 0.05$) | BUT ($p < 0.05$)<br>CFS ($p < 0.05$)<br>SIT ($p < 0.05$)<br>Lid margin scores ($p < 0.05$) | "Intraductal meibomian gland probing seems to provide rapid and lasting symptom relief and significant improvement in symptoms and signs of MGD in patients. Intraductal meibomian gland probing is a safe, effective technique for MGD." |
| 2) MGP + Steroid-Antibiotic Intraglandular Injection | OSDI ($p < 0.05$) | BUT ($p < 0.05$)<br>CFS ($p < 0.05$)<br>SIT ($p < 0.05$)<br>Lid margin scores ($p < 0.05$) | |
| 3) Control: Conventional Treatment (CT) Only | | No significance | |

BUT, tear breakup time; CFS, corneal fluorescein staining; OSDI, Ocular Surface Disease Index; SIT, Schirmer I test.

Data from Dongju Q, Hui L, Jianjiang X. Clinical research on intraductal meibomian gland probing in the treatment of patients with meibomian gland dysfunction. *Chin J Optom Ophthalmol Vis Sci.* 2014;16(10):615-621.

## CONCLUSION

Since its introduction in 2010, intraductal MGP has proven to be an important development in the diagnosis and successful treatment and ongoing management of obstructive MGD. In ten independent studies, all of which included only patients refractory to standard treatments, including three clinical trials, probing was consistently effective in improving objective signs and subjective symptoms of MGD with no side effects.[16] Given this record of efficacy and safety, intraductal MGP merits consideration as a primary treatment for MGD.

## REFERENCES


1. Maskin SL, Alluri S. Expressible meibomian glands have occult fixed obstructions: findings from meibomian gland probing to restore intraductal integrity. *Cornea* 2019;38(7):880-887.
2. Maskin SL, Toland C. Intraductal Meibomian gland probing (MGP) leads to more superficial and accelerated Meibomian gland (MG) basement membrane (BM) differentiation with increased ductal epithelial cell layers (ECL). Poster presented at: *World Cornea Congress; 2022*; Chicago, IL, manuscript in preparation.
3. Maskin SL, Testa WR. Growth of meibomian gland tissue after intraductal meibomian gland probing in patients with obstructive meibomian gland dysfunction. *Br J Ophthalmol.* 2018;102(1):59-68.
4. Maskin SL. Intraductal meibomian gland probing relieves symptoms of obstructive meibomian gland dysfunction. *Cornea* 2010;29(10):1145-1152.
5. Maskin SL, Alluri S. Meibography guided intraductal meibomian gland probing using real-time infrared video feed. *Br J Ophthalmol.* 2020;104(12):1676-1682.
6. Maskin SL, Alluri S. Intraductal meibomian gland probing: background, patient selection, procedure, and perspectives. *Clin Ophthalmol.* 2019;13:1203-1223.
7. Maskin SL, Greenberg EL. Meibomian gland dysfunction, dry eye disease, and unhappy cataract surgery patients. *CRS Today.* 2018;15-17.
8. Maskin SL, Warren NA. *Your Dry Eye Mystery Solved: Reversing Meibomian Gland Dysfunction, Restoring Hope.* Yale University Press; 2022.
9. Maskin SL, Hethorn WR. Meibomian gland probing (MGP) for lid tenderness (LT) & nonfunctioning Meibomian glands in Meibomian gland dysfunction (MGD). Poster presented at: American Academy of Ophthalmology; 2015; Las Vegas, NV.
10. Maskin SL. Meibomian gland probing (MGP): safely providing outflow patency with positive physical proof: concepts, literature review and results. AAO Instructional Course 2018; Chicago, IL.
11. Kheirkhah A, Kobashi H, Girgis J, Jamali A, Ciolino JB, Hamrah P. A randomized, sham-controlled trial of intraductal meibomian gland probing with or without topical antibiotic/steroid for obstructive meibomian gland dysfunction. *Ocul Surf.* 2020;18(4):852-856.
12. Huang X, Qin Q, Wang L, Zheng J, Jin X. Clinical results of intraductal Meibomian gland probing combined with intense pulsed light in treating patients with refractory obstructive Meibomian gland dysfunction: a randomized controlled trial. *BMC Ophthalmol.* 2019;19(1):211.
13. Incekalan TK, Harbiyeli II, Yagmur M, Erdem E. Effectiveness of intraductal meibomian gland probing in addition to the conventional treatment in patients with obstructive meibomian gland dysfunction. *Ocul Immunol Inflamm.* 2019;27(8):1345-1351.
14. Ma X, Lu Y. Efficacy of intraductal meibomian gland probing on tear function in patients with obstructive meibomian gland dysfunction. *Cornea.* 2016;35(6):725-730.
15. Dongju Q, Hui L, Jianjiang X. Clinical research on intraductal meibomian gland probing in the treatment of patients with meibomian gland dysfunction. *Chin J Optometry Ophthalmol Visual Sci.* 2014;16(10):615-621.
16. Warren NA, Maskin SL. Review of literature on intraductal meibomian gland probing with insights from the inventor and developer: fundamental concepts and misconceptions. *Clin Ophthalmol.* 2023;17:497-514.

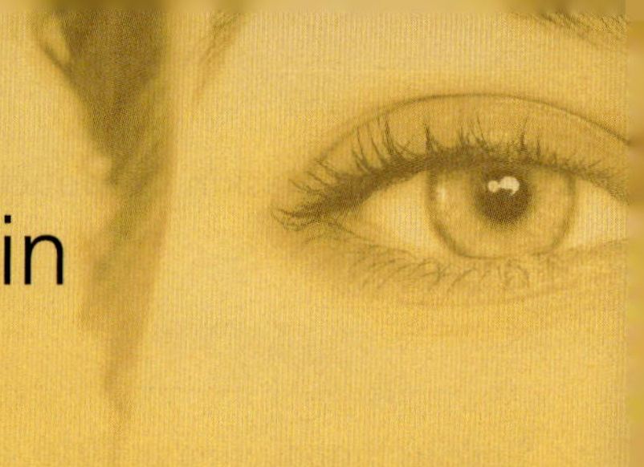

# 19 Radiofrequency in Aesthetics

**Selina R. McGee**

## BACKGROUND

There is a growing demand for less invasive, minimal downtime energy devices that reduce the effects of the aging process of the skin.[1] Utilization of radiofrequency (RF) technology has been on the rise because it can be used on any skin type, and the procedure has minimal to no downtime due to the characteristics and nature of the procedure.[2]

RF works through the tissue resistance of electrical current. The current can be delivered through a monopolar, bipolar, or multipolar device and leads to the formation of heat. Water is a strong conductor of electrical current and is the target chromophore in RF, and therefore gives RF a better safety profile than light-based procedures, such as intense pulsed light (IPL) therapy, which are dependent on skin type because of chromophore targets of oxyhemoglobin and melanin.[3] RF differs from light-based treatments with a laser or IPL, which utilize selective photothermolysis and have limitations in darker skin types.[4]

For a monopolar device, the electrical current flows between the handpiece and a grounding pad. Bipolar devices have two prongs that the electrical current flows between. Based on Ohm's Law, the depth of penetration is half of the distance between the two prongs.[5] Understanding the delivery mechanism of technology will give the user the knowledge needed to utilize different devices.

## INDICATIONS

### Key Indications

- Periorbital rhytids
- Blepharoptosis
- Lateral hooding
- Dermatochalasis
- Ectropion
- Tightening blink

RF works by heating the dermal layer of the skin through the epidermis.[6] The effects of certain temperatures of heat delivered over a given time at a controlled depth have been shown to have immediate effects on collagen.[7] Most studies agree that a target of 40 to 42°C of the epidermis will give the desired result of skin tightening through neocollagenesis.[3] This happens in what is thought to be three phases. Phase I shows collagen type I (80%–85%) and type III (15%–20%) histologically changing structure immediately post RF. The stimulation of the collagen then induces phase II, which activates dermal fibroblasts and mediates collagen denaturation. Phase III follows with the formation of new collagen and elastin, which results in modest skin tightening over a period of months.[2]

The periorbital area can be challenging to address due to the anatomy and thinness of the skin. RF can be helpful in treating this problematic area by stimulating collagen production and helping rejuvenate the periocular area for a more youthful appearance.[8-10] Periorbital rhytids, especially under the eye, can be addressed with RF in a noninvasive way which many patients desire.[11] This area in particular cannot be easily addressed with other options like neurotoxin without unwanted side effects.

Tightening the periorbital skin can have a myriad of benefits. Lateral hooding and mild dermatochalasis can be reduced in a nonsurgical manner with RF. Patients may not be candidates for surgical intervention and/or want a noninvasive procedure. These types of patients can be great candidates for RF. Blepharoptosis can be improved with RF as well. The use of topical oxymetazoline 0.1% has expanded patients' and practitioners' awareness of blepharoptosis. This increased awareness has heightened the demand for noninvasive methodologies to address periorbital concerns.

For patients that struggle with mild ectropion, RF has the potential to tighten the lid in a nonsurgical approach.

Patients that struggle with lid laxity and ineffective blinking can be at risk for meibomian gland dysfunction (MGD) due to the loss of mechanical force. This can contribute to MGD, which in turn can lead to dry eye. Surgical interventions have shown improvement in dry eye symptoms by improving tear drainage and stabilizing the tear film.[12] Although there is no broad evidence to date that supports improving lid laxity with RF to improve MGD and dry eye symptoms, there are several clinical trials studying this effect at the time of publication and there are a number of compelling anecdotal case reports in publication.

Clinical efficacy of RF has been shown with both practitioner and patient appreciating noticeable improvements in skin tightening.[1,13] The remodeling occurs over months and appears to have the most effect at 3 to 6 months post procedure.[1,13]

Patients that desire to have a minimally invasive or noninvasive procedure to reduce the appearance of fine lines and dynamic wrinkles are good candidates.

## CONTRAINDICATIONS AND PRECAUTIONS

### Key Contraindications

- Implanted pacemaker or defibrillator
- Facial implants

**Precautions**

- Pregnancy
- Body dysmorphic disorder
- Wait 3 to 4 weeks post neurotoxin to administer the procedure.
- Metal in the treatment area should be avoided as it is a great conductor of electrical current, and energy could arc, or cause a burn.
- Patients with unrealistic expectations

Patients that have an implanted pacemaker or defibrillator could potentially experience asystole or tachycardia if RF current does interfere with the device.[14] Facial implants can be made of a variety of materials and the use of RF, specifically monopolar energy, could cause heat to be introduced at an undesirable level that has the potential to cause complications or rarely fail.[14] RF has not been studied in pregnancy and therefore is listed as a caution. Patients with body dysmorphic disorder should be approached with caution and if suspected the practitioner should obtain a consult with a mental health professional. Due to the introduction of heat to targeted areas, neurotoxin could potentially migrate and cause unwanted side effects. Therefore, spacing of procedures is important, and 2 to 4 weeks apart is ideal. Due to the nature of RF utilizing certain frequencies, metal should be avoided. Jewelry, metal corneal shields, and any other types of metal should be avoided in and around the treatment area as to not cause an energy arc and subsequent burn. Patients who have unrealistic expectations should be avoided.

## PRETREATMENT PREPARATION

**Key Pretreatment Considerations**

- Results are not guaranteed.
- Treatment typically takes 20 to 25 minutes, depending on the area.
- A series of treatments spaced 2 to 4 weeks apart yields the best results.
- Hydration is key because water is an excellent conductor of the electrical current needed to heat the tissue.
- Informed consent
- Photos of the intended treatment area

### Pretreatment Patient Instructions

- Hydrate! Have the patient drink their own body weight in ounces in the week leading up to the procedure.
- Procedure feels like a hot stone massage if not accompanied by microneedling.
- If microneedling is done alongside RF, then the patient will need 40 to 60 minutes of facial numbing cream prior to treatment. A typical compound for facial numbing cream is 23:7 lidocaine:tetracaine or BLT which is benzocaine:lidocaine:tetracaine at a ratio of 20:4:2, respectively.

## Informed Consent

Patients must sign an informed consent each and every time they undergo a treatment. Do not do lifetime consents. Informed consent should include a description of the procedure in plain language. An example consent form is as follows:

For example: CONSENT TO Radiofrequency (RF) TREATMENT

Radiofrequency (RF) can help stimulate collagen and elastin production through heating of the skin. Treatment with RF can cause a reduction in fine lines or wrinkles through skin tightening. Areas most frequently treated are (a) forehead, (b) crow's feet (lateral areas of the eyes), and (c) midface. Patients may feel heat while the procedure is being performed. The procedure takes about 20 to 25 minutes, and the results last 3 to 6 months. With repeated treatments, the results may tend to last longer.

**RISKS AND COMPLICATIONS**

It has been explained to me that there are certain inherent and potential risks and side effects in any procedure and in this specific instance such risks include but are not limited to (1) posttreatment discomfort, swelling, redness, and bruising; (2) posttreatment bacterial, viral, and/or fungal infection requiring further treatment; and (3) hyperpigmentation may occur in rare instances.

**PREGNANCY, ALLERGIES, AND PACEMAKERS**

I am not aware that I am pregnant, have any significant neurologic disease, or have an implantable device like a pacemaker or defibrillator.

**RESULTS**

I am aware that results may vary from person to person. Full results typically occur in 3 to 6 months. In a very small number of individuals, the treatment does not work as satisfactorily.

I hereby voluntarily consent to treatment with RF for the condition known as fine lines and wrinkles due to skin laxity. The procedure has been explained to me. I have read the above and understand it. My questions have been answered satisfactorily. I accept the risks and complications of the procedure.

________________________________________

Patient Signature Date Witness Signature Date

A note from the counseling practitioner should be included and phrased similar to "I have counseled this patient as to the nature of the proposed procedure, the attendant risks involved, and the expected results." The patient's and doctor's name should be printed and signed with the date as well as a witness (typically a staff member).

## Recording Results

Utilize a standard form for each patient that contains the following:

- Area treated
- Date of treatment

- Energy needed to reach the desired temperature
- Length of treatment at the desired temperature
- Clinical endpoint of erythema, swelling, and change in eyebrow and eyelid height

## Photography

Photos should be obtained before the patient is treated and at every subsequent patient visit. Pretreatment photographs are essential to patient education and comparison posttreatment.

- Take at least three pictures before treatment:
  - Straight on
  - Right side
  - Left side
- Utilize the same background (see Figure 19-1)
  - Blue or black backdrop

## Photography Consent

Because these treatments are being performed on the face, photography informed consent is necessary. An example may read like this:

> I hereby authorize **[physician name]**, of **[name of practice]**, and/or his/her associates or licensees to take preprocedural and postprocedural photographs and slides.
>
> I consent to the use of these images for the purposes of preprocedural planning and postprocedural evaluation by **[physician name]** and/or the staff of **[name of practice]**, and I understand that they shall be made a part of my medical record.

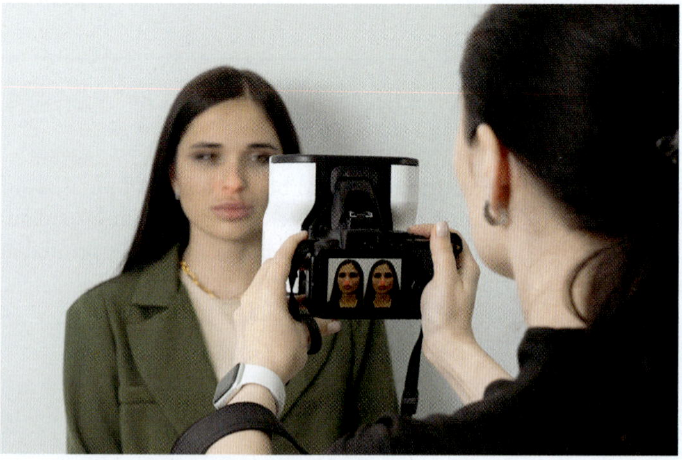

**FIGURE 19-1** Showing uniform background, straight at the patient placed 3 feet away from the patient.

## Equipment Needed/Procedure Checklist

- RF device with appropriate handpieces: 15 mm, 10 mm, 10 mm eye, and 20 mm
- New technology has the temperature gauge built into the handpieces, so no secondary skin temperature device is needed.
- Coupling gel
- Tongue depressors
- 4 × 4 gauze
- Gloves

# PROCEDURE

## Key Procedural Points

- Ensure proper application of RF energy.
- See Table 19-1 for energy settings.
- Target temperature 42°C for 5 minutes in each targeted area.
- A series of treatments will need to be performed 2 to 4 weeks apart for the best results.
- Clear coupling gel for smooth treatments.
- Clinical endpoints
  - Firmness
  - Edema
  - Erythema
  - Elevation
  - Itching

Ensure grounding is in place if utilizing a monopolar device. Application/placement of the grounding pad or plate between the shoulder blades is appropriate. Ensure the patient has no metal on their face. Remove all makeup before applying a thin coupling gel to the treatment area. Ensure gloves are donned, and utilize the handpiece desired for the treatment zone. Utilize gauze to pull the target skin over the bony orbit for the procedure treatment area. Once the treatment area has reached the target temperature and treatment is finished, remove the coupling gel with tongue depressor. Apply postprocedure sunscreen if appropriate (with monopolar devices this is appropriate). If the skin is broken with microneedling, apply the recommended skin care regimen. See Table 19-1 for energy parameters if utilizing TempSure or Pelleve.

**TABLE 19-1** DEPICTING SUGGESTED TREATMENT ENERGIES WITH THE TEMPSURE ENVI OR THE PELLEVE SYSTEM

| HANDPIECE SIZE (MM) | TREATMENT TYPE | RECOMMENDED ENERGY RANGE FOR TEMPSURE (MJ) | RECOMMENDED ENERGY RANGE FOR PELLEVE (MJ) |
|---|---|---|---|
| Small 10 | Eye and periorbital | 15–30 | N/A |
| 10 | Eye and periorbital | 15–35 | 8–15 |
| 15 | Forehead | 20–35 | 15–40 |
| 20 | Cheeks | 40–60 | 25–60 |

# PROCEDURE TECHNIQUE FOR EACH AREA

## Forehead

Figure eight movements are utilized to reach the target temperature. Continue heating and movements until the forehead has been treated for 5 minutes and the clinical endpoint of erythema has been reached. See Video 19-1.

## Periorbital Area

Utilize a pattern of a C, being mindful to move the applicator on the skin overlying the orbital rim. Continue moving the appropriate handpiece until the target temperature is reached and for the desired length of time, ideally 5 minutes. Give trouble spots like the lateral canthal rhytids appropriate attention. See Video 19-2. See Figure 19-2A and B for clinical endpoints.

## Midface

Treating the midface can help enhance how the periorbital area appears. Movements here should be done in a cross-hatch pattern as seen in Video 19-3. Continue moving the appropriate handpiece until the target temperature is reached and for the desired length of time, ideally 5 minutes.

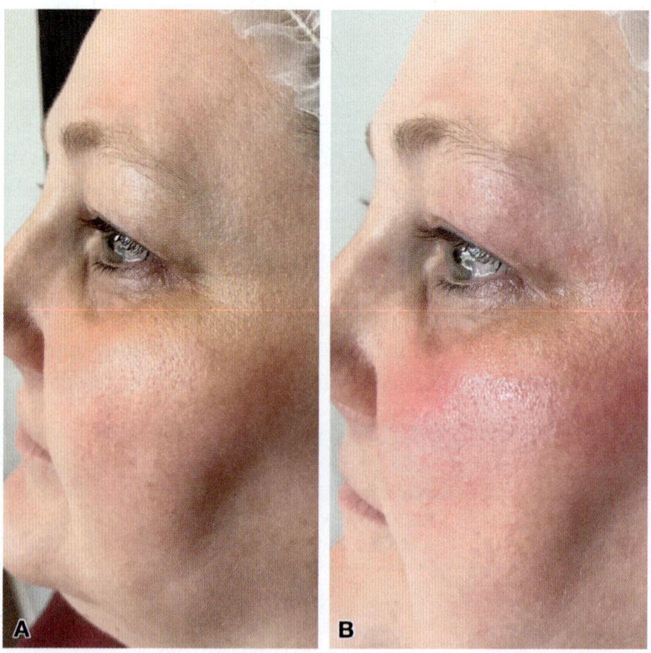


FIGURE 19-2 **A** and **B,** Showing appropriate clinical endpoint before (left) and after (right) radiofrequency (RF) treatment of the periorbital area.

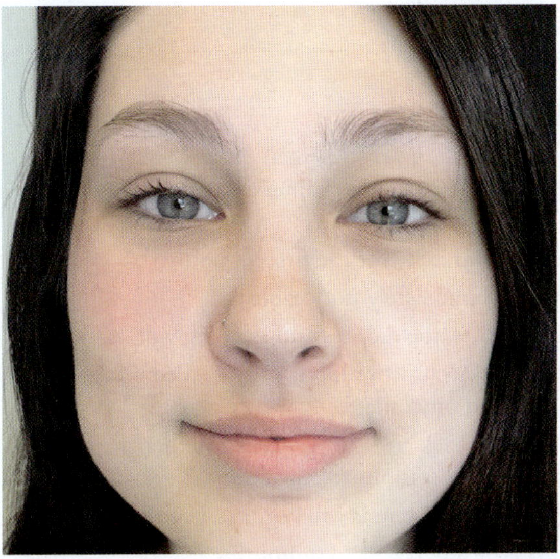

**FIGURE 19-3** Depicting treatment of the right side of the face with normal clinical endpoints of hyperemia and edema.

When performing the procedure for the first time on a patient, it can be helpful to perform the procedure on only the right side of the face as the immediate effect can be more appreciable relative to the untreated side of the face. See Figures 19-3 and 19-4.

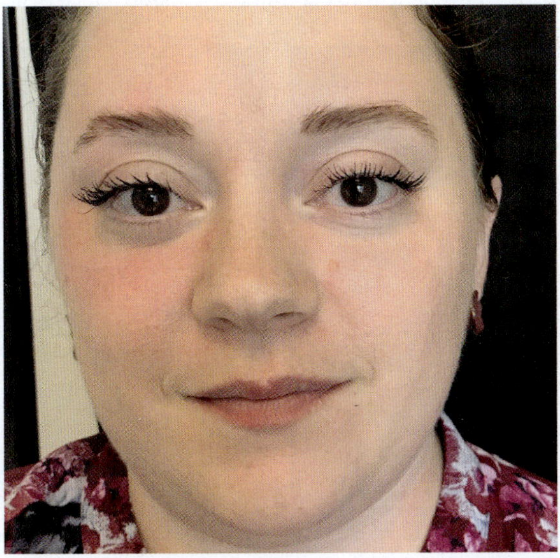

**FIGURE 19-4** Depicting treatment of the right side of the face with anticipated clinical endpoints of hyperemia and edema. Note the elevation of eyebrow and eyelid.

# POSTTREATMENT (FOLLOW-UP SCHEDULE)

## Key Postoperative Considerations

- Application of makeup and sunscreen is perfectly ok unless accompanied by microneedling in which case discontinue them until skin is healed which is typically 2 to 3 days.
- Skin may feel tight and itchy for the first 48 hours.
- Treatment effect is immediately noticeable.
- Over the next 48 hours, the redness and swelling will reduce.
- Posttreatment photo documentation is only needed after the first treatment to show the patient the desired outcome.
- Schedule the patient back in 2 to 4 weeks for their treatment session series. Most patients will need 2 to 4 sessions to reach desired results.
- Neocollagenesis and elastogenesis will begin and continue over the next 3 to 6 months.
- The full benefits typically take 3 to 6 months.

Patients will need a series of treatments to realize the full benefits. Clear expectations are important to document and discuss with the patient for the best results. Once the treatments have been executed, reassess the patient in 3 to 4 months after the last treatment session. Photography is critical to show the patient their improvements at the 3- to 4-month follow-up. One maintenance treatment ideally is done every 6 months to maintain and continue neocollagenesis and elastogenesis. See Figure 19-5A and B for before and after photos of a patient that had four treatments of RF 4 weeks apart. This patient has continued a maintenance treatment every 6 months.

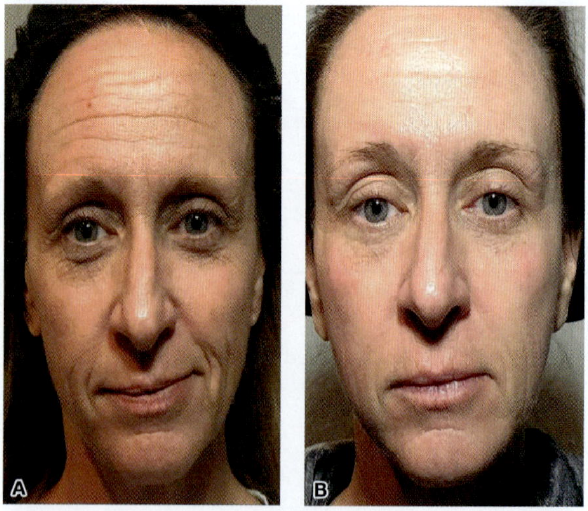


**FIGURE 19-5** **A** and **B,** Showing pretreatment of periorbital rhytids (left) and after four treatments each separated by 4 weeks apart with the TempSure Envi (right).

# POTENTIAL COMPLICATIONS AND THEIR TREATMENT

**Key Potential Complications to Look for:**

- Overtreatment

Overtreatment would potentially look like a burn and fortunately is extremely rare as the patient would not be able to tolerate the heat unless for some reason the patient had reduced sensation. When used on the appropriate patient and with the manufacturer device guidelines, the rate of complications is extremely low. There are currently no documented cases in the literature of periorbital complications.

## VIDEOS OF PROCEDURES

- **Video 19-1**—Demonstrating the pattern of treating the forehead.
- **Video 19-2**—Demonstrating the pattern and treatment of the periorbital region.
- **Video 19-3**—Demonstrating the pattern and treatment of the midface and periorbital region.

# EFFICACY

RF is a relatively safe and noninvasive or minimally invasive way to tighten skin, reducing the appearance of fine lines and wrinkles. Currently, efficacy rates are patient dependent. The multifactorial nature and unique rhytids along with the loss of collagen/elastin from patient to patient make it difficult to establish an exact rate of improvement.

Patients and practitioners typically report a high satisfaction rate with the technology. Eye care providers may be able to help patients with their appearance as well as delay more invasive or surgical procedures depending on the desired outcome. Utilization rates of RF continue to increase year over year as patients desire options that are effective with little to no downtime. Careful knowledge of the technology will ensure proper expectations of the outcomes with RF.

# CODING/BILLING AND MODIFIERS

Currently, there is no CPT code for this procedure.

# REFERENCES

1. Bonjorno AR, Gomes TB, Pereira MC, et al. Radiofrequency therapy in esthetic dermatology: a review of clinical evidences. *J Cosmet Dermatol.* 2020;19(2):278-281. doi:10.1111/jocd.13206
2. Garg S, Vashisht KR, Sushruth PR, Saka DV. Monopolar radiofrequency for reposing drooping fat planes and facial rejuvenation: a prospective study on 30 subjects towards true antiaging. *J Cosmet Dermatol.* 2022;21(4):1489-1500. doi:10.1111/jocd.14255

3. Araújo AR, Soares VP, Silva FS, Moreira Tda S. Radiofrequency for the treatment of skin laxity: myth or truth. *An Bras Dermatol.* 2015;90(5):707-721. doi:10.1590/abd1806-4841.20153605
4. Kołodziejczak A, Rotsztejn H. Efficacy of fractional laser, radiofrequency and IPL rejuvenation of periorbital region. *Lasers Med Sci.* 2022;37(2):895-903. doi:10.1007/s10103-021-03329-7
5. Kruglikov IL. Assessment of mechanical stress induced by radiofrequency currents on skin interfaces. *Biomed Res Int.* 2021;2021:6623757. doi:10.1155/2021/6623757
6. Krueger N, Levy H, Sadick NS. Safety and efficacy of a new device combining radiofrequency and low frequency pulsed electromagnetic fields for the treatment of facial rhytides. *J Drugs Dermatol.* 2012;11:1306-1309.
7. El-Domyati M, el-Ammawi TS, Medhat W, et al. Radiofrequency facial rejuvenation: evidence-based effect. *J Am Acad Dermatol.* 2011;64(3):524-535. doi:10.1016/j.jaad.2010.06.045
8. Carruthers J, Carruthers A. Shrinking upper and lower eyelid skin with a novel radiofrequency tip. *Dermatol Surg.* 2007;33(7):802-809. doi:10.1111/j.1524-4725.2007.33173.x
9. Biesman BS, Baker SS, Carruthers J, Silva HL, Holloman EL. Monopolar radiofrequency treatment of human eyelids: a prospective, multicenter, efficacy trial. *Lasers Surg Med.* 2006;38(10):890-898. doi:10.1002/lsm.20452
10. Taub AF, Tucker RD, Palange A. Facial tightening with an advanced 4-MHz monopolar radiofrequency device. *J Drugs Dermatol.* 2012;11(11):1288-1294.
11. Javate RM, Cruz RT Jr, Khan J, Trakos N, Gordon RE. Nonablative 4-MHz dual radiofrequency wand rejuvenation treatment for periorbital rhytides and midface laxity. *Ophthalmic Plast Reconstr Surg.* 2011;27(3):180-185. doi:10.1097/IOP.0b013e3181fe8e5a
12. Holtmann C, Finis D, Knop E, Borrelli M, Geerling G. Lateral canthal sling procedure for meibomian gland dysfunction? Results of a pilot study. *Curr Eye Res.* 2021;46(10):1489-1494. doi:10.1080/02713683.2021.1896741
13. Suh DH, Ahn HJ, Seo JK, Lee SJ, Shin MK, Song KY. Monopolar radiofrequency treatment for facial laxity: histometric analysis. *J Cosmet Dermatol.* 2020;19(9):2317-2324. doi:10.1111/jocd.13449
14. Pfenninger JL, Fowler GC. *Pfenninger and Fowler's Procedures for Primary Care.* 3rd ed. Elsevier; 2010.

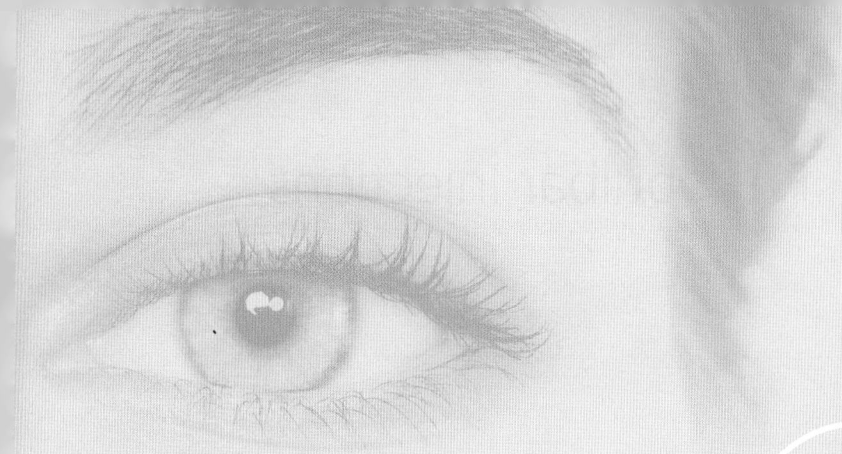

SECTION 4

# Periocular/Orbital Procedures

# 20 Retrobulbar Injections

**Leonid Skorin, Jr**

Management of severe chronic ocular pain in blind and seeing eyes can be an extremely discouraging and frustrating dilemma for the clinician and patient. This type of chronic pain is a complex phenomenon and often multifactorial in etiology. By definition, chronic pain lasts 3 months or longer. It can further be classified by its pathophysiology (Table 20-1). Nociceptive pain results from actual damage or potential tissue-damaging stimuli. The stimuli activate the specialized pain nerve endings known as nociceptors. Nociceptors exist at high levels in the eye and orbit. Nerve terminals originating in the eye, ocular adnexa, and face are connected to the root of the ophthalmic division of the trigeminal nerve (fifth cranial nerve).[1] The pain signal is sent from the eye through the trigeminal nerve to the brainstem nucleus and travels to the somatosensory areas of the brain. Tissue injury also causes the release of chemicals that sensitize or activate the receptors. Neurons then release substance P that stimulates mast cells and blood vessels. The histamine released from the mast cells and bradykinin released from the blood vessels add to the pain stimulus.

Neuropathic pain results from either actual nerve damage or inadequately treated nociceptive pain. There is an abnormal response to the stimulus caused by maladaptive neuronal signals. Neuropathic pain is complex and may be continuous or episodic. Psychogenic pain is physical pain that results from underlying mental, emotional, or behavioral factors.

Superficial ocular pain originates from the cornea or conjunctiva. This pain is usually localized and may be stabbing, burning, or sharp in nature. Blepharospasm and photophobia are often present. Local anesthetic eye drops and simple analgesics can relieve this pain.[2] Deep ocular pain can originate from superficial structures such as the cornea, sclera, iris, and ciliary body, or from lesions of the deep orbital structures and the adjacent sinuses.[2] This pain presents as blunt, dull, severe, occasionally lancinating or throbbing, and usually localized but may be referred.[2] Management of this type of pain is difficult. In patients with severe intractable pain, the underlying cause must be determined and treated. Pain management depends on the level of vision. It is of primary importance to not only preserve vision but also to alleviate pain

**TABLE 20-1 PAIN CLASSIFICATION BY PATHOPHYSIOLOGY**

| |
|---|
| Nociceptive—Triggered by noxious stimuli |
| Neuropathic—Nerves become dysfunctional. |
| Psychogenic—Mental, emotional, behavioral overlay |

where possible.[2] In those with severe intractable pain in a blind or near-blind eye, relief from pain is of primary importance and globe preservation secondary.[3]

Retrobulbar injections have been used to treat blind and painful eyes since the early 1900s, and their results were first published by Gruter.[4] In 1949, Maumenee used retrobulbar injections of alcohol in blind and partially sighted eyes.[5] In a study of 35 patients, he concluded that retrobulbar alcohol injections provided 1 to 3 months of pain relief. Since then, retrobulbar injections of chlorpromazine (Thorazine) and phenols have also been used. Chlorpromazine, first used by French physicians in 1951, was approved by the Food and Drug Administration in the United States in 1954 and has since become the archetypical antipsychotic.[6] It was first used for retrobulbar analgesia in the 1980s by Fiore et al and Bastrikov who reported 83% and 84% reduction in pain, respectively.[7-9] Retrobulbar phenol has also been tried in the management of pain, and the reported success rate is similar to that of alcohol injection.[10]

Therapeutic retrobulbar injection can be a safe alternative to surgery and a good option when medical therapy fails. In most cases, several methods of pain treatment are used in the same patient either concomitantly or sequentially.[2] Enucleation or evisceration is the definitive procedure for chronic and severe ocular pain. Because of psychological, cultural, religious, or aesthetic circumstances, many patients request other means than this surgery to control their pain. In many instances, the eye may look and move normally, compelling the patient to keep their eye.[11] Additionally, surgical procedures such as enucleation and evisceration carry their own risks of morbidity and mortality from anesthesia. Postoperative complications such as superior eyelid sulcus deformity, enophthalmos, socket contracture, restricted implant motility, and implant-associated infections or extrusion may also occur.[12-14] Medical treatment should be considered first in these patients; however, when the eye is disfigured or malignancy involves the globe, surgical treatment would be a better alternative.[14]

## INDICATIONS

### Key Indications

- Trauma
- Glaucoma—end stage (absolute) or neovascular
- Chronic retinal detachment
- Tumor—intraocular, intraorbital
- Cornea—ulcer, decompensation with bulla
- Phthisis bulbi
- Postoperative complications after ocular surgery

A myriad of conditions may lead to a chronically painful eye, the most common being previous trauma.[14] Additional causes include end-stage (absolute) glaucoma, neovascular glaucoma, chronic retinal detachment, intraocular tumor, intraorbital tumor, corneal ulcer, phthisis bulbi, corneal decompensation with bulla formation, healed perforated corneal ulcer with secondary endophthalmitis, intraorbital neuralgia, and postoperative complications after ocular surgery such as uveitis, endophthalmitis, and failed corneal grafts.[2,3,15] Eye pain constitutes a significant problem in patients suffering from the aforementioned conditions. The most common complaint is severe pain in the orbital area, which most frequently extends to the forehead and the temple.[16] Moreover, even though vision is already lost, photophobia usually accompanies the pain.[16]

Topical antiglaucomatous, cycloplegic, steroid agents and bandage contact lenses are the medical treatment alternatives for patients having severe superficial eye pain.[13] For deeper pain, a thorough fundus examination and testing are necessary in every case to rule out an occult intraocular tumor as a source of pain. B-scan ultrasonography, computed tomography, or magnetic resonance imaging should be performed if the fundus is not observable by standard methods.

## CONTRAINDICATIONS

### Key Contraindications

- Unable to successfully perform a retrobulbar injection
- Orbital cellulitis
- Malignancy—ocular, orbital

Retrobulbar injection had been a widely practiced technique providing orbital anesthesia for cataract and other orbital surgery.[2] More recently, the retrobulbar injection was being replaced by extraconal (peribulbar) and sub-Tenon's injections.[17,18] Currently, topical anesthesia has become a popular way to achieve corneal, cataract, and other anterior segment surgical anesthesia.[19]

Retrobulbar injections deposit the injected agent within the muscle cone (intraconal). Substances injected using the peribulbar (extraconal) or sub-Tenon's technique do diffuse into the intraconal area but also result in extensive tissue diffusion outside the muscle cone and may backtrack along the injection route.[2] This can result in additional untoward postinjection complications and less than optimal response to pain relief. Neurolytic agents (alcohol, chlorpromazine, and phenol) should not be injected through the peribulbar or sub-Tenon's routes.[2]

Neurolytic agents can only be used if it is possible to deposit the agent very close to the nerves.[2] Because the retrobulbar injection is performed within the muscle cone that is located within the orbit, any orbital infection would be a contraindication in performing the procedure.

Retrobulbar injection is also contraindicated in patients with active intraocular or intraorbital malignancy. This may be a relative contraindication in special circumstances such as a patient having severe intractable pain unresponsive to all other therapies, unable to endure enucleation or evisceration surgery, and has limited life expectancy. Kumar et al present one such unique case.[2]

# PREOPERATIVE PREPARATION

## Necessary Instrumentation

1. Ophthalmic topical anesthetic (e.g., tetracaine 0.5%, proparacaine 0.5%)
2. Lidocaine 1% or 2% with 1:100,000 epinephrine
3. Alcohol 50%, 70%, 95%, or 100% (absolute) concentration
4. Chlorpromazine 25 or 40 mg/mL
5. Disposable retrobulbar Atkinson-style anesthesia needle—various gauges and lengths available. The most commonly used are 23 gauge × 1½ inch, 25 gauge × 1½ inch, 27 gauge × 1½ inch. The needles can be sharp tipped or blunt tipped. Blunt-tipped needles are more often used for these procedures.
6. Two 3-mL syringes
7. 4 × 4 surgical gauze pads
8. Sterile fenestrated surgical drape
9. Povidone–iodine 5% ophthalmic topical
10. Povidone–iodine 10% swabs for cleaning eyelid and surrounding area
11. Hemostatic mosquito forceps—curved or straight

The methods and instruments needed for retrobulbar injection of alcohol and chlorpromazine are essentially the same. The choice of chemical agent depends on its availability and clinician preference.[2] Alcohol is used in patients whose eyes are completely blind or have no usable vision. After administration of retrobulbar alcohol, any remaining vision is lost. Chlorpromazine can be used in blind and seeing eyes. The results in seeing eyes are promising. In one study, half the seeing eyes treated retained their vision.[9] In another study of five seeing eyes that were treated, vision decreased in two, remained the same in two, and improved in one eye.[20] The improvement was not directly due to the injection of chlorpromazine but can be attributed to subsequent surgeries.[20]

# PROCEDURE

### Key Procedural Considerations

- Patient placed in a supine position
- Topical ophthalmic anesthetic and povidone–iodine 5% applied to the lower cul-de-sac
- Eyelids and periorbital area prepped with povidone–iodine 10%
- Sterile fenestrated drape positioned
- Patient maintains globe in primary position.
- Retrobulbar needle (needle bevel pointing toward the eye) on a 3-mL syringe that contains lidocaine is inserted through the skin at the lateral one-third of the lower lid.

- Retrobulbar needle is advanced parallel to the orbital floor until the needle tip reaches past the globe equator and then it is directed superiorly and medially toward the orbital apex, entering the intraconal space.
- Retract syringe plunger and observe for any blood flashback. If no blood is seen, inject 2 mL of lidocaine slowly into intraconal space.
- Stabilize the needle base and remove the empty 3-mL syringe.
- Wait 2 to 10 minutes for the anesthetic effect.
- Secure the needle base again and place the second 3-mL syringe that contains either alcohol or chlorpromazine, while maintaining the needle in the muscle cone.
- Inject 2 mL of alcohol or chlorpromazine slowly into intraconal space.
- Remove the syringe and needle complex.
- Apply gentle digital pressure with 4 × 4 gauze pads for 30 to 60 seconds.

The administration of therapeutic retrobulbar injection can be done in a clinical office setting or, if the patient is highly anxious, the procedure can be done in a surgical suite under intravenous sedation.

The patient is placed in a supine position, and one drop of topical ophthalmic anesthetic and topical ophthalmic povidone–iodine 5% are applied to the lower cul-de-sac of the treatment eye. The eyelid skin and surrounding area are prepped with povidone–iodine 10%. A sterile fenestrated drape is placed over the patient's face. Ask the patient to look straight up at the ceiling. This positions the globe in primary gaze. The clinician palpates and verifies the space between the globe and the inferolateral orbital rim.[19] The retrobulbar needle, which is attached to a 3-mL syringe that contains lidocaine, is to be inserted through the skin of the lower eyelid at the lateral one-third of the lower lid, just above the inferior rim of the orbit. Prior to insertion of the retrobulbar needle, the clinician may want to gently displace the globe a few millimeters away from the lower orbital rim. This gives more clearance for the retrobulbar needle as it enters the orbital space. The needle bevel should be pointing toward the eye.[19]

Prior to the procedure, two separate 3-mL syringes should be available. The first is filled with 2 mL of lidocaine 1% or 2% with 1:100,000 epinephrine. The second is filled with 2 mL of either alcohol or chlorpromazine.

Retrobulbar injection of alcohol provides analgesia by the destruction of nerve cells.[3] This occurs by extracting phospholipids, cholesterol, and cerebroside and also precipitating mucoprotein and lipoprotein.[2] All the effect is localized to the orbit. The most commonly used alcohol concentration is absolute (100%) ethyl alcohol, but 95% ethyl alcohol has also been used in some studies.[2,15,16] The total volume of these two concentrations to be injected is usually 2 mL.[2,15,16] Another option is to inject 4 mL of 70% alcohol.[5] Retrobulbar injection of alcohol can also be used to alleviate pain and photophobia in seeing eyes. This technique can be used in patients with painful glaucoma with a visual remnant, ciliary body pain in aphakia, or photophobia and blepharospasm after corneal surgery.[21] After the standard retrobulbar injection of anesthetic, 2 mL of 50% ethyl alcohol solution is injected through the same needle. This does not damage the optic nerve.[21]

Retrobulbar chlorpromazine injection is another highly effective treatment for ocular pain and has additional benefits beyond those of alcohol. Although its method of pain control is not well understood, chlorpromazine will cause cell lysis in high concentrations, leading to irreversible changes in the ciliary ganglion and may have an additional membrane-stabilizing effect on the ciliary ganglion.[8,20] Chen et al reported that retrobulbar chlorpromazine injection was found to be a safe and effective form of analgesia when other medications failed and surgery was undesirable.[9] When compared to alcohol, chlorpromazine appears to be more efficacious, has a longer duration of action, and may reduce intraocular pressure.[6-9] There is one study that did not note any significant difference between preinjection and postinjection intraocular pressure with chlorpromazine use.[20]

Chlorpromazine comes in both 25 and 40 mg/mL dosages. Because systemic absorption of this drug may occur after a retrobulbar injection, the 25 mg/mL concentration is recommended.[9,20] Chlorpromazine can be used in both blind and seeing eyes.[9,20] For a comparison of both alcohol and chlorpromazine, see Table 20-2.

The retrobulbar needle is placed on the first 3-mL syringe that is filled with 2 mL of lidocaine. The needle is directed parallel to the orbital floor until the tip reaches the equator of the globe (≈15 mm of needle advancement based on normal axial length).[19] Typically, a "first pop" is felt as the needle passes through the anterior orbital septum.[19] When it is felt that the needle has passed the equator of the globe, the needle is directed superiorly and medially, toward the orbital apex to a distance of 2 cm.[2,19] At this point, a "second pop" is usually felt as the muscle cone is penetrated and the needle enters the intraconal space. Once the intraconal space has been reached, further needle advancement should be stopped.[22] The needle should not be permitted to cross the midsagittal plane of the eye as this increases the risk of optic nerve penetration. Total needle advancement is approximately 25 to 35 mm based on the size of the orbit.[19] In most patients, the needle is too short to reach and penetrate the optic nerve. Prior to injection of the lidocaine, the piston of the 3-mL syringe is retracted partially to confirm that there is no flashback of blood.[16] This prevents the inadvertent injection into a blood vessel or into the subdural space.[16,19]

Two mL of lidocaine can now be injected slowly into the intraconal space (Figure 20-1). An injection of local anesthetic (lidocaine) is necessary prior to the injection of alcohol or chlorpromazine because these agents may produce significant burning pain and discomfort.[23,24] After the first injection is completed, the clinician should secure the base of the retrobulbar needle between their fingers or a hemostatic mosquito forceps. The empty 3-mL syringe can now be removed from the needle while the needle remains in position and

**TABLE 20-2 ASSESSMENT OF RETROBULBAR-INJECTED PHARMACEUTICALS**

| AGENT | DOSE (ML) | CONCENTRATION | DURATION | EFFECT ON INTRAOCULAR PRESSURE | CLINICAL USE |
|---|---|---|---|---|---|
| Alcohol | 2 | 50%, 70%, 95%, 100% | 1–7 mo | No significant effect | Blind eyes |
| Chlorpromazine | 2 | 25 mg/mL, 40 mg/mL | 3 mo to 1 yr | Possible reduction | Blind and seeing eyes |

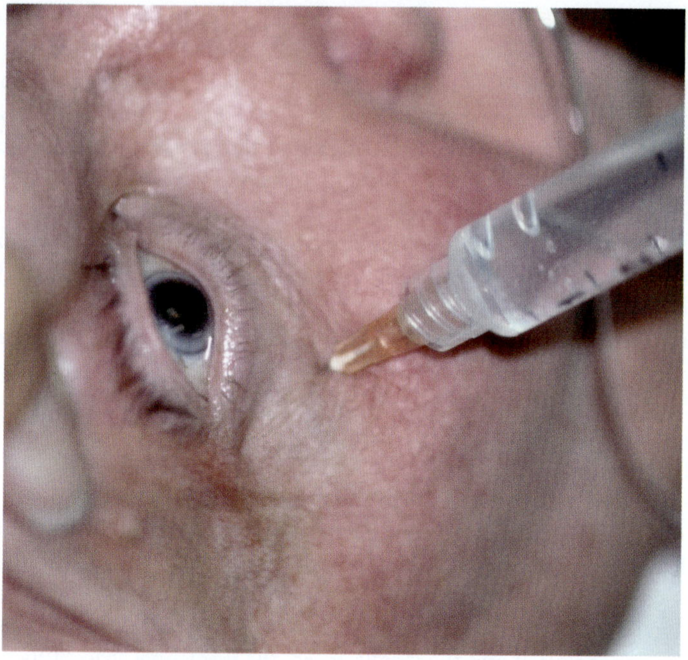

FIGURE 20-1 Needle position in the retrobulbar space (muscle cone) during lidocaine injection and before alcohol injection.

within the intraconal space. The clinician should wait between 2 and 10 minutes for anesthetic effect to result. The second 3-mL syringe with either 2 mL of alcohol or chlorpromazine is now placed onto the retrobulbar needle while the clinician secures the base of the needle with their fingers or the hemostatic mosquito forceps. This prevents the retrobulbar needle from being displaced out of the muscle cone. The 2 mL of alcohol or chlorpromazine is then injected slowly into the intraconal space. The complete syringe and needle complex is then removed from the orbit. Gentle digital pressure with the eyelids closed is applied utilizing a $4 \times 4$ gauze pad for 30 to 60 seconds. This should reduce anterior diffusion of the alcohol or chlorpromazine.[2] A pressure patch can be applied if there is any significant globe proptosis after the procedure.

## POSTOPERATIVE CARE/COMANAGEMENT (FOLLOW-UP SCHEDULE)

### Key Postoperative Considerations

- Continue usual pain medication.
- Recheck in 1 day and 1 week.

Patients are instructed to continue their usual pain medications. Pain relief from the retrobulbar injection can be immediate or can develop more slowly over about 1 week. The patient should return for follow-up in 1 day and 1 week. The eyelids, globe, and orbital area should be assessed for any postoperative complications. Intraocular pressure should be measured.

# POTENTIAL COMPLICATIONS AND THEIR TREATMENT

## Key Potential Complications

- Retrobulbar hemorrhage
- Blepharoptosis
- External ophthalmoplegia
- Eyelid edema and conjunctival chemosis
- Cellulitis
- Corneal epithelial defect
- Loss of consciousness

The most common intraoperative complication is a retrobulbar hemorrhage.[22] This occurs because the retrobulbar injection is a blind stick of a needle behind the eye. If this occurs, the globe becomes progressively proptotic and subconjunctival blood might become evident as the hemorrhage extends anteriorly.[22] It might not be visible, however, until the first postoperative day. Bleeding in a closed space increases orbital pressure and limits further hemorrhage; but, intraocular pressure is elevated and the completion of the procedure must be postponed.[22] No treatment of a retrobulbar hemorrhage is indicated if the eye is blind, as the blood absorbs in a few days. If a retrobulbar hemorrhage occurs in a seeing eye and vision is to be preserved, then the patient should be started on topical intraocular pressure–lowering medications and mannitol (0.5–1.0 g/kg). Intermittent pressure (45 seconds on, 15 seconds off) using one's palm should be applied to the patient's globe as a means of decompression. If conservative medical therapy fails to lower the intraocular pressure, then a lateral canthotomy, and if necessary, a cantholysis of the inferior portion of the lateral canthal tendon should be performed.[25] A retrobulbar hemorrhage can also cause blepharoptosis and external ophthalmoplegia.[3] Recovery from the ptosis and ophthalmoplegia, which can accompany a retrobulbar hemorrhage, usually occurs within 24 hours.[11,24]

Other complications of retrobulbar alcohol injection include blepharoptosis and external ophthalmoplegia with motor nerve infiltration as they enter the orbit through the superior orbital fissure[5,11]; eyelid edema and conjunctival chemosis secondary to tissue reaction[16]; cellulitis[11,15,24]; neurotrophic keratopathy[11,15,24]; and corneal epithelial defect.[11] Some of these complications are more serious than others, but most seem to subside within 12 weeks and leave no lasting effects.[3,24]

Complications reported with chlorpromazine injections include eyelid edema (Figure 20-2) and conjunctival chemosis9,20; sterile orbital cellulitis26; fat necrosis26; blepharoptosis7,9,20; phthisis bulbi7,9,20; external ophthalmoplegia7,9,20; hyphema with nausea

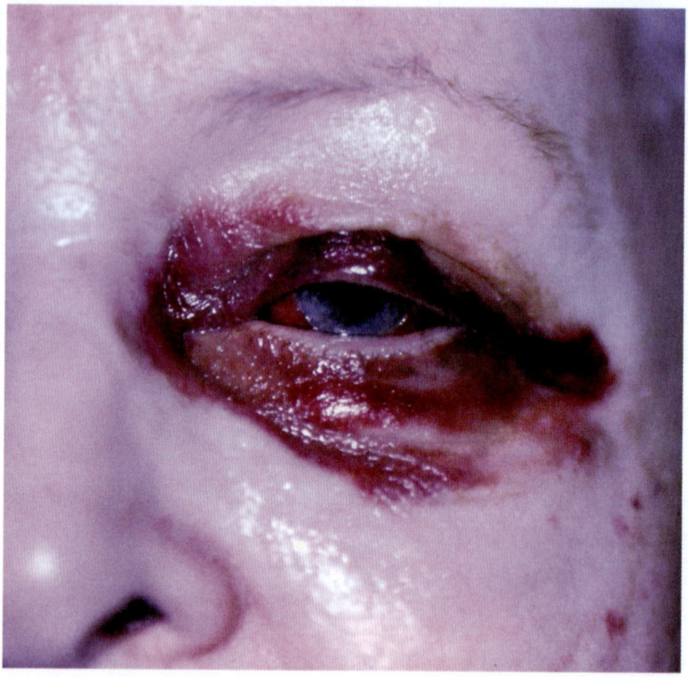

**FIGURE 20-2** Eyelid edema 1 day after retrobulbar chlorpromazine injection. Note that there is also periorbital ecchymosis and a subconjunctival hemorrhage in this patient who is on the blood thinner, warfarin.

and vomiting7,9,20; elevated intraocular pressure7,27; and brief loss of consciousness.[9,20] Because systemic absorption of this drug may occur after a retrobulbar injection resulting in loss of consciousness, the 25 mg/mL concentration instead of the 40 mg/mL concentration is recommended.[9,20] Transient loss of vision may occur, and this is presumably due to the membrane-stabilizing effect of the drug on the optic nerve.[9,20] Most of these complications are transient. In previous studies, only one case was reported as having permanent ptosis and a third nerve stroke.[7]

Retrobulbar injection of any medication carries some general inherent risks. These rare but severe complications (1%–3% risk for each) include retrobulbar hemorrhage (as discussed earlier), optic nerve injury, retinal artery/vein occlusion, globe perforation, oculocardiac reflex, ocular muscle injury, prolonged ptosis, and central nervous system depression.[19]

## VIDEO OF PROCEDURE

**Video 20.1**—Retrobulbar chlorpromazine injection. Retrobulbar injection of 2 mL of lidocaine 1% with 1:100,000 epinephrine using a 3-mL syringe followed by 2 mL of chlorpromazine 25 mg/mL (total 50 mg) using a 3-mL syringe. (Video courtesy of Leonid Skorin, Jr, and Griffin Christenson.)

## EFFICACY

The success of retrobulbar alcohol injections has varied in many studies. Maumenee reported analgesia in only 20% of patients whereas Olurin et al reported a much more significant efficacy of 87%, both over a 3-month period.[5,11] A more recent study by Bhatia et al found that at 1 week after retrobulbar injection of 2 mL of absolute alcohol, 85.7% of patients were pain-free and did not require any additional supportive analgesics.[15] The Bhatia et al study had one patient who had a perforated healed corneal ulcer with secondary endophthalmitis that did not have an adequate initial response.[15] This patient was given a second injection of absolute alcohol after 1 month; but, this second injection did not bring the patient any significant pain relief.[15] The patient ultimately underwent evisceration.[15] Another recent study by Salkaci et al found that 35% of patients who had blind painful eyes due to late-stage neovascular glaucoma had to undergo multiple reinjections of 95% ethyl alcohol in the retrobulbar area because of having therapy-resistant pain.[16] Despite reinjection, 57% still continued to have significant pain and 20% eventually underwent evisceration.[16]

The length of duration for pain relief after retrobulbar alcohol injection also varies, ranging from 2 weeks to 2 years, with an average of 1 to 7 months.[3,9]

It appears that using chlorpromazine 25 mg/mL instead of alcohol is more effective.[7,28] Chlorpromazine efficacy varies from 80% to 90%, lasts 3 months to 1 year, and has the added bonus of sight preservation in more than 50% of seeing eyes.[6-9,20]

## CODING/BILLING

- **CPT code: 67500**—Retrobulbar injection, medication (separate procedure, does not include supply of medication)
- J code for reimbursement of product and is billed by the site of care (office, hospital, ambulatory surgical center, etc.): J3230: billed as 1 unit for every 25 mg/mL of chlorpromazine
- **CPT code: 67505**—Retrobulbar injection of alcohol

Common ICD-10 codes that support this procedure include the following:

- **H57.10** (ocular pain, unspecified eye)
- **S05.9** (unspecified injury to eye and orbit)
- **H40.30X3** (glaucoma secondary to eye trauma, unspecified eye, severe stage)
- **H44.519** (absolute glaucoma)
- **H40.89** (neovascular glaucoma)
- **H33.059** (old total retinal detachment)
- **Z85.840** (personal history of malignant neoplasm of eye)
- **C69.60** (malignant neoplasm of unspecified orbit)
- **H16.009** (unspecified corneal ulcer, unspecified eye)
- **H44.521** (atrophy of globe, right eye)
- **H44.522** (atrophy of globe, left eye)
- **H44.099** (unspecified purulent endophthalmitis, unspecified eye)

# REFERENCES


1. Bron AJ, Tripathi RC, Tripathi BJ. *Wolff's Anatomy of the Eye and Orbit*. 8th ed. Chapman & Hall Medical; 1997:191-205.
2. Kumar CM, Dowd TC, Hawthorne M. Retrobulbar alcohol injection for orbital pain relief under difficult circumstances: a case report. *Ann Acad Med Singap*. 2006;35:260-265.
3. Al-Faran MF, Al-Omar OM. Retrobulbar alcohol injection in blind painful eyes. *Ann Ophthalmol.* 1990;22(12):460-462.
4. Gruter W. Orbital injection of alcohol for the relief of pain in blind eyes. *Ber Dtsch Ophthalmol Ges*. 1918;1:85.
5. Maumenee AE. Retrobulbar alcohol injections: relief of ocular pain in eyes with and without vision. *Am J Ophthalmol.* 1949;32:1502-1508.
6. Scerra C. Chlorpromazine alleviates some eye pain better than alcohol. *Ophthalmol Times*. 1998;23(2):30.
7. Fiore C, Lupidi G, Santoni G. Effet de l'injection retrobulbaire de chlorpromazine dans le glaucoma absolu [Retrobulbar injection of chlorpromazine in the absolute glaucoma]. *J Fr Ophthalmol.* 1980;3:397-399.
8. Bastrikov NI. Symptomatic treatment of terminal painful glaucoma by the retrobulbar administration of aminazine. *Vestn Oftalmol.* 1989;105:47-49.
9. Chen TC, Ahn Yuen SJ, Sangalang MA, et al. Retrobulbar chlorpromazine injections for the management of blind and seeing painful eyes. *J Glaucoma.* 2002;11(3):209-213.
10. Birch M, Strong N, Brittain P, et al. Retrobulbar phenol injection in blind painful eyes. *Ann Ophthalmol.* 1993;25:267-270.
11. Olurin O, Osunthokun O. Complications of retrobulbar alcohol injections. *Ann Ophthalmol.* 1978;10:474-476.
12. Older JJ, Mack WP. Enucleation. In: Levine MR, ed. *Manual of Oculoplastic Surgery*. 4th ed. SLACK Incorporated; 2010:265-272.
13. Shah-Desai SD, Tyers AG, Manners RM. Painful blind eye: efficacy of enucleation and evisceration in resolving ocular pain. *Br J Ophthalmol.* 2000;84:437-438.
14. Custer PL, Reistad CE. Enucleation of blind, painful eyes. *Ophthal Plast Reconstr Surg.* 2000;16(5):326-329.
15. Bhatia J, Narayanadas B, Varghese M, et al. Retrobulbar alcohol injection: a forgotten therapy for management of painful blind eye. *Oman J Ophthalmol.* 2018;11(2):190-191.
16. Salkaci O, Ayyildiz T, Kandemir B, et al. Pain management by retrobulbar alcohol injection in blind painful eyes due to late-stage neovascular glaucoma. *South Clin Ist Euras.* 2017;28(1):17-21.
17. Hamilton RC, Gimbel HV, Strunin L. Regional anaesthesia for 12,000 cataract extraction and intraocular lens implantation procedures. *Can J Anaesth*. 1988;35:615-623.
18. Eke T, Thompson JR. Safety of local anaesthesia for cataract surgery; why we should look again. *Eye*. 2003;17:127-128.
19. Bernardino CR, ed. *The Yale Guide to Ophthalmic Surgery*. Wolters Kluwer; 2011:208-212.
20. Estafanous MF, Kaiser PK, Baerveldt G, Retrobulbar chlorpromazine in blind and seeing painful eyes. *Retina.* 2000;20(5):555-558.
21. Fechner PU, Teichmann KD. *Ocular Therapeutics: Pharmacology and Clinical Application*. SLACK Incorporated; 1998:221-222.
22. Wilson RP. Complications of ophthalmic anesthesia. In: Sherwood MB, Spaeth GL, eds. *Complications of Glaucoma Therapy*. SLACK Incorporated; 1990:133-158.
23. Maza CE. A safer technique for retrobulbar alcohol injections. *Ophthalmic Surg.* 1989;20:823.
24. May DR, May WN. Decreasing discomfort caused by retrobulbar alcohol injection. *Am J Ophthalmol.* 1983;95:262-263.
25. Bahadur GG, Sinskey RM. *Manual of Cataract Surgery*. 2nd ed. Butterworth Heinemann; 2000:13.
26. Margo CE, Wilson T. Orbital cellulitis after retrobulbar injection of chlorpromazine. *Arch Ophthalmol.* 1993;111(10):1322.
27. Indeikina GV. Retrobulbar injections of aminazine during cupping in acute attacks of terminal glaucoma. *Oftalmol Zh*. 1987;21:122-123.
28. Waltz KL, Williams GA, Goldey SH, et al. Alternative to retrobulbar ethanol for blind painful eyes. *Ophthalmology*. 1992;99(suppl):153.


# SUPPLEMENTAL READING


1. Rhen A, Skorin L. Severe pain requires equally severe measures. *Rev Optom.* 2004;141(6):109-112. https://www.reviewofoptometry.com/article/severe-pain-requires-equally-severe-measuresRetrobulbar Injections

# 21 Canthotomy and Cantholysis

**Richard E. Castillo**

Lateral canthotomy/cantholysis is a surgical procedure used to treat ocular emergencies that involve increased pressure within the orbit resulting in orbital compartment syndrome. The procedure involves making a series of small incisions at the lateral canthus of the eyelid (canthotomy followed by cantholysis) to lower an elevated intraorbital pressure, restore perfusion to the affected structures and tissues, and prevent permanent vision loss. Lateral canthotomy/cantholysis is typically performed by ophthalmologists, emergency physicians, or other health care professionals with experience in the procedure. The procedure can be a sight-saving intervention for patients experiencing severe orbital trauma or other eye-related emergencies.

## INDICATIONS

### Key Indications

- Orbital compartment syndrome
- Retrobulbar hemorrhage

The primary indication for emergent lateral canthotomy and cantholysis is orbital compartment syndrome or retrobulbar hemorrhage accompanied by an afferent pupillary defect, ophthalmoplegia, a cherry red macula, optic nerve pallor, optic nerve edema, or severe pain.[1-3] Acute orbital compartment syndrome (AOCS) is a true vision-threatening ophthalmic emergency. AOCS occurs when the intraorbital pressure exceeds the vascular perfusion pressure of the ophthalmic artery. Elevation of intraorbital pressure can result in ischemia, hypoxia, and irreversible vision loss if the elevated intraorbital pressure is not reversed quickly and tissue perfusion restored.[1-4]

Signs of AOCS include[2,3]:

- Proptosis
- Subconjunctival hemorrhage
- Conjunctival chemosis
- Ecchymosis of eyelid
- Resistance to retropulsion of the globe

- Elevated intraocular pressure (IOP)
- Decreased visual acuity
- Ophthalmoplegia
- Afferent pupillary defect
- Optic disc edema
- Central retinal artery pulsation

AOCS is most often seen after trauma; however, there are other less common etiologies that can produce an elevated orbital pressure capable of causing permanent ischemic damage[2-4]:

- Retrobulbar hemorrhage
- Peribulbar or retrobulbar injection
- Orbital infection (with or without abscess)
- Orbital emphysema
- Foreign bodies
- Anatomic anomalies
- Positional edema
- Spontaneous hemorrhage (e.g., Valsalva related)
- Fluid resuscitation (especially after burn injuries)

Because the orbit is a bony cone, rising intraorbital pressure will cause the globe to shift forward along the anterior–posterior axis and become proptotic. However, at the limit of its travel along the anterior–posterior axis, the globe will be constrained by the medial and lateral canthal ligaments and their attachments to the superior and inferior tarsi, limiting the range of its anterior movement.[3] The intraorbital pressure may then rise precipitously. Releasing the lateral canthal ligament via the canthotomy/cantholysis procedure will functionally expand the volume of the orbit by removing the anterior constraints on the globe, thus lowering the intraorbital pressure and ideally restoring perfusion to the intraorbital contents.[4-6]

## CONTRAINDICATIONS

As a vision-saving and organ-salvage procedure, there are few, if any, absolute contraindications to performing an emergent canthotomy in the setting of orbital compartment syndrome, especially within the context of facial trauma.

Relative contraindications include[4,5]:

- Lack of patient consent
- Inexperienced practitioner
- Conditions mimicking AOCS and retrobulbar hemorrhage
  - Thyroid orbitopathy
  - Idiopathic orbital inflammatory syndrome
  - Space-occupying lesions of the orbit
- A ruptured globe would also be a relative contraindication

# PREOPERATIVE PREPARATION

- Signed (or verbal) informed consent is obtained where possible.
- Preoperative note is documented and includes:
  - Diagnosis is confirmed (e.g., *orbital compartment syndrome secondary to retrobulbar hemorrhage*), including operative site.
  - Allergies and current medications are documented.
  - Proposed procedure: *lateral canthotomy with cantholysis [state eye]*
  - Anesthesia given is documented (e.g., *lateral infiltrative block was administered via subcutaneous injection of 2 mL of lidocaine 2% with epinephrine 1:100,000 along the lateral orbital rim*).
- Operative site is marked and prepared in standard fashion with povidone–iodine (or alternative in the case of iodine allergy).
- A "time-out" is called prior to starting procedure whereby patient identification, diagnosis, procedure, and operative site are confirmed by all present.

## Instrument Tray

- Small (mosquito) straight hemostatic forceps
- Blunt-tipped Wescott-style scissors (or any small tissue scissors may suffice)
- 0.3-mm tissue forceps (or any heavy-toothed forceps may suffice)
- 1% or 2% lidocaine with epinephrine 1:100,000 (unless contraindicated). Otherwise, 1% or 2% lidocaine without epinephrine
- 3-mL syringe for anesthetic
- 27 gauge × 1½ needle
- Sterile gauze 4 × 4
- Sterile saline (0.9%)
- Surgical drapes
- Skin prep (povidone–iodine or substitute)
- Sterile gloves
- Wound dressing material

# PROCEDURE

## Lateral Canthotomy and Cantholysis

The lateral palpebral ligament (*Ligamentum palpebrae laterale*), sometimes referred to as the lateral canthal tendon, passes from the lateral edges of the superior and inferior tarsal plates to the marginal (Whitnall's) tubercle on the zygomatic bone along the lateral orbital margin (Figure 21-1).

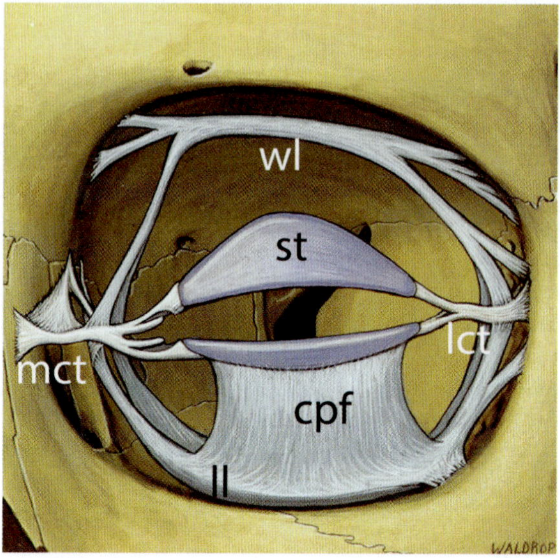


**FIGURE 21-1** Anatomy of the lateral canthal tendon (lct) and its attachments. The lateral canthal tendon, sometimes referred to as the lateral canthal ligament (ligamentum palpebrae laterale), passes from the lateral edges of the superior and inferior tarsal plates to the marginal (Whitnall's) tubercle on the zygomatic bone along the lateral orbital margin. Whitnall's ligament (wl) is observed superior to the superior tarsus (st). The medial canthal tendon (mct; medial palpebral ligament) is depicted here as well, along with the capsulopalpebral fascia (cpf) below the inferior tarsal plate. (Reprinted with permission from Dutton J, Proia A, Tawfik H. *Comprehensive Textbook of Eyelid Disorders and Diseases*. Wolters Kluwer; 2023:23; Figure 3.12.)

## SURGICAL STEPS[2,6-8]

Step 1: Confirm diagnosis and obtain informed consent (where possible).

Step 2: Administer local anesthesia via a lateral block (infiltration of the tissue along the zygomatic arch). Then, infiltrate the lateral one-third of the lower eyelid. Always aim the needle tip away from the globe.

**Note: In the setting of trauma, tissue edema, and tissue hypoxia, local anesthesia may not be very effective.**

Step 3: Utilizing a small (mosquito) straight hemostatic forceps, open the jaws and insert the lower jaw into the lateral canthus in the space between the eyelid and the globe, directing the tip of the instrument toward the lateral orbital rim, until you come to a natural stop at the bone of orbital rim. Clamp and lock the hemostatic forceps for 3 minutes. This will achieve crush hemostasis of the soft tissue and provide a track to follow for the next step.[8-10]

Step 4: Perform the lateral canthotomy—using a blunt-tipped Westcott-style scissors, incise full-thickness along the hemostat track you just created in Step 3 (Figure 21-2). Carry the incision to the orbital rim.

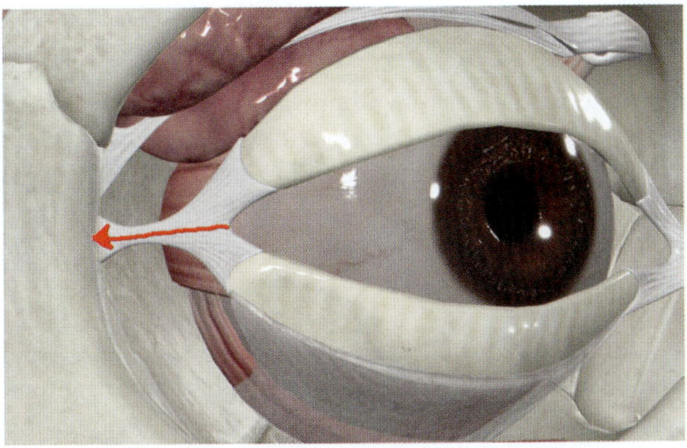

**FIGURE 21-2** Using a small scissors cut along the crimped track created by the hemostatic forceps (along the red arrow) from the lateral canthus up to the boney lateral tubercle (orbital rim), splitting the sideways "Y"-shaped ligament and transforming it from a "Y" into a "V."

Step 5: Perform the cantholysis[2,6-8,10,13,14]

5a: Grasp the lower lid with tissue forceps and pull up, holding the lower lid under tension.

5b: Insert the lower jaw of a small open tissue scissors into the space between the back of the eyelid and the globe, pressing the tip of the lower jaw of your scissors against the lateral orbital rim (the same location in which you had previously placed the hemostatic forceps, ideally, up against Whitnall's tubercle, Figure 21-1). You will come to a natural stop at the orbital rim, with the inner blade touching the orbital rim and the outer blade on the outside of the eyelid.

5c: Maintaining the point of contact between the inner tip of the blade and the lateral orbital rim, rotate the entire scissors along an inferior-medial arc such that the tip of the outer blade is pointed toward the ipsilateral outer corner of the mouth.

**IMPORTANT: Maintain the inner blade pressed up against the lateral orbital rim, while maintaining the lower lid on upward traction with your forceps.**

5d: Again, with the lower lid under traction, perform a full-thickness incision (in the direction of the ipsilateral outer corner of the mouth) with the scissors. Extend the incision up to the inferior orbital rim. When performed correctly, you will feel a pop in the hand that is holding the lower lid when you transect the lower arm of the lateral canthal ligament that you split during the preceding canthotomy procedure.

**Note: You should be cutting through the inside margin of the canthotomy incision as you advance toward the lower orbital rim. You should not be cutting through the actual lower lid margin itself.**

**5e:** Verify that the procedure has been successfully completed, by assessing the eye with digital pressure (or a portable tonometer if available). The eye that was once firm should now be soft and amenable to retropulsion. **DO NOT perform if there is a possibility of a ruptured globe.**

Note: It is the cantholysis and not the canthotomy that relieves the intraorbital pressure. The canthotomy allows one to preserve the integrity of the lower eyelid margin by enabling the cantholysis procedure without cutting through the eyelid margin.

## POSTOPERATIVE CARE (FOLLOW-UP SCHEDULE)

- A successful procedure is confirmed by improved visual acuity, resolution of a previously detected afferent pupillary defect, and decrease in IOP to below 40 mm Hg.[11,13,14]
- Note that proptosis and extraocular motion testing are less reliable indicators of procedure success.[14]
- Do not attempt to reconstruct the canthus until further assessment confirms resolution of the ocular compartment syndrome and the IOP is noted to be stable within the normal range.[10]
- Hemostasis should be achieved with direct pressure to the wound or with minimal cautery.
- A dressing should be applied to the wound along with appropriate topical antibiotic, and the wound should be gently cleaned (irrigated with sterile saline), the dressing changed, and antibiotic ointment reapplied daily.
- Imaging (e.g., a computed tomography scan of the orbit) is advisable when available to confirm and monitor the amount of blood in the orbit.[9,11-13]
- At a minimum, visual acuity, ocular motility, pupillary reflexes, some measure of IOP, and an evaluation of the optic nerve head should be documented if a comprehensive ocular examination is not practical immediately following the procedure.
- A comprehensive ocular exam should be performed at the first opportunity.
- Follow-up examinations should be scheduled based on the patient's progress.
- Reconstruction may be considered once the patient is stable.

## POTENTIAL COMPLICATIONS[2,5,7-9,11,14]

- Failure of the lateral canthotomy/cantholysis to bring the intraorbital pressure down must be recognized and addressed expeditiously if salvageable vision is to be retained.
  - If the inferior cantholysis does not bring about the proper release, then a superior cantholysis may be attempted.
  - Emergent transfer to a facility for orbital decompression surgery would be warranted if the situation is not reversed and stabilized via the canthotomy/cantholysis procedure.
- Iatrogenic injury to the globe during the procedure
- Ptosis secondary to iatrogenic damage to the levator if a superior cantholysis is attempted
- Damage to the lacrimal gland and lacrimal artery if a superior cantholysis is attempted
- Ectropion if extensive dissection is performed during the inferior cantholysis
- Bleeding and hematoma formation secondary to surgical manipulation
- Infection

## VIDEO OF PROCEDURE

**Video 21-1**—Lateral canthotomy/cantholysis demonstration on a model being performed on the left eye.

## EFFICACY

In a study performed by Yung et al to determine which procedure, canthotomy, canthal tendon disinsertion, or cantholysis produced the largest reduction in IOP after simulated orbital hemorrhage, canthotomy alone yielded a mean IOP reduction of 14.2 mm Hg, lateral canthal tendon disinsertion alone yielded a mean IOP reduction of 19.2 mm Hg, whereas cantholysis yielded a mean IOP reduction of 30.4 mm Hg.[15] There was a statistically ($p < 0.05$) greater reduction in IOP with cantholysis than that produced by canthotomy or canthal tendon disinsertion alone.[15] The study concluded that cantholysis in acute orbital hemorrhage may produce significantly greater reduction in IOP, and thus in intraorbital pressure, allowing for better perfusion of orbital tissues than either lateral canthotomy or canthal tendon disinsertion.[15]

## CODING AND BILLING

- **CPT code: 67715**—Canthotomy
  Common ICD-10 codes that support this procedure include the following:
- **T79A9XA**—Traumatic compartment syndrome other sites, initial encounter
- **T79A0XA**—Compartment syndrome, unspecified, initial encounter
- **H05.23**—Hemorrhage of orbit
- **H05.231**—Hemorrhage of right orbit
- **H05.232**—Hemorrhage of left orbit
- **H05.233**—Hemorrhage of bilateral orbit

## REFERENCES

1. Murali S, Davis C, McCrea MJ, Plewa MC. Orbital compartment syndrome: pearls and pitfalls for the emergency physician. *J Am Coll Emerg Physicians Open*. 2021;2(2):e12372.
2. Lim CS, Malick H, Berry-Brincat A. Emergency canthotomy and cantholysis—factors affecting confidence among ophthalmic trainees in the United Kingdom. *Ind J Ophthalmol*. 2021;69(9):2385-2388.
3. Haubner F, Jägle H, Nunes DP, et al. Orbital compartment: effects of emergent canthotomy and cantholysis. *Eur Arch Otorhino*. 2015;272(2):479-483.
4. Kitaguchi Y, Takahashi Y, Sabundayo MS, Kakizaki H. Bony orbital decompression following lateral canthotomy and cantholysis for traumatic orbital compartment syndrome. *J Craniofac Surg*. 2019;30(1):231-234.
5. Oester AE Jr, Fowler BT, Fleming JC. Inferior orbital septum release compared with lateral canthotomy and cantholysis in the management of orbital compartment syndrome. *Ophthalmic Plast Reconstruct Surg*. 2012;28(1):40-43.
6. Sun MT, Chan WO, Selva D. Traumatic orbital compartment syndrome: importance of the lateral canthomy and cantholysis. *Emerg Med Australas*. 2014;26(3):274-278.
7. Welkoborsky HJ, Graß SK, Küstermeyer J, Steinke KV. Orbital decompression: Indications, technique, results. *HNO*. 2017;65(12):1023-1038.
8. Yoon MK, McCulley TJ. Orbital disease in neuro-ophthalmology. *Neurol Clin*. 2010;28(3):679-699.
9. Belliveau MJ, Johnson D. Orbital compartment syndrome after head trauma. *Lancet. Neurol*. 2015;14(2):136-137.
10. Lima V, Burt B, Leibovitch I, et al. Orbital compartment syndrome: the ophthalmic surgical emergency. *Surv Ophthalmol*. 2009;54(4):441-449. doi:10.1016/j.survophthal.2009.04.005

11. Shek KC, Chung KL, Kam CW, Yau HH. Acute retrobulbar haemorrhage: an ophthalmic emergency. *Emerg Med Australasia*. 2006;18(3):299-301.
12. Gerbino G, Ramieri GA, Nasi A. Diagnosis and treatment of retrobulbar haematomas following blunt orbital trauma: a description of eight cases. *Int J Oral Maxillofac Surg*. 2005;34(2):127-131.
13. Goodall KL, Brahma A, Bates A, Leatherbarrow B. Lateral canthotomy and inferior cantholysis: an effective method of urgent orbital decompression for sight threatening acute retrobulbar haemorrhage. *Injury*. 1999;30(7):485-490.
14. Oester AE Jr, Sahu P, Fowler B, Fleming JC. Radiographic predictors of visual outcome in orbital compartment syndrome. *Ophthalmic Plast Reconstruct Surg*. 2012;28(1):7-10.
15. Yung CW, Moorthy RS, Lindley D, et al. Efficacy of lateral canthotomy and cantholysis in orbital hemorrhage. *Ophthalmic Plast Reconstruct Surg*. 1994;10(2):137-141.

# 22 Brow Ptosis Repair

**Audrey E. Ahuero**

Numerous surgical techniques have been used to address brow ptosis or descent of the brow. Surgeons have individual preferences and variations on techniques. Several of these procedures can be performed under local anesthesia. More extensive forehead lifting surgeries that typically require intravenous sedation or general anesthesia are outside the scope of this chapter but include coronal brow lift, endoscopic brow lift, pretrichial brow lift, posttrichophytic brow lift, fat grafting of the brow, and temporal brow lift. Some surgeons will occasionally perform temporal brow lifting under local anesthesia.[1,2] Additional information on these techniques may be found in the list of supplemental readings.[2-9]

Nonsurgical options that can be performed in the office that may help improve brow ptosis include botulinum toxin injections (neuromodulators), soft tissue fillers,[10] radiofrequency tightening and laser resurfacing.[4,5] Injection of botulinum toxin type-A in the brow depressors, specifically, the procerus, corrugator muscles, depressor supercilii, and orbicularis oculi muscles, can provide elevation of the brow, typically lasting 3 to 5 months.[2,4,9] In certain appropriate patients, soft tissue fillers may be used to volumize the temples and brow region to improve the brow contour. Minimally invasive procedures include thread lifting and tattooing.[11] Brow tattoo does not correct the underlying brow ptosis but helps disguise undesirable brow contour.

The most common brow procedures performed in the office setting are the direct brow lift and internal browpexy (otherwise referred to as the transblepharoplasty browplasty).[12] In the presence of brow ptosis, the surgeon has several options depending on goals and patient preference. If the patient prefers to avoid an incision near the brow, the brow can be elevated slightly and stabilized using a browpexy in the setting of concomitant upper blepharoplasty. If a brow incision is not bothersome and more elevation is desired or longer lasting stabilization is needed, direct brow lifting would be more optimal.[13]

The direct brow lift provides the most lift per millimeter of excised tissue and provides excellent lateral brow elevation.[2] It is suitable for any degree and pattern of brow ptosis and works well for both involutional and paretic brow ptosis.[14,15] It may leave a scar above the brow and is best suited for males with thick brows to hide the incisions better or older patients with deep rhytids. Because it is a quick procedure, it is optimal for patients who are not healthy enough for anesthesia or lengthier surgeries. It also has significant versatility in addressing brow asymmetry.[9] The midforehead lift provides better medial brow elevation but is used infrequently because of the unpredictable forehead scar.[16] It is used almost exclusively in men, and they must have deep forehead furrows.[14] Sensation above the wound is often compromised, and the degree of lift may be limited if inadequate mobilization of the forehead tissue occurs.[14] The browpexy is suitable for smaller degrees of brow ptosis affecting mainly the lateral 2/3 of the brow in any age group.[3,14,15] External browpexy techniques have also been described.[17]

# INDICATIONS

### Key Indications

- Paralytic brow ptosis
- Involutional brow ptosis

The brow is an essential facial feature for conveying emotion.[16] Upward slanting eyebrows convey surprise or sadness, downward slanting eyebrows suggest anger, flat or sagging brows denote fatigue, and properly arching brows convey happiness.[16] Women tend to have a higher, more arched brow located above the superior orbital rim, whereas men usually have a straight brow that is located perpendicular to the nose at the superior orbital rim.[3,4,16] There are some structural differences between ethnicities.[16]

The eyebrow may droop because of involutional change or as a result of facial nerve palsy.[14] Facial nerve palsy (or paresis) can occur owing to a variety of etiologies and is typically unilateral.[9] Involutional change is more often bilateral, although it may be asymmetric (Figure 22-1). Gravity causes sagging of underlying structural foundations of the face, which leads to descent of the brow. The reduced number of deep attachments of the muscle plane of the eyebrow to the frontal-bone periosteum in the lateral brow region results in earlier and greater ptosis of that portion of the brow.[3,16] In some situations, the brow ptosis is more of a hereditary feature, but most often it is due to the aging process, with loss of tissue elasticity and loss of adipose tissue volume.[9] The drooping brow then combines with aging skin that has lost elasticity to allow the upper eyelid tissue to hang over the eyelid margin, which can obstruct the superior visual field.[16] Patients often attempt to elevate the brows by activating the frontalis

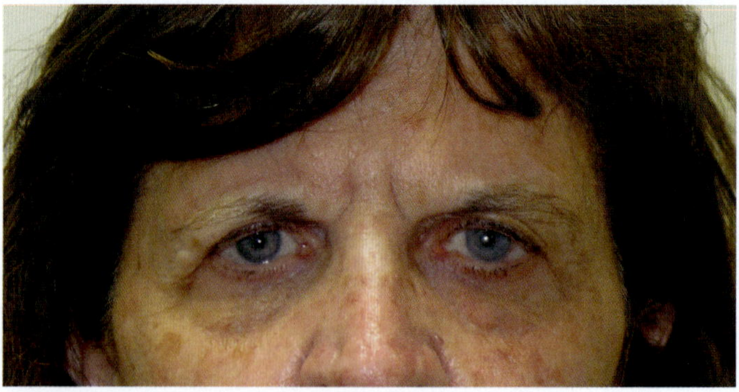

**FIGURE 22-1** Patient with involutional brow ptosis.

muscle, which can create deep horizontal furrows in the forehead. There is a lack of frontalis fibers temporally, which limits the improvement of lateral brow ptosis with frontalis muscle contraction. It is essential to determine whether brow ptosis is present when contemplating upper eyelid blepharoplasty to formulate an appropriate treatment plan. Eyebrow ptosis can lead to redundancy of upper eyelid tissue, which can cause dermatochalasis centrally, lateral hooding, and medial tissue draping.[16] Simple excision of eyelid tissue without addressing the underlying structural brow defect can lead to an unsatisfactory result and unhappy patient.[16] If upper blepharoplasty is performed in the setting of uncorrected brow ptosis, the brow may descend further, with the result that the brow hair ends up on the lashes.[16] Once the underlying structure has been restored, an optimal upper blepharoplasty result may be achieved by the removal of any remaining excess tissue. In some cases (though fairly rare), only the brow ptosis requires correction.

One situation where brow ptosis may be unmasked is in the setting of upper eyelid ptosis repair. If the patient has been recruiting their brows to compensate for eyelid ptosis and an eyelid ptosis repair is performed, the brow may relax, and the upper eyelid appearance would be suboptimal. Brow ptosis may be temporarily induced by excessive or imprecise placement of botulinum toxin in the frontalis muscle, which is the elevator of the brow.[2]

Brow surgery can either be functional or cosmetic. Restoration of normal structure is usually considered "functional" surgery, whereas the same techniques may be employed for purely cosmetic purposes or correction of asymmetry. Compromised visual field may be documented by formal visual field testing. There are three categories of indications for brow and forehead lifting procedures:

1. Improve the patient's visual function
2. Rejuvenate the upper third of the face
3. Rehabilitation of facial nerve paralysis[9]

Brow ptosis repair may be performed unilaterally, particularly in the setting of facial nerve palsy or trauma.

Some young patients may demonstrate eyebrow ptosis related to underlying facial structure, which is an inherited characteristic and may be more difficult to correct with standard eyebrow procedures.[16]

## CONTRAINDICATIONS

### Key Contraindications

- History of severe scarring, that is, keloids (direct brow lift)
- Active infection (herpes zoster, cellulitis)
- Lagophthalmos
- Severe dry eye
- Unrealistic patient expectations
- Active thyroid eye disease

- Very recent facial nerve palsy
- Pregnancy

**Relative Contraindications**

- Alopecia of eyebrow (direct brow lift)
- Dry eye symptoms
- Unable to hold anticoagulants/significant bleeding history
- Recent botulinum toxin treatment
- Taking medications that can interfere with healing—isotretinoin (Accutane), sirolimus (Rapamune), and so on
- Patients with a history of thyroid eye disease, proptosis, keratitis sicca, and facial nerve palsy are at increased risk for exposure keratoconjunctivitis postoperatively.[16]

## INFORMED CONSENT CONSIDERATIONS

### Key Informed Consent Adverse Events Listed

- Bleeding
- Infection
- Scarring
- Asymmetry
- Numbness
- Bruising
- Trouble closing the eyes
- Inability to wear contact lenses
- Tearing
- Dry eye
- Vision changes: vision loss, double vision, blindness
- Local anesthesia problems: vision loss, bleeding, damage to eye or surrounding structures
- Need for further procedures
- Upper facial paralysis

## PREOPERATIVE PREPARATION

Patients should be carefully evaluated to ensure that they are a good candidate for surgery and to determine the best surgical plan. A thorough history is crucial, including patient complaint (and whether functional or cosmetic), type of impairment (visual: impaired visual field;

sensory: headaches or brow ache; motor: difficulty opening eyes caused by heaviness of lid/brow),[9] duration of symptoms, history of dry eye (may be relative or absolute contraindication), prior surgery (of brow, forehead, or eyelid), medications (especially anticoagulants), history of bleeding/bleeding disorders, allergies, trauma, scarring history, facial nerve palsy, blepharospasm or hemifacial spasm, and ability to follow postoperative instructions.

Physical examination should include best corrected visual acuity as well as measurements of the structural position of the brow (arch, position and supraorbital ridge, symmetry, hair quality, mobility, and skin quality) and upper eyelid, specifically, margin reflex distance 1(MRD1), grade of dermatochalasis, pupil-to-brow distance, brow laxity, facial nerve strength and symmetry, lagophthalmos, presence or absence of Bell's phenomenon, and assessment of the ocular surface via slit lamp as well as tear production. Look for any facial scars to determine healing ability and evidence of prior surgery. When evaluating the brow, ensure that the patient is not subconsciously recruiting the frontalis muscle to elevate the brows. Photographic documentation and any visual field testing (if indicated) should be performed with and without eyebrow elevation. Blood pressure should be checked to ensure it is properly controlled in order to minimize bleeding risk.

Following proper history and physical examination, a discussion regarding surgical planning as well as goals and expectations is imperative. Any abnormalities and asymmetries should be reviewed. A mirror will help facilitate this conversation.[16] Options for correction of brow ptosis (surgical and nonsurgical) should be discussed as well as whether any redundant upper eyelid skin should be addressed at the same time. Risks of the proposed treatment should be reviewed with the patient by the surgeon. A discussion regarding cessation of blood thinners is important, and instructions regarding holding prescribed blood thinners should be provided by the patient's cardiologist, if applicable. Ensure that the patient's goals are realistic and that expectations are properly managed.

On the day of the procedure, informed consent should be obtained, allergy history confirmed, photographs taken, visual acuity tested, and vitals recorded, including temperature, blood pressure, and pulse. It should be confirmed that the patient has held blood thinners as directed, and the recommendation regarding resuming the blood thinners should be reviewed. Written postoperative instructions should be provided. If topical anesthetic cream is desired, such as lidocaine 2.5% and prilocaine 2.5% (EMLA), this should be carefully applied (avoiding the ocular surface) 1 hour prior to the procedure.

Appropriate instrumentation should be placed in a sterile fashion on a Mayo stand in the procedure room. A marking pen, gloves, topical anesthetic drops (proparacaine 0.5% burns less than tetracaine 0.5%), protective corneal shields with lubricant, 4 × 4 gauze, smooth Adson forceps (if concomitant blepharoplasty to be performed), an alcohol swab, and 5% ophthalmic povidone iodine should be placed on a Mayo stand separate from the sterile instruments. Local anesthetic in a 3-mL syringe with a 30-gauge, ½″ needle, consisting of either 1% or 2% lidocaine with 1:100,000 epinephrine mixed 1:1 with 0.25%, 0.5%, or 0.75% bupivacaine (Marcaine) may be buffered with bicarbonate 8.4% or bacteriostatic saline (containing 0.9% benzyl alcohol)[2] (Figure 22-2).

On a separate sterile setup, there should be sterile towels, sterile corneal eye shields with lubricant and a corneal eye shield remover, 4 × 4 gauze, cotton-tipped applicators, a No. 15 Bard-Parker blade on a handle, a monopolar (bovie) electrocautery handpiece with a needle tip

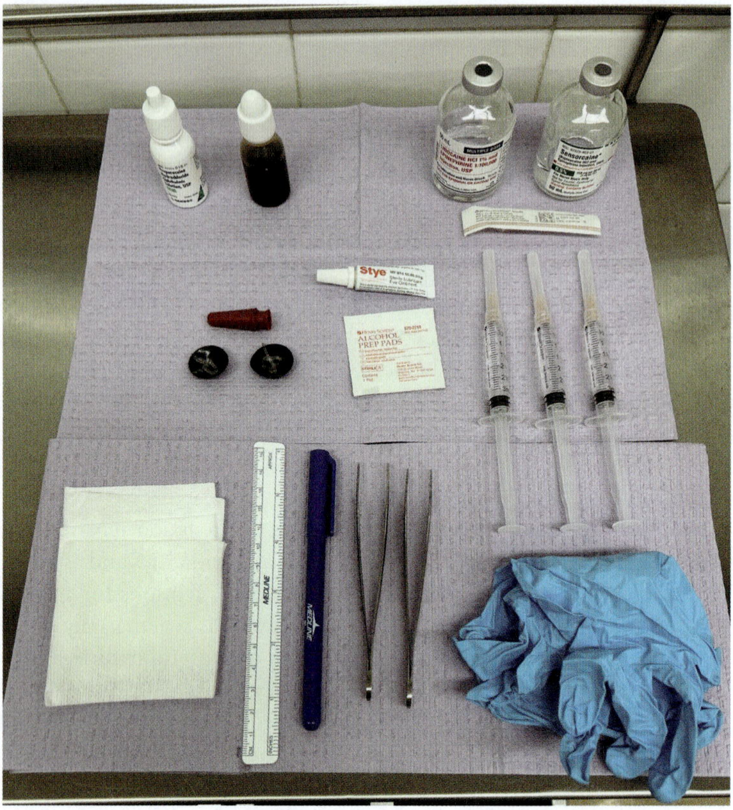


**FIGURE 22-2** Instrument setup for the preprocedure prep (marking and local).

or high-temperature battery cautery, Westcott scissors (blunt or sharp depending on surgeon preference), Bishop-Harmon forceps, 0.5 forceps, Adson forceps, and a Castroviejo needle driver.

For a direct brow lift, a 5-0 polyglactin (Vicryl), 5-0 chromic gut, or 4-0 Monocryl suture will be needed for deep closure and a 5-0 nylon or 5-0 Prolene suture for the skin (Figure 22-3).

For a browpexy, 5-0 or 6-0 nylon or Prolene suture and a Freer periosteal elevator or Adson forceps as well as a rake or Desmarres retractor are additionally needed (Figure 22-4).

## PROCEDURE

### Direct Brow Lift

This surgical technique is most optimal in patients who have thicker eyebrows (Figures 22-5 and 22-6). The proposed incision should be marked with the patient sitting upright. The marking technique is sometimes referred to as the "lift and drop" technique.[9] The lower line

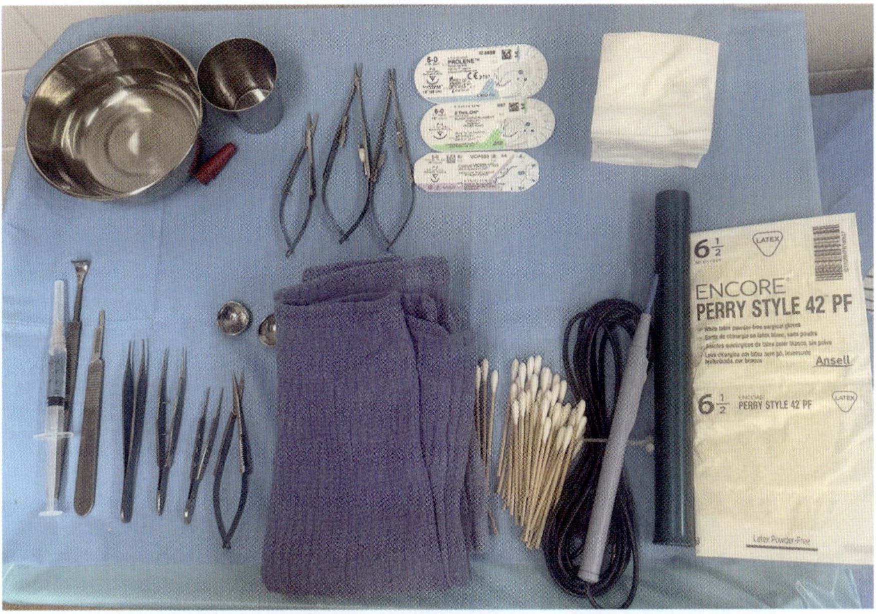


**FIGURE 22-3** Instrument setup for direct brow lift.

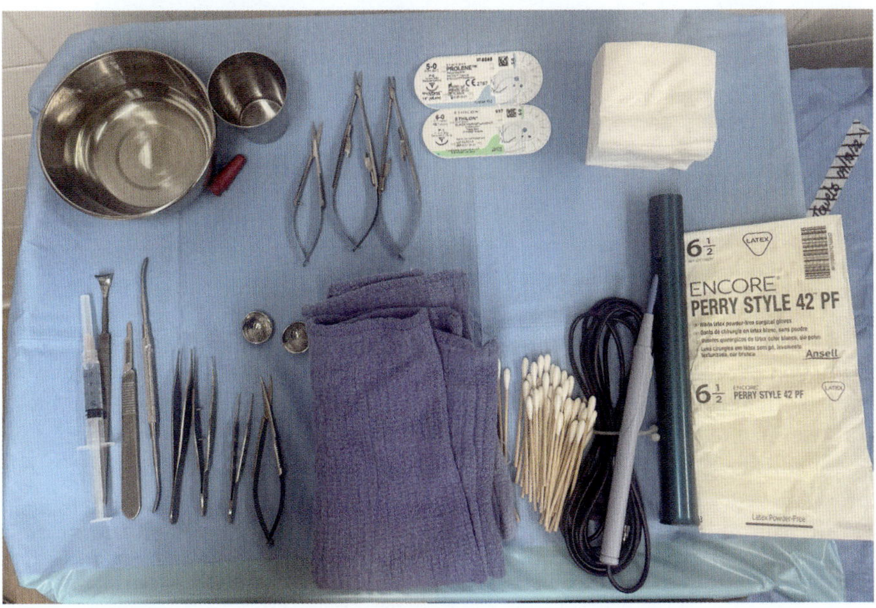


**FIGURE 22-4** Instrument setup for browpexy.

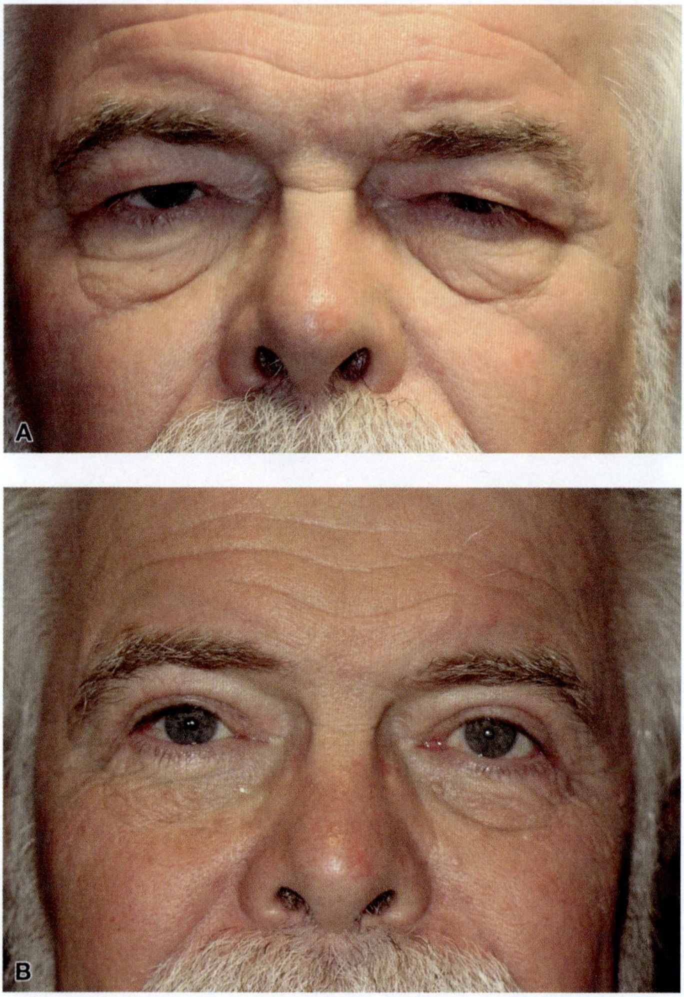


**FIGURE 22-5** **A** and **B,** Patient before and 4 months after direct brow lift (with upper blepharoplasty).

of the incision should lie just within or slightly above the most superior row of brow hairs. The medial extent of the incision should not extend to the head of the brow. The brow is then manually elevated to the desired position, and the marking pen is held at that location and the brow released. The pen is then located at the superior incision line, and the point is marked. The process is repeated along the brow until the entire superior line is created in an elliptic shape.[16] Measure at least three or four points above the eyebrow. Connect the dots forming an ellipse with the medial and lateral portions tapering to join the lower line[9] (Figure 22-7). If a blepharoplasty is to be performed at the same time, the patient's lid crease is marked bilaterally with the patient supine. The upper blepharoplasty incisions are measured and marked once

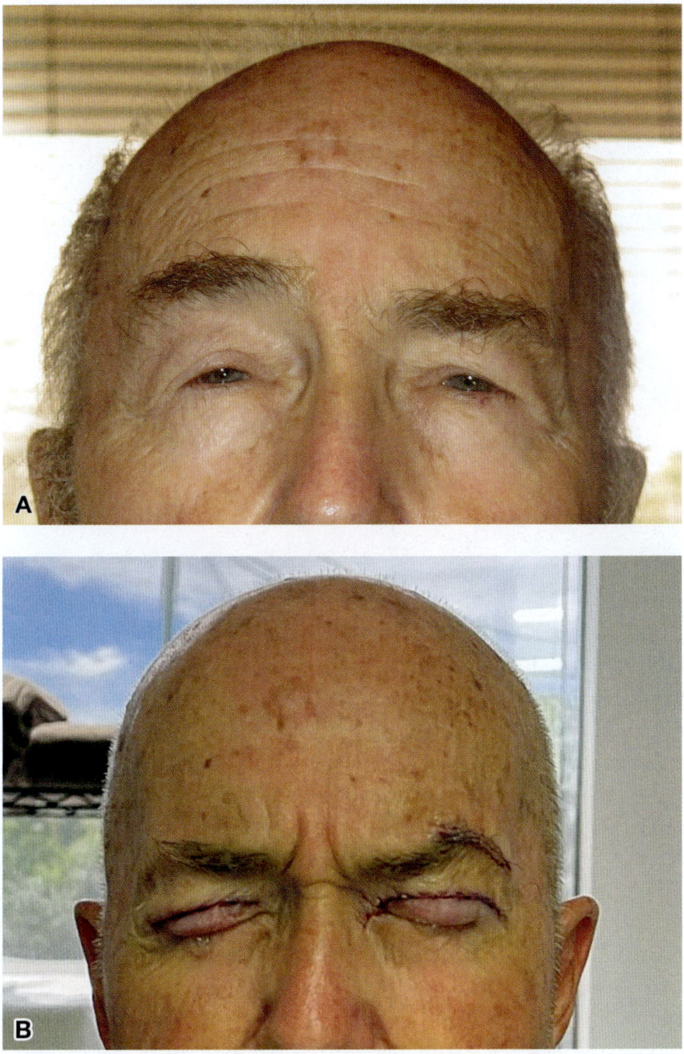

FIGURE 22-6 A and B, Patient before and immediately after unilateral direct brow lift (left) (with upper blepharoplasty).

the brow is in its new elevated position in order to avoid overcorrection, but the eyelid crease may be marked in advance.

Topical ophthalmic anesthetic is instilled. Protective corneal shields are placed. The surgical area is injected with local anesthetic. The patient is prepped and draped in the usual sterile ophthalmic fashion. After allowing approximately 10 minutes for epinephrine vasoconstriction, the incision is made with a No. 15 Bard-Parker blade. Along the inferior incision line, the blade may be beveled medially to parallel the brow hair follicles.[2] The incision is carried to the level of the frontalis muscle-deep to the subcutaneous tissue with the frontalis muscle visible

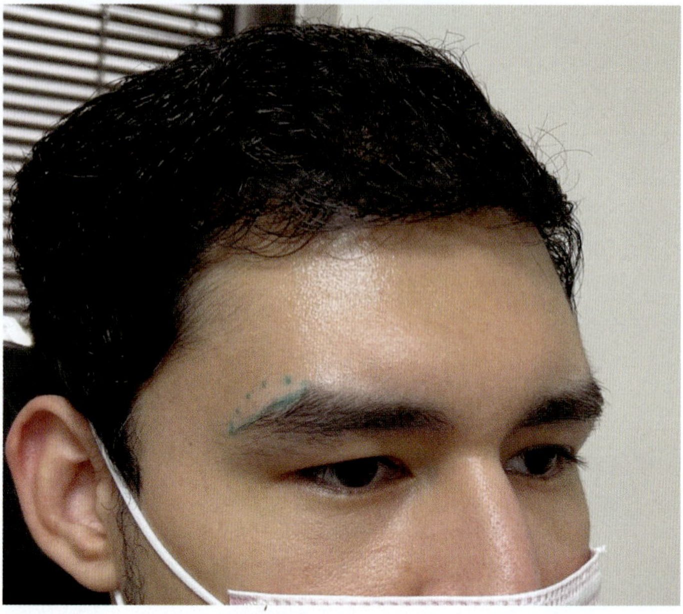

FIGURE 22-7 Direct brow lift marking.

(excise skin and subcutaneous fat stopping at the frontalis muscle).[2,14] Care is taken to be aware of the supraorbital nerve and vessels and limiting any deeper dissection in this region to avoid damaging these structures.[14] Take care not to extend the temporal incision more than 1 cm lateral to the tail of the brow to avoid damaging the frontal nerve.[3] The tissue crescent is excised with Westcott scissors, small tenotomy scissors, monopolar cautery, or high-temperature handheld cautery depending on surgeon preference. The wound is closed in a layered fashion in two to three layers based on brow mobility and skin thickness.[9] The deeper tissue is closed with buried, interrupted 5-0 polyglactin, 4-0 Monocryl, 5-0 chromic gut or nonabsorbable suture at the level of the frontalis and a second layer in the superficial subcutaneous tissue. If one deeper layer of closure is performed, ensure that the needle passes through the dermis on both sides of the wound as well as the deeper tissues to avoid creating a dead space that will result in an obvious sunken skin scar.[14] If the patient has paralytic brow ptosis, some surgeons will incorporate the periosteum along the superior aspect of the wound in their deeper closure.[14] The skin is closed in a mattress fashion to evert the wound edges using 5-0 (or occasionally 6-0) nylon or Prolene. Some surgeons will close the skin with a subcuticular or continuous interlocking suture.[14] The position of the brow is overcorrected more in patients with paralytic brow ptosis.[3]

## Browpexy

Browpexy slightly lifts and stabilizes the brows and is therefore not ideal for patients with severe brow ptosis. This technique best serves patients with mild-to-moderate lateral brow ptosis (Figures 22-8 and 22-9). It is a very useful technique for many patients, however, and

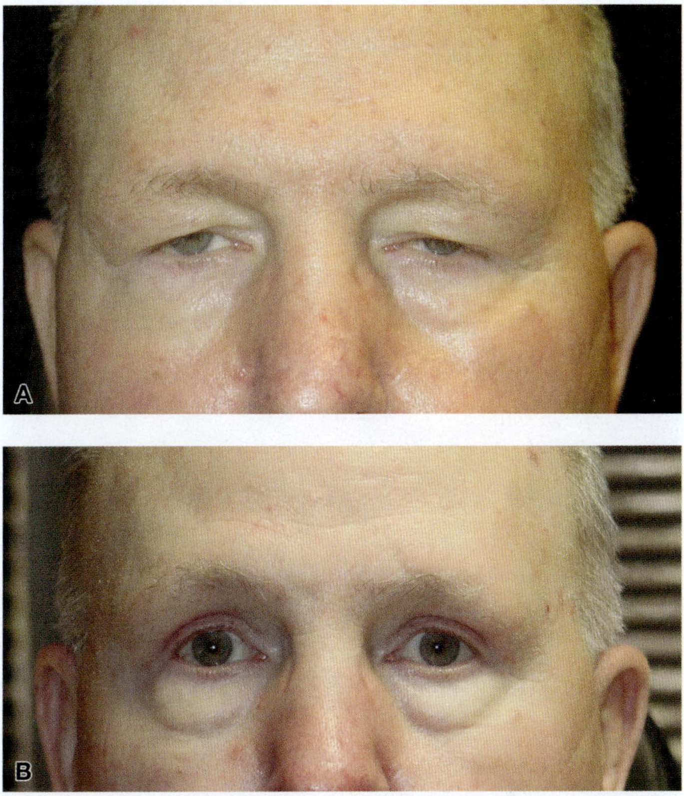


FIGURE 22-8 **A** and **B**, Patient before and 2 months after bilateral browpexy (with upper blepharoplasty).

is typically done at the time of upper blepharoplasty. The main advantage is the lack of an additional incision or scar. It may also be used to contour the subbrow fat in especially full brows.[9] The portion of the brow to be secured is marked with the patient seated upright. The upper eyelid skin is then measured and marked using a pinch technique with the patient supine (Figure 22-10). The supraorbital notch and peak of the brow arch are also marked by some surgeons.[16]

The upper eyelid and brow tissue is then injected with local anesthetic. The patient's face is prepped and draped in the usual sterile ophthalmic fashion. After allowing 10 minutes for epinephrine vasoconstriction, the marked eyelid tissue is then removed in standard upper blepharoplasty fashion. Dissection is then performed posterior to the orbicularis along the surface of the septum at the superior aspect of the blepharoplasty incision and carried upward to 1 to 2 cm above the superior orbital rim using needle-tipped cautery or tenotomy scissors. The dissection plane is located between the orbicularis muscle and the septum (preseptal plane) in the eyelid up to the orbital rim at the arcus marginalis, then extended down anterior to the periosteum for approximately 1.5 to 2 cm above the superior orbital rim. Blunt dissection is performed in a preperiosteal plane using cotton-tipped applicators, the back of an Adson

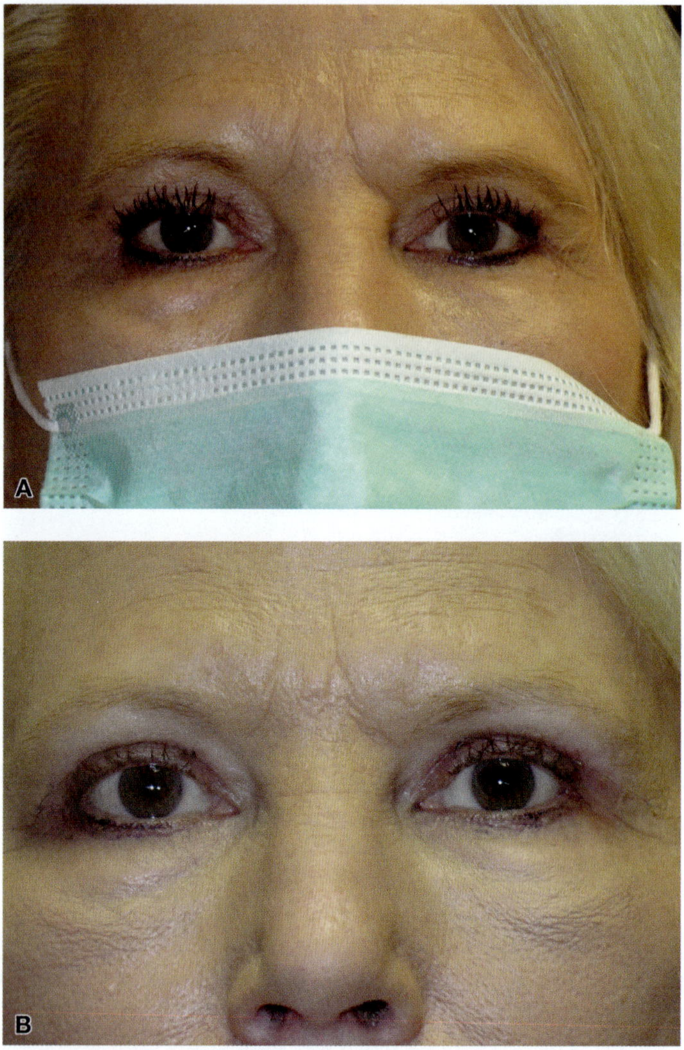

FIGURE 22-9 **A** and **B**, Patient before and 7 days after unilateral browpexy (left) (with upper blepharoplasty).

forceps, or the blunt side of a Freer to clear an area for fixation where previously marked.[3] If necessary, the brow fat can be sculpted.[3,14,16] Care is taken to remain lateral to the neurovascular bundle. A 5-0 nonabsorbable suture is then used to secure the brow to the periosteum in a horizontal mattress fashion. Some surgeons pass the suture through the skin initially at a point immediately inferior to the brow hairs, then a horizontal bite through the soft tissue and frontal-bone periosteum at the desired height (typically, 1–1.5 cm above the rim or 1 cm above the brow fat[14]), and then through the soft tissue or muscle layer of the flap; the transcutaneous end is then pulled through and tied down.[14] Other surgeons omit the pass through the skin and simply pass a horizontal bite through the soft tissue and periosteum at the desired height,

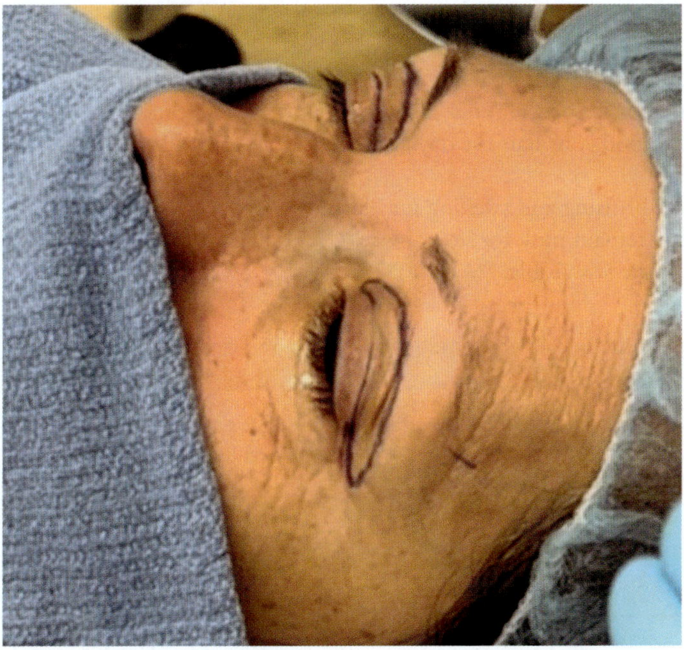

FIGURE 22-10 Browpexy marking.

then through the soft tissue and muscle layer. This will suspend the soft tissue of the brow (retroorbicularis oculi fat [ROOF] and subcutaneous tissue) to the underlying brow periosteum 1 to 1.5 cm above the rim. With both techniques, it is important to avoid passing the last pass too deeply through the muscle in the flap, which would be too superficial to the skin to avoid dimpling the skin. 1 to 3 similar sutures are placed total along the brow, with care taken to avoid the supraorbital complex and sentinel vein depending on the degree of elevation and securing needed and contour desired. The blepharoplasty incision is then closed in the standard fashion.[16] Some surgeons would use an Endotine for transblepharoplasty fixation of the brow tissue as opposed to suture.[3]

# POSTOPERATIVE CARE (FOLLOW-UP SCHEDULE)

## Follow-Up

- Suture removal is scheduled typically 7 to 8 days following surgery. After suture removal, patients are seen again approximately 6 to 8 weeks later.

Our postoperative regimen is as follows, but this may vary depending on surgeon preference:

- Apply ophthalmic antibiotic ointment to the incisions three times a day.
- Apply plain petroleum jelly three times a day instead of antibiotic ointment if history of contact dermatitis.
- Some surgeons apply a pressure dressing headband.

- Apply cold packs (or frozen peas) wrapped in a cloth to the operative site.
- Sleep with head elevated for 2 to 3 nights.
- Avoid bending over or lifting heavy things (over 8 lbs.) for 1 week.
- No swimming, gym, or strenuous athletic activity for 1 week.
- You may shampoo your hair the day after surgery. Do not allow the water to spray directly into your face.
- Be aware that bruising and swelling may last up to 2 weeks.
- Incisions may remain pink for several weeks, and the scar may take up to 3 months to mature and become less visible.

**WARNINGS**

If you are experiencing severe pain, rapid swelling or protrusion of the eye, dimming or loss of vision, persistent bleeding not controlled with cold compresses, please call IMMEDIATELY.

## POTENTIAL COMPLICATIONS AND THEIR TREATMENT

Bleeding is best controlled by prevention with controlling blood pressure and holding blood thinners (per cardiology recommendation if prescribed). If excessive bleeding occurs and does not stop with applying cold and pressure to the area or a hematoma forms, the wound may be opened and bleeding controlled and hematoma evacuated. Fortunately, bleeding from these procedures rarely becomes retrobulbar (Figure 22-11).

Undercorrection is common because the brows tend to descend again.[14] Additional brow lifting procedures may be performed if indicated.

The scars from direct brow lifting may be obvious[14] and are more common with the medial extent of the incision, so limiting the incision may mitigate this. Scar revision, laser and off-label 5-fluorouracil, or steroid injections are potential treatment options. Meticulous primary closure to prevent the issue, applying scar gel, sun avoidance, and massaging the wounds

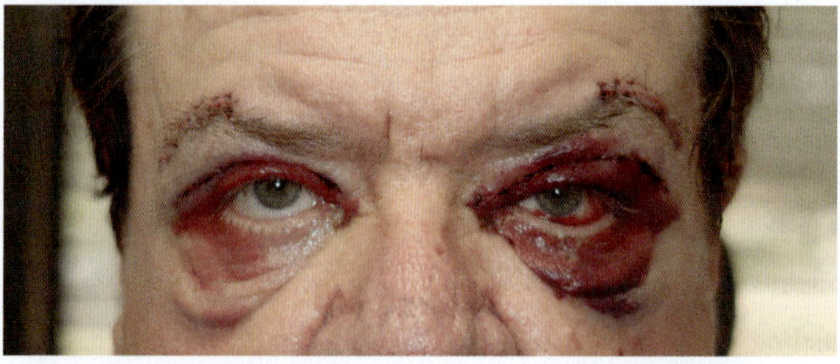

**FIGURE 22-11** Complication of hemorrhage (left) after direct brow lift with blepharoplasty.

postoperatively help to best control the healing process. Granuloma formation may occur owing to the use of braided absorbable sutures.[15]

A serious complication would be nerve damage. Care should be taken to avoid the frontal branch of the facial nerve because damage to this nerve may cause prolonged paresis or permanent paralysis of the eyebrow and forehead.[3] The position of this nerve can be estimated by drawing a line from the tragus of the ear to 1 cm above the tail of the eyebrow.[3] Damage to the supraorbital nerve would result in numbness or paresthesia of the forehead, which is potentially permanent. Prevention is key by identifying and avoiding the supraorbital nerve, especially with cautery.[14]

Browpexy may provide inadequate elevation, and dimpling of the brow may occur.[14] Massage of the area can soften dimpling, or a revision can be performed and the offending suture removed.

Infection is best prevented by thorough povidone iodine prep but may be treated with oral antibiotics and warm compresses if infection does occur postoperatively.

## VIDEOS OF PROCEDURES

### Direct Brow

**Video 22-1**—This video demonstrates a direct brow lift. First, proparacaine or tetracaine ophthalmic drops are instilled, and protective corneal shields with lubricant ointment are placed. Local anesthetic is infiltrated in the previously marked area above the brow. The anesthetic in this case is 1% lidocaine with epinephrine mixed 1:1 with 0.5% bupivacaine with epinephrine. This may be buffered with sodium bicarbonate or preserved saline.

The patient's face is prepped with povidone iodine, draped, and the corneal shields replaced. Approximately 10 minutes elapse prior to making the initial incision to allow for optimal hemostasis.

Attention is directed to the brow markings. An incision is made along the previously marked lines using a No. 15 Bard-Parker blade. The lower mark is incised first to optimize visualization. The blade is beveled parallel to the brow cilia follicles. The upper line of the ellipse is then incised.

Westcott scissors are used to initiate the dissection of the flap in the proper plane. Bishop-Harmon or Adson forceps are used to hold the flap under gentle traction.

The flap, consisting of skin and subcutaneous fat, is dissected with monopolar cautery with a needle tip on cut blend two setting, with care taken to avoid excessive thermal energy on the remaining skin edge. Westcott scissors, straight iris scissors, tenotomy scissors, or high-temperature battery cautery may all be used to dissect the flap as well.

Care is taken to avoid violating the frontalis muscle, so do not dissect deeper than the subcutaneous fat.

Hemostasis is obtained with monopolar cautery.

The deeper tissues are closed with buried interrupted 5-0 polyglactin sutures, with care taken to make deep enough passes to avoid a dead space, which can contribute to depressed scarring. Some surgeons close the deeper tissues in two layers. The dermis is engaged to eliminate any skin tension. Usually, 6 to 10 sutures are needed to provide adequate deeper support.

The skin is then closed with interrupted horizontal mattress sutures using 5-0 nylon, but Prolene may be used as well. This suture technique provides generous eversion of the wound edges. I place the tied ends at the top of the incision line to facilitate easier suture removal because they can blend in with the brow hair. A number of different types of sutures and techniques are used for the skin closure.

A blepharoplasty may then be performed if desired. The same procedure was then performed on the other side.

**Video 22-2**—This video demonstrates a Unilateral Direct Brow Lift with an aerial view. The technique is the same as the prior video.

Protective shields are placed.

Local anesthetic is injected.

The face is prepped with povidone iodine and new shields placed.

The incision is made with a No. 15 blade, with the inferior limb incised first. Care is taken to achieve the proper depth to avoid going too deep.

The flap is initiated with Westcott scissors. The flap, which consists of skin and subcutaneous fat, is then dissected and removed with monopolar cautery and Westcott scissors.

Hemostasis is obtained with monopolar cautery.

The deeper tissues are closed with buried interrupted 5-0 polyglactin sutures. Several buried sutures are needed to properly close the deeper tissues.

This skin closure differs from Video 22-1 because 5-0 Prolene was used on skin here, although the same horizontal mattress technique was used.

An upper blepharoplasty was then performed bilaterally.

## Browpexy

**Video 22-3**—This video depicts the browpexy technique. First, protective corneal shields are placed. Local anesthetic is infiltrated in the marked upper eyelid and lateral brow areas. The anesthetic in this case is 1% lidocaine with epinephrine mixed 1:1 with 0.5% Marcaine with epinephrine.

I place my finger on the superior orbital rim and inject down to the periosteum in the marked lateral brow area, typically 0.5 to 1 mL. Ten minutes elapse before making the initial incision to allow for optimal hemostasis.

The face is prepped. First, the upper blepharoplasty is performed. Attention is directed to the lateral brow, and dissection is performed initially in a preseptal plane until above the superior orbital rim. The dissection is then carried down to a preperiosteal plane.

Blunt dissection is performed using cotton-tipped applicators and the back of an Adson forceps. Care is taken to avoid dissecting more medially to avoid the supraorbital and supratrochlear complexes. Brow fat may be sculpted at this time.

On this left side, the 5-0 nylon suture is passed through the periosteum at the desired height.

The suture is tested to ensure that the periosteal bite is sufficiently secure.

This is followed by a pass through the soft tissue, with care taken to avoid passing too close to the skin to avoid dimpling.

Several sutures may be passed in this fashion.

The same procedure is then performed on the right side. First, there is the preseptal dissection, followed by the preperiosteal dissection. On this side, a Freer periosteal elevator is used to perform the preperiosteal blunt dissection. I make sure to use the blunt end of the Freer in order to preserve the periosteum.

The suture is passed through the periosteum at the desired height and checked. The sentinel vein on this side is especially prominent and is avoided during the suture pass through the soft tissue.

The upper blepharoplasty incision is then closed in the usual fashion with 6-0 nylon.

The lateral skin closure demonstrates the lack of dimpling of the secured brow tissue.

**Video 22-4**—This video demonstrates the technique for transcutaneous placement of the browpexy suture.

The upper blepharoplasty is performed. Attention is directed to the lateral brow, where the preseptal dissection is performed with the monopolar cautery.

The preperiosteal dissection is initiated with the monopolar cautery and performed with a Freer periosteal elevator.

Dissection is continued until a sufficient area has been exposed.

The 5-0 nylon suture is passed transcutaneously at the level of the inferior brow cilia, full-thickness through the skin and soft tissue. The suture is then passed through the periosteum at the appropriate height. The final pass is through the soft tissue at the level of the transcutaneous pass. The transcutaneous end is then pulled through to tie internally.

The blepharoplasty incision is then closed in the usual fashion.

**Video 22-5**—This video demonstrates a browpexy with the use of a caliper to determine optimal placement of the browpexy suture.

An upper blepharoplasty is performed.

Lateral preseptal dissection is performed with monopolar cautery.

Preperiosteal blunt dissection is performed with the back of an Adson forceps.

A Desmarres retractor is placed, and the caliper set to 15 mm is used to confirm the proper height for the browpexy.

The nylon suture is passed through the periosteum at the desired height 15 mm above the orbital rim, as designated by the caliper.

The nylon suture is then passed through the soft tissue and tied. Care is taken to avoid a deep pass, which could result in dimpling.

## EFFICACY

Direct brow lift surgery provides a reliable method for treating involutional or paralytic brow ptosis with a predictable outcome and high patient satisfaction in appropriately selected patients.[18] Butler et al. concluded that unilateral direct brow lifting in paralytic brow ptosis provided excellent symmetry (0–1.5 mm difference) in 71% of brows.[19]

Cohen et al. reviewed browpexy results and found overall excellent results with a high degree of patient satisfaction.[20] A study by Kaderli demonstrated adequate elevation of the brow with internal and external browpexy techniques and a statistical difference from patients who underwent standard blepharoplasty alone, which was sustained during long-term follow-up.[21] Mokhtarzadeh et al. supported these findings with their subsequent study, demonstrating a statistically significant elevation for both internal and external browpexy compared with standard blepharoplasty but no statistically significant difference between the internal versus external techniques themselves.[22] Zandi et al compared internal browpexy versus temporal brow lift and found the internal browpexy to provide a more significant sustained improvement in brow position compared with temporal brow lifting.[23] Nemet et al asserted that browpexy adds to the success and longevity of upper blepharoplasty, but patients with significant ptosis, heavy brow tissue, significant medial brow ptosis, and postfacial palsy would not be good candidates.[24]

## CODING/BILLING AND MODIFIERS

ICD-10 codes:

- Other specified disorders of eye and adnexa
  - **H57.811** (brow ptosis, right)
  - **H57.812** (brow ptosis, left)
  - **H57.813** (brow ptosis, bilateral[25])

Current Procedural Terminology (CPT) codes:

- Direct Brow lift: 67900 with modifier −50 if bilateral. Repair of brow ptosis; supraciliary, midforehead, or coronal approach.

Browpexy:

- The Category I code for Repair of brow ptosis; supraciliary, midforehead, or coronal approach (67900) does not pertain to a procedure performed through an eyelid incision, according to the ICD-10 definition of "approach."[26]
- The preferred CPT code is 67999 (unlisted procedure, eyelids).
- Another option is the addition of the −22 modifier to the blepharoplasty code.[26]

## REFERENCES


1. Bidros RS, Salazar-Reyes H, Friedman JD. Subcutaneous temporal browlift under local anesthesia: a useful technique for periorbital rejuvenation. *Aesthet Surg J.* 2010;30(6):783-788.
2. Hartstein ME, Massry GG, Holds JB, eds. *Pearls and Pitfalls in Cosmetic Oculoplastic Surgery.* Springer Science + Business Media; 2015.
3. Nerad JA. *Techniques in Ophthalmic Plastic Surgery: A Personal Tutorial.* Saunders Elsevier; 2010.
4. Zins JE. Coombs DM. Endoscopic brow lift. *Clin Plast Surg.* 2022;49(3):357-363.
5. Azizzadeh B, Massry G. Brow and upper eyelid surgery: multispecialty approach. *Clin Plast Surg.* 2012:1–240.
6. Dunn T, Hohman MH. Pretrichial brow lift. *StatPearls [Internet].*2022. Accessed September 1, 2022. https://www.statpearls.com/ArticleLibrary/viewarticle/18664
7. Dayan SH, Perkins SW, Vartanian AJ, Wiesman IM. The forehead lift: endoscopic versus coronal approaches. *Aesthet Plast Surg.* 2001;35(1):35-39.
8. Chen WPD, Kahn JA, McCord CD, eds. *The Color Atlas of Cosmetic Oculofacial Surgery.* Elsevier; 2010.
9. Jian-Amadi A. Oculofacial plastic surgery education center: brow lift. *American Academy of Ophthalmology* [Internet]. 2022. Accessed August 27, 2023. https://www.aao.org/oculoplastics-orbit
10. Fagien S, ed. *Putterman's Cosmetic Oculoplastic Surgery.* Elsevier; 2008.
11. Nasir W, Aguilera SB, Weiss E. Non-surgical eyebrow rejuvenation techniques: a review. *J Drugs Dermatol.* 2021;20(9):970-978.
12. Kersten RC, Codere F, Dailey RA, et al. Orbit, eyelids and lacrimal system. Basic and clinical science course. *Am Acad Ophthalmol.* 2006;7:234-241.
13. Jawad BA, Raggio BS. Direct brow lift. *StatPearls [Internet].* 2022. Accessed September 1, 2022. https://www.statpearls.com/articlelibrary/viewarticle/20546/
14. Collin JRO, Tyers AG. Section C: brow ptosis. *Colour Atlas of Ophthalmic Plastic Surgery.* 3rd ed. Butterworth, Heinemann, Elsevier; 2007:241-257.
15. Tyers AG. Brow lift via the direct and trans-blepharoplasty approaches. *Orbit.* 2006;25(4):261-265.
16. Seiff SR. Eyebrow ptosis and blepharoplasty. In: Stewart WB, ed. *Surgery of the Eyelid, Orbit and Lacrimal System.* Volume 2. American Academy of Ophthalmology; 1994:2-12.
17. Massry, GG. The external browpexy. *Ophthalmic Plast Reconstr Surg.* 2012;28(2):90-95.
18. Booth AJ, Murray A, Tyers AG. The direct brow lift: efficacy, complications, and patient satisfaction. *Br J Ophthalmol.* 2004: 88(5):688-691.
19. Butler DP, Nagendran S, Malhotra R. Revisiting the direct brow lift in patients with facial palsy: 4 key modifications. *Ophthalmic Plast Reconstr Surg.* 2021;37(2):179-182.
20. Cohen, BD, Reiffel AJ, Spinelli HM. Browpexy through the upper lid (BUL): a new technique of lifting the brow with a standard blepharoplasty incision. *Aesthet Surg J.* 2011;31(2):163-169.
21. Kaderli A, Katircioglu Y, Ozdemir ES, Kaderli ST. Long-term comparison of the efficacies of internal and external browpexy combined with blepharoplasty. *Arq Bras Oftalmol.* 2020;83(3):185-189.
22. Mokhtarzadeh A, Massry GG, Bitrian E, Harrison AR. Quantitative efficacy of external and internal browpexy performed in conjunction with blepharoplasty. *Orbit.* 2017;36(2):102-109.
23. Zandi A, Ranjbar-Omidi B, Pourazizi M. Temporal brow lift vs internal browpexy in females undergoing upper blepharoplasty: effects on lateral brow lifting. *J Cosmet Dermatol.* 2018;17(5):855-861.
24. Nemet AY. Brow ptosis: is transblepharoplasty internal browpexy suitable for everyone? *J Craniofac Surg.* 2019;30(8):2425-2428.
25. Buck CJ. *Buck's 2019 ICD-10-CM For Physicians.* s.l. Elsevier, 2019:843.
26. Freeman N. Coding, billing and practice management. *ASOPRS Forum.* [Online]. Published June 13, 2018. Accessed September 1, 2022. https://asoprsforum.org

# 23 Neurotoxin Injections

**Selina R. McGee**

Alan Scott began utilizing botulinum neurotoxin A (BoNT-A) as a therapeutic agent to treat strabismus and blepharospasm in the late 1980s. Decades later, there are well over 100 therapeutic and cosmetic indications.[1] Injection of BoNT-A is the most commonly performed cosmetic procedure to treat facial wrinkles.[2]

BoNT-A works by inhibiting the release of acetylcholine at the neuromuscular junction.[2] Repetitive contraction of the underlying facial muscles leads a wrinkle (rhytid) to form in the overlying skin. When BoNT-A is injected in small amounts into dynamic muscles, this relaxes the muscle that smooths the skin overlying it and reduces the wrinkle effectively. It takes about 2 weeks to see the full effects of BoNT-A and lasts a median of 4 months.[2] At the time of this publication, there are five commercially available BoNT-A products. AbobotulinumtoxinA (Dysport Galderma), onabotulinumtoxinA (Botox, Allergan, an AbbVie Company), incobotulinumtoxinA (Xeomin, Merz), daxibotulinumtoxinA (Daxxify, Revance), prabotulinumtoxinA (Jeuveau, Evolus).[3,4] There doesn't appear to be differences in safety or efficacy if units are adjusted accordingly. One study does show that abobotulinumtoxinA has a faster onset of action with a median of 2 to 3 days[5] and daxibotulinumtoxinA appears to have a possible longer duration of action with a median duration of 24 weeks.[6] Dilution, dosage, and injection points are the most important considerations for desirable patient outcomes.

## INDICATIONS

### Key Indications

- Patients that desire to have a minimally invasive procedure to reduce the appearance of fine lines and dynamic wrinkles
- Patients that desire functional relief of benign essential blepharospasm (BEB) and/or benign hemifacial spasm

BoNT-A is indicated for the temporary reduction of dynamic wrinkles. Typical injection sites for cosmetic BoNT-A are the glabella complex, the lateral canthal rhytids, and frontalis muscle in the periocular regions. Our discussions will be limited to these three areas.

## CONTRAINDICATIONS AND PRECAUTIONS

### Key Contraindications

- Patients who have unrealistic expectations should be avoided
- History of neuromuscular disorders such as myasthenia gravis, amyotrophic lateral sclerosis, or Lambert–Eaton syndrome
- Those who are taking certain muscle relaxants and antibiotics such as aminoglycosides
- Pregnant or breastfeeding women
- Those with infection or inflammation at the proposed site of injections and bleeding disorders

### Key Precautions

- Severe elastosis
- Preexisting conditions that may be worsened by treatment, like dry eye disease or midfacial paresis
- History of lower eyelid blepharoplasty
- Body dysmorphic disorder
- Stable or progressive muscular dystrophic conditions causing blepharoptosis
- Already-compromised function of orbicularis oculi

## PRETREATMENT CONSIDERATIONS

The following should be discussed with patients prior to performing neurotoxin treatment:

- Results are not guaranteed.
- Bruising at the injection site can occur. Due to potential for bruising, don't do the treatment within 2 weeks of an important event.
- Headaches may occur.

## PRETREATMENT PATIENT INSTRUCTIONS

Discontinue the following 3 to 5 days prior to treatment:

- Aspirin
- Ibuprofen
- Omega-3 fatty acids

- Ginger
- *Ginkgo biloba*
- Ginseng
- Garlic
- Alcohol
- Green tea

If patients are using prescription aspirin or blood thinners, don't discontinue use unless permitted by the ordering physician.

## Informed Consent

Patient must sign each and every time they have an injection. Do not do lifetime consents.

Informed consent should include a description of the procedure in plain language.

See the following example consent form:

## CONSENT TO BOTULINUM TOXIN "A" TREATMENT

Botox, a neurotoxin, is produced by the bacterium Clostridium serotype A. Botox can relax the muscles on areas of the face and neck that cause wrinkles associated with facial expressions. Treatment with Botox can cause your facial expression lines or wrinkles to be reduced. Areas most frequently treated are (a) glabellar area of frown lines, located between the eyes; (b) crow's feet (lateral areas of the eyes); and (c) forehead wrinkles. Patients may feel a slight burning sensation while the solution is being injected. The procedure takes about 15 to 20 minutes, and the results last 3 to 6 months. With repeated treatments, the results may tend to last longer.

## RISKS AND COMPLICATIONS

It has been explained to me that there are certain inherent and potential risks and side effects in any invasive procedure and in this specific instance, such risks include but are not limited to (1) posttreatment discomfort, swelling, redness, and bruising; (2) posttreatment bacterial, viral, and/or fungal infection requiring further treatment; (3) allergic reaction; (4) minor temporary drop of eyelid(s) in approximately less than 1% of injections, which usually lasts 2 to 3 weeks; (5) occasional numbness of the forehead lasting up to 2 to 3 weeks; (6) transient headache; and (7) flu-like symptoms may occur.

## PREGNANCY, ALLERGIES, AND NEUROLOGIC DISEASE

I am not aware that I am pregnant, have any significant neurologic disease, or have any allergies to the toxin ingredients, or to human albumin.

# RESULTS

I am aware that when small amounts of purified botulinum ("BOTOX") are injected into a muscle, it causes weakness or paralysis of that muscle. This appears in 3 to 4 days and usually lasts 3 to 6 months but can be shorter or longer. In a very small number of individuals, the injection does not work as satisfactorily or for as long as usual. I understand that I will not be able to "frown" while the injection is effective but that this will reverse after a period of months at which time retreatment is appropriate. I understand that I must stay in the erect posture and that I must not manipulate the area of the injection for the 4 hours postinjection period.

I hereby voluntarily consent to treatment with Botulinum Toxin Type A injection for the condition known as facial dynamic wrinkles. The procedure has been explained to me. I have read the above and understand it. My questions have been answered satisfactorily. I accept the risks and complications of the procedure.

| Patient Signature | Date | Witness Signature | Date |
|---|---|---|---|

A note from the counseling practitioner should be included and phrased similar to "I have counseled this patient as to the nature of the proposed procedure, the attendant risks involved, and the expected results." The patient's and doctor's name should be printed and signed with the date as well as a witness (typically a staff member).

## Documentation

Utilize a standard form for each patient that contains the following:

- Specific product
- Date of injection
- Dilution
- Expiration date
- Lot number

Utilize the standard image to record the number of units and placement. See the example in Figure 23-1.

## Photography

Photographs should be obtained before the patient is treated and at every subsequent patient visit. Pretreatment photographs are essential to patient education and comparison postinjection. Have the patient overly exaggerate the movements you ask them to make: raising the forehead, making a frown, and smiling a full smile.

- Take at least three pictures before at rest and in motion with each of the aforementioned muscle movements.
  - Straight on
  - Right side
  - Left side

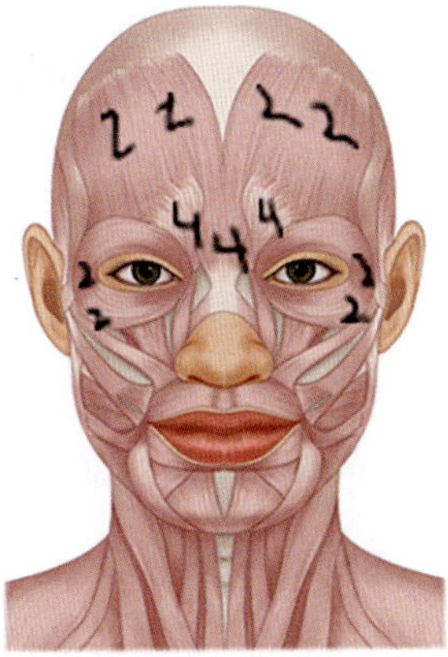

| |
|---|
| Name: Patient Name |
| Date: 02-11-2023 |
| Product: Botox |
| Dilution: 100 unit bottle/2.5 mL for 4 units/0.1 mL |
| Expiration Date: 04/2025 |
| Lot Number: C25547687 |

FIGURE 23-1 Example of a neurotoxin treatment form with documentation.

- Utilize the same background
  - Blue or black backdrop (Figure 23-2)

## Photography Consent

Because these treatments are being performed on the face, photography informed consent is necessary. An example may read as:

I hereby authorize **[physician name]**, of **[name of practice]**, and/or his/her associates or licensees to take preprocedural, and postprocedural photographs, slides.

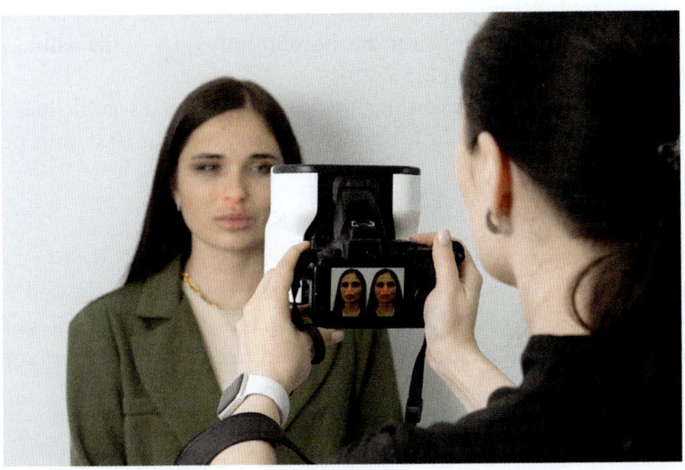

FIGURE 23-2 Depicts a uniform background and straight ahead view. Patient is positioned 3 feet away from the camera.

I consent to the use of these images for the purposes of preprocedural planning and postprocedural evaluation by **[physician name]** and/or the staff of **[name of practice]**, and I understand that they shall be made a part of my medical record.

## Equipment Needed

Utilize a 20-gauge needle and 3-mL syringe to draw up 0.9% bacteriostatic saline (which will be injected into the botulinum toxin vial).

Utilize a 27-gauge needle to inject the saline into the botulinum toxin vial (thus reconstituting the botulinum toxin powder). Draw up this reconstituted solution in a smaller 1-mL syringe. This gives you the capability of having 0.1 mL = 4 units.

- Go *slow*!!
- The vial should have a vacuum seal. If a vacuum seal is not present, do not use the vial as it has been compromised.
- Do not shake or agitate the solution—gently roll the vial.
- Let any alcohol, which is used to clean the skin, completely dry after utilizing it on the patient's face and also on the vial tops so as not to denature the product.

See images of the product list in Figures 23-3 to 23-5.

Utilize a 30-gauge needle (or a higher gauge needle) to inject the botulinum toxin for increased patient comfort.

## Reconstitution and Storage

Utilize the manufacturer's and Food and Drug Administration (FDA)-recommended dilution rates. For onabotulinumtoxinA, incobotulinumtoxinA, and prabotulinumtoxinA, the dilution rates are 2.5 mL into a 100-unit vial with 0.9% sodium chloride, which results in 4.0 units per 0.1 mL dose. For daxibotulinumtoxinA, the dilution rates for a 100-unit vial are double that of onabotulinumtoxinA, so 8.0 units per 0.1 mL dose. These dilution rates give you 4 or 8 (for daxibotulinumtoxinA) units, respectively, per 0.1 mL dose, which has migration about the size of a nickel. Therefore, 2 or 4 (for daxibotulinumtoxinA) units will have migration of approximately the size of a dime (Figure 23-6).

AbobotulinumtoxinA diluted according to the manufacturer's guidelines for a 100-unit bottle at 3.0 mL of 0.9% sodium chloride diluent added results in 10.0 units per 0.1 mL dose.

## Storage

Store reconstituted medication in refrigerator between 2 and 8°C. Best practices are to use it within 7 hours of dilution, but there was a consensus paper that showed it can be stored for up to 4 weeks with 87% potency utilizing preserved or bacteriostatic saline preferably.[7] The stored medication should be clear, colorless, and free of particulate matter before being administered.

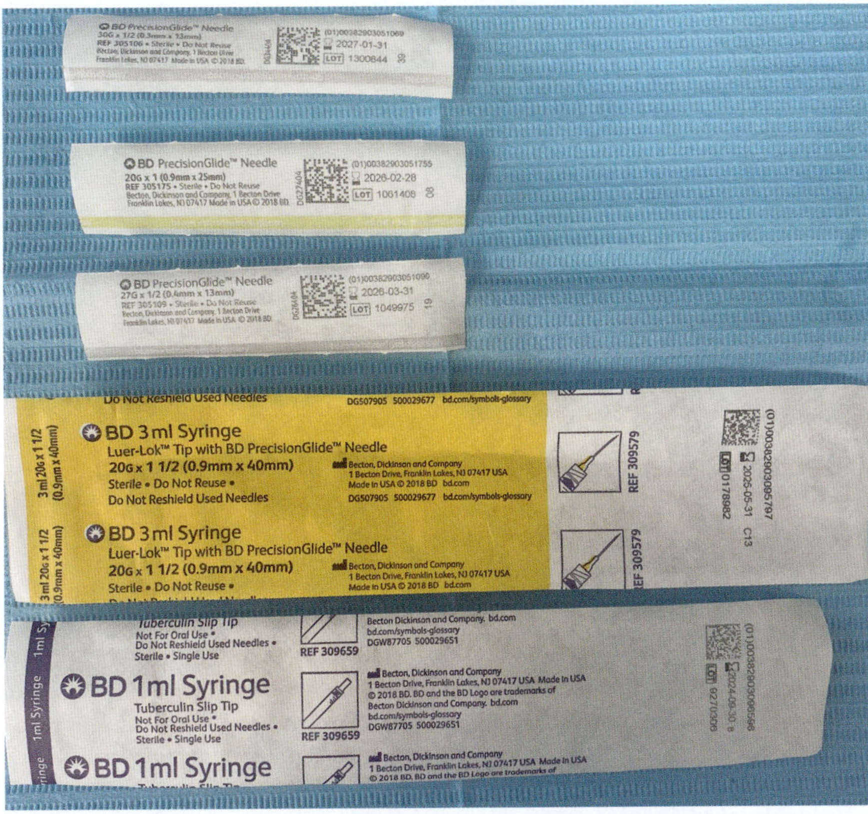


**FIGURE 23-3** Syringes and needles appropriate for neurotoxin injections.

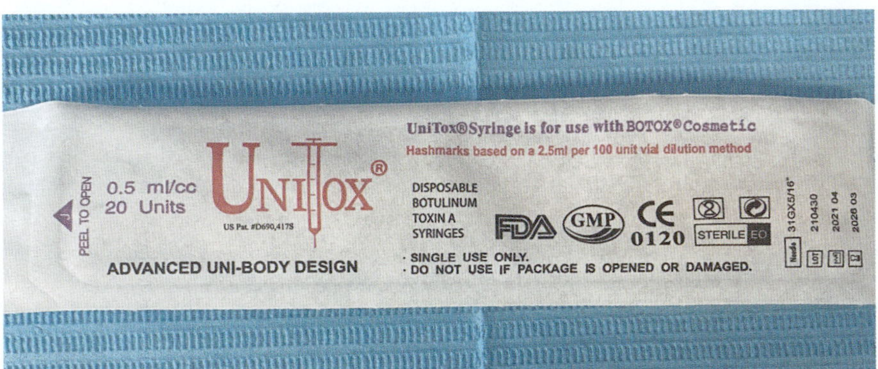


**FIGURE 23-4** Unique neurotoxin specific syringe that holds 20 units of neurotoxin.

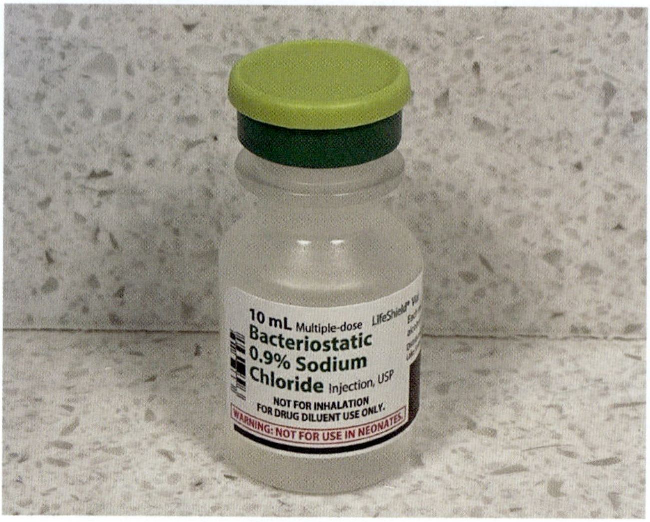


**FIGURE 23-5** Bacteriostatic 0.9% sodium chloride that may be used to reconstitute neurotoxin for injection.

## Anatomy Review

The muscles that are commonly injected for desired periorbital results are the procerus and corrugators which make up the glabella complex, the frontalis, and the orbicularis oculi. The frontalis is an elevator whereas all the rest are depressors. Taking into effect the action of the muscles allows the practitioner to relax the action, thereby reducing the muscle contraction and reducing the overlying skin rhytid. Figure 23-7 shows the muscle action of either depression or elevation. Figure 23-8 shows the names of specific musculature.

# PROCEDURE

## Glabella

There is significant variation in individuals in the strength and size of the glabellar complex muscles. Men have a larger glabellar complex than women. The glabellar complex muscles are

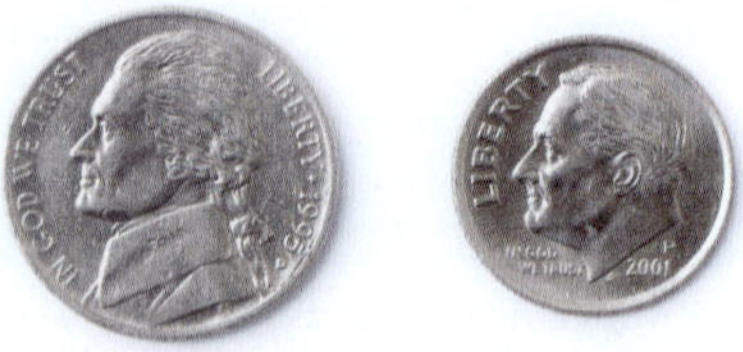

**FIGURE 23-6** The migration areas of 4 units (nickel-size) and 2 units (dime-size) when diluted to 0.1-mL dose with bacteriostatic saline.

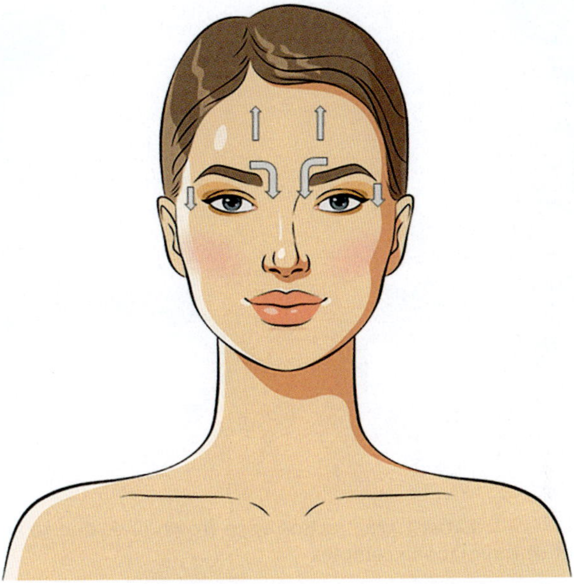

**FIGURE 23-7** Specific muscle movement of frontalis (elevator), orbicularis oculi (depressor), and glabella complex (depressors).

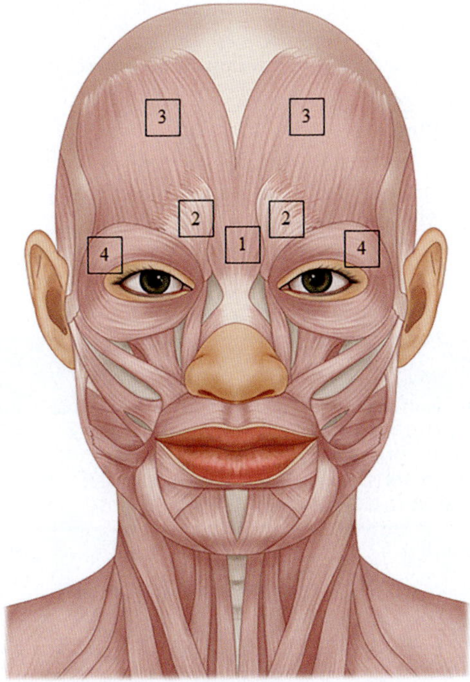


**FIGURE 23-8** Musculature labeled 1: procerus, 2: corrugators, 3: frontalis, and 4: orbicularis oculi.

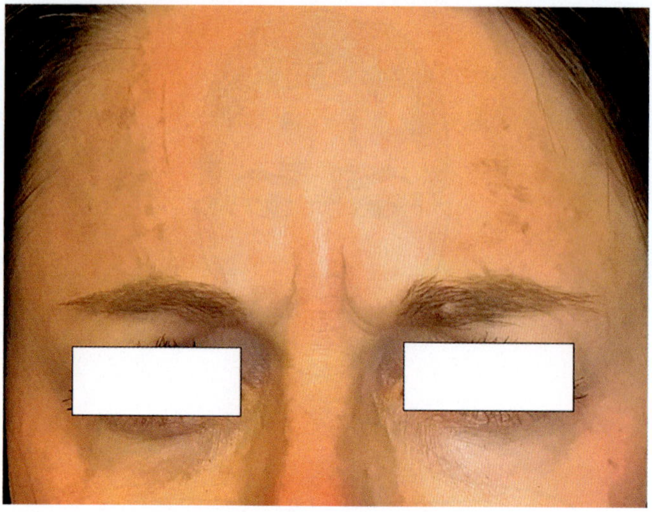

**FIGURE 23-9** Patient preinjection with frown lines due to movement of the glabella complex.

used almost solely for facial expression. The symptom that patients sometimes use to describe this is they want "help with their frown lines" or "11s" (Figure 23-9).

- Muscles targeted
  - Corrugator, procerus, orbicularis oculi, depressor supercilii.
- Pearls for injecting
  - Utilize the pinch technique.
  - It is an intramuscular injection.
  - Four units per injection site (typical) and 8 units per injection site for daxibotulinumtoxinA.
  - Injection can be as little as three sites and as little as 2 units for smaller muscles (Table 23-1).

**TABLE 23-1** INJECTION NUMBER OF SITES AND VOLUMES FOR GLABELLA LINES

| FACIAL AREA | ONABOTULINUMTOXINA, INCOBOTULINUMTOXINA PRABOTULINUMTOXINA WOMEN/MEN (# OF UNITS) | ABOBOTULINUMTOXINA WOMEN/MEN (# OF UNITS) | DAXIBOTULINUMTOXINA WOMEN/MEN (# OF UNITS) |
|---|---|---|---|
| Glabellar lines | 4–6/6–8 (each site) | 10–13/10–15 (each site) | 8–12/12–16 (each site) |
| # of injections | 3–7 sites/3–5 sites | 3–7 sites/3–5 sites | 3–5 sites/3–5 sites |
| Type of injection | Intramuscular | Intramuscular | Intramuscular |
| Total # of units | 12–40 units | 50–105 units | 40–80 units |

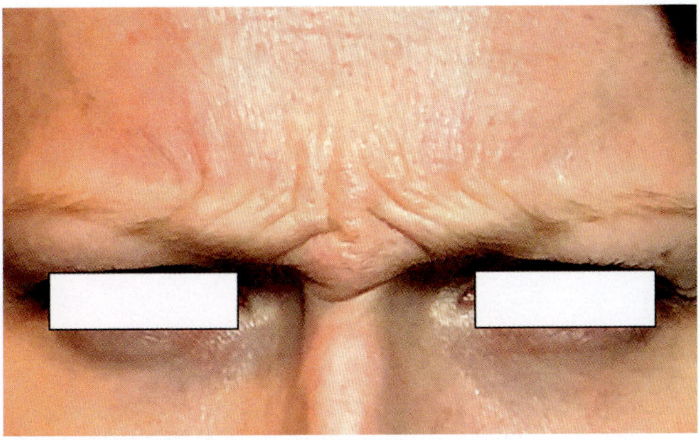

FIGURE 23-10 Glabella complex region preinjection.

Figure 23-10 depicts a strong glabella complex region preinjection, and Figure 23-11 depicts the glabella complex region 2 weeks postinjection.

## Frontalis

The frontalis muscle is an elevator. Patients often utilize this muscle to "recruit" other muscles that need elevation. Be careful to not inject too low on the forehead as to induce brow droop. A good rule of thumb is to inject only 1 to 2 finger widths above the supraorbital rim. Figure 23-12 illustrates the line to not inject below.

- Muscle targeted
  - Frontalis.
- Pearls for injecting
  - Two unit per injection emphasizing symmetry—multiple injections (Table 23-2).
  - Look for vasculature before injection to avoid hematoma formation.

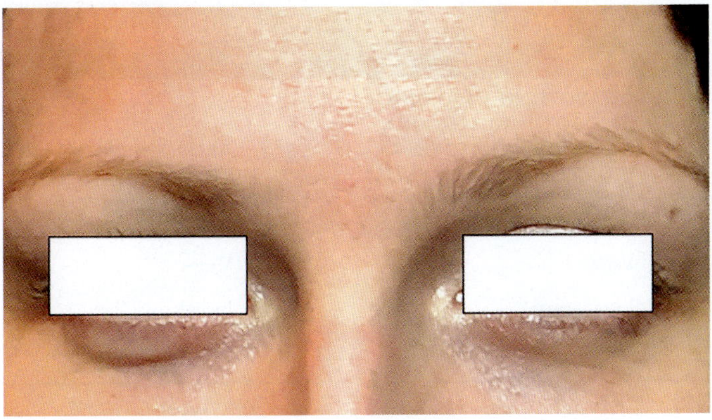

FIGURE 23-11 Glabella complex region 2 weeks postinjection.

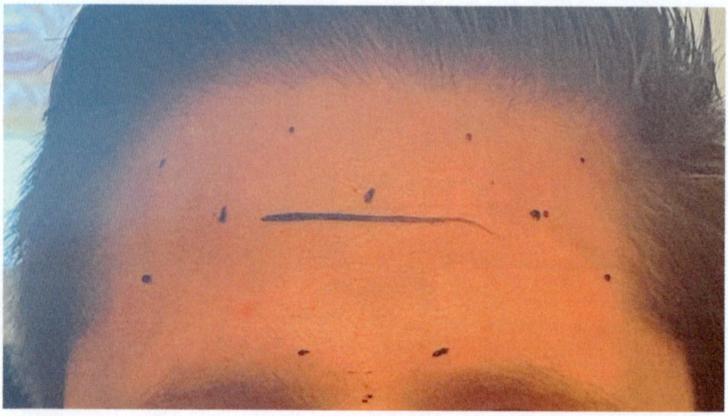

**FIGURE 23-12** Marking pen used to illustrate the line that is two-finger width above the superior orbital rim. Possible injection sites for glabella region and frontalis are also shown. Injections of the frontalis muscle placed below this illustrative line may cause brow droop.

- Injection pattern is discretionary, and placement is targeted to where rhytids occur (Figure 23-13).
- Fibers of the frontalis muscle extend above the corrugator muscle. This is why a brow may droop if the injections are administered too superficially. No injection should be given 1 cm above the supraorbital ridge (not the eyebrow) starting at midpupil (Figure 23-14).
- Notice that the end of the corrugator muscle ends at midpupil where the levator is the most superficial. See Figure 23-14. Injections in the glabella area should never extend past the midline of the pupil where neurotoxin can easily migrate into the levator and could induce ptosis.

**TABLE 23-2 INJECTION NUMBER OF SITES AND VOLUMES FOR FRONTALIS MUSCLE**

| FACIAL AREA | ONABOTULINUMTOXINA, INCOBOTULINUMTOXINA PRABOTULINUMTOXINA WOMEN/MEN (# OF UNITS) | ABOBOTULINUMTOXINA WOMEN/MEN (# OF UNITS) |
|---|---|---|
| Traverse rhytids | 2–4 (each site) | 5–10 (each site) |
| # of injections | Varies | Varies |
| Type of injection | Intradermal | Intradermal |
| Total # of units | 10–40 units | 25–100 units |

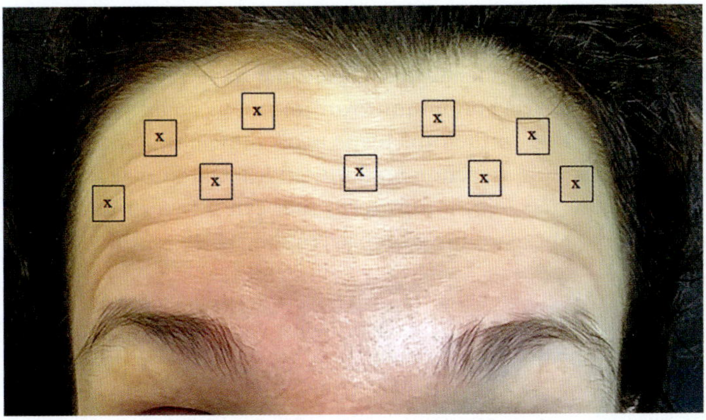


FIGURE 23-13 Possible injection sites for frontalis muscle treatment.

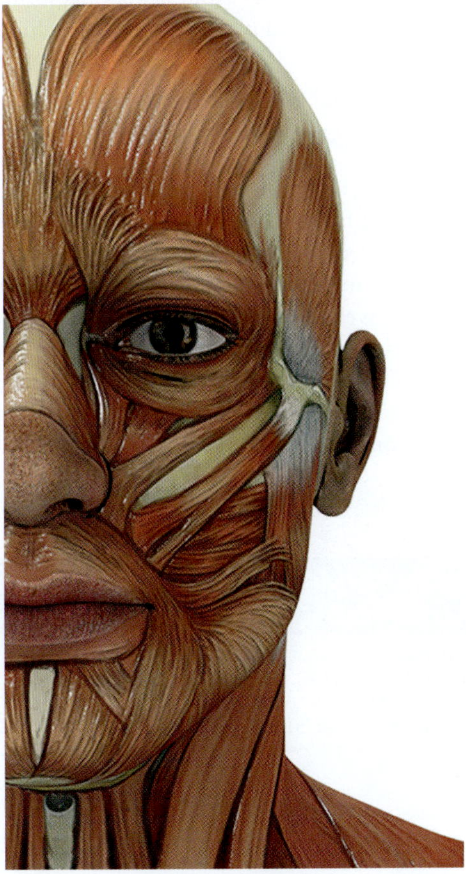

FIGURE 23-14 Note that the end of the corrugator muscle ends at midpupil where the levator is the most superficial.

## Lateral Canthal Rhytids

The orbicularis oculi is a depressor muscle responsible for eye closure. Patients with dry eye disease should be educated that botulinum toxin injections could potentially make their dry eye disease worse. Weakening of the orbicularis oculi muscle can change the blink response. This is dependent on dilution, injection amount, and injection placement of the botulinum toxin.[8] There are different fan injection patterns that can be administered in the lateral canthus. Each individual patient's fan injection pattern should be adjusted to where their rhytids occur (Table 23-3).[9,10]

- Muscles targeted
  - Lateral portion of the orbicularis oculi.
- Pearls for injecting
  - Two units per injection emphasizing symmetry—multiple injections.
  - Needle should always be pointing away from the orbital rim with the bevel pointing up.
  - Look for vasculature before injection to avoid hematoma formation.
  - Injection pattern is discretionary, and placement is where rhytids occur (Figure 23-15).

## Benign Essential Blepharospasm and Benign Hemifacial Spasm

Both BEB and idiopathic hemifacial spasm are abnormal muscle movements. Both involve the eyelids (orbicularis oculi) and facial nerve innervation (cranial nerve 7). These abnormal muscle spasms cannot be controlled and are not caused by a structural pathologic condition like nerve compression secondary to a tumor. These muscle spasms can become so bothersome that vision and productivity, as well as psychosomatic impacts, can be greatly disturbing to those afflicted. Functional blindness can occur due to not being able to keep the eyes open long enough to see adequately. BoNT-A can be a very effective way to manage both blepharospasm and hemifacial spasm. Reconstitution and dilution rates are the same as for cosmetic injections. See the previous discussion on reconstitution.

**TABLE 23-3** INJECTION NUMBER OF SITES AND VOLUMES FOR LATERAL CANTHAL RHYTIDS

| FACIAL AREA | ONABOTULINUMTOXINA, INCOBOTULINUMTOXINA, PRABOTULINUMTOXINA WOMEN/MEN (# OF UNITS) | ABOBOTULINUMTOXINA WOMEN/MEN (# OF UNITS) |
|---|---|---|
| Crow's feet | 2–4 (each site) | 5–10 (each site) |
| # of injections | 2–5 on each side | 2–5 each side |
| Type of injection | Intradermal | Intradermal |
| Total # of units | 8–30 units | 20–100 units |

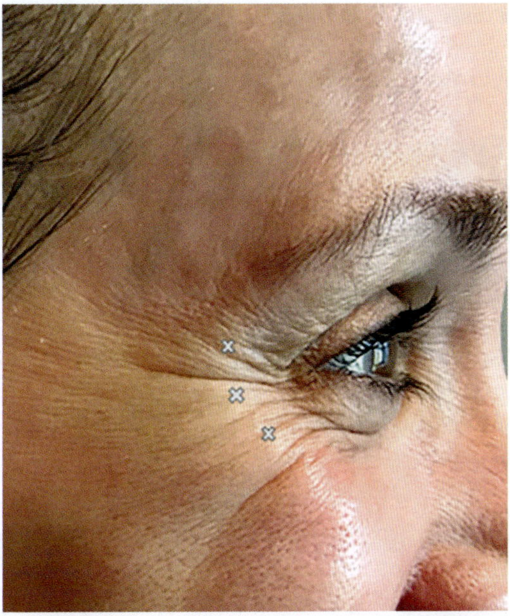

**FIGURE 23-15** Possible injection sites to treat lateral canthal rhytids.

The placement of botulinum toxin injections in the preseptal or the pretarsal portion of the orbicularis oculi are both effective (Figure 23-16). Each location utilizes 1 to 2 units per injection site.[11,12] Both also have different rates of complications. Pretarsal injection sites can have a higher rate of lagophthalmos, whereas injections in the preseptal portion of the orbicularis oculi can have higher rates of ptosis.[11,12] It's important to discuss the complications with patients and provide informed consent as to which areas to inject, that the effects are temporary, and that they will most likely need repeat injections. Both injection sites are efficacious and have high rates of patient satisfaction.[11,12]

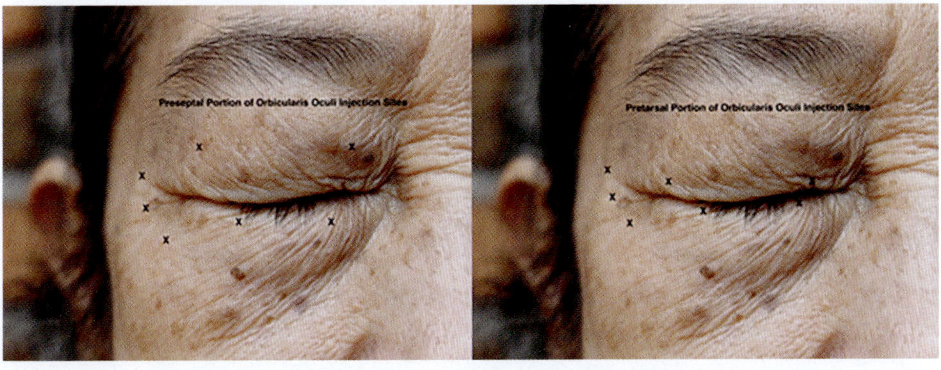


**FIGURE 23-16** Injection sites for benign essential blepharospasm (BEB) can be placed in the following depicted areas. Preseptal injections (left image) and pretarsal injections (right image).

In hemifacial spasm cases, the same injection sites, as would be administered for blepharospasm injection, are utilized. In addition, injection into the zygomaticus major, zygomaticus minor, and risorius would also need to be performed (Figure 23-17).

## Other Uses in Eye care for Neurotoxin

BoNT-A has also been utilized in treating other ocular conditions like refractory dry eye disease and filamentary keratitis.[13,14] For example, in patients with Sjogren's syndrome, it has been shown to reduce lacrimal drainage secondary to the decreased function of the orbicularis oculi, which decreases the action of the canaliculi pumping tears from the front surface.[15] Mechanistically, if the disease process is due to overaction of a muscle, then BoNT-A could temporarily offer relief. There continues to be exploration of different uses for BoNT-A that plague patients due to aqueous deficiency, excessive mechanical friction of the eyelids, and ocular surface disease. More research and case reports are continuing to be explored and published, which offers exciting high-level thinking!

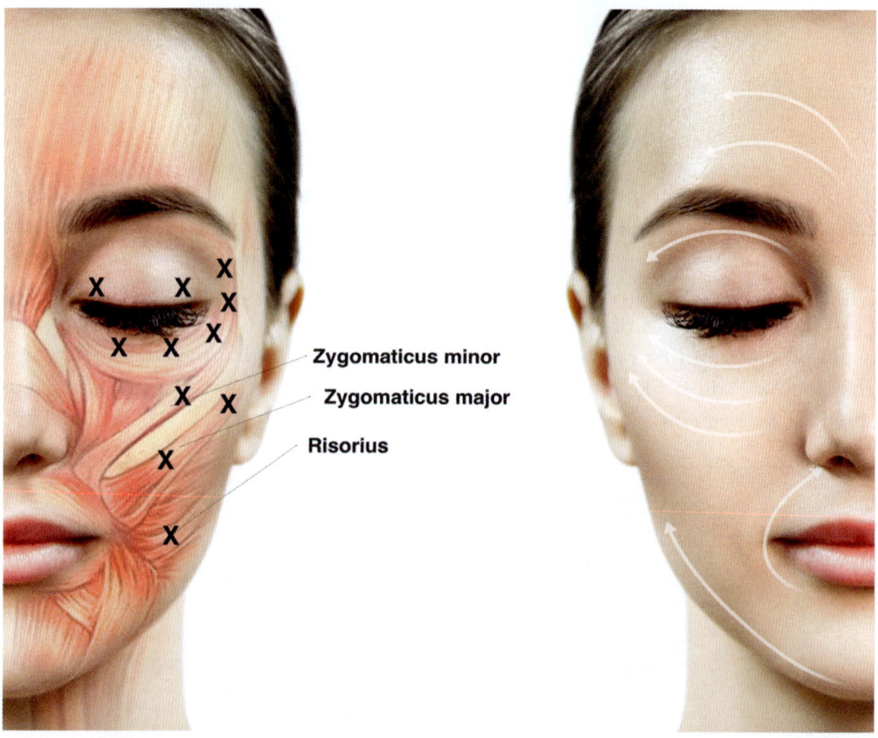


**FIGURE 23-17** Botulinum toxin injection sites for hemifacial spasm.

# POSTTREATMENT CARE AND FOLLOW-UP SCHEDULE

**Key Posttreatment Considerations**

- Avoid lying down for several hours following treatment.
- Avoid manipulation of the area the first 4 hours after procedure.
- No hats, sweatbands, or scarves that could inadvertently displace neurotoxin from intended injection site

**Note:** These measures should minimize the possibility of eyelid ptosis.

- Treatment effect may take 3 to 8 days to appear. Full results occur at 2 weeks.
- The benefits may last 3 to 6 months, and the average is 4 months.
- A touch-up may be necessary in 2 weeks.

If this is the patient's first injection, then follow-up in 2 weeks is recommended to ensure desired results. The patient may be retreated at 2 weeks if touch-ups are needed. Otherwise, patients may follow up in 90 days for continued therapy.

# POTENTIAL COMPLICATIONS AND THEIR TREATMENT

- Blepharoptosis
  - Almost always due to the patient rubbing the site of injection
  - Typically only lasts 1 to 2 weeks

Can utilize apraclonidine 0.5% or 0.1% oxymetazoline to activate Müller's muscle, which can help with ptosis. As the neurotoxin becomes less effective, the ptosis will resolve. Patient reassurance is key.

## Forehead complications

- Brow ptosis/heaviness
  - Know why the wrinkles are really there: meaning are they using the frontalis to recruit because they have brow ptosis, blepharoptosis, or dermatochalasis.
  - Treat brow depressors.
  - Use lower dosing and/or higher frontalis muscle placement with future treatments.
- Mephisto sign
  - Need full paralysis of frontalis above lateral orbicularis where it's the strongest.
  - Foreheads wider than 12 cm are more at risk.

## Lateral canthal rhytids complications

- Diplopia
- Worsening or causing dry eye syndrome
- Ectropion

## VIDEOS OF PROCEDURES

**Video 23-1**—This video demonstrates the injection of the glabella complex with onabotulinumtoxinA.

**Video 23-2**—Botox for the glabella region injected into the procerus and corrugators.

**Video 23-3**—Treatment of glabellar furrows. Utilize the pinch technique to localize each muscle that is to be treated. A total of five intramuscular injections of 4 units per injection site of reconstituted (4 units/0.1 mL) onabotulinumtoxinA (Botox Cosmetic) are administered in the glabellar complex. One intramuscular injection is administered into the Procerus muscle. Each corrugator/depressor supercilii receives two individual intramuscular injections. The depressor supercilii muscle is located just below the corrugator muscle. When botulinum toxin is administered into the region of the corrugator muscle, it simultaneously weakens the depressor supercilii muscle as it lies in close proximity and can be conceptualized as a single functional unit. The patient should be asked to frown, animating their central brow depressors. This highlights the glabellar furrows or lines that are also known as the "number 11s." Each intramuscular injection is given into the center or "belly" of the muscle and not into the furrow (wrinkle). Do not administer any injections below the orbital rim so as to minimize eyelid ptosis. (Video courtesy of Leonid Skorin Jr)

# EFFICACY

BoNT-A is a relatively safe and minimally invasive way to temporarily treat a multitude of conditions including age-related dynamic wrinkles, blepharospasm, and hemifacial spasm. Patients typically report a high satisfaction rate and may have improved psychological perception of appearance when being treated for age-related dynamic wrinkles. Patients with BEB or benign hemifacial spasm can have a marked improvement in quality of life. Friction issues of the eyelids can be temporarily relieved by relaxing the orbicularis oculi, resulting in a variety of improvements to the ocular surface. Utilization rates of BoNT-A continue to increase year over year and can be quite efficacious in an eye care clinician's trained hands.

# REFERENCES

1. Scott AB. Development of botulinum toxin therapy. *Dermatol Clin.* 2004;22(2):131-133, *v.* doi:10.1016/s0733-8635(03)00019-6
2. Small R. Botulinum toxin injection for facial wrinkles. *Am Fam Physician.* 2014;90(3):168-175.
3. Camargo CP, Xia J, Costa CS, et al. Botulinum toxin type A for facial wrinkles. *Cochrane Database Syst Rev.* 2021;7(7):CD011301. doi:10.1002/14651858.CD011301.pub2
4. Carruthers JD, Fagien S, Joseph JH, et al; SAKURA 1 and SAKURA 2 Investigator Group. DaxibotulinumtoxinA for injection for the treatment of glabellar lines: Results from each of two multicenter, randomized, double-blind, placebo-controlled, phase 3 studies (SAKURA 1 and SAKURA 2). *Plast Reconstr Surg.* 2020;145(1):45-58. doi:10.1097/PRS.0000000000006327
5. Nestor M, Cohen JL, Landau M, et al. Onset and duration of abobotulinumtoxinA for aesthetic use in the upper face: a systematic literature review. *J Clin Aesthet Dermatol.* 2020;13(12):E56-E83.
6. Solish N, Carruthers J, Kaufman J, et al. Overview of daxibotulinumtoxinA for injection: a novel formulation of botulinum toxin type A. *Drugs.* 2021;81(18):2091-2101. doi:10.1007/s40265-021-01631-w
7. Carruthers J, Fagien S, Matarasso SL; Botox Consensus Group. Consensus recommendations on the use of botulinum toxin type a in facial aesthetics. *Plast Reconstr Surg.* 2004;114(6 suppl):1S-22S. doi:10.1097/01.PRS.0000144795.76040.D3

8. Ho RW, Fang PC, Chang CH, et al. A review of periocular botulinum neurotoxin on the tear film homeostasis and the ocular surface change. *Toxins (Basel)*. 2019;11(2):66. doi:10.3390/toxins11020066
9. Kane MA. Classification of crow's feet patterns among Caucasian women: the key to individualizing treatment. *Plast Reconstr Surg*. 2003;112(5 suppl):33S-39S. doi:10.1097/01.PRS.0000082192.45787.B6
10. Carruthers, A. *Botulinum Toxin: Procedures in Cosmetic Dermatology Séries*. 3rd ed. Saunders;2012:85-109.
11. Lolekha P, Choolam A, Kulkantrakorn K. A comparative crossover study on the treatment of hemifacial spasm and blepharospasm: preseptal and pretarsal botulinum toxin injection techniques. *Neurol Sci*. 2017;38(11):2031-2036. doi:10.1007/s10072-017-3107-2
12. Sanguandikul L, Apinyawasisuk S, Jariyakosol S, Hirunwiwatkul P, Chongpison Y. Complications of preseptal versus pretarsal botulinum toxin injection in benign essential blepharospasm: a randomized controlled trial. *Am J Ophthalmol*. 2021;232:9-16. doi:10.1016/j.ajo.2021.04.029
13. Gumus K, Lee S, Yen MT, Pflugfelder SC. Botulinum toxin injection for the management of refractory filamentary keratitis. *Arch Ophthalmol*. 2012;130(4):446-450. doi:10.1001/archophthalmol.2011.2713
14. Choi EW, Yeom DJ, Jang SY. Botulinum toxin A injection for the treatment of intractable dry eye disease. *Medicina (Kaunas)*. 2021;57(3):247. doi:10.3390/medicina57030247
15. Bukhari AA. Botulinum neurotoxin type a versus punctal plug insertion in the management of dry eye disease. *Oman J Ophthalmol*. 2014;7:61-65. doi:10.4103/0974-620X.137142

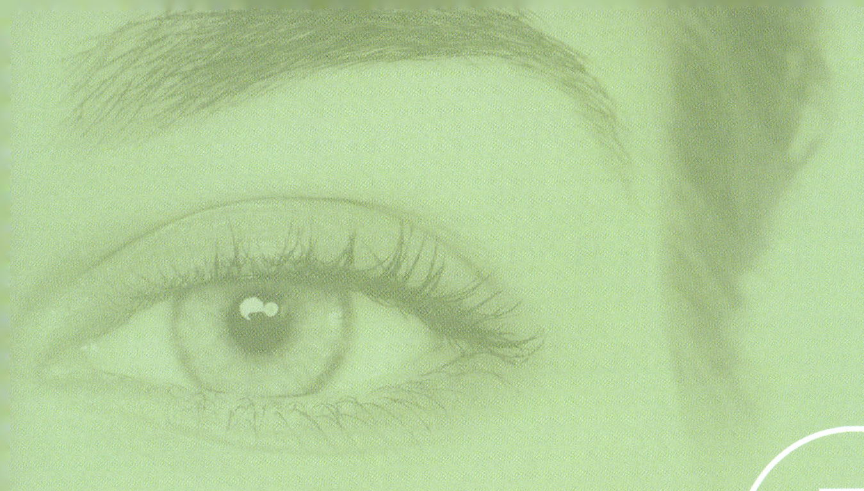

SECTION 5

# Cornea and Conjunctiva

# 24 Corneal and Conjunctival Foreign Body Removal

**Joseph L. Shetler**

Removing corneal and conjunctival foreign bodies (FBs) can be one of the most rewarding aspects of the eye care profession. When handled professionally and efficiently, this procedure not only preserves sight, and can restore significant comfort in a short period of time, but also generates thankful, loyal, and referring patients.

## INDICATIONS

### Key Indications

- Foreign body (FB) sensation resulting from corneal and conjunctival FBs
- Ocular pain
- Tearing
- Photophobia
- History of ocular trauma

Although it is certainly possible for a foreign object to become embedded in the cornea or conjunctiva without the patient's direct knowledge, it is highly unlikely. The history of the incident is usually the primary indication that the patient has an FB in the cornea or conjunctiva. When taking the history, it is extremely important to acquire a complete understanding of the mechanism of trauma if possible. Was the patient working under a car, chipping wood, or riding a four-wheeler through a field of corn? In most cases, the patient can give a highly descriptive assessment of the event. Determining the approximate speed of the projectile will give an indication as to the risk of an intraocular FB. Was the material organic or inorganic? This information will lend itself to grading the risk of infection and heighten or diminish the concern of an accompanying rust ring. The approximate length of time the FB has been present in the cornea or conjunctiva is also very pertinent information. It is also prudent to inquire as to the eyewear, if any, the patient was utilizing at the time of the incident. Whether the patient had a safety eyewear and what action was taken after the injury may play a role in the choice of the course of action as well as legal ramifications such as worker's compensation that may need to be adjudicated after the incident.

In an effort to provide holistic care and protect the patient's systemic health, a good history should also include inquiring about the last tetanus booster. If the last booster was more than 10 years prior, or the patient did not receive all booster shots, refer for additional booster shots after the procedure is completed.[1] Figure 24-1 shows a typical corneal metallic FB that displayed all the primary key indicators.

## CONTRAINDICATIONS

### Key Contraindications

- Identified or suspected intraocular FB
- Penetration of the globe
  - Positive Seidel sign
  - Asymmetric intraocular pressure (IOP)
  - Abnormally shaped pupil
  - Asymmetrical anterior chamber depth (most often a shallow anterior chamber depth)
- Magnetic resonance imaging (MRI) is contraindicated in the event of metallic FB.
- Uncooperative patient

The overall theme of contraindications to proceeding as an in-office procedure is the depth of the FB. The vast majority of corneal FBs will be located in the epithelial layer and rarely penetrate Bowman's membrane that acts as a defensive barrier due to its tough consistency.[2]

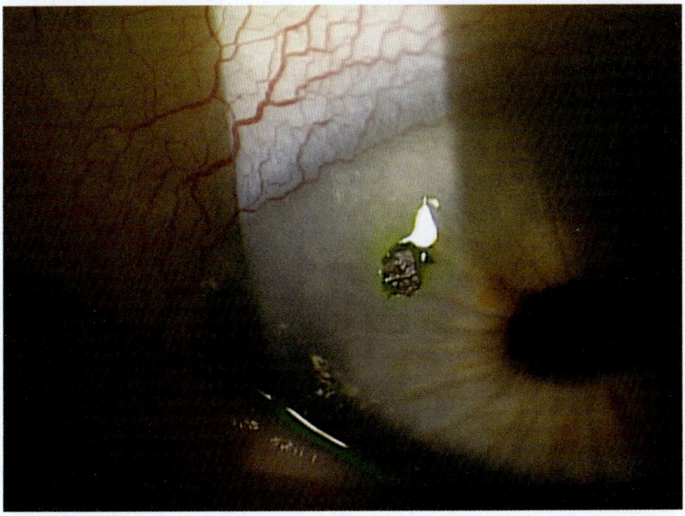

**FIGURE 24-1** This metallic corneal foreign body was accompanied by all the key indicators. (Photo courtesy of Dr. C. Tejchma.)

As described in more detail in the preoperative assessment section, it behooves the clinician to fully investigate the suspected FB to have a complete understanding of the location, both on the clock dial of the cornea and the depth into the corneal surface. Any suspected globe perforation would be a contraindication to an in-office procedure. Ocular signs that indicate the FB has possibly penetrated beyond the cornea include an abnormally low IOP (<8 mm Hg), a peaked pupil, a shallow anterior chamber, and/or a positive Seidel sign. A positive Seidel sign demonstrating aqueous humor leaking via a corneal penetrating injury is visualized in Figures 24-2 and 24-3.

The composition of the FB will also determine the diagnostic tests available to locate intraocular FBs. Metal containing FBs may heat up or move during the MRI scanning process and therefore an MRI is contraindicated in the case of suspected metallic FBs.[3] In the case of a suspected intraocular metallic FB, an x-ray or computed tomography (CT) scan of the orbit may be the diagnostic test of choice.[4]

As with virtually any in-office medical procedure done under local or topical anesthetic, patient cooperation is crucial to achieving a successful outcome. Patients are frequently particularly anxious about this procedure. Visual impairment is a leading concern among patients and in many cases their anxiety may lead them to fear the worst-case scenario. It is imperative that the clinician deliver a truthful prognosis with a touch of empathy. In most cases, calm reassurance from a confident and competent clinician will quell the patient's fears and concerns, and they will calmly be able to cooperate fully during the procedure. Understanding the patient's desire for information and education is critical. Some patients will be better participants in their own care and more cooperative if they understand each step very thoroughly, at the other end of the spectrum is the patient who desires only a basic understanding and relies on trust in the doctor–patient relationship and "just wants it out." In rare instances when the reassuring

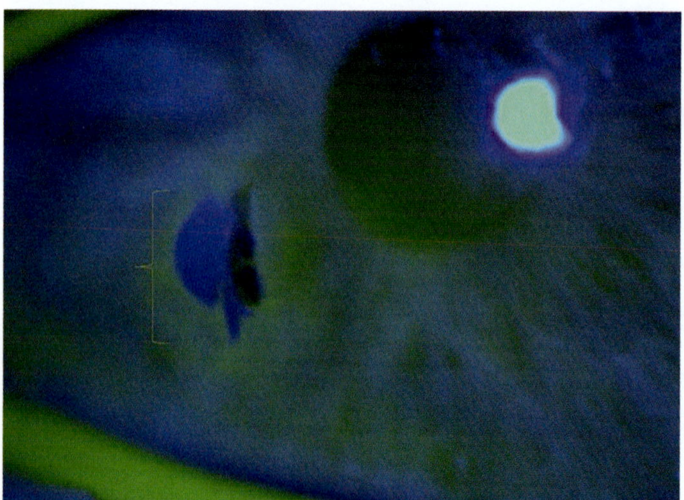

**FIGURE 24-2** Note the small area of black fluid (highlighted with the bracket). The area of black fluid is the aqueous humor leaking from the eye. (© Paul M. Barney, O.D.)

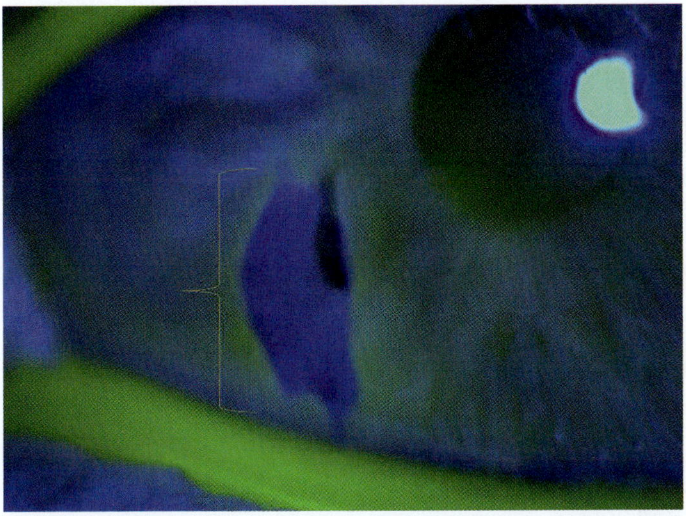

**FIGURE 24-3** In this photo taken seconds after Figure 24-2, the positive Seidel sign is larger showing more leakage. Note the black area of fluid is larger than in the previous photo. (© Paul M. Barney, O.D.)

and calming demeanor of the attending doctor does not allay the patient's fear and garner cooperation, the in-office procedure may become more complex in terms of necessary anesthesia and surgical environment. This is a very rare scenario.

# INFORMED CONSENT CONSIDERATIONS

**Key Informed Consent Adverse Events**

- Eye infection
- Eye inflammation
- Ocular hemorrhaging
- Corneal scarring
- Temporary loss of vision
- Permanent loss of vision
- Failure to achieve desired results
- The need for further procedures and/or additional surgeries

Regardless of how uncomplicated or complex a procedure may be, informed consent is an important part of the process and should not be taken lightly. Informed consent serves several purposes. The foremost purpose is to remind the clinician of the importance of patient education. Prior to completion of the consent form, the clinician must take time to educate the patient about the potential risks and benefits of the procedure, potential complications, and alternative treatment options; discuss the procedural steps in very understandable terms; and answer any questions the patient may have. This education will help to set realistic expectations of the anticipated outcome as well as make the patient aware of improbable outcomes that may require additional care and services. In the litigious environment that medicine is practiced in, it is extremely important to document the discussion of risks versus benefits of the procedure in the confines of the consent form.

# PREOPERATIVE EVALUATION

## Key Preoperative Considerations

- *History: "The how, what, when, and where"*
  - How did this happen?
  - What foreign substance is believed to be in the eye?
  - Where did this occur?
  - Has the patient had prior ocular surgeries? (i.e., Lasik)
- *Slit-lamp evaluation*
  - Identifying the origin of the FB
  - Metallic/nonmetallic
  - Toxic/nontoxic
  - Depth and location of FB
  - Observe for signs of intraocular penetration
  - Positive Seidel sign
  - Asymmetric IOP
  - Shallow anterior chamber depth
  - Peaked pupil and associated iris trauma

Although entrance testing is similar to many ocular conditions, the preoperative evaluation revolves around a thorough history and an extensive slit-lamp examination. Each inquiry should include the typical questions of how, what, when, and where. How did this happen, what does the patient suspect is in their eye, when did it occur, and where did it occur? These questions are critical to providing subjective clues to what will be found objectively during the slit-lamp examination.

The how question should give the clinician a reasonable idea of the force of the projectile and heighten or decrease the concern about intraocular FBs. A grinding wheel rotating at 8,000 revolutions per minute is more likely to result in an intraocular FB, compared to a seed kicked up from a weed trimmer.

What foreign substance does the patient believe they have in their eye? If a metallic FB is suspected, an MRI will not be part of the diagnostic workup due to induced injuries that could occur with the MRI and metallic FB combination. If the answer to the what question leads to suspecting vegetative matter, the astute clinician will recognize the patient may be more likely to present with an infection and more frequent follow-up appointments may be indicated to monitor for the development of an infection.

The answer to the when question can play a substantial role in concerns about other sequelae that may be developing. Approximately 4 to 6 hours is all the time required for the fluid of the cornea to begin to decompose an iron FB and rust to begin to leach into the surrounding tissue and initiate the formation of a rust ring.[5] The risk of infection and inflammation also increases with the length of time the FB has been present in the cornea or conjunctiva.

The answer to the where question could be one of the most sought-after notations in the record to evaluate worker's compensation and insurance issues. The notation should not only accurately record where the incident occurred but also if the patient reported wearing safety glasses at the time of injury. According to The National Institute for Occupational Safety and Health (NIOSH), 2000 American workers have job-related eye injuries yearly and it is estimated 90% of those injuries could be prevented or be less severe if the correct eye protection was used.[6]

It is also pertinent to inquire what other ocular surgeries the patient has undergone. Prior corneal surgeries, particularly Lasik, can be overlooked clinically but can impact prognosis and healing. Penetration into the flap interface can play a role in the overall outcome. Epithelial ingrowth may also be stimulated in this scenario.

The clinician needs to specifically ask the patient if they have had anything removed from their eye in the past. Certain professions such as auto mechanics, welders, and sawmill employees have a higher propensity to having ocular FBs, and this will give the clinician a "heads up" as to the possibilities of residual corneal scars from prior FBs. Thorough documentation is critical, as many of these incidents will occur at work and may involve other legal or insurance concerns.

Entrance testing such as pupillary testing, extraocular motilities, confrontation fields, and best corrected visual acuities should be conducted if the patient is able to cooperate. Pupil irregularities, asymmetrical IOPs, or shallow anterior chamber depth are possible indicators of penetrating FBs. Visual acuities prior to any procedure are critical for postoperative prognosis as well as medicolegal liability reasons. Having knowledge of any preexisting reasons for vision decrease such as amblyopia, prior ocular injuries, or corneal scarring to account for decreased vision other than the current FB concern is important. If the patient's glasses were broken during the incident, unavailable, or their contact lenses have been removed, pinhole acuity testing is mandated.

Patients with a corneal FB and to a lesser extent a conjunctival FB will often be in significant pain, display photophobia, and may be unable to participate in entrance testing. A protocol for the office should be developed to address these situations. In the vast majority of cases, the use of topical ophthalmic proparacaine 0.5% will temporarily alleviate the pain and allow for the completion of entrance testing prior to the slit-lamp evaluation. Technicians should be educated to take a "no touch" approach to avoid further injury or movement of the FB.[7] Checking IOPs should be avoided until the initial slit-lamp evaluation is completed to ensure safety and an intact globe.

A thorough history and entrance testing are customarily followed by a comprehensive slit-lamp examination. Initially, the clinician should take a "fly-over" view and assess the overall status of the eye to get the lay of the land. Initiation of the FB removal without a thorough assessment of the situation objectively could lead to regrets and poor outcomes. The red flags the clinician should carefully review are signs of globe penetration, corneal laceration, inflammation, and infection. After instillation of proparacaine, the clinician should assess the cornea and surrounding tissue without fluorescein stain. The clinician should thoroughly investigate the FB, including the size, depth, and origin if possible. A meticulous view of the cornea will assist in ruling in or out full-thickness lacerations. Keep in mind that it is possible to have a penetrating corneal FB that has self-sealed. The clinician should carefully evaluate the FB's origin and correlate the slit-lamp view with the patient's history of the incident. Some of the common categories of foreign substances include toxic metallic FBs such as iron, copper, mercury, aluminum, nickel, zinc, and lead, as opposed to nontoxic metallic FBs such as gold, silver, platinum, and tantalum. A corneal or conjunctival FB can originate from a variety of nonmetallic sources with toxic potential. Some of the most common are vegetative matter, fabric, insulation, and dry wall. Nontoxic elements include glass, porcelain, and some plastics.[8]

Assessment of the depth of the FB is critical to successful medical decision-making. Close examination under high magnification and the use of the optic section will assist the clinician in determining FB depth and making a well-informed clinical decision. Anterior segment OCT (AS-OCT) can help determine the depth in unclear cases. An AS-OCT can lend additional insight and clearly identify the layers of penetration.[9] The anterior chamber and iris must also be assessed for gross or subtle changes prior to proceeding. Iritis is a potential complication when removing a corneal FB; therefore, assessment of anterior chamber inflammation prior to the removal is critical. This initial assessment will play a role in determining postoperative medications as well as pain and visual concerns. Evidence of preoperative iritis should be clearly graded and documented.

The clinician should then continue inward from the anterior chamber and carefully assess the iris and observe the pupil status. Iris tears and abnormally shaped or irregularly responsive pupils are indicators of possible intraocular FBs. After understanding the overall status of the globe and the patient's systemic health and potentially complicating issues, the clinician should complete the comprehensive slit-lamp evaluation by instilling sodium fluorescein. With the use of the cobalt blue filter and the fluorescein stain, the clinician can accurately assess the extent of the tissue damage. Is the stain isolated to the area of the FB, or does it track in from the side indicating the path of the FB before it came to rest? Horizontal entry will heighten the concern of a recurrent corneal erosion and must be dealt with appropriately. It is also important to assess all areas of stain, paying particular attention to telltale signs of superior vertical tracking, which is indicative of an FB under the upper lid, or in rarer cases, inferior vertical tracking raising concern about an FB in the inferior cul-de-sac. An overall diffuse stain or significant punctate staining surrounding the area of the wound may indicate corneal toxicity. The stain should also be used to evaluate for a Seidel sign, noted as positive when fluorescein is diluted by aqueous humor leaking onto the corneal surface. This can be visualized by a cascading stream of dark, nonstaining fluid within the bright green stain seen on the ocular surface (Figures 24-2 and 24-3).

After evaluating all the key indicators for global penetration or laceration, if in the clinician's judgment, the risk is high for a penetrating wound, referral to a corneal specialist is in order. Known penetration behind the lens depositing a foreign object into or near the retina is an immediate referral to a retinal specialist for an operating room procedure. If either of these scenarios is suspected, the globe should be stabilized with a fox shield and the patient transported to the appropriate eye surgeon for probable intraocular surgery. The patient should be advised not to eat or drink in preparation for the possibility of ocular surgery. If the clinician suspects a retained FB within the globe but key indicators are not conclusive, an orbital radiograph, B scan, or CT may prove to be diagnostic.

In the vast majority of corneal and conjunctival FB cases, extensive imaging will not be necessary as the entire FB will be readily apparent. Analyzing the depth of the FB as well as the nature of the injury also plays a role in determining if it is in the patient's best interest to proceed. It is possible to have an inert FB that has not penetrated the cornea but has approached or encroached on Bowman's membrane and re-epithelization may have already begun. In this case, it might be more prudent to monitor the FB than remove it.

Prior to doing the final preparation to remove the corneal FB, take a final slit-lamp fly-over view, being cognizant that a patient can have more than one corneal and/or conjunctival FB. Inspect for multiple FBs. After evaluating the globe carefully and arriving at the conclusion the FB has not penetrated the full thickness of the cornea, proceed with lid eversion to be certain there is not an additional FB lodged under the upper lid. In the case of vertical tracking on the cornea or conjunctiva without identifying any other foreign substance, a particle under the upper lid may be the primary offending agent. Keep in mind the patient has two eyes. It may be easy to identify the offending substance in the eye the patient was complaining about initially and miss a corresponding FB in the fellow eye that was not as painful.

It is now advisable to assess anterior angles and check IOPs. After this, dilation may occur depending on the case and nature of the FB. In some instances, it is an efficient use of both the doctor's and patient's time to instill dilating agents prior to FB removal, so after the FB is removed, the iris will be dilated adequately to allow an inspection of the vitreous and retina. The dilating agent will have the additional secondary effect of temporarily eliminating ciliary spasm, beginning iritis prevention and pain management.

# PROCEDURE

## Key Procedural Points

- Corneal and conjunctival FB removal instruments of choice:
  - Saline irrigation
  - Sterile cotton swab
  - Jeweler's forceps
  - Magnetized spud
  - Standard "golf club" spud
  - Loop
  - 18-, 20-, 25-, 27-, or 30-gauge needle (25-gauge preferred)

- Upper eyelid FB removal
  - Evert the upper eyelid.
  - Utilize saline irrigation, cotton swab, or a jeweler's forceps to dislodge the palpebral conjunctiva FB.
  - Remove dislodged FB with cotton swab or jeweler's forceps.
- Corneal FB
  - Approach the FB tangentially.
  - Flick the FB out with a spud or 25-gauge needle.
  - Assess if a rust ring is present, and if so, utilize an Alger brush to remove the rust ring.

The actual procedure for removing the FB will be driven by the preoperative assessment. The FB may have been located under the superior lid, indicated not only by the presence of the FB but also by the vertical superficial fluorescence staining tracking from the upper limbus toward the visual axis. This conjunctival FB removal from underneath the upper eyelid is often the least complicated but very rewarding in terms of patient comfort. After reapplying a drop of topical ophthalmic anesthetic (e.g., proparacaine 0.5%), evert the upper lid. In many cases, the FB is not embedded, but only adheres to the palpebral conjunctiva due to mucoid matter pasting it against the soft tissue. This can often be removed simply by sterile saline irrigation. Evert the upper lid and vigorously rinse the offended area. This will typically dislodge the FB, but it may wash it to the lower cul-de-sac where it is floating uninhibited. If this is the case, be certain to remove the foreign substance completely by irrigation, by grasping it with a jeweler's forceps, or by swiping with a sterile cotton swab that the object will adhere to.

The particle is usually dislodged successfully with short strokes tangential to the plane of the eyelid. The other acceptable option is to simply pluck the FB off the conjunctiva with a jeweler's forceps. Always approach tangentially with the instrumentation to avoid inadvertently penetrating the tissue. Very little tissue trauma occurs with the removal of an FB trapped under the upper lid, and patients will experience almost instant relief.

As any craftsman knows, a significant step in achieving the desired outcome is choosing the appropriate tool. The same adage is certainly true in removing embedded corneal and conjunctival FBs. The depth of the FB, location, composition, and patient cooperation will all play a role in selecting the proper instrument for removal. The instrument chosen will be determined by the task at hand as well as personal preference. If the identified FB is metallic, consider using a magnetized spud. The advantage of the magnetized spud is that the clinician can often lift out a very superficial metallic FB with minimal tissue damage. The spud edge is readily available to scrape and penetrate deeper into the cornea if the magnetic aspect does not readily lift out the foreign matter. The other advantage of the magnetized spud is its ability to gather flakes of metallic material with a swipe around the affected area or in the inferior cul-de-sac and leave the wound field and palpebral area clean of debris without requiring additional instrumentation or irrigation[5] (Figure 24-4).

A standard spud "golf stick" may be the instrument of choice (Figure 24-5). The blunt edge of the spud dramatically reduces the risk of corneal perforation. Although applying direct

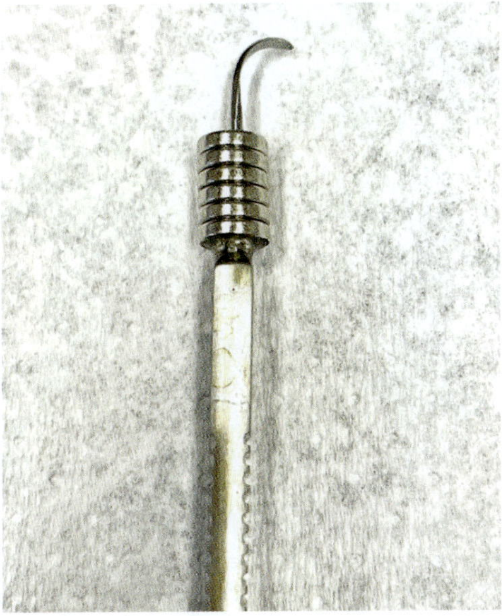

**FIGURE 24-4** A magnetized curved tip spud is an excellent choice for removing a superficial metallic foreign body and collecting the metallic flakes.

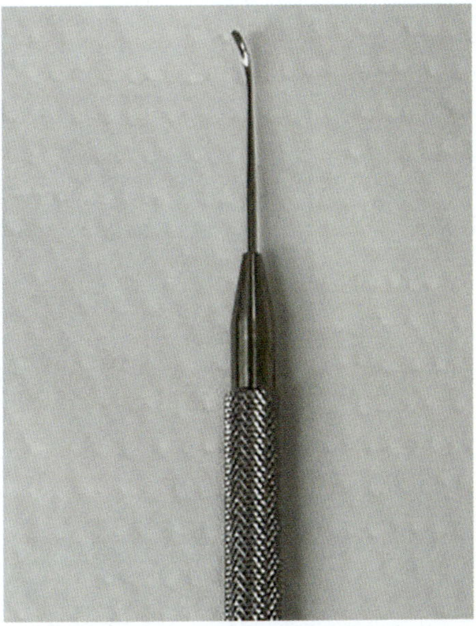

**FIGURE 24-5** A standard spud is often the instrument of choice due to its blunt edge, but in many cases may cause more tissue disruption than a 25-gauge needle.

perpendicular pressure on the cornea is contraindicated, the physician does not need to be overly concerned about penetrating the cornea with the blunt edge of the spud when approached tangentially as it requires considerable pressure to penetrate the stroma.[8] Caution is always the order of the day. If the FB is of vegetative matter and simply adhered to the cornea tightly enough that it will not dislodge with irrigation, the use of jeweler's forceps or a standard golf spud may lift the foreign material off the cornea with little or no additional epithelial damage (Figure 24-6).

Although not used as often as the spud, there may be occasions when the loop is the best choice. A wire loop is mounted on the tip of a pencil-like instrument (Figure 24-7). The loop does not have a sharp edge and is highly flexible. The loop enhances the safety of the procedure as corneal penetration is virtually impossible, but the drawback is that the clinician is unable to remove tissue or penetrate any depth of the cornea to assist in FB removal. The two primary factors driving the choice of a loop are depth of the FB and the patient cooperation. Due to the rounded circular aspect of the loop and its flexibility, it may be the instrument of choice when working with a child or minimally cooperative patient who has a superficial corneal or conjunctival FB.

Despite the choices of specialty instruments such as the magnetized spud, standard golf spud, or the loop, the standard needle due to its accessibility and familiarity in the clinician's hands is the most often selected instrument. Although a standard gauge needle of 18, 20, or 25 may be chosen, the 25 gauge is the go-to needle size. A 25-gauge 5/8″ needle provides adequate strength and is short enough to avoid flexure[4] (Figure 24-8). Typically, less surrounding

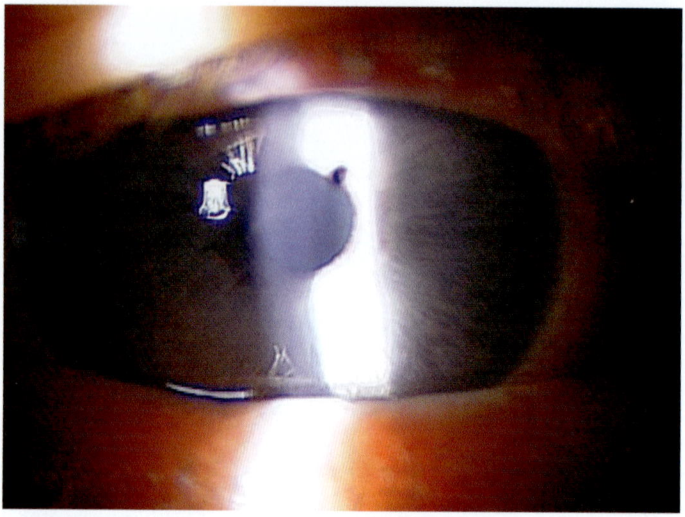

**FIGURE 24-6** A nonmetallic foreign body that was removed in its entirety with a standard golf spud (see Video 24-2).

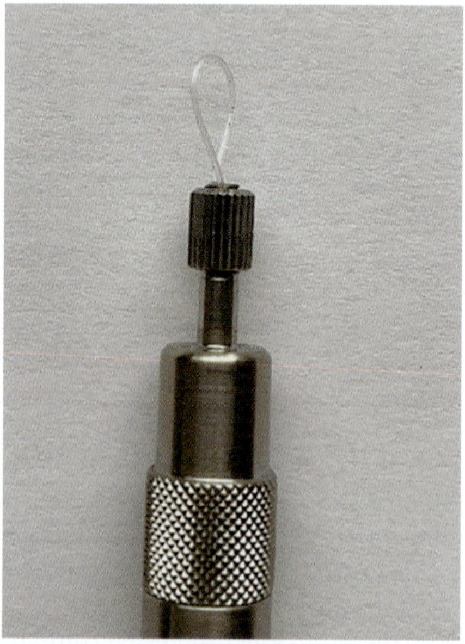

**FIGURE 24-7** The loop on the end of this pencil-shaped instrument is often the instrument of choice for superficial foreign bodies or in cases of uncooperative patients.

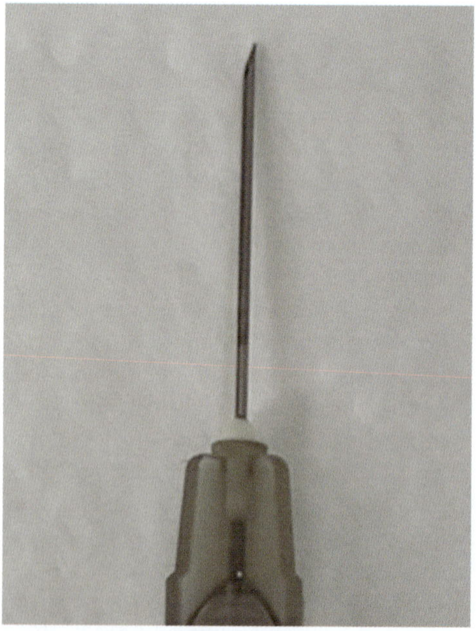

**FIGURE 24-8** A 25-gauge 5/8″ needle is still often the instrument of choice to "flick" the foreign body out with minimal collateral damage.

tissue is damaged when using a needle as opposed to a spud. Although the blunt edge of the spud reduces the risk of perforation, in the hands of a steady practitioner, the needle is often preferred, and the risk of perforation is minimal. If the FB has a metallic component or if the preoperative slit-lamp examination has identified a rust ring, an Alger brush should be readily available to the practitioner once the evacuation procedure begins.

Before starting the surgical procedure, the following steps should be completed:

- The consent form is signed, and the patient has been properly educated regarding the risks versus benefits of the procedure. The clinician should review possible complications, including scarring and residual visual impairment.
- A sterile cotton tip applicator may initially be seen as the instrument of choice due to the lack of a sharp edge; however, it may drive the FB deeper and disrupt significant epithelial tissue, which may impair healing. Often it will not dislodge the offending agent successfully, making it contraindicated except in cases of an adhered palpebral conjunctival FB.
- The patient's cornea should be anesthetized to make the procedure as pain and movement free as possible. This often requires reinstallation of topical ophthalmic proparacaine 0.5%, depending on the length of time for the preoperative evaluation and the patient's pain tolerance. It is advisable to anesthetize the fellow eye to improve patient cooperation and fixation.
- Although rarely necessary after the proper use of an anesthetic agent, a patient with an exceptionally strong blink reflex may require a lid speculum to ensure the lids do not interfere with the procedure.
- The patient's blood pressure should be taken prior to initiating the procedure. According to the American Heart Association, the patient is considered to be in a hypertensive crisis if the blood pressure is 180/120 mm Hg or higher and it may be prudent to defer the procedure until the blood pressure is reduced.
- All instruments should be sterilized and remain in the sterile tray until needed or in an appropriate sterile environment.
- Be certain both the patient and clinician are seated comfortably and in the appropriate position, so the clinician has a complete vertical range with the slit lamp, which will aid in the removal of the foreign object.
- Low to moderate magnification is typically the most appropriate setting for removing the FB, and a final inspection on higher magnification is often warranted. A wide parallelepiped of moderate-intensity illumination will give the best view with a minimal amount of fine-tuning to stay in focus.[2]
- For educational, documentation, and medicolegal purposes, it is advisable to take anterior segment photos of the FB prior to removal.

The patient is seated behind the slit lamp comfortably, the appropriate instrument has been selected, the patient is anesthetized, consent form is signed, and it is time to begin the procedure. Be certain to reeducate the patient about the importance of fixation and encourage them to keep their forehead pressed against the forehead rest of the slit lamp. The use of a fixation target for the nonaffected eye will minimize eye motion and serve to decrease anxiety. Regardless of the instrument selected to remove the offending object, it should be held as a pencil in the dominant hand, allowing the other hand to be free to make minor slit-lamp adjustments as well as assist in holding eyelids open. An elbow rest may be utilized if the clinician desires to create a steadier hand. However, the procedure is often finished in such a short amount of time an elbow rest is rarely necessary. The clinician resting their fourth and fifth fingers on the patient's cheek is usually satisfactory in achieving the necessary stability.

The FB should be approached tangentially to decrease the risk of corneal perforation (Figure 24-9). The desired approach is to enter at the temporal peripheral edge of the FB with a depth just slightly deeper than the FB. Do not be overly alarmed if, as you remove the corneal FB, some wrinkling of the cornea becomes evident. This is temporary due to the light pressure applied by the instrument to the cornea and will typically resolve when the pressure is removed. It is not a sign of perforation. A subtle flicking motion is usually adequate to free the offending object that can then be lifted off the cornea with a jeweler's forceps or moistened sterile cotton swab. Often a sterile saline rinse will clean the injured area of any residual foreign material rinsing it completely from the eye.

After the initial removal of the FB, it is recommended that the clinician view the evacuated area to assess loose epithelial tissue. Although not common, it may be necessary to remove unattached, loose epithelial tissue to help prevent posttrauma recurrent erosion. This is not typically required, and the clinician should avoid being overly aggressive in removing loose irregular epithelial tissue. This removal is best done with a jeweler's forceps.

In the case of a metallic FB removal, assess if additional steps are necessary to remove the rust ring. This evaluation is best conducted with higher magnification than used for the actual FB removal. If the slit-lamp investigation after the removal of a metallic FB identifies a rust ring, a secondary procedure to remove the rust should be conducted using an ophthalmic drill, often referred to as an Alger brush (Figure 24-10). The Alger brush has varying size burrs that can be attached. A 0.5-mm round tip is the usual choice for superficial rust ring removal, as it is the smallest size but typically large enough to adequately remove the rust while minimizing tissue damage. These are available in single-use packages as well as products designed to be sterilized for use for multiple procedures. The Alger brush is engaged simply by spinning the base of the burr with the clinician's thumb and is stopped by applying pressure at the same location, effectively halting the motion. Other designs have an on-and-off switch at the bottom

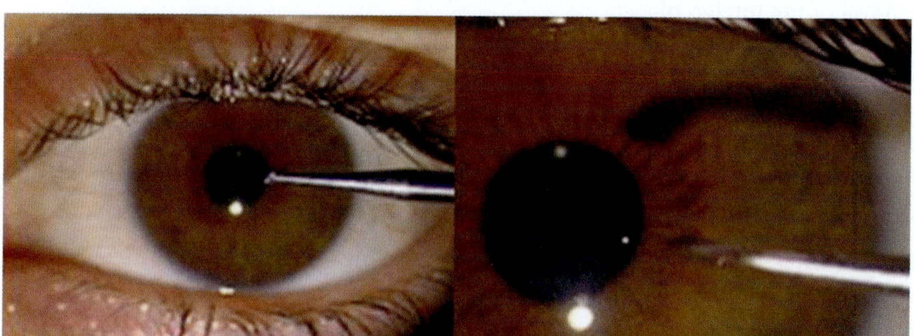

**FIGURE 24-9** Regardless of the tool used, the instrument should be held like a pencil and the cornea should be approached tangentially to prevent inadvertent perforation. In this figure, both the Alger brush (left) and spud (right) are being held appropriately with the desired tangential approach.

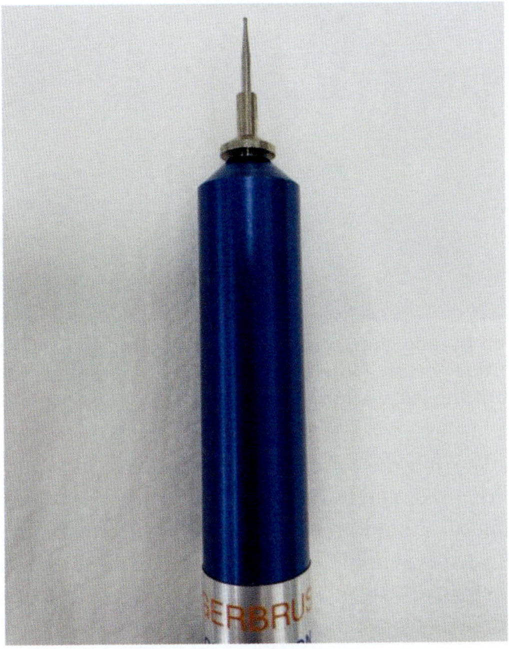


**FIGURE 24-10** The Alger brush is the instrument of choice to remove residual corneal rust rings.

end of the brush. The Alger brush only spins in one direction, and the burrs are oriented to clean rust out in that direction. It may be advantageous in the case of a deep rust ring to manipulate the Alger brush, so it is approaching the rust from the other direction. This is done by switching the Alger brush to the other hand, which will effectively reverse the direction of the spinning.[9] This technique will aid in cleaning out the rust more thoroughly due to the reversed angle of the brushes. Mild pressure will be required to remove the rust, and therefore, slight wrinkling of the cornea can be seen similar to what occurs when removing the FB with a spud. The battery-powered Alger brush is a very low-power motor and has a clutching mechanism that is designed to stop rotating with the calibrated resistance of Bowman's membrane. This is designed to prevent penetration of Bowman's membrane, but be aware if Bowman's membrane has already been penetrated by the FB, the clutch mechanism will not function. Caution is advised to prevent removing excessive tissue, resulting in permanent scarring and consequential permanent visual reduction.[10] The drill will make a soft whirring noise when in operation, and the patient should be reassured about the normalcy of this sound.

The clinician's goal should be to remove the rust ring in its entirety, compromising and disrupting the minimal amount of tissue to decrease potential residual scarring (Figure 24-11). A rust ring will retard healing and may contribute to recurrent corneal erosions. Occasionally, when dealing with a large deep rust ring, it may be wise to leave a portion of the rust at the base of the excavation due to the risk of removing excessive tissue. This rust may spontaneously resolve or migrate toward the epithelium and may be removed at a second visit.[11] This is not a desirable approach. The goal should be to remove the rust in its entirety at the onset; however,

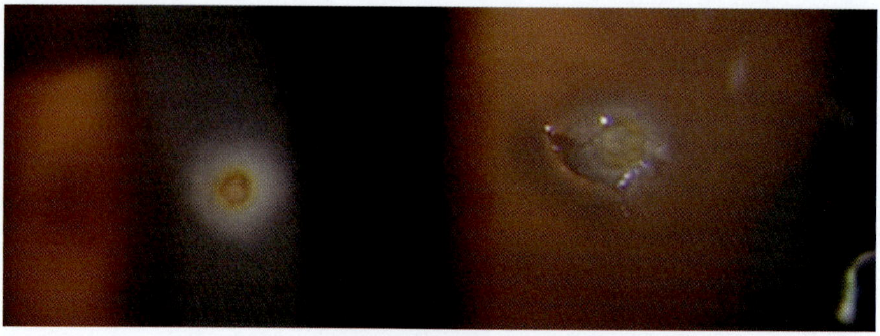

**FIGURE 24-11** A side-by-side comparison before the removal of the rust ring and after removal using an Alger brush. Note the small and acceptable amount of siderosis remaining in the pit of the excavation. (Photo courtesy of Dr. S. Johnson.)

this is not always possible. After the patient has been reeducated about the need to remove the rust, appropriately anesthetized, and both the clinician and patient are comfortably positioned at the slit lamp, the clinician should proceed to remove the remaining siderosis.

The patient's nonaffected eye should be directed toward a fixation target. It is advisable that the clinician stabilize their arm with an elbow rest, pivoting the instrument toward the patient and balancing it appropriately by resting the fourth and fifth fingers against the patient's cheek. Initial alignment is often smoother outside the oculars of the slit lamp. Once the Alger brush is fairly close to the eye, the clinician should look in the oculars to finalize the position of the Alger brush to be ready for rust ring removal. Removal is best accomplished at low to moderate magnification and moderate illumination. The Alger brush is held like a pencil just as was done for the actual FB removal with the spud or a needle. Engage the motor and approach the rust ring tangentially, using the side of the burr. Gentle pressure will be necessary, and corneal wrinkling in the area immediately surrounding the rust ring will be visible and is normal. The clinician will observe the rust-colored tissue being removed as the burr spins. It will likely take multiple touches with the Alger brush to remove most or all of the rust ring. Each touch of the Alger brush to the rust ring should take just a second or two, and it is advisable to allow the patient to blink in between touches of the Alger brush to the cornea. If excessive pressure is required or an orange tinge at the bottom of the crater-like defect remains, the clinician should reassess the situation to determine whether it is best to leave residual rust to avoid excessive scarring or deep penetration. This is also a good time to debride loose and unattached epithelium to promote solid adherence and decrease the risk of corneal erosion.

In rare instances, the patient may be overly alarmed by the sound of the burr or the whirling aspect. In those cases, the clinician may opt for a manual burr. The rust ring is approached tangentially as with the Alger brush, but the clinician manually rotates the burr between their thumb and forefinger to remove the rust. This is not the preferred method but may serve as a backup if the use of the Alger brush is contraindicated due to patient anxiety or poor cooperation.

Prior to declaring the procedure complete, it is advisable to irrigate the area to remove any dislodged debris. In the case of a metallic FB, a final sweep with a magnetized head (Figure 24-12) will collect the residue that was created by the Alger brush. The clinician should

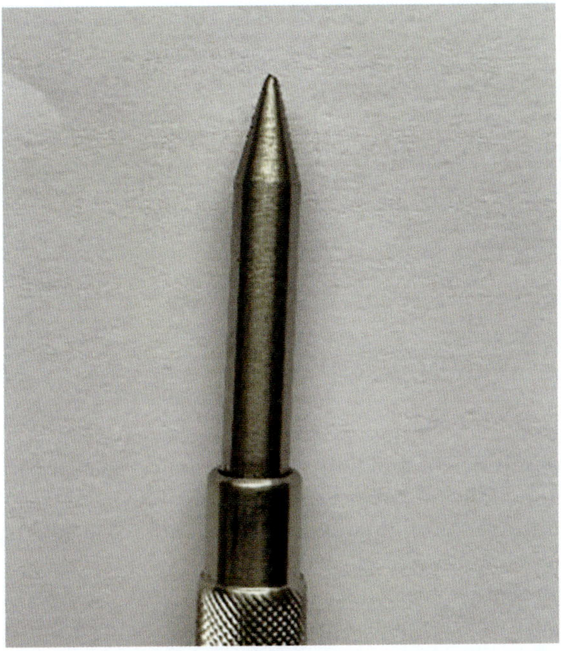

FIGURE 24-12 The cone-shaped head is magnetized and works well to remove metallic flakes generated during rust ring removal.

do a final visual sweep under both low and high magnification to be certain the invasive substance has been removed. As a caution, review for any FBs that may not have been identified initially and be certain no residual particles have taken residence in the lower cul-de-sac. Reinstill fluorescein and reinspect the stained area to fully identify how much epithelial tissue was removed during the FB and rust ring removal process. It is also a good chance to review the area for a Seidel sign to rule out a small corneal perforation, which is highly unlikely. Anterior segment photography is advised after removal, with and without fluorescein.

In many cases, a dilating agent such as 1% tropicamide was instilled prior to the procedure and the patient will now be adequately dilated. With the eye dilated, examine the vitreous and retina for a possible intraocular FB.[12] Identification of an FB in or near the retina would mandate an immediate referral to a retinal specialist.

## POSTOPERATIVE CARE (FOLLOW-UP SCHEDULE)

### Key Postoperative Considerations

- Postoperative drops:
  - Broad-spectrum topical ophthalmic antibiotic

- Pain control
  - Topical ophthalmic cycloplegic (e.g., cyclopentolate) as indicated
  - Pressure patching or bandage contact lens as indicated
  - Topical ophthalmic NSAIDs
  - Oral NSAIDs or oral narcotics (rarely needed)
- Patient education:
  - Safety eyewear
  - Risk of complications
  - Visual prognosis
- Return to the clinic within 24 to 48 hours

As corneal infection is one of the most significant potential complications, a prescription for a broad-spectrum topical antibiotic, such as moxifloxacin QID, should be written for the patient. The length of time the antibiotic should be used can be modified depending on the follow-up presentation, but it is typically written for 7 days.

The Bhaktapur eye study evaluated the benefit of the use of prophylactic antibiotic ointment in corneal ulcer prevention. Of the 442 patients studied, none of the 284 patients who were treated prophylactically within 18 hours of the injury developed a corneal ulcer. Of those who presented 18 to 24 hours after injury, 3.7% developed an ulcer and 28.6% of those seen between 24 and 48 hours after the injury developed corneal ulceration.[13] In summary, maximum benefit is obtained if a prophylactic antibiotic is started within the initial 18-hour window.

After reviewing the dilated fundus, the clinician should make an evaluation as to the necessity of an additional cycloplegic agent. The use of in-office cyclopentolate 1% ophthalmic solution will temporarily paralyze the ciliary muscle and provide the patient with additional comfort as well as serve as a preventative measure for potential traumatic iritis. If anterior chamber cells and flare were identified prior to the removal, the clinician should prescribe cyclopentolate BID or TID until dosage modification is indicated at follow-up visits. In the vast majority of cases, the in-office instillation of cyclopentolate is adequate.

Pressure patching has become more controversial and not used routinely although it is still a simple way to reduce pain and manage photophobia.[1] Pressure patching is contraindicated if the offending agent is vegetative or highly unsterile. Pressure patching is also not advised for contact lens wearers. If patching is indicated, it should be used only minimally. For example, if a superficial FB is removed in the morning, the patch should be removed at bedtime. Afternoon patches should be removed by the next morning. Another alternative is the application of an approved bandage contact lens. This is not without risk and may promote infection or the contact lens may become dislodged and require additional emergency care. The same contraindications for pressure patching also apply to bandage contact lenses. The use of a bandage contact lens (or pressure patching) is a case-by-case decision depending on the size of the FB, size of the epithelial defect after FB removal, patient pain tolerance, and clinician preference.

Any corneal wound that is covered with a bandage contact lens or pressure patch should have a topical ophthalmic antibiotic such as moxifloxacin or gatifloxacin instilled in office prior to placing the bandage contact lens or pressure patching. A covered wound needs to be reevaluated within 24 hours as the coverage can promote infection. The general rule of thumb should be to leave the wound uncovered (if possible) and instruct the patient to remain in a dimly lit environment and wear sunglasses inside and out unless the level of pain and/or size of the epithelial defect dictates the necessity of a bandage contact lens or pressure patching.

The patient should not wear contact lenses unless being used as a bandage contact lens and monitored appropriately. It is imperative the patient is not given proparacaine or similar anesthetic drops once the procedure is completed. Proparacaine significantly retards healing and prevents the patient from experiencing subjective pain that may warrant additional emergency care.

Pain is often better managed with a topical nonsteroidal anti-inflammatory such as ketorolac up to four times daily. Alternatively, oral nonsteroidal anti-inflammatories or oral narcotics could be considered in severe cases, although it is exceedingly rare to need to prescribe oral pain medications after ocular FB removals. Topical steroids should not be used initially as they can slow healing and decrease natural immunity. An exception to this would possibly be in the case of a central FB in the visual axis of the cornea. In this case, a steroid could be considered earlier to minimize the chance of scarring in the visual axis, which could be detrimental to vision.

The patient should be given the appropriate instructions to care for the wound. The patient should be cautioned not to rub their eye, along with a brief educational explanation regarding corneal erosion. The use of preservative-free artificial tears and topical lubricating ointment can also aid in pain management and promote healing. They should be reminded of their visual prognosis. It is also a good time to discuss safety eyewear and actions necessary to prevent additional ocular trauma. A follow-up appointment should be scheduled for 24 to 48 hours. In the case of a small superficial peripheral corneal wound with a low risk of infection or inflammation, a 5- to 7-day follow-up is sufficient.

Prior to scheduling the patient for follow-up, it is advisable to acquire an anterior segment photo of the excavated area with and without fluorescein, which will prove beneficial in education and documentation.

Any reusable instrumentation should be disinfected according to Centers for Disease Control and Prevention (CDC) recommendations. After gently brushing off any residual tissue and gently rinsing and cleaning the tools, the instruments should be autoclaved. If an autoclave is not available, a 15-minute soak in 1:10 diluted bleach or a 20-minute soak in glutaraldehyde will adequately sterilize instrumentation.[14]

At the 24- to 48-hour follow-up visit, the patient will typically report slight improvement in discomfort. Visual acuities may still be affected depending on how central the corneal FB was and the amount of corneal stromal edema present. Best corrected acuities or pinhole acuities should be assessed. The pupil shape and response should be within normal limits unless the patient has been instructed to continue a cycloplegic drop.

The slit-lamp evaluation should include an assessment of the excavated area. The primary concerns are infection and inflammation, which may inhibit healing. The clinician should carefully assess the wound area and judge the percentage of corneal re-epithelization. The epithelial layer generally heals quickly, and the clinician should be able to visualize a trend toward epithelial coverage. The wound should be carefully inspected for any remaining FB. In the case of a deep rust ring, the clinician will need to assess the remaining rust and residual discolored tissue. In many cases, the remaining rust will dissipate without further concern and no additional action will be required (see Figure 24-11). If the rust ring has risen to the corneal surface over time and can be removed with minimal tissue damage, it should be lifted out with forceps or a gentle touch of the Alger brush. The wound should be inspected with and without fluorescein. When the fluorescein is instilled, it is an excellent time to look for a Seidel sign to ensure that there is no full-thickness corneal penetration (see Figures 24-2 and 24-3). IOP should be taken and should be within normal limits. An inspection of the anterior chamber specifically evaluating for cells and flare that are a telltale sign of iritis should always be conducted. Assuming re-epithelization is occurring appropriately, no signs of infection or inflammation are present, and no additional concerns about residual foreign material or corneal penetration are present, the patient should then continue the broad-spectrum antibiotic for 5 to 7 days and be reevaluated in 1 week prior to returning to standard care.

## POTENTIAL COMPLICATIONS AND THEIR TREATMENT

### Key Potential Complications

- Infection of the wound area
- Inflammation (Iritis)
- Recurrent corneal erosion (RCE)
- Nonhealing or slow-healing wound
- Postoperative scarring
- Vision loss
- Ocular pain

The use of properly sterilized instrumentation and prophylactic antibiotics will minimize the development of corneal infections. Increased injection, redness, pain, and discharge are indicators of a corneal infection. Developing infiltrates and excessive discharge are also indicative of an infection, and a culture is often warranted in these situations. Corneal infiltrates should be considered nonsterile until proven otherwise by the culture results. Infiltrates should be treated aggressively with antibiotics and evaluated every 24 hours until progress is seen. The origin of the offending matter is also critical. Fungal infections should be considered in the case of trauma from plant matter. Do not hesitate to make an immediate referral to a corneal specialist in the case of a nonresolving infectious wound.

A minimal to moderate amount of inflammation is common and will typically resolve in 3 to 4 days without additional treatment. The anterior chamber should be carefully inspected to determine if anterior chamber cell and flare exist, indicating an active or ensuing iritis. If iritis is a concern, the patient should be placed on a cycloplegic agent such as cyclopentolate 1% BID or TID depending on the severity of the condition. Although anterior chamber inflammation calls for a steroid drop, it should be used with the utmost caution. It is not advisable to use a steroid to treat the iritis and corresponding inflammation until the cornea has re-epithelialized, especially if the initial FB was organic in nature. Monitor the healing of the cornea daily, so that a steroid drop such as prednisolone acetate 1% can be on board as soon as possible without putting the healing process at risk. After the cornea has healed, this can be managed as a standard iritis episode.

If the cornea appears to be healing appropriately at the initial follow-up visit, but the patient contacts the office weeks to months later complaining of increased pain, possible decreasing vision, and photophobia, the concerns about corneal erosion escalate. The concern heightens even more if the patient reports noticing this pain upon awakening. The clinician should be aware of the complication of initial or recurrent corneal erosion and take all initial steps to lessen the chances of a recurrent corneal erosion developing. Debriding loose tissue initially to give the new epithelial growth a firm foundation to adhere to will assist in preventing erosions. Keeping the eye heavily lubricated with preservative-free artificial tears throughout the day and ophthalmic ointment lavishly applied at night will play a positive role in preventing erosion. It is advisable to continue the artificial tears and ointment up to a month or longer in the case of significant epithelial damage to promote a solid healing process. Advise the patient not to rub their eyes when they itch during the healing process to prevent inadvertently disrupting the new epithelial growth. Even with the best of education and preventative care, a corneal erosion can still develop and be a painful and frustrating complication of a corneal FB removal. If the cornea does not appear to be healing properly at the initial evaluation or if epithelial slough off is noted at additional follow-ups, the efforts to keep the cornea heavily lubricated, especially at night, should be increased. After an antibiotic has been on board for 24 to 48 hours and no evidence of infection is evident, a bandage contact lens should be considered to promote healing and decrease the risk of recurrent corneal erosion. It is advisable to follow these patients every 24 hours until the cornea shows improvement and the epithelial layer is restored.

In the case of a nonhealing or slowly healing wound of the cornea, the primary question that needs to be asked is why. It is prudent to treat the underlying cause rather than the symptoms. Do not forget the eye is the window into overall systemic health and a slow-healing wound may have underlying systemic causes. Is the patient diabetic, and if so, are they well controlled? Encourage good diabetic control in an effort to promote corneal healing. Not only is the patient with diabetes at risk of slower healing, they are also at a greater risk of infection. This problem is magnified in the case of a person with poorly controlled diabetes and opens the door to good diabetic education and the ocular complications that often go hand in hand with poor control. Sjögren's syndrome is accompanied by dry eye and punctate staining, and may be another underlying cause for poor corneal healing. Systemic and ocular diseases such as dry eye and Meibomian gland dysfunction that compromise the corneal integrity can also contribute to slow-healing, recurrent corneal erosion, and corneal ulceration. In these cases, the underlying cause should be addressed. Carefully reevaluating the wound and cornea to be certain that there is not a secondary FB or substantial rust ring is important in the case of a slow healing wound. It is important to keep a broad-spectrum topical ophthalmic antibiotic on board until the epithelium is regenerated and the wound is closed. Although rarely necessary in corneal FB removal cases, an amniotic membrane could be considered to promote healing and decrease scarring.

Postoperative scarring is typically not a concern following a superficial corneal FB removal, or even a peripheral FB that has penetrated Bowman's membrane and entered the stroma, but all measures to reduce scarring that will have a long-term visual effect should be taken. The location of the corneal scar is critical to evaluating the risk of visual impact. Both the depth and position should be considered. In cases where Bowman's membrane is breached, a small focal scar is expected. Generally, even if the visual axis is involved, the intensity of the scar will diminish with time and rarely has a visual impact. If the clinician anticipates a nonvision-threatening scar, the patient should be educated about the scar, preferably by photography, and reassured the scar is visible to an eye care provider with the appropriate instrumentation but is not casually visible and will not create a vision problem. Over time, the intense focal scar will generally become a mild haze in the stroma visible during a slit-lamp evaluation. In the event of a central scar that may have more than a transient effect on vision, steroid drops after the epithelial layer has been restored may be used to reduce scarring. Amniotic membranes could also be considered in cases where significant central scarring is a concern. In cases of significant scarring that remains after approximately 6 months, surgical intervention may become the most viable option. This time period will serve to allow the cornea to stabilize and the vision to be consistent and no longer improving.[10]

Ocular pain, especially in the case of a slow-healing wound, requires additional investigation to identify the etiology. Treating the underlying cause is the most prudent way to manage pain. Is the pain due to a recurrent erosion, a smoldering iritis, or even extreme patient sensitivity? Pain management is important, but can often be handled with education. In most cases, the pain is most severe in the first 24 hours after FB removal and abates quickly. Cycloplegic agents and limiting light into the eye with the use of sunwear protection typically manage the pain. In more severe cases, bandage contact lenses, over-the-counter ibuprofen, and topical nonsteroidal anti-inflammatory agents will help get the patient over the pain threshold during the first few hours.[7] Rarely is anything additional required. The use of oral narcotics for pain should be prescribed infrequently and with the utmost caution as they are rarely necessary.

## VIDEOS OF PROCEDURES

**Video 24-1**—Removal of a metallic foreign body (FB) with a 25-gauge needle, followed by the use of an Alger brush to remove the remaining rust ring: This video shows the removal of a metallic FB. The patient presenting was a healthy 30-year-old who had been grinding metal approximately a day and a half ago. The patient had a prior history of having metallic FBs in the cornea. This depicts a classic metallic FB with a surrounding rust ring. The patient's visual acuities were unaffected, and pain was described as constant and moderate in intensity. The initial FB was removed with a 25-gauge needle under topical anesthetic. The primary FB proved to be very superficial and was easily removed with the needle. After the FB was dislodged, it took up residence in the lower cul-de-sac and was removed from the eye with a sterile cotton swap. An Alger brush was used to remove the residual rust ring. Note the cornea appears to indent while the rust is being removed as some pressure must be applied to adequately remove the rust. The most stubborn area of rust required the burr be operated by the other hand so the blades of the burr spin in an opposite direction and aid in excavating more rust. It is well within standard of care to leave a slight amount of discolored tissue in the pit of the rust as demonstrated by this video. The patient was placed on ophthalmic tobramycin and a follow-up was conducted in 1 week. (Courtesy of Dr. Nate Lighthizer.)

**Video 24-2**—Removal of an organic foreign body (FB) with a curved spud. This video demonstrates the removal of a nonmetallic corneal FB. This patient had been cleaning his woodstove 2 days prior to reporting to the clinic with symptoms. The patient had the classic symptoms of tearing and corneal FB sensation and reported the pain as mild. His vision was unaffected and demonstrated no findings of a penetrating injury. A corneal FB was noted superior temporal to the pupillary axis and recorded as superficial. The upper lids were everted, and no palpebral conjunctival FBs were located. The FB, presumably organic from cleaning the stove, was removed with a simple wrist flick using an FB spud. The area of tissue disruption was minimal, and the wound was superficial with no evidence of infection. The patient was placed on topical tobramycin solution QID and advised to return if he was not symptom free in 3 days. (Courtesy of Dr. Matthew Krein.)

## EFFICACY

Efficacy is defined as the ability to produce a desired or intended result. For the purpose of evaluating efficacy, the discussion is limited to superficial corneal and conjunctival FBs that have not penetrated the cornea. As with many medical procedures, efficacy is dependent on the appropriate diagnosis and timely competent treatment. It is the author's opinion based on numerous clinical encounters that removing corneal and conjunctival FBs is an extremely efficacious procedure, benefiting the patient both in function and comfort. Complications, although rare, must be managed promptly and appropriately to promote efficacy.

## CODING/BILLING AND MODIFIERS

Billing and coding for ocular FBs:

The codes commonly used in ophthalmic practice for the removal of a corneal or conjunctival, nonperforating FB are as follows:

- **65205**—Removal of FB, external eye; conjunctival superficial[15]
- **65210**—Removal of FB, external eye; conjunctival embedded (includes concretions), subconjunctival or scleral nonperforating[15]
- **65220**—Removal of FB, external eye; corneal, without slit lamp[15]
- **65222**—Removal of FB, external eye; corneal, with slit lamp[15]

Included in the global surgical fee is the initial evaluation preceding the removal procedure as well as the initial bandage contact lens (if necessary), and these services are not billed separately from the surgical procedure Current Procedural Terminology (CPT) code. A −25 modifier may accompany a 99XXX code only if another problem unrelated to the surgical procedure is to be addressed at the same visit. These codes should be correlated with the appropriate -RT or -LT modifier to identify which eye was affected by the FB. If FBs are identified in each eye, they should be reported as two separate procedures, with the −52 modifier attached to the code for the second eye. If one eye has multiple FBs, only one global surgical code can be submitted unless FBs are located in both the cornea and conjunctiva, in which case both surgical codes can be reported separately with a −51 modifier.[4,16]

ICD-10 options:

- **T15.00XA**—FB in cornea, unspecified eye, initial encounter
- **T15.00XD**—FB in cornea, unspecified eye, subsequent encounter
- **T15.00XS**—FB in cornea, unspecified eye, sequela
- **T15.10XA**—FB in conjunctiva, unspecified eye, initial encounter
- **T15.10XD**—FB in conjunctiva, unspecified eye, subsequent encounter
- **T15.10XS**—FB in conjunctiva, unspecified eye, sequela
- **T15.01XA**—FB in cornea, right eye, initial encounter
- **T15.01XD**—FB in cornea, right eye, subsequent encounter
- **T15.01XS**—FB in cornea, right eye, sequela
- **T15.11XA**—FB in conjunctiva, right eye, initial encounter
- **T15.11XD**—FB in conjunctiva, right eye, subsequent encounter
- **T15.11XS**—FB in conjunctiva, right eye, sequela

- **T15.02XA**—FB in cornea, left eye, initial encounter
- **T15.02XD**—FB in cornea, left eye, subsequent encounter
- **T15.02XS**—FB in cornea, left eye, sequela
- **T15.12XA**—FB in conjunctiva, left eye, initial encounter
- **T15.12XD**—FB in conjunctiva, left eye, subsequent encounter
- **T15.12XS**—FB in conjunctiva, left eye, sequela

The global period for these FB removal procedures is 0 day; therefore, all follow-up visits should be billed with the appropriate 99XXX code. The initial follow-up would be billed with the ICD-10 code T15.00XD, and the D would be replaced by an S to bill for additional follow-ups that may be medically necessary.

## REFERENCES


1. Filips RF, Kattouf VM. *Clinical Pearls for Optometry*. 2nd ed. Anadem Publishing; 2006.
2. Casser L, Fingeret M, Woodcome HT, Schilling SP, Tilberry SC. *Atlas of Primary Eyecare Procedures*. 2nd ed. Appleton & Lange; 1997.
3. Gunenc U, Maden A, Knynak S. Magnetic resonance imaging and computed tomography in the detection and localization of intraocular foreign bodies. *Doc Ophthalmol*. 1992;81:369-378.
4. Pate CB. Be an ocular foreign body fixer. *Rev Optom*. 2019;156(4):60-65. Accessed October 5, 2022. https://www.revieweducationgroup.com/ce/be-an-ocular-foreign-body-fixer
5. Shetler J, Lighthizer N. Foreign body removal in 12 steps. *Rev Optom*. 2015;152(12):22-29. Accessed October 5, 2022. https://www.reviewofoptometry.com/article/foreign-body-removal-in-12-steps
6. Centers for Disease Control and Prevention. Eye safety. Accessed September 30, 2010. www.cdc.gov/niosh/topics/eye
7. Koetting C. Foreign body removal start to finish: these patients are in need of help—quickly. Here's how to prepare your office. *Rev Optom*. 2020;157(4):30-34. Accessed October 5, 2022. https://www.reviewofoptometry.com/article/foreign-body-removal-start-to-finish
8. Langston DP, ed. *Manual of Ocular Diagnosis and Therapy*. 4th ed. Little Brown & Co; 1996.
9. Hendricks B. Clinical pearls in corneal foreign body removal. *Rev Optom*. 2022;159(4):32-41. Accessed October 5, 2022. https://www.reviewofoptometry.com/article/clinical-pearls-in-corneal-foreign-body-removal
10. Bronner A. No insult to injury: managing foreign body removal. *Rev Optom*. 2017;154(1):47-54. Accessed October 5, 2022. https://www.reviewofoptometry.com/article/no-insult-to-injury-managing-foreign--body-removal
11. Gerstenblith AT, Rabinowitz MP. *The Wills Eye Manual: Office and Emergency Room Diagnosis and Treatment of Eye Disease*. 6th ed. Lippincott Williams & Wilkins; 2012.
12. Rhee DJ, Pyfer MF. *The Wills Eye Manual: Office and Emergency Room Diagnosis and Treatment of Eye Disease*. 3rd ed. Lippincott Williams & Wilkins; 1999.
13. Upadhyay MP, Karmacharya P, Koirala K, et al. The Bhaktapur eye study: ocular trauma and antibiotic prophylaxis for the prevention of corneal ulceration in Nepal. *Br J Ophthalmol*. 2001;85(4):388-392.
14. Tyhurst KN, Hettler DL. Infection control guidelines—an update for the optometric practice. *Optometry*. 2009;80(11):613-620.
15. American Medical Association. *CPT 2022 Professional Edition*. American Medical Association; 2021.
16. Wright A, Burns C. Coding and billing how-to: corneal foreign body visits. *Rev Optom Bus*. Published May 3, 2017. Accessed October 12, 2022. https://www.reviewob.com/coding-corneal-foreign-body-dos-donts/#:~:text=The%20ICD%2D10%20diagnosis%20code,%2C%20left%20eye%2C%20initial%20encounter

# 25 Corneal Debridement

Sophia Leung • Jason Ellen

## BACKGROUND

Corneal debridement for corneal opacities and lesions has been documented since the early 1950s. This procedure involves the manual dissection, surgical excision, or removal of the superficial corneal layers without tissue replacement. Typically, the epithelial layer is removed while preserving Bowman's layer.[1,2] Diamond burr polishing to smoothen underlying layers (Bowman's layer or anterior stroma if Bowman's layer is missing) and remove defective epithelial tissue or persistent abnormalities is strongly recommended following corneal debridement.[1,3] Alternative nomenclature for this procedure includes superficial keratectomy, epithelial debridement, and epithelial basement membrane debridement.[1]

Goals of corneal debridement can be diagnostic or therapeutic. Diagnostically, corneal debridement facilitates obtaining tissue for biopsies, with minimal damage to adjacent tissue. This is applicable in suspicious corneal lesions or growths. Therapeutic goals include improving corneal transparency without significantly changing corneal topography. This allows improved visual acuities, as well as alleviates ocular surface discomfort and other symptoms associated with certain corneal surface diseases.[2,4]

## INDICATIONS

**Key Indications**

- Epithelial basement membrane dystrophy (EBMD)
- Recurrent corneal erosions (RCE)
- Salzmann nodular degeneration
- Infectious keratitis
- Band keratopathy
- Suspected ocular surface neoplasia (diagnostic indication)

## Epithelial Basement Membrane Dystrophy

- Poor epithelial layer attachment because of abnormal basement membrane structure causes higher risk of RCE, symptoms of intermittent blurred vision, and ocular surface discomfort.[5] In the context of preoperative cataract surgery consideration, untreated or undiagnosed EBMD can result in inaccurate intraocular lens (IOL) calculations and postoperative corneal healing issues.[3]
- The goal of corneal debridement in EBMD is to remove the unhealthy or poorly adhered epithelium, optimize the Bowman's layer, and allow regeneration of new firmly attached epithelial tissue for a healthy and smooth ocular surface.[1,3] Inclusion criteria for studies reporting on this procedure for EBMD include negative fluorescein staining within the central 6 mm of the cornea, suggestive patient symptoms, and/or measurable astigmatism attributable to the corneal surface.[2]

## Recurrent Corneal Erosions

- This condition is characterized by a recurring disruption of epithelial attachment to the underlying Bowman's layer. Trauma and corneal dystrophies such as EBMD are the most common etiologies.[1,5]
- Treatment goals are similar to EBMD. Some studies have also reported good success with anterior stromal puncture performed simultaneously with corneal debridement, including with visual axis involvement.[2,6]

## Salzmann Nodular Degeneration

- Salzmann nodules appear as blue/white-gray nodules formed anterior to Bowman's layer with thinned and defective overlying epithelium. The basement membrane is disrupted, leading to irregular proliferation, migration, and deposition of disorganized extracellular matrix at the basement membrane and Bowman's layer junction.[7,8] Salzmann nodular degeneration often coexists with EBMD and is also associated with post-LASIK, other ocular surface diseases, and Crohn's disease in recurring bilateral cases. It is also associated with Meibomian gland dysfunction in up to 53% of cases.[2,7,8]
- Treatment goals of corneal debridement aim to remove the nodules, restore healthy epithelial tissue, improve ocular surface comfort, and stabilize fluctuating refractive error changes.

## Infectious Keratitis

- Corneal debridement in infectious keratitis can be in both a diagnostic and therapeutic capacity. In corneal ulcers that are large, chronic, extending into the deeper stroma, unresponsive to empirical therapy, or suspicious of fungal or amoebic activity, corneal culturing is imperative. Debridement allows the removal of epithelial layers for proper tissue sampling.[4]
- Poor healing epithelium in a slow-healing corneal ulcer or active viral infection, such as *Herpes simplex* dendritic keratitis, may benefit from having devitalized tissue removed to promote healing.[4] This must be performed with appropriate therapeutic antimicrobial treatment under close observation.

## Band Keratopathy

- Calcific deposition in the corneal layers occurs from chronic ocular or systemic disease, particularly inflammatory conditions. Band keratopathy presents as a horizontal calcium band that starts at the nasal and temporal cornea, with a clear lucid space between the limbus and calcium deposition.[4,9] EDTA chelation has been largely reported on being effective in removing corneal calcium deposits. However, chelation in isolation can be slow and limited to superficial areas of calcification. Studies now report that a combination of corneal debridement, diamond burr polish, and EDTA chelation has higher success in the treatment of band keratopathy.[4]

## Suspected Ocular Surface Neoplasia

- This is a diagnostic application of corneal debridement. Removed tissue is sent for biopsy. Several authors report that any doubt in diagnosis based on clinical appearance alone warrants diagnostic corneal debridement for cytologic and histopathologic investigation. Clinicians performing this procedure should be comfortable with proper biopsy and tissue collection protocols. Comanagement or referral to corneal specialists should be considered.[2,4]

# CONTRAINDICATIONS

**Key Contraindications**

- Pterygium
- Bullous keratopathy
- Other corneal dystrophies and scarring

## Pterygium

- Abnormal epithelial and fibrovascular tissue growth leads to corneal invasion across the limbus. This can impair vision and result in recurrent inflammation. Although the exact pathogenesis remains unclear, altered epithelial cell proliferation and vascularization triggered by ultraviolet (UV) exposure, viral infections, and hereditary predisposition have been discussed.
- Surgical removal techniques include bare sclera excision, conjunctival autograft, conjunctival transpositional flap, and amniotic membrane (AM) grafting. Although corneal debridement alone may be able to remove the pterygium tissue away from the cornea, it is insufficient as treatment goals include decreasing recurrences, which have been reported as high as 90%.[10]

## Bullous Keratopathy

- Coalesced fluid accumulates in the epithelium and subepithelium, commonly caused by endothelial dysfunction or significant inflammation. Advanced age, history of ocular trauma, or ocular surgeries risking endothelial cell loss and damage have been implicated. Corneal grafting or transplants are the primary treatment of choice. Corneal debridement has been considered a treatment option in several studies, but it should only be considered with endothelial keratoplasty, which would not be performed in an office-based setting.[1]

## Other Corneal Dystrophies and Scarring

- OCT-guided phototherapeutic keratectomy is typically the primary treatment of choice for corneal dystrophies and scars, depending on the depth of stromal involvement. Manual corneal debridement may be considered for scars and lesions no deeper than the anterior stroma. However, this requires a delay in treatment of at least 6 to 12 months after the initial corneal consult to allow for scar regression without surgical intervention. Caution for surgical dissection of deeper corneal layers is paramount for risk of ectasias, perforation, and significant topographical alterations.[4]

# PREOPERATIVE PREPARATION

Informed consent via paper or electronic means should address the risks, benefits, and potential complications of the procedure in plain language. This should include a simple explanation of the corneal debridement procedure, its indications and purpose, and potential alternative treatments. Typical postoperative expectations and adverse effects should be listed. A statement outlining that the counseling physician discussed the procedure, risks involved, and expected results should be included, with signatures from the patient, the counseling physician, and a witness (typically a staff member).

## Equipment Required[2-4] (Figure 25-1)

- Slit-lamp *or* surgical microscope in a minor surgical suite
- Topical ophthalmic anesthetic (0.5% proparacaine)
- Topical ophthalmic antibiotic (0.5% moxifloxacin)
- Buffer saline solution (BSS) (multiple bottles)
- Povidone–iodine 10% swab stick (Betadine) application
- Sterile drape
- Lid speculum
- Surgical blade (diagnostic)
  - #57 or #64 Blade
  - No. 15 Bard-Parker blade
- Foreign body spud or Kimura spatula
- Amoils rotary brush (*optional*)
- Forceps (nontoothed or microtoothed)

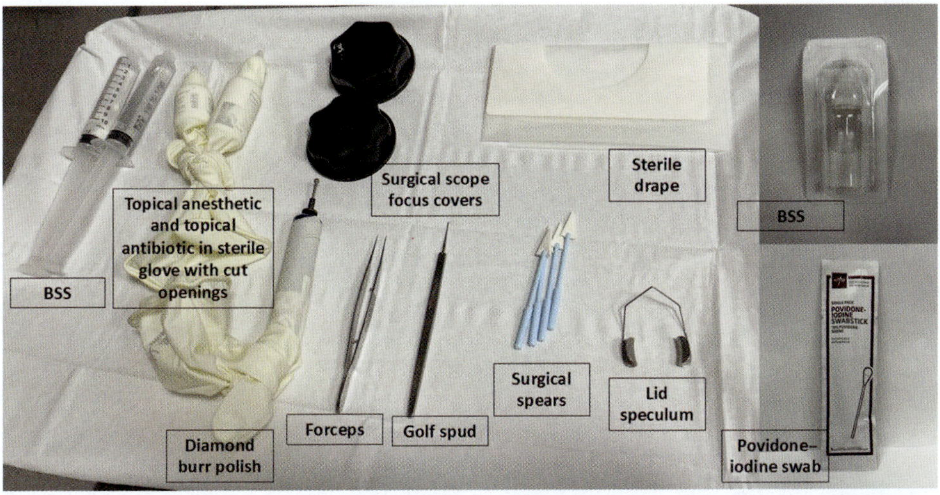


**FIGURE 25-1** A majority of the equipment used in procedure videos shown here. BSS, buffer saline solution.

- Surgical spear sponges (Weck-cel)
- Sterile cotton swabs
- EtOH 20% (*optional*)
- Alcohol well (*optional*)
- Cotton corneal light shield (*optional*)
- Diamond burr
- Bandage contact lens (BCL)
- Amniotic membrane (AM)

## THE PROCEDURE[1,2,4,7,11,12]

1. Clean the eyelid and lashes of the affected eye with standard povidone–iodine 10% swab stick (Betadine).
2. Instill topical ophthalmic anesthetic and apply a sterile drape.
3. Insert eyelid speculum in the affected eye.
4. *Optional: alcohol delamination*
    a. Apply 20% EtOH to the cornea using an alcohol well or a saturated cotton corneal light shield for 40 seconds.
    b. Absorb EtOH from alcohol well with surgical spear sponges or remove saturated light shield using forceps.
5. Using a dry surgical spear sponge, surgical blade, foreign body spud, or Amoils rotary brush, remove weakened epithelium (Figure 25-2).
    a. Leave at least 1 mm of peripheral epithelium at the limbus. Edges of the debrided area can be cleaned up using forceps.
6. Irrigate with BSS to remove epithelial debris.

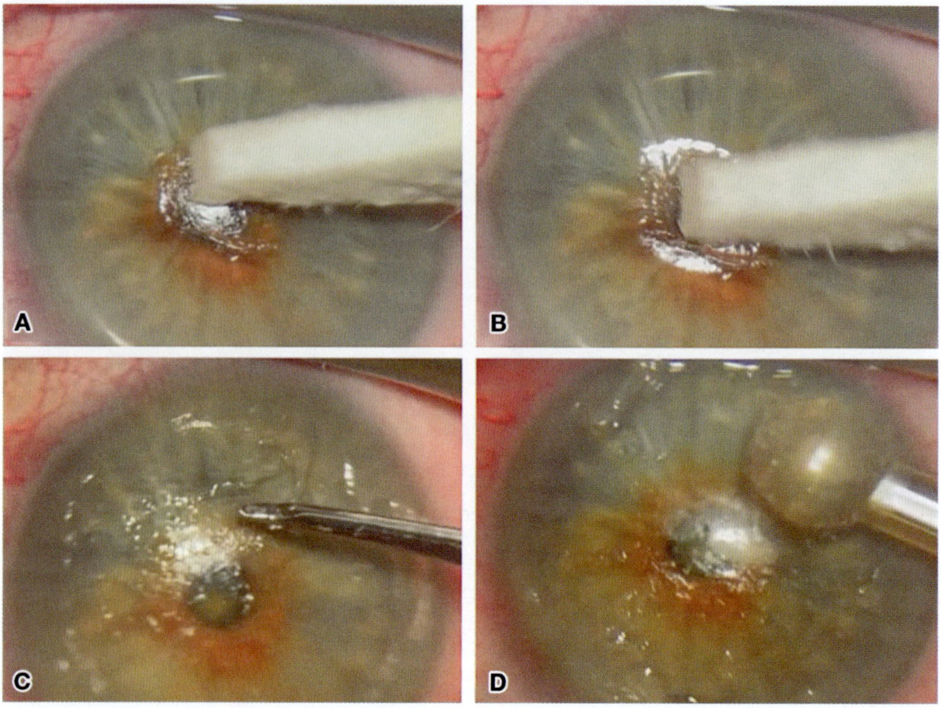


FIGURE 25-2 Corneal debridement procedure shown. **A,** Loose epithelium is removed with a surgical spear. **B,** Depression of cornea shown. **C,** Golf spud is used to further remove tissue and smoothen out layers. **D,** Diamond burr polishing of Bowman's layer to remove persistent epithelial attachments is shown.

7. *Recommended: diamond burr polishing*
   a. Perform diamond burr polishing by making gentle uniform circular movements no more than 30 seconds at a time to avoid too much pressure. Rotations of the diamond burr head should be directed toward the visual axis to avoid limbal cell damage.
8. Instill topical ophthalmic antibiotic after the procedure.
9. Insert BCL in the treated eye for pain management and wound coverage.
   a. Consider AM placement for improved surface healing.
10. Remove the lid speculum being careful not to dislodge or disturb the BCL or AM device.

## FOCAL DEBRIDEMENT (WHEN TREATING A PORTION OR SECTION OF THE CORNEA)

1. Clean the eyelid and lashes of the affected eye with standard povidone–iodine 10% swab stick (Betadine).
2. Instill topical ophthalmic proparacaine and apply a sterile drape as necessary.
3. Insert eyelid speculum in the affected eye as necessary.
4. Test for area of loose tissue with a dry surgical spear sponge or sterile cotton swab.

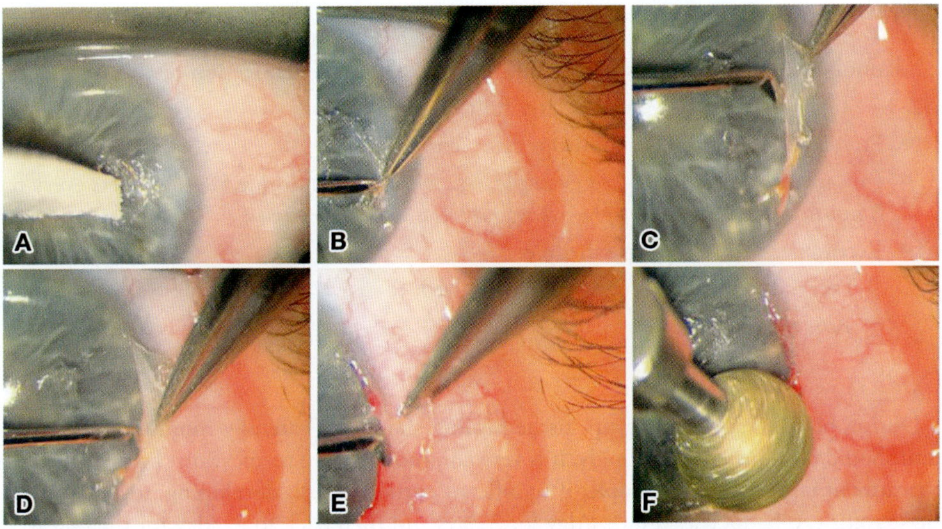


**FIGURE 25-3** Salzmann nodule removal. **A,** Loose epithelium adjacent to Salzmann nodule removed with surgical spear. **B,** Salzmann nodule grasped with forceps and a golf spud is used to detach Salzmann nodular tissue from layers below. **C,** "Peeling" motion is made with forceps. **D,** Salzmann nodular removal is performed to the limbus if limbal area involved. **E,** Care is taken to avoid extending past limbus. **F,** Diamond burr polishing of Bowman's layer to remove persistent epithelial attachments is shown.

5. Debride areas of loose epithelium with a surgical spear sponge (Weck-cel), surgical blade, or foreign body spud.
   a. Salzmann nodules can be removed by grasping the edge of the nodule with microtoothed or nontoothed forceps and separating it from underlying layers using a flat-edge spatula or foreign body spud (Figure 25-3).
   b. Granular or calcific depositing, as found in various corneal dystrophies, can be peeled off with a blunt blade or surgical spear sponge in a continuous plane. Sharp dissection may be required if peripheral or surrounding tissue cannot be shaved off or if a smooth surface beneath the lesion is otherwise not possible.
6. Clean up edges of debrided area with forceps, clearing away rolled edges.
7. Insert BCL for pain management and wound coverage. Consider AM application for improved surface healing.
8. Remove lid speculum, being careful not to dislodge or disturb the BCL or AM.

# POSTOPERATIVE CARE/COMANAGEMENT (FOLLOW-UP SCHEDULE)

### Key Postoperative Considerations[2-4]

- Topical ophthalmic antibiotic drops QID (Avoid topical antibiotics that have propensity for corneal precipitation such as ciprofloxacin.)

- Topical steroid drops (e.g., prednisolone acetate 1% ophthalmic suspension or loteprednol 0.5% ophthalmic solution) TID (unless concern for infection or corneal melting)
  - Taper steroids over 3 weeks after fully epithelialized
- Preservative-free lubrication drops every 2 to 3 hours
- Pain medication (orals)—for example, tramadol hydrochloride 50 mg tablets every 6 to 8 hours as needed. *Proper prescribing protocols must be followed.*
- Recommended follow-up schedule:
  - Every few days until fully re-epithelialized, then every 1 to 2 weeks for stability
  - 1, 4, then at 8 weeks

During postoperative follow-up, tissue healing should be carefully monitored, and treatment should be adjusted accordingly. It is very common to have medication changes according to treatment response. For example, if significant corneal haze is developing, topical ophthalmic steroids can be increased to 6×/day for 2 days and then back to 4×/day for the first week. If a cryopreserved AM is used, a topical steroid may not be necessary. However, if a dehydrated AM with a BCL is used, then a topical ophthalmic steroid is still recommended to prevent hypoxia-induced corneal infiltrates.

If corneal tissue healing seems delayed or poor, consider decreasing the topical ophthalmic steroids to 2×/day and adding topical ophthalmic cyclosporine. Certain advanced dry eye disease medications such as autologous serum eye drops or plasma-rich plasma drops, for example, could be continued if tissue healing is poor.

Studies have reported that 81% of patients are typically fully epithelialized at the 1-week postoperative visit.[1] Patients should be made aware that vision will be blurred during healing and that significant ocular pain is expected for the first 1 to 3 days. Patients should also be advised to stay out of dry and/or dusty environments and consider refrigerating their preservative-free lubrication drops for comfort.

## POTENTIAL COMPLICATIONS AND THEIR TREATMENTS

### Key Potential Complications

- Corneal haze
- Ocular pain
- Delayed epithelial healing
- Microbial keratitis (rare)

Corneal haze is the most common complication, reported in up to 26% of cases of corneal debridement with diamond burr polish. Without diamond burr polishing, corneal haze was reported in up to 35% of cases. However, the level at which corneal haze is considered visually significant is minimally reported. Although prophylactic use of mitomycin C is routinely used with tissue ablation, it is rarely used with corneal debridement. This is mainly because corneal debridement is relatively much more superficial than tissue ablation, and the potential risks of mitomycin C do not outweigh the potential benefit. There are presently no randomized controlled trials comparing the use of mitomycin C in superficial keratectomies versus superficial keratectomies with diamond burr polishing. AMs, on the other hand, have been reported to be successful in reducing scarring and corneal haze. Extending topical steroids with a slow taper to encourage haze reduction may be warranted on a case-by-case situation[1-3,13-15] (Figure 25-4).

Ocular pain is commonly reported and can persist for a few days. Informing patients of expected discomfort after the procedure can help manage expectations. Prescribing pain

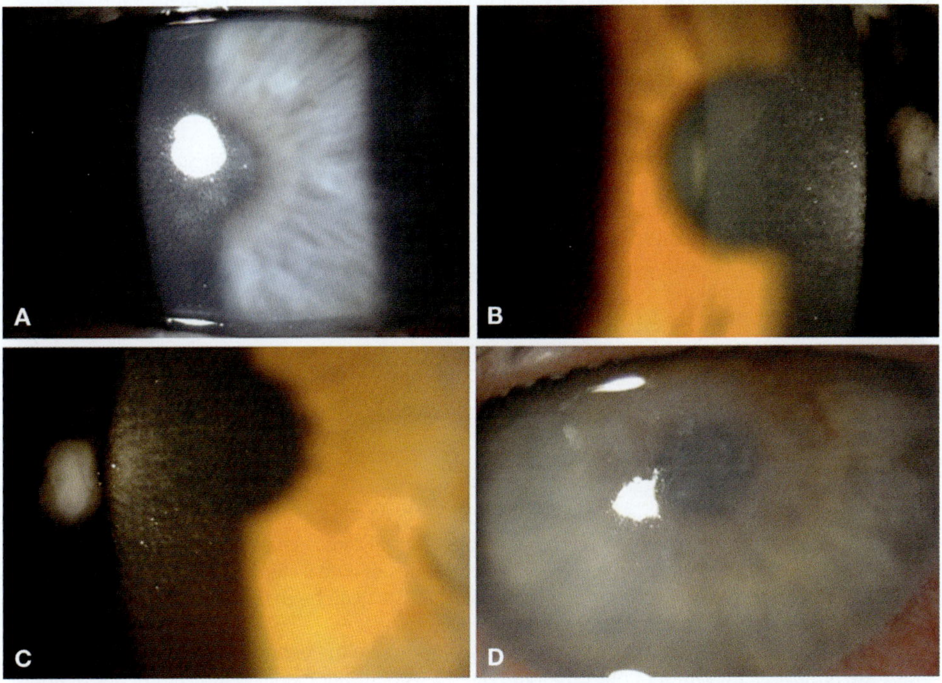


**FIGURE 25-4** Examples of different levels of corneal haze after corneal debridement. **A,** An appropriate level of corneal haze 48 hours after a simple focal corneal debridement is shown. A standard topical steroid taper was sufficient here. **B,** Shown here is an appropriate level of corneal haze at 1 week following a superficial keratectomy with diamond burr polishing. A standard topical steroid taper was also sufficient here. **C,** This is an example of mild persistent corneal haze that was present at 1 month following a superficial keratectomy with diamond burr polishing. In this case, topical ophthalmic steroids were extended at BID for 1 week, then QD for 1 week. The residual corneal haze was slightly less and not visually significant at the end of the taper schedule. **D,** An excessive amount of corneal haze with stromal keratitis is shown here. Corneal debridement was performed for culturing and to remove necrotic tissue in a patient with *Acanthamoeba* keratitis. Topical treatment including a combination of antiparasitic medications and steroids was adjusted on a follow-up to follow-up basis based on treatment response. Topical ophthalmic steroids were carefully decreased over 14 months.

medications responsibly can help with pain control.[1] Delayed epithelial healing, RCE, and recurrences of the treated condition have been reported as well. These cases may require alternative therapies including specialty contact lenses or more aggressive therapy such as deep anterior lamellar keratoplasties or partial tarsorrhaphies if corneal scarring or persistent epithelial defects develop.[3]

Microbial keratitis is a rare but possible complication. Topical antibiotics may need to be adjusted quickly should infection be suspected. In patients who have had a history of recurring herpetic keratitis, prophylactic oral antivirals may be necessary.

## VIDEOS OF PROCEDURES

**Video 25-1**—Corneal debridement + Diamond burr polish (DBP) + amniotic membrane (AM) insertion (epithelial basement membrane dystrophy [EBMD]).

Prior to the procedure, the patient is fully numbed with topical ophthalmic anesthetic drops, lids and lashes cleaned with standard povidone–iodine 10% swab stick (Betadine), and draped for a sterile environment. Topical ophthalmic antibiotic drops should be instilled prior to starting the procedure.

This video shows loose epithelium gently debrided using a dry surgical spear sponge, leaving behind roughly 1 to 1 ½ mm of tissue from the limbus. Special care is taken to remove any redundant epithelial layers and basement membrane islands. Clumps of debrided epithelial tissue are seen being removed with a surgical spear sponge. Rolled edges at the edge of the debridement zone are shown being cleaned up with a foreign body golf spud.

The diamond burr polishing is shown with smooth circular motions. Rotations of the diamond burr are made away from the limbus, toward the center. Any residual islands of epithelial tissue or defective basement membrane are removed at this step.

A cryopreserved AM is shown being inserted into the patient's eye after corneal debridement and diamond burr polishing.

**Video 25-2**—Salzmann nodule removal + DBP + cryopreserved AM insertion.

This video shows loose epithelium around a Salzmann nodule being debrided. Then, forceps are used to grasp the edge of the Salzmann nodule, lifting it away while using a foreign body golf spud to detach the nodule from the underlying layers.

Salzmann nodules can often extend to the limbus. Special care is taken not to tear conjunctival tissue. Provided that there are neighboring areas or sources of limbal stem cells, focal debridement to the limbus can be performed, as it is here. Wescott scissors can be used to cut the tissue as well. This could have been an option here.

Diamond burr polishing is shown next over the areas where the debridement and Salzmann nodules were removed. Smooth motions no more than 30 seconds are made, being careful not to apply too much pressure onto the cornea and being careful not to disrupt the limbal area too much. An AM is inserted following the procedure.

**Video 25-3**—Salzmann nodule removal + DBP + dehydrated AM and BCL insertion.

This video shows a large Salzmann nodule being debrided using a golf spud and forceps. Another area of the cornea affected by EBMD is also shown being debrided. Diamond burr polishing is performed, including gentle polishing at the limbus where the Salzmann nodule was previously located.

A dehydrated AM disc is placed onto the cornea and carefully rehydrated to allow for proper positioning and covering. A BCL is then inserted overtop.

**Video 25-4**—Corneal debridement + DBP (gelatinous drop-like corneal dystrophy).

This patient had a gelatinous drop-like corneal dystrophy appearance, which affected the entire cornea, resulting in significant ocular surface discomfort and decreased visual acuity.

The patient was fully numbed with topical ophthalmic anesthetic drops, lids and lashes cleaned with standard povidone–iodine 10% swab stick (Betadine), and draped for a sterile environment. Topical ophthalmic antibiotic drops were instilled prior to starting the procedure.

A lid speculum is shown being inserted onto the eye. The corneal debridement begins with loose epithelium overlying the gelatinous nodules being easily removed by a foreign body golf spud. Interestingly, sheet-like layers of tissue are observed and are seen being peeled away in large sections at a time. Circular motions are made to guide the debridement, being careful to leave 1 to 1 ½ mm of tissue from the limbus intact. Forceps are used to guide this process along, with a technique similar to Salzmann nodule removal.

After the initial epithelial layer and nodules are removed, any areas of redundant basement membrane are further removed by using a foreign body golf spud to debride any residual islands. Nodular material near the limbus is also smoothed out or removed to reduce recurrence as much as possible.

After a few drops of buffer saline solution is instilled to keep the ocular tissue moisturized, diamond burr polishing is shown, with the rotation of the diamond burr rotating away from the limbus, or rather, toward the center of the cornea.

## EFFICACY

For *EBMD and RCE*, corneal debridement with diamond burr polishing has recurrence rates of 0% to 11.1%. Corneal debridement alone resulted in 24% recurrence rates, whereas phototherapeutic keratectomy (PTK) resulted in 27% recurrence rates with significant changes in refractive error.[2,13,14] In a small study, corneal debridement with diamond burr polish followed by cryopreserved AM application resulted in 67% of corneas healed without any staining, with 100% of patients treated having no residual symptoms at the 1-month follow-up.[3] Other studies have reported a statistically significant improvement in corneal and refractive astigmatism. No statistical difference has been reported for techniques with or without alcohol delamination.[2,4,13]

For *Salzmann nodular degeneration*, 90% to 100% of patients treated reported subjective improvement and 78% to 100% of patients had decreased corneal astigmatism. Recurrence rates of 22% have been reported, with some requiring repeat debridement over 5 years of follow-up.[1,2,14]

In *band keratopathy*, corneal debridement with EDTA chelation resulted in significant improvement in clinical signs and symptoms in 72% to 100%, according to multiple studies. Visual acuity improvement of two or more lines was reported in 35%, whereas 8% lost two lines of visual acuity. Recurrence rates were reported in several studies to be 0% to 17% for corneal debridement with EDTA chelation, and 12.5% to 28% without EDTA chelation.[1,2,16]

## CODING AND BILLING

- **65435**—Removal of corneal epithelium with or without chemocauterization, 0 day global period.

Corneal debridement is considered a minor procedure. A minor surgical procedure already includes the office visit, meaning that it should not be billed in conjunction with a same-day office visit (unless the office visit was unrelated to the decision to perform the minor surgery). Corneal procedures cannot be billed on the same day as 92071 (fitting of a contact lens for ocular surface disease) or 65778 (placement of AM; without sutures).[17,18]

Common ICD-10 codes that support the removal of corneal epithelium include (right eye used as an example)[19]:

- **H16.011**—Central corneal ulcer, right eye
- **H16.021**—Ring corneal ulcer, right eye
- **H16.041**—Marginal corneal ulcer, right eye
- **H16.061**—Mycotic corneal ulcer, right eye
- **H16.121**—Filamentary keratitis, right eye
- **H18.421**—Band keratopathy, right eye
- **H18.43**—Other calcareous corneal degeneration
- **H18.441**—Keratomalacia, right eye
- **H18.451**—Nodular corneal degeneration, right eye
- **H18.461**—Peripheral corneal degeneration, right eye
- **H18.49**—Other corneal degeneration
- **H18.611**—Keratoconus, stable, right eye
- **H18.831**—Recurrent erosion of cornea, right eye
- **S05.01XA**—Injury of conjunctiva and corneal abrasion without foreign body, right eye, initial encounter
- **T26.61XA**—Corrosion of cornea and conjunctival sac, right eye, initial encounter

## ACKNOWLEDGMENT

Special thanks to Dr. Cedrick Mah for assisting with equipment photos.

## REFERENCES


1. Salari F, Beikmarzehei A, Liu G, Zarei-Ghanavati M, Liu C. Superficial keratectomy: a review of literature. *Front Med.* 2022;9:915284. doi:10.3389/fmed.2022.915284
2. Bae SS, Chan CC. Superficial keratectomy: indications and outcomes. *Can J Ophthalmol.* 2018;53(6):553-559. doi:10.1016/j.jcjo.2018.01.030
3. Yeu E, Hashem O, Sheha H. Treatment of epithelial basement membrane dystrophy to optimize the ocular surface prior to cataract surgery. *Clin Ophthalmol.* 2022; 16:785-795. doi:10.2147/OPTH.S356421
4. McGrath LA, Lee GA. Corneal epithelial debridement for diagnosis and therapy of ocular surface disease. *Clin Exp Optom.* 2015;98(2):155-159. doi:10.1111/cxo.12213
5. Meghpara B, Hammersmith KM. Anterior corneal dystrophies. In: Mannis M, Holland E, eds. *Cornea: Fundamentals, Diagnosis, and Management.* 5th ed. Elsevier Inc; 2022:701.e1-711.
6. Itty S, Hamilton SS, Baratz KH, Diehl NN, Maguire LJ. Outcomes of epithelial debridement for anterior basement membrane dystrophy. *Am J Ophthalmol.* 2007;144(2):217-221. doi:10.1016/j.ajo.2007.04.024
7. Paranjpe V, Galor A, Monsalve P, Dubovy SR, Karp CL. Salzmann nodular degeneration: prevalence, impact, and management strategies. *Clin Ophthalmol.* 2019;13:1305-1314.
8. Roszkowska AM, Aragona P, Spinella R, Pisani A, Puzzolo D, Micali A. Morphologic and confocal investigation on Salzmann nodular degeneration of the cornea. *Investig Ophthalmol Vis Sci.* 2011;52(8):5910-5919. doi:10.1167/iovs.11-7789
9. Kwon YS, Song YS, Kim JC. New treatment for band keratopathy: superficial lamellar keratectomy, EDTA chelation and amniotic membrane transplantation. *J Korean Med Sci.* 2004;19(4):611-615. doi:10.3346/jkms.2004.19.4.611
10. Nuzzi R, Tridico F. How to minimize pterygium recurrence rates: clinical perspectives. *Clin Ophthalmol.* 2018;12:2347-2362. doi:10.2147/OPTH.S186543

11. McGrath LA, Lee GA. Techniques, indications and complications of corneal debridement. *Surv Ophthalmol.* 2014;59(1):47-63. doi:10.1016/j.survophthal.2013.03.004
12. Teus MA, de Benito-Llopis L, Alió JL. Mitomycin C in corneal refractive surgery. *Surv Ophthalmol.* 2009;54(4): 487-502. doi:10.1016/j.survophthal.2009.04.002
13. Vo RC, Chen JL, Sanchez PJ, Yu F, Aldave AJ. Long-term outcomes of epithelial debridement and diamond burr polishing for corneal epithelial irregularity and recurrent corneal erosion. *Cornea.* 2015;34(10):1259-1265. doi:10.1097/ICO.0000000000000554
14. Maharana PK, Sharma N, Das S, et al. Salzmann's nodular degeneration. *Ocul Surf.* 2016;14(1):20-30. doi:10.1016/j.jtos.2015.08.006
15. Arranz-Marquez E, Katsanos A, Kozobolis VP, Konstas AGP, Teus MA. A critical overview of the biological effects of mitomycin C application on the cornea following refractive surgery. *Adv Ther.* 2019;36(4):786-797. doi:10.1007/s12325-019-00905-w
16. Najjar DM, Cohen EJ, Rapuano CJ, Laibson PR. EDTA chelation for calcific band keratopathy: results and long-term follow-up. *Am J Ophthalmol.* 2004;137(6):1056-1064. doi:10.1016/j.ajo.2004.01.036
17. Corcoran Consulting Group. Reimbursement for amniotic tissue. Published 2022. Accessed August 29, 2022. https://www.corcoranccg.com/products/faqs/amniotic-tissue/.
18. Rumpakis J. Minor procedures, major rules. *Rev Optom.* Published 2020. Accessed August 29, 2022. https://www.reviewofoptometry.com/article/minor-procedures-major-rules
19. American Medical Association. *CPT 2021 Professional Edition.* American Medical Association; 2020.

# 26 Anterior Stromal Puncture

Sophia Leung

## BACKGROUND

Anterior stromal puncture (ASP) focuses on the anterior portion of the cornea: namely the epithelium, basement membrane, Bowman's layer, and anterior stroma. In a healthy cornea, the epithelial cells are firmly adherent to their fellow neighboring cells by tight junctions and desmosomes. The basal layer of the epithelium adheres to the underlying basement membrane less tightly, via hemidesmosomes. These hemidesmosomes link to anchoring fibrils composed of type VII collagen, which then penetrates through the basement membrane and Bowman's layer, forming anchoring plaques with the stromal collagen below.[1]

The goal of ASP is to strengthen the adherence of the corneal epithelium to the underlying stroma by mimicking naturally occurring anchoring plaques at the epithelial–stromal interface. By creating punctures into the anterior stroma and inducing localized subepithelial fibrosis, stronger attachment of the epithelium to the stroma is theoretically achieved.[2,3] Two key facts are known so far about the puncture site. Firstly, a puncture depth of 0.1 mm is sufficient to cause a fibrotic reaction.[2] Knowing that the corneal epithelium is roughly 50 μm thick, this means a puncture depth of roughly twice the epithelial layer is sufficient. Secondly, achieving a break in Bowman's layer at the puncture site is essential to stimulate more secure epithelial anchoring. Histologic studies have shown that the breaks in Bowman's layer lead to its collagen fibrils bowing anteriorly and forming hook-like projections into the epithelium. However, although these breaks are considered crucial for stronger epithelial bonds, it does not guarantee its adhesion due to other structural and pathophysiologic factors.[4]

## INDICATIONS

### Key Indications

- Epithelial basement membrane dystrophy
- Recurrent corneal erosions
- Recalcitrant bullous keratopathy
- Chronic microcystic edema

## Epithelial Basement Membrane Dystrophy

- Epithelial basement membrane dystrophy (EBMD) occurs when a defective basement membrane leads to poor adhesion of the overlying epithelium and redundant basement membrane. Poor healing of the epithelium can result in symptoms of transient blurry vision, ocular surface discomfort, and recurrent corneal erosions. Clinical signs include map, dot, and fingerprint lines at the corneal surface. Alternative treatment options include conservative topical treatment (lubrication, anti-inflammatory medications) or surgical intervention (manual corneal debridement, phototherapeutic keratectomy).[5,6]

## Recurrent Corneal Erosions

- Recurrent corneal erosions (RCE) can result from intrinsic or acquired injury. Studies report that trauma (i.e., traumatic corneal abrasions) makes up 45% to 64% of the etiology of RCE, whereas EBMD was found to make up 26% to 29% of RCE etiologies. Symptoms can include blurred vision, transient pain that can present upon awakening, or pain that lasts several hours or days and can disrupt sleep. Clinical signs include epithelial microcysts, broken and loose epithelium, and abrasions. Treatment options are similar to that of EBMD, with the addition of bandage contact lens application for acute pain control.[5]

## Recalcitrant Bullous Keratopathy and Chronic Microcystic Edema

- Bullous keratopathy results from coalesced fluid accumulation forming on the epithelium and subepithelium. Typically, this is caused by endothelial dysfunction, but significant inflammation can also be causative. Other risk factors include advanced age, history of ocular trauma, and history of ocular surgeries that risk endothelial cell loss or damage (i.e., glaucoma surgeries, corneal surgeries and graft failures, cataract surgeries, and vitreoretinal surgeries requiring silicone oil). Primary treatment methods include corneal grafting or transplants. However, it has been hypothesized that the fibrotic reaction induced by ASP strengthens the junctional complexes between epithelial cells. This theoretically hinders fluid retention in the subepithelial space, leading to the disappearance of corneal blistering or microcystic edema. It is imperative to note that currently there are limited studies on this.[4,7]

# CONTRAINDICATIONS

**Key Contraindications**

*Absolute:*

- Microbial keratitis
- High risk or likelihood of corneal perforation

*Relative:*

- Neurotrophic keratitis

- Central location—Due to recurrence concerns and the risk of visually significant scarring, other procedures with higher efficacy may be warranted.
- Significant corneal scarring (herpetic keratitis, proud nebulae in keratoconus)[8]
- Blepharitis—Lid hygiene should be established prior to the procedure.

The presence or high suspicion of microbial keratitis is an absolute contraindication for ASP. Microbial keratitis must be treated and fully resolved prior to considering ASP to minimize the risk of postoperative infection. A very thin cornea or one that has a high risk of perforation is not a good candidate for ASP. The level of indentation, although small, could surpass the threshold of a very thinned and unhealthy cornea. Examples of this include but are not limited to patients with post-laser-assisted in situ keratomileusis (LASIK) ectasia, a history of corneal melt, and a history of microbial keratitis with necrosis.

Neurotrophic keratitis is a relative contraindication due to the risk of poor or lack of healing ability. This is because the expected fibrotic reaction induced by ASP may not behave as anticipated and can result in prolonged damage or persistent epithelial defects instead. Other treatment methods such as recombinant human nerve growth factors, scleral lenses, and tarsorrhaphies may be better options.

Centrally involved corneal conditions have a higher visual impact if scarring persists, whether after ASP or from recurring epithelial defects or erosions. Therefore, procedures like corneal debridement or superficial keratectomy with diamond burr polishing may be more appropriate for cases where the central cornea and/or larger areas are involved. If a patient is more prone to corneal scarring, such as in cases like herpetic keratitis or proud nebulae (elevated scarring) in advanced keratoconus, ASP may not be appropriate, depending on disease stability and size of the area needed to be treated. The risk of the respective condition progressing and corneal scarring worsening must be carefully weighed against the potential benefit of induced fibrosis and epithelial growth.

## PREOPERATIVE PREPARATION

Informed consent via paper or electronic means should address the risks, benefits, and potential complications of the procedure in plain language. This should include a simple explanation of the ASP procedure, its indications and purpose, and potential alternative treatments. Typical postoperative expectations and adverse effects should be listed. A statement outlining that the counseling physician discussed the procedure, risks involved, and expected results should be included, with signatures from the patient, the counseling physician, and a witness (typically a staff member).

### Equipment Required[2,4,5,7] (Figure 26-1)

- ASP needle *or* bent 25G to 28G needle
  - Use the plastic needle cover to bend the tip of the needle (roughly 5/8 inches) being careful not to blunt or dull the needle tip.

    *Caution to avoid using a cystotome by accident*
- 1-mL syringe to use as a handle
- Lid speculum
- Bandage contact lens
- Slit lamp with cobalt blue filter

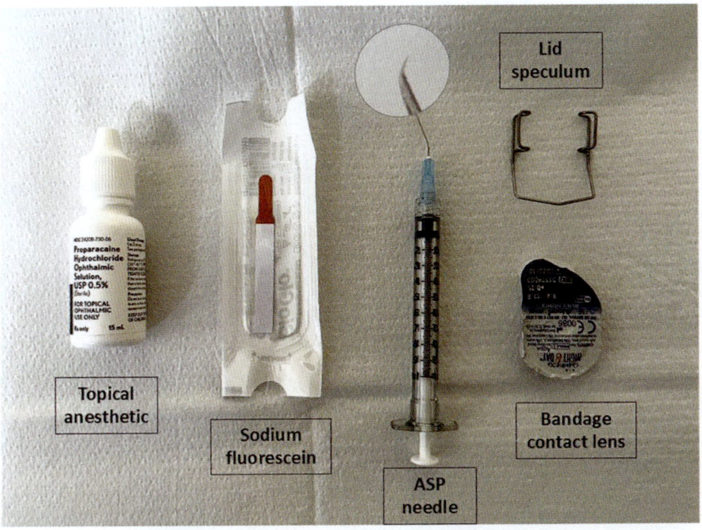


**FIGURE 26-1** Specific equipment from recommended equipment list shown here. ASP needle tip is magnified to show bent angle. ASP, anterior stromal puncture.

- Sodium fluorescein
- Topical ophthalmic anesthetic (i.e., 0.5% topical proparacaine drops)
- Topical ophthalmic antibiotic drops (i.e., moxifloxacin 0.5%)

## THE PROCEDURE[2,4,5,7]

1. Plan the area of treatment by assessing for signs of loose epithelium or area(s) of RCE (Figure 26-2).
   - Do not debride loose epithelial tissue prior to performing the ASP procedure if performing ASP.
2. Instill 1 drop of topical ophthalmic 0.5% proparacaine or equivalent in the affected eye.
3. Optional: Insert lid speculum to control blink reflex.
4. Using either an ASP needle or bent needle tip attached to a 1-mL syringe, position the needle tip perpendicular to corneal surface.
5. Create micropunctures by gently indenting the affected epithelium directly at a perpendicular angle (as opposed to a tangential entry).
   - Sufficient pressure to feel resistance against the stroma should be applied. This is roughly 5% to 10% stromal depth.
   - ASPs should be less than 1 mm apart.
   - An area of roughly 3 mm × 3 mm would require about 20 to 40 ASPs.
6. Apply fluorescein and use cobalt blue light to visualize "bubbles" that represent adequate Bowman's layer break and stromal contact (Figure 26-3).
   - Small circular bubbles should be seen at the subepithelial level, and triangular-shaped micropockets are seen at the intrastromal level which denote sufficient depth achieved.
7. Instill 1 drop of topical ophthalmic antibiotic in the treated eye.
8. Place a bandage contact lens over the cornea of the treated eye.

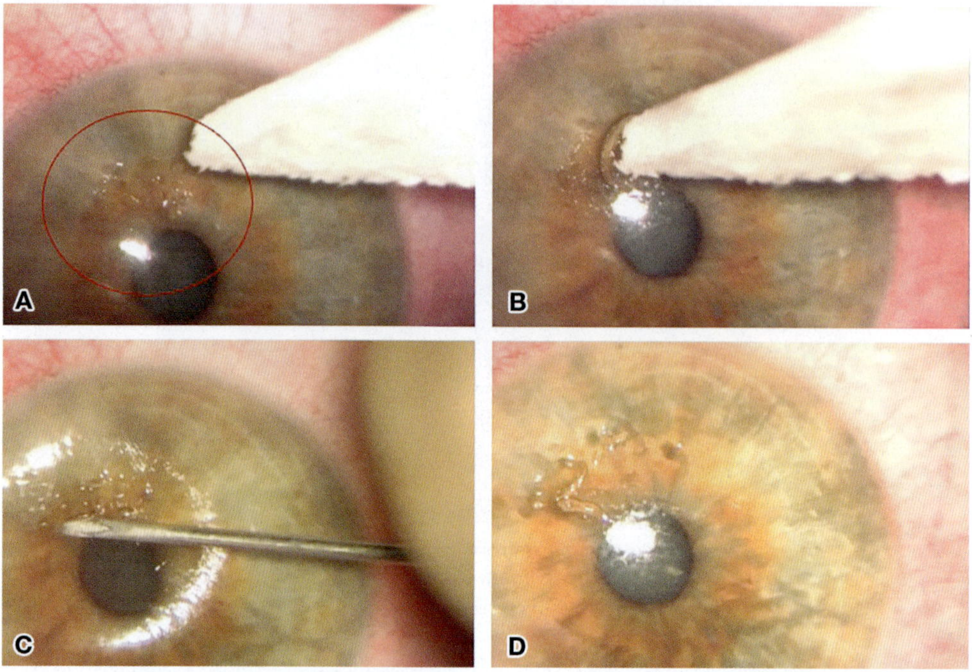


**FIGURE 26-2** **A,** Area of loosened tissue shown prior to testing with a surgical spear. **B,** Very loose epithelium identified after testing with surgical spear. **C,** Anterior stromal puncture (ASP) with indentation of roughly 5% to 10% stromal depth shown. **D,** Area of ASPs roughly 1 mm apart shown.

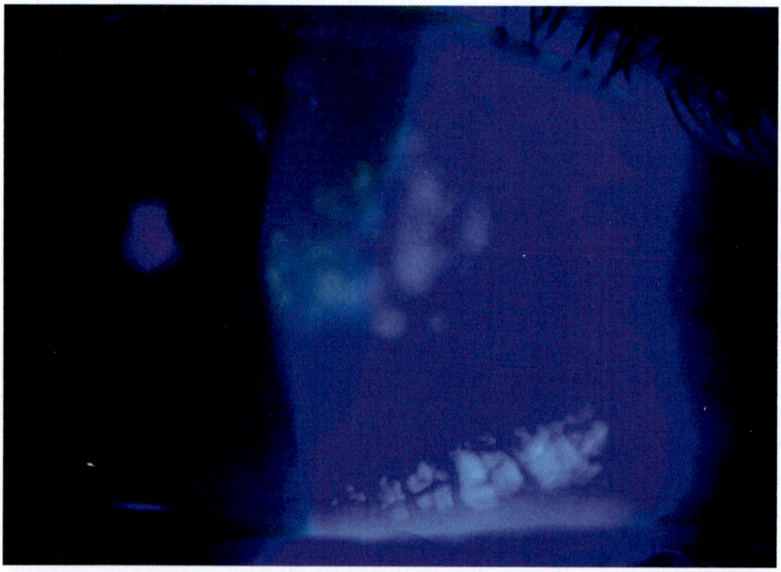

**FIGURE 26-3** Fluorescein and cobalt filter showing bubbles and fluorescein staining at areas of epithelium puncture and basement membrane stimulation immediately after anterior stromal puncture.

# POSTOPERATIVE CARE/COMANAGEMENT (FOLLOW-UP SCHEDULE)

## Key Postoperative Considerations

- Topical ophthalmic antibiotic drops four times a day (QID) while healing
- Topical ophthalmic steroid drop QID with optional taper
- Bandage contact lens kept in for 6 weeks (replaced as necessary during follow-up)
- Preservative-free artificial tears with ointment overnight after bandage contact lens removal
- Optional oral pain medication as needed (but often not required)
- Recommended weekly follow-up schedule to be adjusted per clinical assessment

Because there is intentional epithelial disruption, topical ophthalmic antibiotic coverage is required. Examples include moxifloxacin 0.5% ophthalmic solution 4×/day or a tobramycin 0.3%/dexamethasone 0.1% ophthalmic suspension 4×/day for a week while the treated epithelium is healing. A bandage contact lens is recommended to remain for further corneal healing and stability, and replaced when necessary, based on follow-up assessments. Topical ophthalmic steroids can be tapered over the course of the first month or two while the bandage contact lens is still in place. Typically, a bandage contact lens is sufficient for pain management. In rare cases, oral pain medications may be required, but patients should be made aware that they will have discomfort within the first 24 to 48 hours after the procedure.[2]

# POTENTIAL COMPLICATIONS AND THEIR TREATMENTS

## Key Potential Complications

- Mild ocular discomfort or pain
- Recurrence of symptoms

Overall, ASP is relatively safe and has minimal adverse effects.[2,5] In most cases, further management is less likely due to complications but rather due to treatment failure or the recurrence of symptoms. Seventeen percent of treated patients have been reported to require retreatment.[2] Watering and occasional ocular pain were reported in 20% and 7%, respectively.[4]

Nonvisually significant corneal scars have been reported in 71% of patients in one study. Risk of postoperative infection, visually significant corneal haze or scarring, and postoperative refractive shifts have not been reported.[2,5]

## VIDEOS OF PROCEDURE

**Video 26-1**—Anterior stromal puncture (ASP).

In this video, the eye has already been prepped with topical ophthalmic antibiotics and topical ophthalmic anesthetic, and the lid speculum has already been placed.

A dry surgical spear sponge is shown testing the cornea for surrounding poor adhesion to determine the area of treatment. Many times, the area of loose epithelium is greater than the specific area of erosion. As shown in the video, the epithelium slides very easily from the underlying layers.

ASPs are shown being made using an ASP needle held firmly. The anterior cornea is depressed with moderate pressure, making sure that the ASP needle penetrates the stromal surface. The punctures are roughly ¼ to 1 mm apart.

**Video 26-2**—Anterior stromal puncture (ASP; performed at slit lamp)

This is a video of the ASP procedure performed at the slit lamp. The eye had been prepped with topical ophthalmic antibiotics, topical ophthalmic anesthetics, and in this case, no lid speculum was used.

A dry surgical spear sponge is used to test the cornea for loose epithelium. ASPs are shown being made using a bent 25G needle tip. The punctures are roughly ¼ to 1 mm apart. Small air bubbles can be seen with white light and under cobalt blue light after fluorescein staining to show the epithelium puncture and basement membrane activation.

# EFFICACY

In the treatment of RCE, studies have reported 63% to 94% of treated patients achieving success, defined by no recurrences of macroerosions.[1,2] Around 40% of patients were still symptomatic but with milder severity in multiple studies.[2,3] Eighty-three percent of patients in one study were reported as not requiring any further surgeries or procedures.[2] Whether history of trauma is a predictor of ASP success or not is still inconsistently reported.

Where EBMD was also present, clinical signs persisted postoperatively in 71% of treated patients, but this did not correlate with persistent symptoms.[2]

In the treatment of bullous keratopathy, small sample sizes where treatment was performed while waiting for penetrating keratoplasty reported roughly 70% of treated patients with ASP achieving resolution of symptoms. Complete regression of epithelial bullae and edema was reported in 36% of treated patients, and partial regression was reported in 62%; 40% of treated patients proceeded to require penetrating keratoplasty, without any direct complications caused by history of ASP being performed.[4] It is important to highlight that the inclusion criteria were patients who had failed conservative therapies and were awaiting penetrating keratoplasty, and therefore clinicians must consider the application of ASP carefully in such cases.

# SPECIAL CONSIDERATIONS

## Advantages over Other Procedures[2]

- Focal area treatment allowing for quicker healing and with less discomfort compared to larger epithelial defects from other treatments
- No chemicals or delaminating agents required

- Minimal adverse effects
- Repeatable
- Can be performed in patients who have had refractive surgeries
- Does not prevent or complicate further treatments or surgeries

## Disadvantages over Other Procedures[2]

- Other procedures may have higher efficacy.
- Adjunctive medical management may still be necessary.

## Alternative Procedure Using an Nd:YAG Laser[3]

Instill topical ophthalmic 0.5% proparacaine in the affected eye.

1. Set energy setting of Nd:YAG laser to 0.3 to 0.6 mJ with 0 µm offset.
2. Focus on corneal subepithelium or superficial stroma in the affected area.
3. Place shots less than 1 mm apart.
4. Postoperative care:
   - Topical ophthalmic lubrication drops at least QID in the treated eye
   - Topical ophthalmic antibiotic drops and topical ophthalmic steroid drops at therapeutic dosages
   - Topical ophthalmic antibiotic or lubrication ointment every night at bedtime (QHS)
5. Reported follow-up schedule (according to Tsai et al[3]):
   - 1 week
   - 4 weeks
   - 3 months
   - 6 months

It is imperative to note that this is not the primary or traditional technique of performing anterior stromal puncture. This method is included to present an alternative method that may be considered. Efficacy has been reported to be 85% of treated patients having no recurrence of macroerosions at 15 months. However, only 50% of patients in one study were found to be completely symptom free and 15% had persistent symptoms that required further treatment. Authors reported that in all patients, the frequency of corneal erosions and pain severity improved significantly. No adverse reactions such as corneal haze or endothelial damage were reported.[3]

# CODING AND BILLING

- **65600-RT/LT**—Multiple punctures of the anterior cornea, 90 days global period
- **992XX-57**—Same-day office visit

Anterior stromal puncture is considered a major procedure. A same-day office visit can be separately reported using the modifier −57. Corneal procedures cannot be billed on the same day as 92071 (fitting of a contact lens for ocular surface disease).[9,10]

Common ICD-10 codes that support anterior stromal puncture include (right eye used as an example)[11]:

- **H17.01**—Adherent leukoma, right eye
- **H17.11**—Central corneal opacity, right eye
- **H17.811**—Minor opacity of cornea, right eye
- **H17.821**—Peripheral opacity of cornea, right eye
- **H17.89**—Other corneal scars and opacities
- **H18.11**—Bullous keratopathy, right eye
- **H18.421**—Band keratopathy, right eye
- **H18.43**—Other calcareous corneal degeneration
- **H18.441**—Keratomalacia, right eye
- **H18.451**—Nodular corneal degeneration, right eye
- **H18.461**—Peripheral corneal degeneration, right eye
- **H18.49**—Other corneal degeneration
- **H18.831**—Recurrent erosion of cornea, right eye
- **H53.2**—Diplopia
- **H59.89**—Other postprocedural complications and disorders of the eye and adnexa, not elsewhere classified

## ACKNOWLEDGMENT

Special thanks to Dr. Cedrick Mah for assisting with equipment photos and to Dr. Jason Ellen for contributing a procedure video.

## REFERENCES

1. Nishida T, Saika S, Morishige N. Cornea and sclera: anatomy and physiology. In: Mannis M, Holland E, eds. *Cornea*. 4th ed. Elsevier; 2017:1-22.
2. Avni Zauberman N, Artornsombudh P, Elbaz U, Goldich Y, Rootman DS, Chan CC. Anterior stromal puncture for the treatment of recurrent corneal erosion syndrome: patient clinical features and outcomes. *Am J Ophthalmol.* 2014;157(2):273-279.e1. doi:10.1016/j.ajo.2013.10.005
3. Tsai T-Y, Tsai T-H, Hu F-R, Hou Y-C. Recurrent corneal erosions treated with anterior stromal puncture by neodymium: yttrium–aluminum–garnet laser. *Ophthalmology*. 2009;116(7):1296-1300. doi:10.1016/j.ophtha.2009.01.037
4. Sridhar MS, Vemuganti GK, Bansal AK, Rao GN. Anterior stromal puncture in bullous keratopathy: a clinicopathological study. *Cornea*. 2001;20(6):573-579.
5. Meghpara B, Hammersmith KM. Anterior corneal dystrophies. In: Mannis M, Holland E, eds. *Cornea: Fundamentals, Diagnosis, and Management*. 5th ed. Elsevier Inc; 2022:701.e1-711.
6. Yeu E, Hashem O, Sheha H. Treatment of epithelial basement membrane dystrophy to optimize the ocular surface prior to cataract surgery. *Clin Ophthalmol.* 2022; 16:785-795. doi:10.2147/OPTH.S356421
7. Li G, Zheng J, Gong J, et al. Efficacy of anterior stromal puncture surgery with corneal bandage lens for bullous keratopathy. *Int J Med Sci*. 2019;16(5):660-664. doi:10.7150/ijms.31669
8. Kang SY, Park YK, Song J-S, Kim HM. Anterior stromal puncture for treatment of contact lens-intolerant keratoconus patients. *Graefe's Arch Clin Exp Ophthalmol.* 2011;249(1):89-92. doi:10.1007/s00417-010-1423-9
9. Rumpakis J. Minor procedures, major rules. *Rev Optom*. Published 2020. Accessed August 29, 2022. https://www.reviewofoptometry.com/article/minor-procedures-major-rules
10. Rumpakis J. RCE: code correctly, again and again. *Rev Optom*. Published 2019. Accessed August 29, 2022. https://www.reviewofoptometry.com/article/rce-code-correctly-again-and-again
11. American Medical Association. *CPT 2021 Professional Edition*. American Medical Association; 2020.

# 27 Amniotic Membrane Placement

**Sophia Leung**

## BACKGROUND

The application of amniotic membranes dates back to 1910 and has since been used for a multitude of conditions including open wound coverings, diabetic ulcers, trauma, and burn injuries.[1] The amniotic membrane is the innermost layer of the placental tissue surrounding a fetus and acts as a protective barrier.[2,3] It has pro-epithelialization, anti-angiogenic, anti-inflammatory, and anti-fibrotic properties.[1,4-7] Antimicrobial properties have also been reported, but studies are inconsistent. It is more likely that the physical barrier aspect of amniotic membrane tissue acts, in part, as a defense against microbial infection.[8]

Derived from the innermost layer of the placenta, amniotic membranes have three notable layers: epithelium, basement membrane, and stroma.[5,9] The epithelial layer maintains a microenvironment of stem cells, with components that reduce inflammation and neovascularization. The basement membrane provides a scaffolding for cell migration, cell growth, and promotes proper cell differentiation. The stroma suppresses inflammatory cascades and inhibits myofibroblast differentiation, reducing scarring. Certain complexes, such as the heavy chain hyaluronic acid Pentraxin 3 (HC-HA/PTX3) complex, inhibit pro-inflammatory cells and suppress T cells. The amniotic membrane matrix also traps and induces apoptosis of inflammatory cells to minimize the immunologic response. This is significant because amniotic membranes have an extremely low propensity for rejection.[1,5,8,9]

All amniotic tissue donors are screened for transmissible diseases prior to the amniotic membrane being harvested during elective cesarean delivery, under a sterile environment. The tissue is then further treated with broad-spectrum antibiotics after collection.[5] Currently, there are three main forms of amniotic membranes for office-based application. Amniotic grafts requiring suturing or placement in a surgical setting will not be discussed in this chapter.

### Sutureless Cryopreserved Amniotic Membrane

- A cryopreserved amniotic membrane graft is attached to a dual polycarbonate ring with an inner diameter of 16 mm and an outer diameter of roughly 21 mm. There is typically an epithelial side and a stromal side to the amniotic membrane, fixed by its attachment to the conformer ring. Different products available may have different ring heights or multilayered amniotic tissues for various conditions and severity. These must be stored frozen. The shelf life of cryopreserved amniotic membranes is generally 2 years.[1,5]

- All preservation methods, including cryopreservation, significantly decrease the amount of soluble factors for biological activity compared to fresh amniotic membrane tissue.[3] However, some studies have reported that cryopreservation retains the architecture and key complexes, like HC-HA/PTX3, most similarly to fresh amniotic tissue.[1]
- Food and Drug Administration (FDA) approved for wound protection, wound healing, and anti-inflammation.[4,10]

## Dehydrated Amniotic Membrane

- Air-dried, heat-dried, or freeze-dried amniotic tissue is stored at room temperature and available in various sizes. Different thicknesses, orientation (epithelial side vs. stromal side), and shapes are available. Shelf life of dehydrated amniotic membranes is generally 3 to 5 years.[5]
- Studies have reported that dehydration significantly compromises the amniotic membrane structure, and heat-drying specifically can result in minimal to no retention of key soluble factors. However, recent studies have shown that newer dehydration methods retain growth factors and other complexes better than cryopreservation. Pretreatment with chemical compounds such as trehalose and trisaccharide raffinose that protect cellular structure during dehydration has been reported to allow the dehydrated amniotic membrane to be even more resemblant of fresh amniotic membrane than any other preservation method.[1,3]
- FDA approved for wound covering only.[4,10]

## Amniotic Membrane Extract Eye Drop

- Several methods of extraction exist with varying yields. Although the structural properties of amniotic membranes are completely lost, studies have reported an increased retention of HC-HA/PTX3 matrix. However, clinical data on the efficacy of the various extraction methods are limited, and the shelf life of the various preparations has not been fully studied.[9] As such, this will only be minimally discussed in this chapter.

# INDICATIONS

### Key Indications

- Corneal erosions
- Persistent epithelial defects
- Neurotrophic keratitis
- Severe or recalcitrant corneal inflammation
- Partial limbal stem cell deficiency
- Preoperative care (refractive corneal and cataract surgery)
- Postoperative care (superficial keratectomy and corneal debridement)

## Corneal Erosions

- Caused by either intrinsic or acquired injury, treatment aims to optimize the epithelial layer and its adherence to the layers below to decrease the frequency of erosions. Recurrent corneal erosions often require epithelial debridement. Application of amniotic membranes, especially after epithelial debridement or superficial keratectomy, has been reported to be beneficial.[4,5,10]

## Persistent Epithelial Defects

- Defined as a defect failing to epithelialize within 10 to 14 days from the initial corneal trauma or insult, persistent epithelial defects benefit from having a scaffold for epithelial cell migration and growth. Anti-inflammatory properties of amniotic membranes aim to reduce scarring as the defect heals.[6,11]

## Neurotrophic Keratitis

- Decreased sensory feedback from the corneal surface leads to impaired wound healing, and vulnerability to degeneration, ulceration, inflammation, and secondary infection. Causes include viral infections, corneal surgery, diabetes mellitus, and other conditions that can affect the trigeminal nerve. Exposure to growth factors and complexes that promote healing and reduce inflammation is imperative.[5,6,10]
- The Mackie Classification System categorizes neurotrophic keratitis into the following three stages:
  - *Stage 1*: neurotrophic keratopathy with punctate staining, corneal scarring, neovascularization but no epithelial defect
  - *Stage 2*: neurotrophic keratopathy with epithelial defects but no stromal ulceration
  - *Stage 3:* Stromal ulcer is present.[6]
- Stage 1 and 2 neurotrophic keratitis would benefit most from amniotic membrane application.[6]

## Severe or Recalcitrant Corneal Inflammation

- Whether primary or secondary, chronic and persistent corneal inflammation often leads to irreversible scarring. Amniotic membranes reduce reliance on topical and oral anti-inflammatory treatment in certain cases, thereby reducing the adverse risks associated with those treatment modalities. Commonly encountered conditions that result in recalcitrant corneal inflammation are as follows:
  - Dry eye disease[12]
  - Ocular chemical and/or thermal burn injuries
  - Autoimmune-related ocular surface disease (i.e., Sjogren's syndrome, acute phases of Stevens–Johnson syndrome)
  - Symptomatic bullous keratopathy
  - Band keratopathy
  - Filamentary keratitis[5,13]

## Partial Limbal Stem Cell Deficiency

- Leading to poor corneal healing, epithelial irregularity, and occasional neovascularization, limbal stem cell deficiency treatment focuses on reestablishing of stem cells at the corneoscleral limbus. Causes include viral infection and significant inflammation.[4,5]

## Preoperative Care: Prior to Corneal-Based Refractive Surgery (i.e., Photorefractive Keratectomy (PRK), Laser-Assisted in Situ Keratomileusis (LASIK)) and Elective Cataract Surgery for Optimize Intraocular Lens (IOL) Selection

- Studies have reported 60% to 80% of routine cataract patients having ocular surface disease and dry eye syndrome despite being asymptomatic. Optimizing the ocular surface prior to surgery may improve surgical outcomes and refractive target accuracy.[13,14]

## Postoperative Care: Superficial Keratectomy and/or Corneal Debridement

- To reduce corneal haze and scarring after corneal debridement, many authors recommend amniotic membrane application after such procedures are performed.[10]
- Anecdotally, when the central corneal or visual axis is involved, cryopreserved amniotic membranes may be preferable to dehydrated amniotic membranes.

# CONTRAINDICATIONS

**Key Contraindications**

- Active infectious keratitis (relative contraindication)
- Total limbal stem cell deficiency (relative contraindication)
- Lid and aperture restriction
- Poor compliance with drops or follow-up schedule

## Relative

- Active infectious keratitis
  - Whether bacterial, viral, fungal, or parasitic, it is recommended that amniotic membrane application only be considered after adequate anti-infectious control is initiated and the infectious keratitis is stabilized. Close monitoring is paramount.[6]
- Total limbal stem cell deficiency
  - Amniotic membrane alone is insufficient in total limbal stem cell deficiency. Advanced stages will often require autologous or allogenic limbal stem cell transplantation.[15] When measuring the area of healing, amniotic membrane transplantation achieved more

healing compared to in-office application. However, sutureless amniotic membranes require lower costs, no operating room, and shorter absorption time. Clinicians must evaluate its application on a case-by-case basis.[10]

### Absolute

- Lid and aperture restriction (i.e., partial or complete tarsorrhaphy)
  - Structural restrictions prevent proper insertion and placement of amniotic membranes
- Poor compliance with drops or follow-up schedule

## PREOPERATIVE PREPARATION

### Equipment Required: Sutureless Cryopreserved Amniotic Membrane (Figure 27-1)

- Cryopreserved amniotic membrane package—removed from freezer and thawed to room temperature
- At least two bottles of buffer saline solution (BSS)
- Topical ophthalmic anesthetic (i.e., 0.5% proparacaine)
- Surgical tape
- Sterile gloves

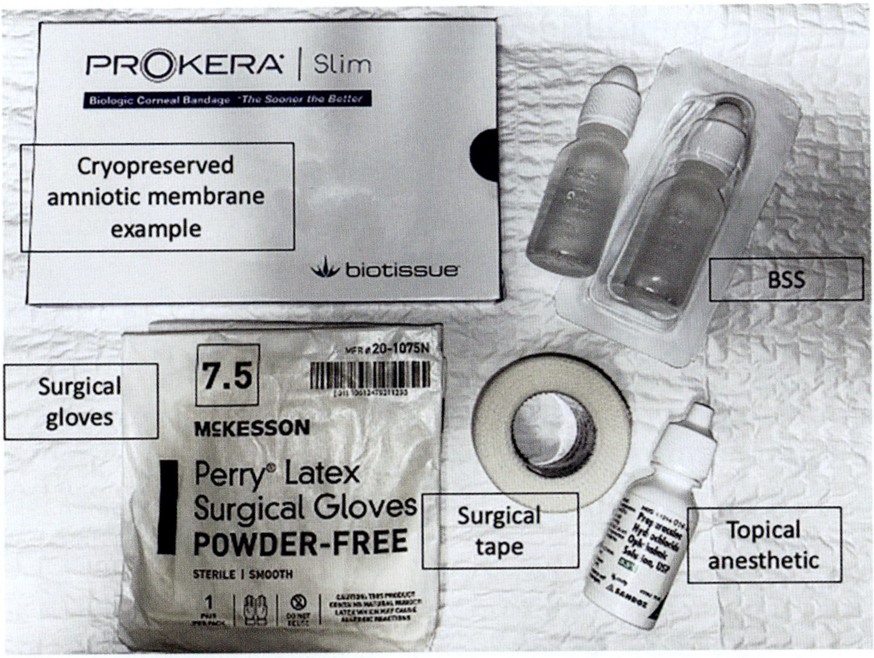


**FIGURE 27-1** Equipment needed for cryopreserved amniotic membrane insertion. BSS, buffer saline solution.

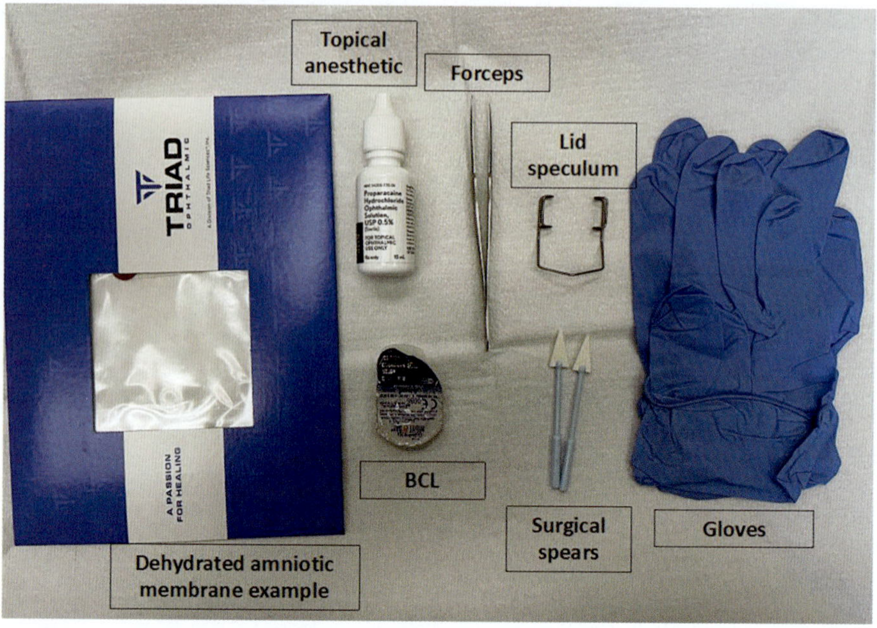


FIGURE 27-2 Equipment needed for dehydrated amniotic membrane insertion. BCL, bandage contact lens.

## Dehydrated amniotic membrane (Figure 27-2)

- Dehydrated amniotic membrane package
- Bandage contact lens (BCL)
- Nontoothed forceps
- Surgical spear sponges (Weck-Cel)
- Topical ophthalmic anesthetic (i.e., 0.5% proparacaine)
- Lid speculum
- Sterile gloves

# THE PROCEDURE

## Amniotic Membrane Insertion: Sutureless Cryopreserved Amniotic Membrane[5,13,14]

1. Open package (thawed to room temperature) and open pouch.
2. Put on sterile gloves.
3. Remove plastic cartridge from the opened pouch.
4. Without removing the small plastic retainer holding the amniotic membrane in its well, drain preservation fluid (Figure 27-3).
5. Rinse the amniotic membrane with sterile saline to remove glycerol. (Two bottles of BSS are recommended.)

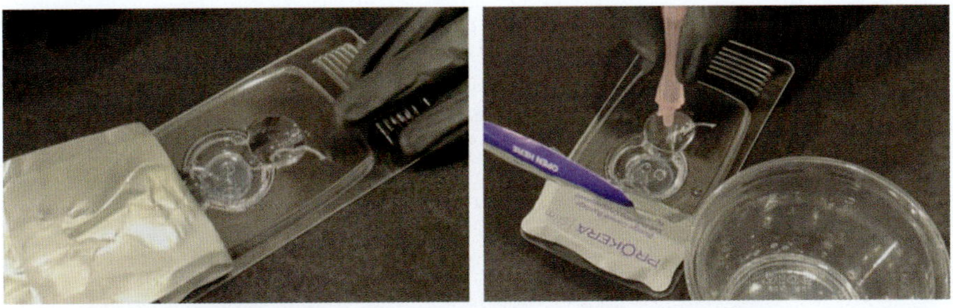


**FIGURE 27-3** Cryopreserved amniotic membrane package opening and rinsing shown. Note the plastic retainer in place over the amniotic membrane tissue.

6. Instill one drop of topical ophthalmic anesthetic into the affected eye.
7. Remove cryopreserved amniotic membrane by holding the ring.
8. Instruct the patient to look down (Figure 27-4).
9. Gently lift the upper eyelid, and insert superior edge of the ring under the upper eyelid.
10. Instruct the patient to look up.

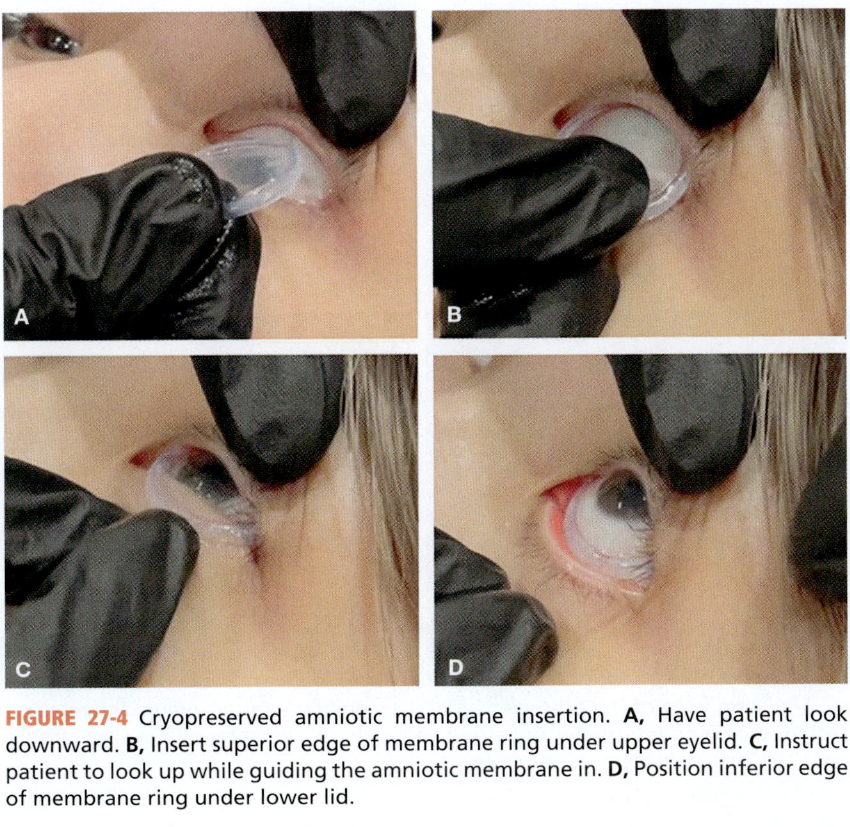


**FIGURE 27-4** Cryopreserved amniotic membrane insertion. **A,** Have patient look downward. **B,** Insert superior edge of membrane ring under upper eyelid. **C,** Instruct patient to look up while guiding the amniotic membrane in. **D,** Position inferior edge of membrane ring under lower lid.

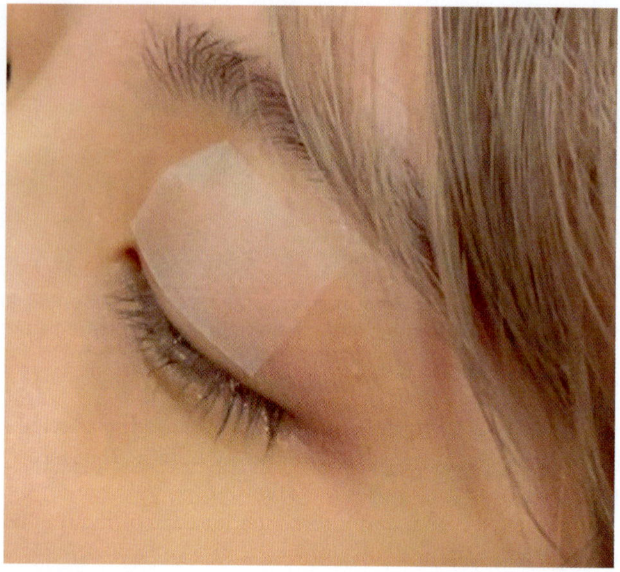

**FIGURE 27-5** One example of lid taping to partially immobilize lid movement for better comfort.

11. Place the inferior edge of the ring into the eye.
12. Optional: For comfort, apply tape for a temporary tarsorrhaphy (Figure 27-5).
13. Optional: Examine the patient behind the slit lamp to ensure accurate amniotic membrane placement (Figure 27-6).

*In the proper orientation (concave ring curvature facing toward the eye), the stromal side of the amniotic membrane faces the cornea.*

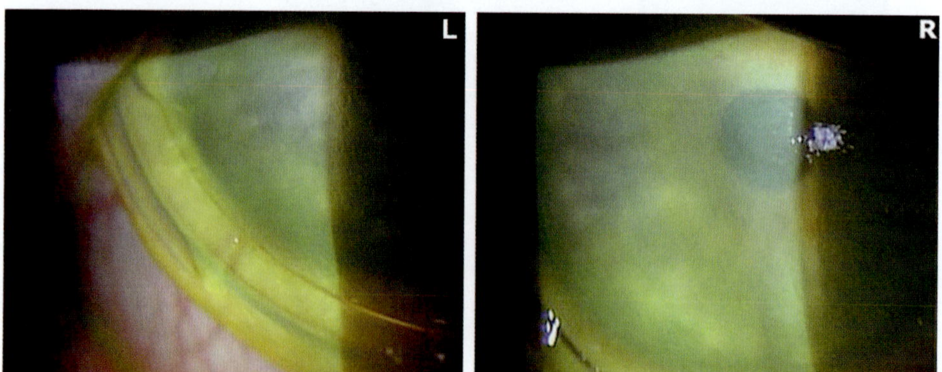


**FIGURE 27-6** Ring edge of cryopreserved amniotic membrane (after sodium fluorescein [NaFl] instillation) shown on left photo. Cryopreserved amniotic membrane (after NaFl instillation) over central cornea shown on right photo.

## Dehydrated Amniotic Membrane: Method 1: Direct Amniotic Membrane Disc Application to the Cornea (Figure 27-7)

1. Instill topical ophthalmic anesthetic into the affected eye.
2. Insert lid speculum into the affected eye to control blink reflex.
3. Using nontoothed forceps, carefully remove the dehydrated amniotic membrane disc from the inner package.
4. Dry off the cornea slightly with a dry surgical spear sponge (Weck-Cel).
5. Place dehydrated amniotic membrane disc onto the ocular surface, either in the center of the cornea or overlying the affected area.

   *Watermarks to identify the orientation of the amniotic membrane are product dependent. Consult the specific company of the product being used to determine how to identify the epithelial side from the stromal side.*

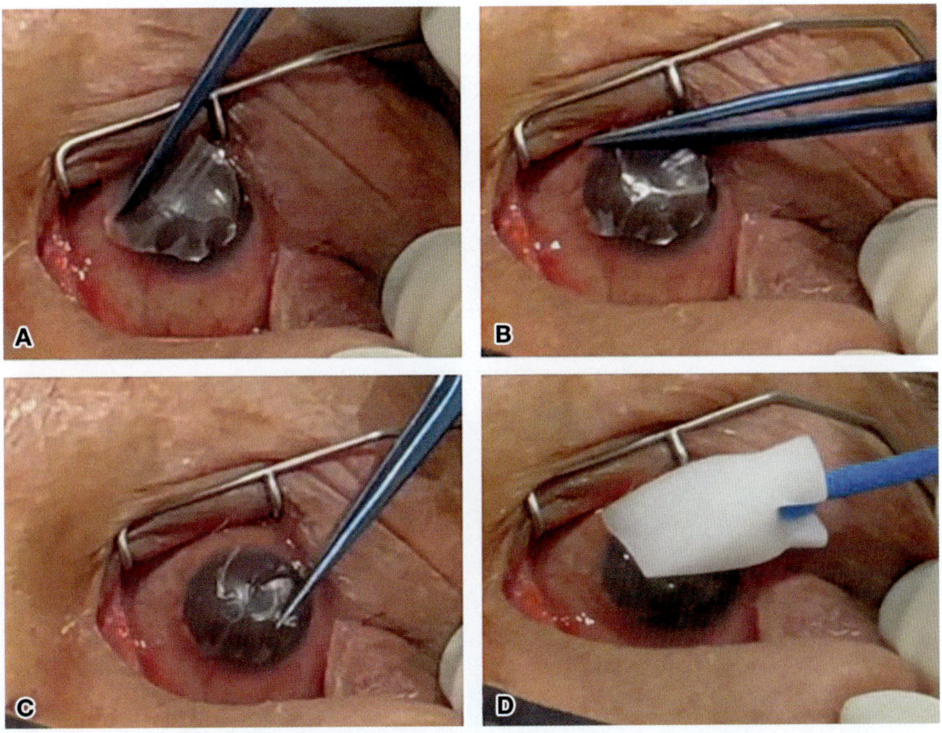


**FIGURE 27-7** Dehydrated amniotic membrane insertion—direct to cornea method. **A,** Amniotic membrane is placed directly onto the cornea. **B,** Smoothening of the dehydrated amniotic membrane disc on the cornea can be performed with either forceps or surgical spears. **C,** Repositioning can be done with sufficient rehydration. **D,** A bandage contact lens is placed directly overtop the amniotic membrane and cornea.

6. Smooth out the amniotic membrane disc with forceps or a dry surgical spear sponge (Weck-Cel) immediately after placement (Figure 27-8).
7. Optional: Add one or two drops of sterile saline to rehydrate the disc. Do not overhydrate as the disc will slide out of position.
8. Add a BCL overtop of the disc.
9. Carefully remove the lid speculum, and check for proper positioning of the amniotic membrane disc under the BCL.[5,11]

## Method 2: Combining Amniotic Membrane Disc with a BCL Prior to Application to the Ocular Surface* (Figure 27-9)

1. Instill topical ophthalmic anesthetic into the affected eye.
2. Prepare BCL onto a wet surgical spear sponge (Weck-Cel) or clean finger and/or sterile glove. Slightly dry BCL with a dry surgical spear sponge (Weck-Cel).
3. Using nontoothed forceps, carefully remove dehydrated amniotic membrane disc from inner package.
4. Place amniotic membrane disc into the center of the BCL.
   **Note watermarks or orientation of disc. Watermarks that should be legible when assessing at the slit lamp should be placed downward or facing the BCL.*
5. Smooth out any wrinkles of the amniotic membrane disc with dry surgical spear sponge (Weck-Cel).
6. Instruct the patient to look straight ahead (Figure 27-10).
7. Place the BCL and amniotic membrane disc combination onto the affected eye directly.[5,11]
8. Assess the patient under the slit lamp to ensure accurate insertion and placement of the amniotic membrane and BCL (Figures 27-11 to 27-13).
   **Anecdotally, this method is more convenient because it can be done without any assistance. However, the amniotic membrane disc is more prone to slippage and wrinkling with this method.*

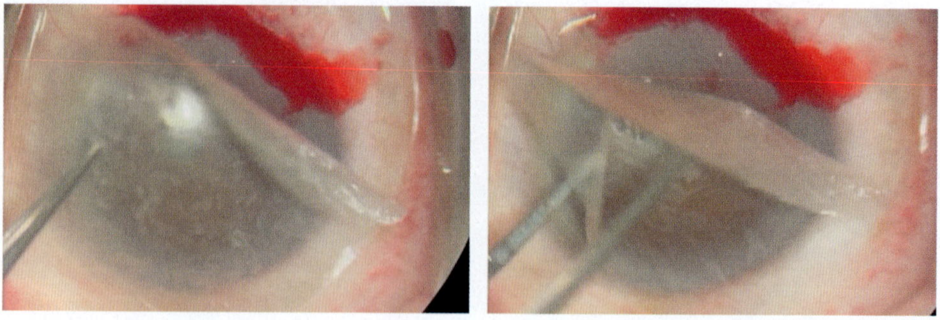

**FIGURE 27-8** Dehydrated amniotic membrane insertion—direct to cornea method. The dehydrated amniotic membrane has a tendency to curl once it nears the cornea, as shown here on the left photo. This is because of the heat disparity. The membrane should be swiftly and smoothly placed onto the cornea and then smoothened out, to avoid the disc folding onto itself during application.

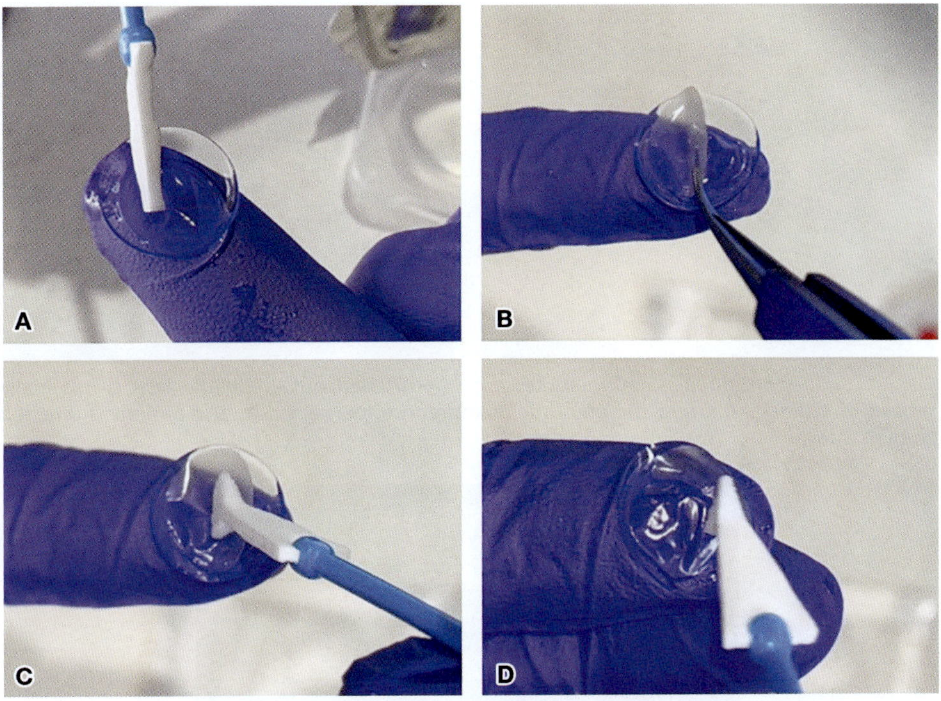


**FIGURE 27-9** Dehydrated amniotic membrane preparation—direct to bandage contact lens (BCL) method. **A,** The BCL is dried slightly with a surgical spear. **B,** The dehydrated amniotic membrane disc is placed onto the BCL. **C,** A surgical spear is used to smoothen the dehydrated amniotic membrane disc. **D,** Repositioning is possible with the dehydrated disc—slight rehydration may be required.

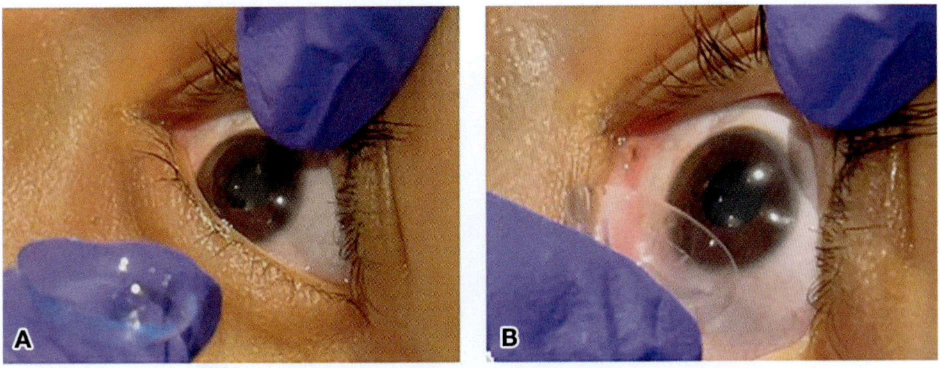


**FIGURE 27-10** Dehydrated amniotic membrane (dAM) insertion—direct to bandage contact lens (BCL) method. **A,** Instruct the patient to look straight ahead. **B,** BCL + dAM combo is applied directly to the anesthetized cornea.

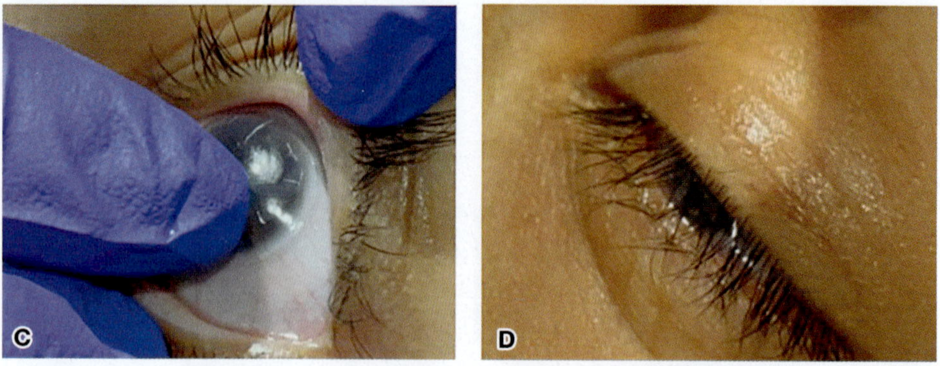


**FIGURE 27-10** (*continued*) **C,** Air bubbles are smoothened out while the lens is minimally moved, avoiding displacing the amniotic membrane underneath. **D,** The patient is directed to blink slowly.

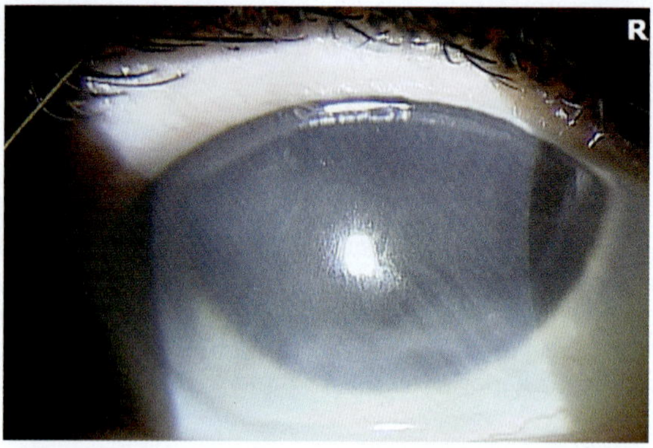


**FIGURE 27-11** Example of a 12-mm dehydrated amniotic membrane disc under a bandage contact lens (BCL) with good centration.

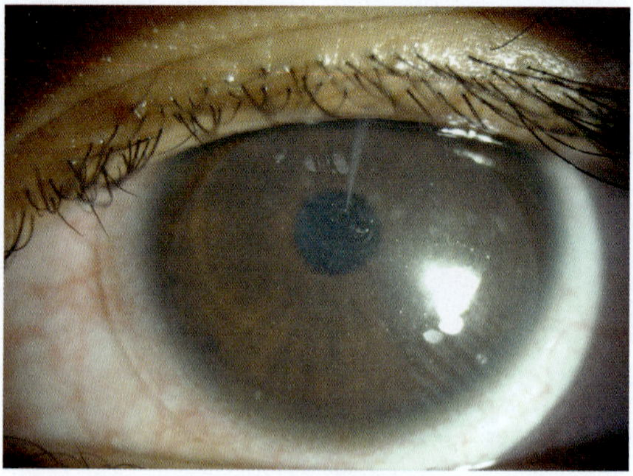

**FIGURE 27-12** An example of a 10-mm dehydrated amniotic membrane disc under a bandage contact lens (BCL) with slight inferior decentration.

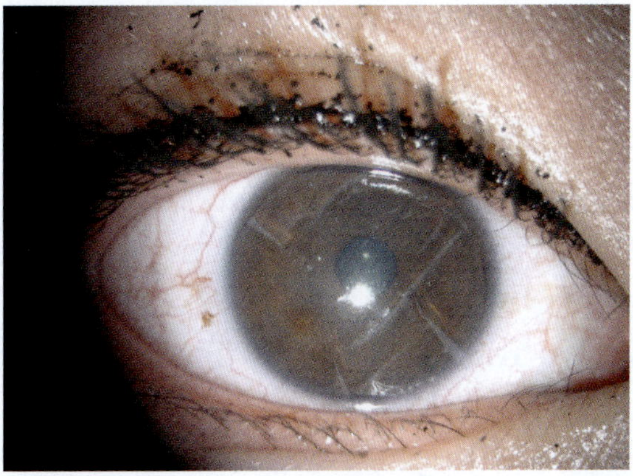

**FIGURE 27-13** An example of a 12-mm dehydrated amniotic membrane disc under a bandage contact lens (BCL). Because the dehydrated amniotic membrane is a flat tissue applied to a curved cornea, wrinkles may not always be avoidable, but should be minimized.

# POSTOPERATIVE CARE/COMANAGEMENT (FOLLOW-UP SCHEDULE)

## Sutureless Cryopreserved Amniotic Membrane

- Topical ophthalmic antibiotic drops QID
- Preservative-free lubrication drops as needed
- Follow up every few days to monitor for amniotic tissue absorption.
- Can remove amniotic membrane with ring to assess cornea more clearly at follow-ups as needed[13]
  - The amniotic membrane can be reinserted if there is still remaining tissue for further treatment response.
- Topical ophthalmic steroid drops can be discontinued or decreased depending on treatment response at follow-up appointments.

## Dehydrated Amniotic Membrane

- Topical ophthalmic antibiotic drops QID
- Topical ophthalmic steroid drops BID–TID depending on the inflammatory state of the ocular surface
- Preservative-free lubrication drops at least QID
- Follow up every 1 to 3 weeks for monitoring amniotic tissue absorption or BCL replacement as necessary.[11]

## Amniotic Membrane Removal: Sutureless Cryopreserved Amniotic Membrane (Figure 27-14)

1. Instill topical ophthalmic anesthetic in the affected eye.
2. Instruct patient to look up.
3. With nontoothed forceps, carefully grab the inferior portion of the conformer ring.
4. Instruct the patient to slowly look down, removing the ring as the patient looks downward in motion.

## Dehydrated Amniotic Membrane (Figure 27-15)

1. Instill topical ophthalmic anesthetic in the affected eye.
2. Instruct patient to look downward or upward (depending on clinician preference).
3. With nontoothed forceps, carefully grab the edge of the BCL.
4. Instruct the patient to look straight (or in the opposite direction of initial gaze) while lifting the BCL away from the eye.

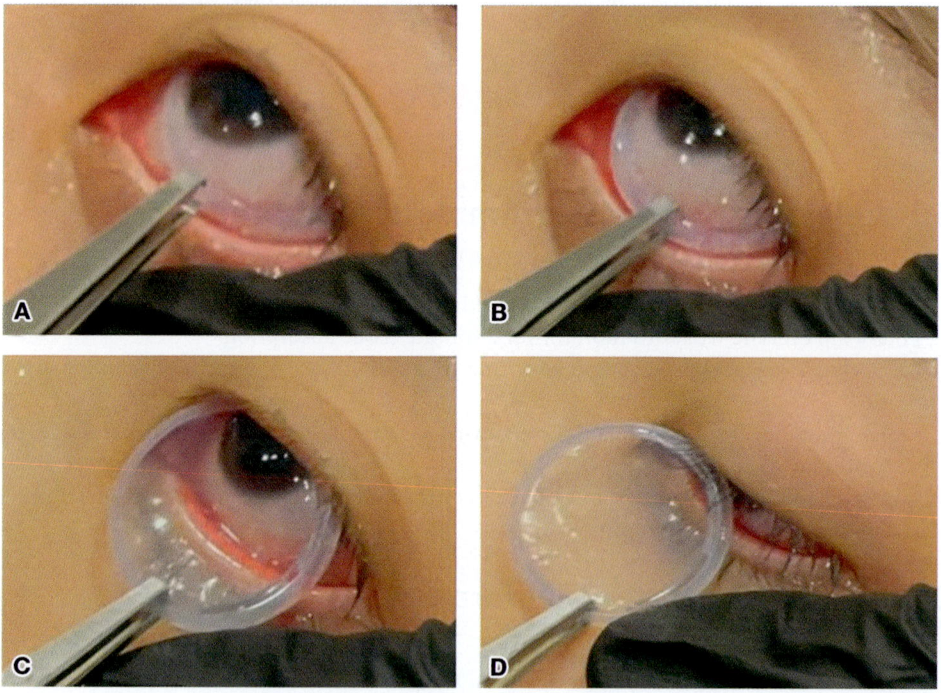


**FIGURE 27-14** Cryopreserved amniotic membrane removal. **A,** Direct patient to look upward. **B,** Grasp the inferior edge of the amniotic membrane ring. If the tissue is fully absorbed, only the ring will remain. **C,** Instruct the patient to look downward as the ring is removed from the eye. **D,** Remove the ring in a smooth motion as the patient looks down.

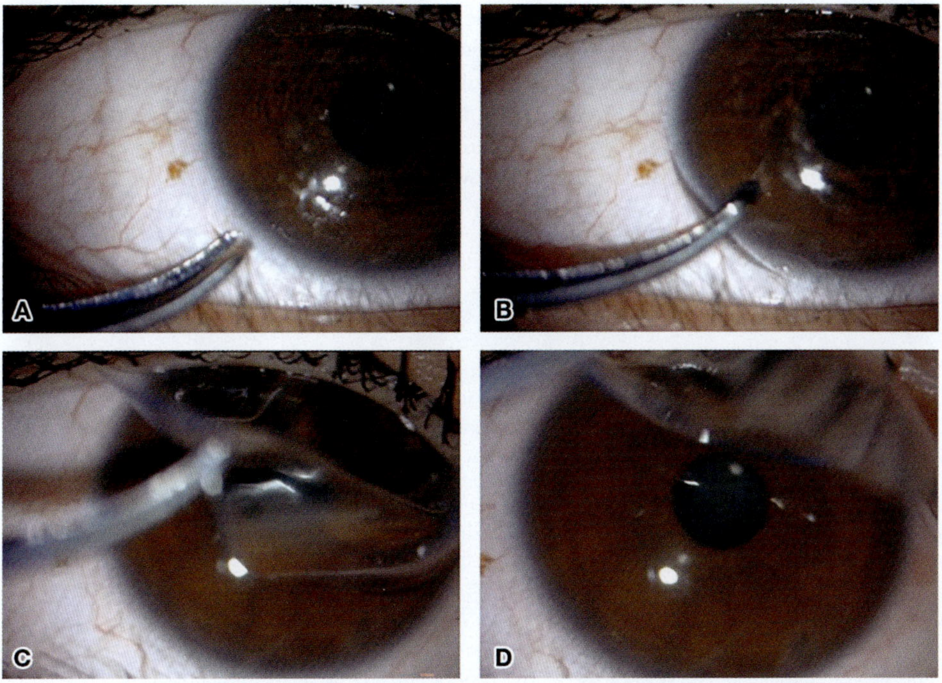


**FIGURE 27-15** Dehydrated amniotic membrane (dAM) + bandage contact lens (BCL) removal. **A,** The patient is directed to look upward. **B,** Forceps are used to grasp the edge of the BCL. **C,** The BCL is carefully lifted away from the cornea. **D,** The patient is directed to look straight as the rest of the BCL is removed.

# POTENTIAL COMPLICATIONS AND THEIR TREATMENTS

### Key Potential Complications

- Spontaneous extrusion/membrane falls out (cryopreserved amniotic membranes)
- Patient discomfort (cryopreserved amniotic membranes)
- Amniotic membrane disc movement (dehydrated amniotic membranes)
- Inflammatory infiltrates (dehydrated amniotic membranes)
- Contaminated amniotic membranes (extremely rare)

The most common complication with cryopreserved amniotic membranes is spontaneous extrusion, reported in 20% of cases.[4] The most commonly reported adverse effect is discomfort due to the size of the ring. This has been reported in roughly 17% to 30% of cases, with some improvement in comfort and stability from eyelid taping or a temporary tape tarsorrhaphy. Roughly about 4% to 6% of patients required early removal of the device before full absorption.[4,6,14,16]

With dehydrated amniotic membranes, the disc can move shortly after application. This can be adjusted if caught early enough. Otherwise, a replacement is necessary. Because a BCL is necessary with the dehydrated amniotic membrane disc, inflammatory infiltrates have been reported but large-scale studies are limited. Anecdotally, the author has found that adding a topical ophthalmic anti-inflammatory drop during the postoperative period is beneficial.

Risk of contaminated tissue is extremely low. One study reported an incidence of 1.6% to 8% for Gram positive isolates, but this was for cryopreserved amniotic membranes in a surgical setting.[8]

## VIDEOS OF PROCEDURES

**Video 27-1**—Cryopreserved amniotic membrane insertion and removal.

In this video, a cryopreserved amniotic membrane is first rinsed thoroughly with buffer saline solution (BSS) to remove the glycerol solution. Then, it is inserted by having the patient look downward while the upper edge of the amniotic membrane is inserted under the upper lid. The patient is directed to look upward, and the lower lid is moved down to allow the insertion of the lower edge of the ring. To decrease discomfort, lid taping is done to immobilize the upper lid. The removal of the cryopreserved amniotic membrane is then shown. The patient is directed to look upward, and the lower edge of the amniotic membrane ring is carefully grabbed with forceps. The patient is directed to look downward as the ring is carefully removed.

**Video 27-2**—Dehydrated amniotic membrane (direct to cornea) + bandage contact lens (BCL).

In this video, a dehydrated amniotic membrane is first cut to match the desired shape based on the area or epithelial defect being treated. This patient had a large slightly nasal but centrally involved nonhealing epithelial defect. After the eye is fully anesthetized and the lid speculum is placed, the amniotic membrane is carefully placed directly to the cornea and smoothened out. A BCL is then carefully placed with the patient looking straight ahead, being careful not to disrupt or displace the amniotic membrane.

**Video 27-3**—Dehydrated amniotic membrane (direct to cornea) + BCL.

In this video, a dehydrated amniotic membrane is placed directly onto a treated cornea. It is rehydrated slightly with a drop of BSS for easier movement and centration. A BCL is placed over top of the amniotic membrane, and air bubbles are smoothened out.

**Video 27-4**—Dehydrated amniotic membrane (direct to BCL).

A BCL is shown being prepared by placing it on the forefinger and drying lightly with a surgical spear. A dehydrated amniotic membrane is shown being removed from the packaging and placed directly onto the BCL. A surgical spear is used to smoothen the amniotic membrane disc along the BCL surface. For the insertion, the patient looks straight forward and the BCL + amniotic membrane (AM) is placed directly onto the cornea.

**Video 27-5**—Dehydrated amniotic membrane (direct to BCL).

A dehydrated amniotic membrane disc is carefully placed with the edge of the disc touching the BCL first. A surgical spear is used to smoothen the disc onto the BCL. In the same video, another example of a dehydrated amniotic membrane being prepared onto a BCL is shown; a smaller disc is shown here. For the insertion, the patient is directed to look straight ahead, the BCL + dehydrated AM disc combination is placed directly onto the eye. The patient is instructed to keep their gaze straight ahead while air bubbles are moved out of the way manually.

## EFFICACY

Amniotic membranes have variable efficacy based on the conditions treated as well as the preservation method of the device used. The efficacy between different dehydrated amniotic membranes may also vary; comparison studies of the various dehydrated amniotic membranes commercially available are limited.

In *epithelial defect and corneal wound healing*, longer exposure to amniotic membranes led to better epithelial defect healing.[6] In persistent epithelial defects, dehydrated amniotic membrane discs were reported to achieve resolution in 90% of cases, with roughly 2 weeks required for full absorption of the tissue.[11]

With cryopreserved amniotic membranes in *neurotrophic ulcers*, 40% of patients were successfully treated, 18% had partial improvement, and 27% had recurrent erosions and filaments. Three of five patients in that study that required additional therapy and treatment fully healed.[6] In advanced stages of neurotrophic keratitis, amniotic membranes are not sufficient in isolation.

In treating *ocular surface inflammation*, cryopreserved amniotic membranes were found to reach complete success (reduction in signs and symptoms) in 40% of patients, partial success in 30%, but cicatrizing complications were not necessarily prevented. Inclusion criteria of conditions that caused ocular surface inflammation in this study included adenoviral membranous keratoconjunctivitis, exposure keratopathy, epithelial basement membrane dystrophy (EBMD), persistent epithelial defects, postpenetrating keratoplasty and neurotrophic ulcers, limbal stem cell deficiency, severe dry eye syndrome, and bullous keratopathy.[6]

In *chemical and thermal burns*, cryopreserved amniotic membranes were found to achieve complete healing in 60% of patients, though the sample sizes are small.[6]

For *dry eye disease* specifically, both cryopreserved and dehydrated amniotic membranes show strong efficacy. Cryopreserved amniotic membranes improved visual acuity in 60% of cases, improved corneal staining scores in 88%, improved corneal sensitivity, corneal nerve density, and decreased Standard Patient Evaluation of Eye Dryness (SPEED) scores.[4,12-14] Dehydrated amniotic membranes were also found to statistically improve punctate epithelial erosions and variably improve visual acuity across multiple studies.[11,17]

Studies reporting the efficacy of amniotic membrane extract eye drops are limited. Currently, its use seems most effective in conjunction with advanced topical therapy or amniotic membrane transplantation for epithelial wound healing, limbal stem cell deficiency, and acute chemical burns. Further studies are underway for a better understanding of its application in ocular disease management.[9]

## CODING AND BILLING

- **65778-RT/LT**—Placement of amniotic membrane on the ocular surface; without sutures, 0 day global period

Modifier −79 can be used if the procedure was performed for a reason unrelated to prior surgery.

This is considered a minor procedure. A minor surgical procedure already includes the office visit, meaning that it should not be billed in conjunction with a same-day office visit. The only rare exception to this would be if E&M service was unrelated to the decision to perform the minor surgery; modifier −25 would be used in this case.[18]

According to Centers for Medicare and Medicaid Services, 92071 (fitting of a contact lens for ocular surface disease) and 65435 (performing debridement) cannot be billed with the same day 65778 (placement of self-retained amniotic membrane).[19]

Common ICD-10 codes that support the placement of amniotic membranes on the ocular surface without sutures include (right eye used as an example)[20]:

- **H11.011**—Amyloid pterygium of right eye
- **H11.021**—Central pterygium of right eye
- **H11.031**—Double pterygium of right eye
- **H11.041**—Peripheral pterygium, stationary, right eye
- **H11.051**—Peripheral pterygium, progressive, right eye
- **H11.061**—Recurrent pterygium of right eye
- **H11.811**—Pseudopterygium of conjunctiva, right eye
- **H11.821**—Conjunctivochalasis, right eye
- **H16.011**—Central corneal ulcer, right eye
- **H16.021**—Ring corneal ulcer, right eye
- **H16.031**—Corneal ulcer with hypopyon, right eye
- **H16.041**—Marginal corneal ulcer, right eye
- **H16.051**—Mooren's corneal ulcer, right eye
- **H16.061**—Mycotic corneal ulcer, right eye
- **H16.071**—Perforated corneal ulcer, right eye
- **H16.121**—Filamentary keratitis, right eye
- **H16.141**—Punctate keratitis, right eye
- **H16.231**—Neurotrophic keratoconjunctivitis, right eye
- **H18.11**—Bullous keratopathy, right eye
- **H18.411**—Arcus senilis, right eye
- **H18.421**—Band keratopathy, right eye
- **H18.441**—Keratomalacia, right eye
- **H18.451**—Nodular corneal degeneration, right eye
- **H18.461**—Peripheral corneal degeneration, right eye
- **H18.511**—Endothelial corneal dystrophy, right eye
- **H18.521**—Epithelial (juvenile) corneal dystrophy, right eye
- **H18.531**—Granular corneal dystrophy, right eye
- **H18.541**—Lattice corneal dystrophy, right eye
- **H18.551**—Macular corneal dystrophy, right eye
- **H18.591**—Other hereditary corneal dystrophies, right eye
- **H18.731**—Descemetocele, right eye
- **H18.821**—Corneal disorder due to contact lens, right eye
- **H18.831**—Recurrent corneal erosion, right eye
- **L51.1**—Stevens–Johnson syndrome
- **Q13.1**—Absence of iris

- **S05.01XA**—Injury of conjunctiva and corneal abrasion without foreign body, right eye, initial encounter
- **S05.01XD**—Injury of conjunctiva and corneal abrasion without foreign body, right eye, subsequent encounter
- **T26.11XA**—Burn of cornea and conjunctival sac, right eye, initial encounter
- **T26.21XA**—Burn with resulting rupture and destruction of right eyeball, initial encounter
- **T26.31XA**—Burns of other specified parts of right eye and adnexa, initial encounter
- **T26.61XA**—Corrosion of cornea and conjunctival sac, right eye, initial encounter
- **T26.71XA**—Corrosion with resulting rupture and destruction of right eyeball, initial encounter
- **T26.81XA**—Corrosions of other specified parts of right eye and adnexa, initial encounter
- **T81.31XA**—Disruption of external operation (surgical) wound, not elsewhere classified, initial encounter

## SPECIAL CONSIDERATIONS: CHOOSING THE ORIENTATION OF THE AMNIOTIC MEMBRANE

The orientation of cryopreserved amniotic membranes is fixed as the device is inserted into the eye. Dehydrated amniotic membranes, on the other hand, are available in different options of orientation, depending on the company. For example, some dehydrated amniotic membrane options include the following:

- Epithelium on one side, stromal tissue on the other
- Stromal tissue on both sides with a layer of epithelial cells in the center (basically two dehydrated amniotic membranes sandwiched together)
- Epithelium on both sides with a stromal layer in the center (the opposite of the previous point)

This allows the clinician to decide on the orientation of the dehydrated amniotic membrane disc being placed onto the eye.[21]

Studies are limited in the efficacy of office-based dehydrated amniotic membrane orientation choice at this time. However, histologic studies have suggested that orientation may play a role in the transplantation of amniotic membranes. Ocular surface re-epithelialization by host tissue has been found to occur preferentially on the basement membrane and epithelial side, though still possible on the stroma. When prioritizing providing a substrate for wound healing and re-epithelialization, it may be beneficial to have the amniotic membrane transplanted with the epithelial side facing externally (away from cornea).

On the other hand, the stromal matrix can trap and induce apoptosis in inflammatory cells to help downregulate the inflammatory response. In the presence of significant acute inflammation, the stromal portion of the membrane could protect the ocular surface from pro-inflammatory cells and mediators (from the conjunctiva, lids, or tear film). To take advantage of this, the amniotic membrane transplanted with the stromal side facing externally (away from cornea) may be preferred.[8] Again, while evidence of orientation-based efficacy for in-office dehydrated amniotic membranes is limited at this time, it may be possible that this might affect office-based amniotic membrane placement in the future.

This section has been included to simply provide clinicians with some suggestions at this time, given the commercial availability of different amniotic membrane products.

# REFERENCES


1. Cooke M, Tan E, Mandrycky C, He H, O'Connell J, Tseng S. Comparison of cryopreserved amniotic membrane and umbilical cord tissue with dehydrated amniotic membrane / chorion tissue. *J Wound Care*. 2014;23(10):465-476. doi:10.12968/jowc.2014.23.10.465
2. Paolin A, Cogliati E, Trojan D, et al. Amniotic membranes in ophthalmology: long term data on transplantation outcomes. *Cell Tissue Bank*. 2016;17(1):51-58. doi:10.1007/s10561-015-9520-y
3. Allen CL, Clare G, Stewart EA, et al. Augmented dried versus cryopreserved amniotic membrane as an ocular surface dressing. *PLoS One*. 2013;8(10):e78441. doi:10.1371/journal.pone.0078441
4. Pachigolla G, Prasher P, Di Pascuale MA, McCulley JP, McHenry JG, Mootha VV. Evaluation of the role of ProKera in the management of ocular surface and orbital disorders. *Eye Contact Lens Sci Clin Pract*. 2009;35(4):172-175. doi:10.1097/ICL.0b013e3181a66a12
5. Rojas MJ, Yeu E. Indications for and uses of amniotic membrane: clinic. In: Mannis MJ, Holland EJ, eds. *Cornea: Fundamentals, Diagnosis, and Management*. 5th ed. Elsevier Inc; 2022:1497.e1-1500.
6. Suri K, Kosker M, Raber IM, et al. Sutureless amniotic membrane ProKera for ocular surface disorders. *Eye Contact Lens Sci Clin Pract*. 2013;39(5):341-347. doi:10.1097/ICL.0b013e3182a2f8fa
7. Morkin MI, Hamrah P. Efficacy of self-retained cryopreserved amniotic membrane for treatment of neuropathic corneal pain. *Ocul Surf*. 2018;16(1):132-138. doi:10.1016/j.jtos.2017.10.003
8. Malhotra C, Jain AK. Human amniotic membrane transplantation: different modalities of its use in ophthalmology. *World J Transplant*. 2014;4(2):111-121. doi:10.5500/wjt.v4.i2.111
9. Murri MS, Moshirfar M, Birdsong OC, Ronquillo Y, Ding Y, Hoopes PC. Amniotic membrane extract and eye drops: a review of literature and clinical application. *Clin Ophthalmol*. 2018;12:1105-1112. doi:10.2147/OPTH.S165553
10. Zhou TE, Robert M-C. Comparing ProKera with amniotic membrane transplantation: indications, outcomes, and costs. *Cornea*. 2022;41(7):840-844. doi:10.1097/ICO.0000000000002852
11. Mimouni M, Trinh T, Sorkin N, et al. Sutureless dehydrated amniotic membrane for persistent epithelial defects. *Eur J Ophthalmol*. 2022;32(2):875-879. doi:10.1177/11206721211011354
12. John T, Tighe S, Sheha H, et al. Corneal nerve regeneration after self-retained cryopreserved amniotic membrane in dry eye disease. *J Ophthalmol*. 2017;2017:1-10. doi:10.1155/2017/6404918
13. Starr CE, Gupta PK, Farid M, et al. An algorithm for the preoperative diagnosis and treatment of ocular surface disorders. *J Cataract Refract Surg*. 2019;45(5):669-684. doi:10.1016/j.jcrs.2019.03.023
14. McDonald MB, Sheha H, Tighe S, et al. Treatment outcomes in the DRy Eye Amniotic Membrane (DREAM) study. *Clin Ophthalmol*. 2018;12:677-681. doi:10.2147/OPTH.S162203
15. Haagdorens M, Van Acker SI, Van Gerwen V, et al. Limbal stem cell deficiency: current treatment options and emerging therapies. *Stem Cells Int*. 2016;2016:1-22. doi:10.1155/2016/9798374
16. Kaisey M, Solomon AJ, Luu M, Giesser BS, Sicotte NL. Incidence of multiple sclerosis misdiagnosis in referrals to two academic centers. *Mult Scler Relat Disord*. 2019;30:51-56. doi:10.1016/j.msard.2019.01.048
17. Parikh AA, Yalamanchili S, Gemmel D, Erzurum S. Dehydrated extracellular membranes in the treatment of severe dry eye. *Invest Ophthalmol Vis Sci*. 2019;60(9):6754.
18. Rumpakis J. Minor procedures, major rules. *Rev Optom*. Published 2020. Accessed August 29, 2022. https://www.reviewofoptometry.com/article/minor-procedures-major-rules
19. Corcoran Consulting Group. Reimbursement for amniotic tissue. Published 2022. Accessed August 29, 2022. https://www.corcoranccg.com/products/faqs/amniotic-tissue/.
20. American Medical Association. *CPT 2021 Professional Edition*. American Medical Association; 2020.
21. Labtician. Lab Amnio dehydrated amniotic membrane. Published 2022. Accessed November 8, 2022. https://www.labtician.com/product/labamnio/

# 28 Autologous Serum

**Pamela Theriot • Bryan E. Lusk**

## BACKGROUND

The concept of using autologous serum tears (AST) or autologous serum eye drops (ASED) as a treatment is based on the biochemical similarities between an individual's serum and natural tears (NT).[1] These similarities include antimicrobial factors, electrolytes (sodium, potassium, chloride, bicarbonate, magnesium, and calcium), fibronectin, cytokines, vitamins A and C, proteins (lysozyme, lactoferrin, albumin, and immunoglobulins), epithelial growth factors (EGF), and nerve growth factor (NGF).[2-7] These components are all similar to those of NTs but found in higher concentrations in ASTs.[2-6] It is the higher concentrations of these epitheliotrophic factors in ASTs that have been shown to increase the power to heal the ocular surface.[1,3] In one study, the use of 50% ASTs was an effective medical treatment to heal persistent epithelial defects (PED) that were recalcitrant to conventional medical therapy.[8]

## INDICATIONS

### Key Indications

- Keratoconjunctivitis sicca (KCS)/dry eye disease (DED)[1,2,6,9]
- Persistent epithelial defects (PED)[1,2]
- Punctate epithelial erosions (PEE)[1]
- Sjögren syndrome (SS)[1,2,5,10]
- Graft-versus-host disease (GVHD)[1,2]
- Recurrent corneal erosions (RCE)[5,6]
- Neurotrophic keratopathy (NK)[1,6]
- Superior limbic keratoconjunctivitis (SLK)[1]
- Ocular cicatricial pemphigoid (OCP)[1]
- Mooren's ulcer[1]
- Filtering blebs after trabeculectomy[1,5]
- Post-keratorefractive surgery[1,5]

- Chemical burns[5,6]; Stevens–Johnson syndrome[1,2,5]
- Limbal stem cell deficiency[2]
- Tissue necrosis after orbital implants[5]

ASTs are often used as a second line of treatment when other methods have failed to resolve corneal defects. ASTs are used in these more common diagnoses when the severity level is moderate to severe: DED, PED, PEE, and RCE. Adding ASTs to the treatment regimen in conjunction with other dry eye treatment therapies has a significant and faster improvement of signs and symptoms.[2] Often patients can use ASTs for acute phases of the disease and stop the treatment once their flare has resolved.

ASTs are fast and effective in treating cases of moderate to severe DED. In two separate case studies, PED was treated with 20% AST dosed 6 to 10 times per day. In both studies, 60% of the patients had complete resolution of their signs and symptoms within 1 month.[11,12]

In patients with more severe diagnoses such as GVHD, Stevens–Johnson syndrome, limbal stem cell deficiency, and neurotrophic keratitis, AST treatment may be recommended earlier in the treatment protocol. Higher concentrations of ASTs and a more frequent dosing regimen is a common practice to control the disease. There may also be a need to continue using the treatment in the long term.[2]

Long-term efficacy and safety have been demonstrated in a trial by Lee and Chen. Their patients utilized 20% ASTs, and the patients were followed for 6 to 55 months. Results demonstrated 73.9% had a complete resolution of signs and 76% had a complete resolution of symptoms. There were no adverse events noted during the treatment period.[13]

## CONTRAINDICATIONS

### Key Contraindications

- HIV
- Hepatitis B
- Hepatitis C
- Syphilis
- Taking systemic immunosuppressive therapies (not necessarily a contraindication, but rather warrants closely monitoring if using ASTs)

Contraindications for ASTs should include any history of blood-borne infectious disease that could pose a risk to those preparing the solution or those assisting the patient in handling the solutions. These include HIV, hepatitis B and C, and syphilis.[14]

Studies have shown that patients who are undergoing systemic immunosuppressive therapies (such as cyclosporine or mycophenolic acid) have relevant concentrations of the medication detected on their ocular surface when utilizing ASTs. The effects of these systemic medications on the ocular surface, whether they are potentially beneficial or adverse, are not yet completely understood.[15] Close monitoring of these patients is indicated while taking systemic immunosuppressive therapy and utilizing ASTs.

## PREOPERATIVE PREPARATION

Advise the patient to eat a good meal and drink lots of water before arriving at the blood draw station. Six 8.5-mL vials of blood will be drawn during the session. The patient should sign an informed consent form detailing the nature of the procedure, potential risks and complications, and alternative treatment options prior to the procedure.

### Venipuncture Setup (Figure 28-1)

- Latex exam gloves
- 20-mL syringe
- Four to six red top vacutainers
- Alcohol wipe
- Butterfly needle
- Phlebotomy tourniquet
- Band-Aid
- Felt-tip marker

### Autologous Serum Tears Preparation Setup (Figure 28-2)

- Latex exam gloves
- Sterile exam gloves
- Laminar flow hood
- Sterile drape
- Sterile pipettes
- Vacutainer tubes full of centrifuged blood
- Sterile saline
- 4 to 12 sterile eye drop bottles 3- to 5-mL size
- Ziplock bags

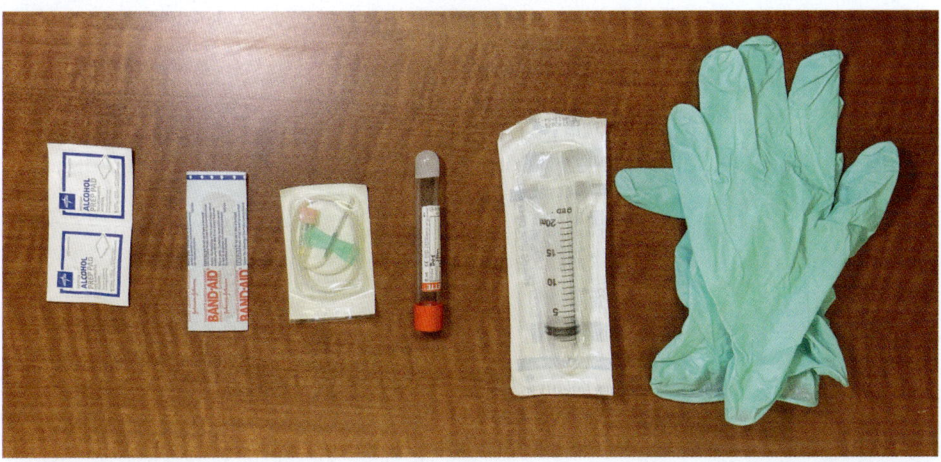


**FIGURE 28-1** Equipment needed to perform venipuncture. All items should be kept within arm's reach, and collection tubes should be labeled accurately with the patient's name and date.

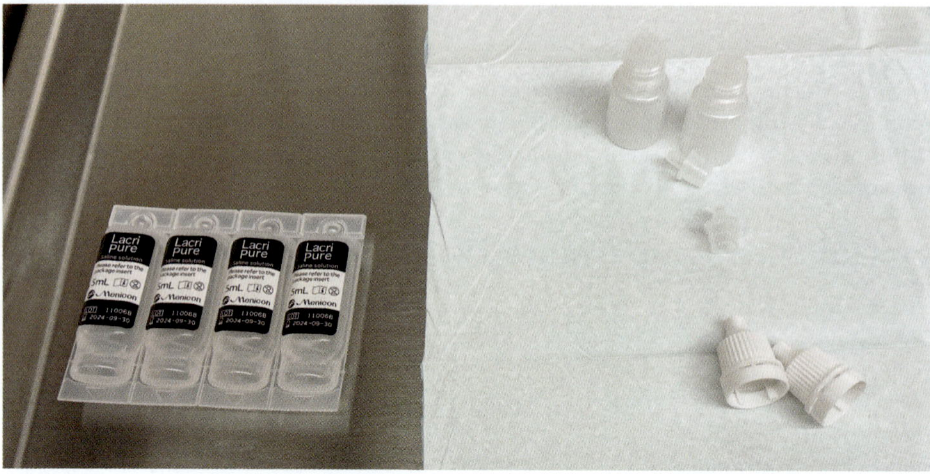


**FIGURE 28-2** Equipment needed for AST preparation. It is important to maintain the sterility of the preparation site. Gather all of the equipment before starting the procedure to reduce the possibility of introducing bacteria into the sterile field. Affix the labels to the eye drop bottles once they are filled with AST and securely capped. The patient will transport the AST bottles in a cooler or insulated bag.

- Ice
- Labels
- Felt-tip markers
- Patients should provide an insulated bag or cooler.

# PROCEDURE

## Venipuncture Procedure

- Label the vacutainers with the patient's name, date of birth, and date and time of blood draw.
- Draw six 8.5-mL vacutainers of blood.
- Allow the blood to clot for 2 hours at room temperature.

Label the vacutainer tubes with the patient's name, date of birth, and date and time of the blood draw. A registered nurse or licensed phlebotomist draws the patient's blood to fill six 8.5-mL vacutainers.[14] Allow the blood to clot at room temperature in the red top vacutainer tubes for a minimum of 2 hours. After 2 hours, you are ready to centrifuge the blood.[16,17]

## Centrifuge Setup

- Place the vacutainer tubes into the centrifuge (Figure 28-3).
- Counterbalance any vacutainers that are not completely full with an equal portion of water in an empty vacutainer (Figure 28-4).

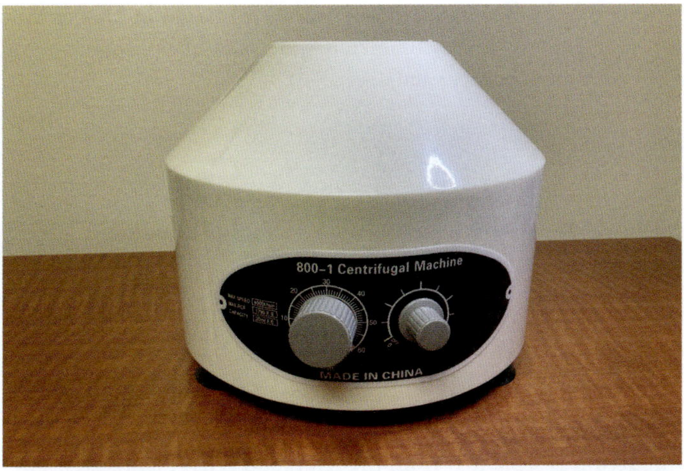


**FIGURE 28-3** The centrifuge device. The dial on the left side sets the time in minutes, from 0 to 60 minutes. The dial on the right side sets the speed of the rotation in RPM (rounds per minute). The model shown is adjustable from 0 to 4,000 RPM.

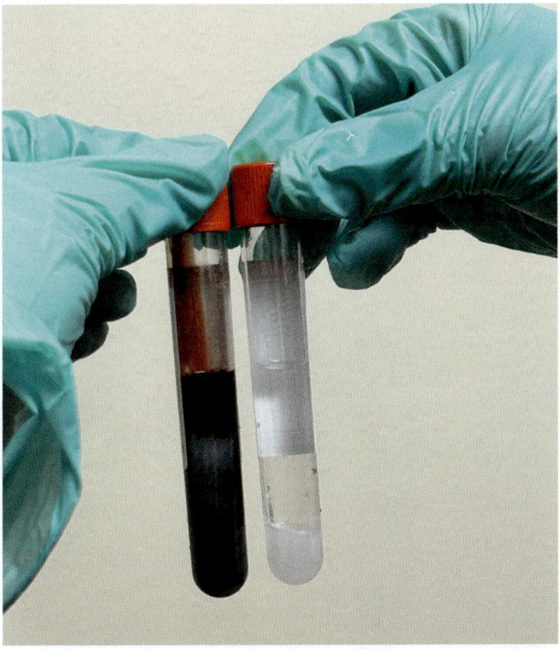

**FIGURE 28-4** Water counterbalance. When working with a vacutainer tube that isn't completely filled with blood, it is important to counterbalance the tube to ensure proper functioning of the centrifuge. Simply fill an empty vacutainer with the same amount of water as the partially filled blood tube. Set the two tubes across from each other within the well of the centrifuge. This will ensure the well remains balanced and the tubes spin at a steady speed.

Place the vacutainer tubes full of blood directly across from one another and ensure they are counterbalanced. If one vacutainer isn't completely full, create the proper counterbalance with an equal portion of water in an empty vacutainer.

## Centrifugation

- Close the lid.
- Set the speed dial to 2,000 or up to 4,000 RPM (rounds per minute).
- Set the timer for 15 minutes.

Close the lid and set the speed to at least 2,000 RPM or up to 4,000 RPM for 15 minutes.[16]

## Postcentrifugation

- Remove the vacutainers.
- Observe that the serum is separated from the red blood cells (Figure 28-5).

Remove the vacutainers from the centrifuge, and observe the serum is separated from the spun-down red blood cells.

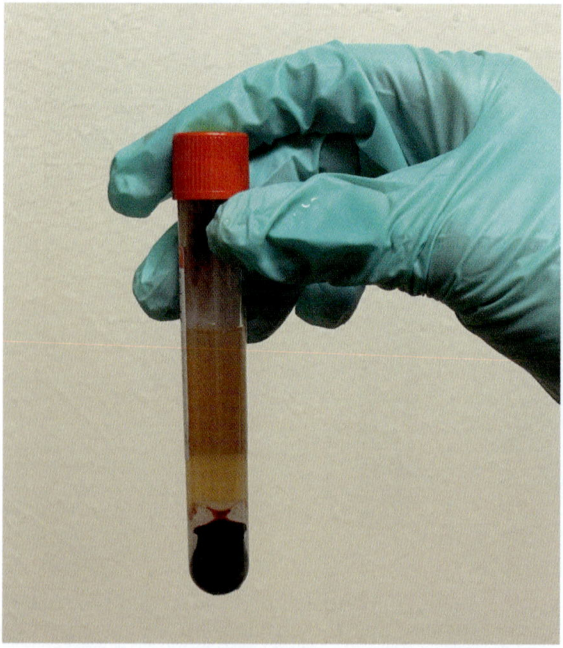

**FIGURE 28-5** Once the blood is spun down, the vacutainer will be filled with the serum at the top (clear yellowish liquid) and red blood cells at the bottom of the tube.

## Autologous Serum Tears Preparation Step-by-Step Instructions

- Set up a sterile field in the laminar flow hood.
- Use a sterile pipette to draw off 1 mL of serum.
- Place the serum into the sterile eye drop bottle.
- Add 1 mL of sterile saline solution to yield 2 mL of 50% serum.
- Place the dropper cap and lid onto the eyedrop bottles.
- Label bottles with the patient's name and the date.
- Patient should transport the bottles with a bag of ice.

Each 8.5-mL tube of blood yields approximately 4 mL of serum.[14] Serum is platelet poor and should have a yellow color. Set up a sterile field in the laminar flow hood (Figures 28-6 and 28-7).

Use a sterile pipette to draw off 1 mL of serum from the vacutainer tube and place it into the sterile eye drop bottle (Figure 28-8).

Use a new sterile pipette for each tube to bottle transfer to reduce the probability of contamination. Afterward, add 1 mL of sterile saline solution to yield 2 mL of 50% serum.

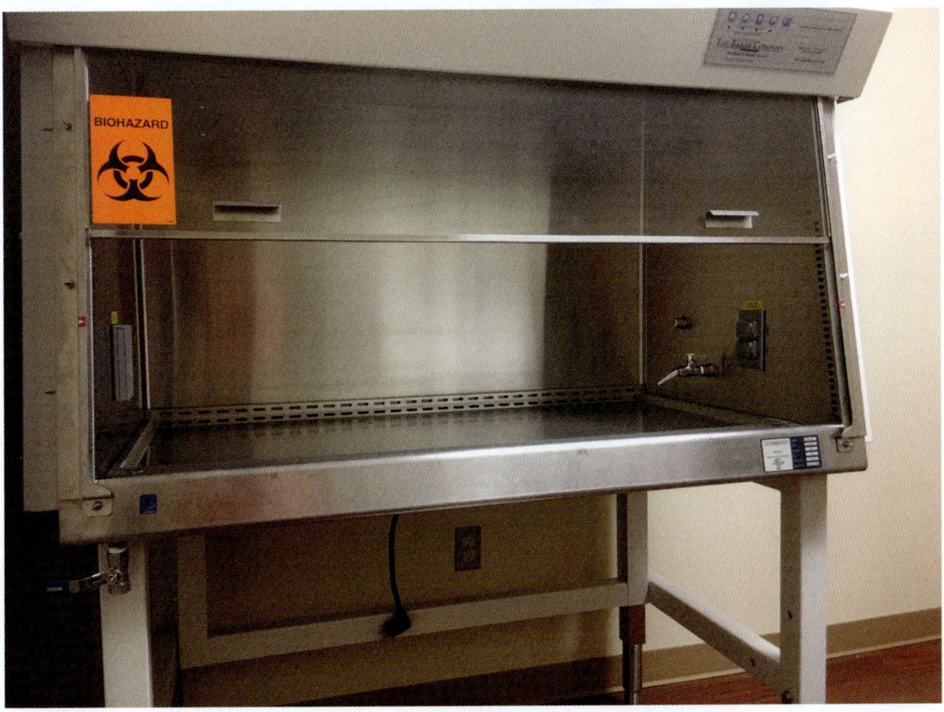


**FIGURE 28-6** Laminar flow hood. The hood is utilized to protect the AST preparation environment from dust, debris, and other airborne contaminants. The flow hood maintains a constant flow of high efficiency particulate air (HEPA)-filtered air over the workspace. Using a hood is a great way to ensure the quality of the AST and reduce the incidence of introducing bacteria into the eye drop bottles. AST, autologous serum tears.

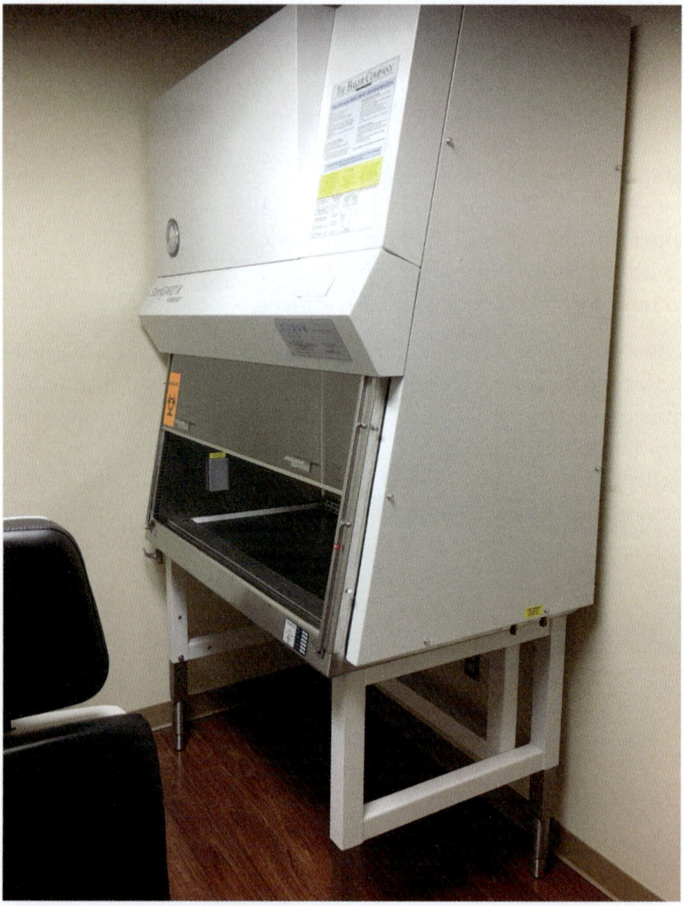

**FIGURE 28-7** Laminar flow hoods are often used when working with biological samples. They may also be referred to as clean benches, cell culture hoods, or tissue culture hoods. They provide a sterile work environment.

The amount of serum can be varied to produce 20% to 50% solutions, as desired. Place the dropper tip and lid onto the eyedrop bottles (Figure 28-9). Label them with the patient's name and the date and give them to the patient with a bag of ice.

Advise the patient to transport them in a cooler or insulated bag when not being stored at home. Once the patient is home, instruct them to store all vials in a freezer until ready to use. One bottle should be removed from the freezer at a time for use and kept in the refrigerator between applications. ASTs can remain in the refrigerator for 5 days after which time they should be discarded.[3]

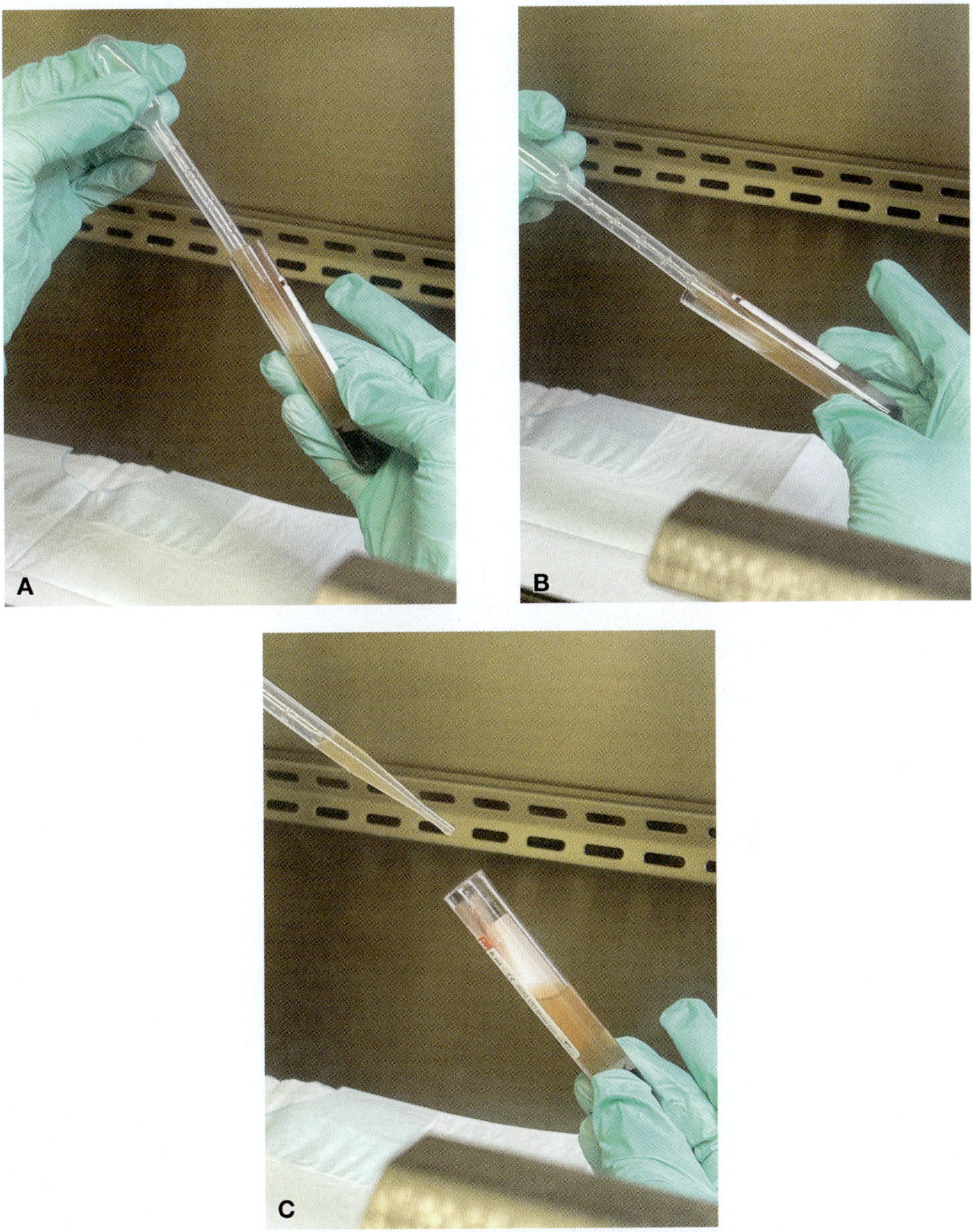


**FIGURE 28-8** Blood serum. Note that blood serum is a clear yellowish liquid. This portion of the blood is rich in proteins and does not contain any white blood cells, red blood cells, platelets, or clotting factors. **A,** Insert the sterile pipette into vacutainer tube without touching the outside of the tube. **B,** Draw up only the serum into the pipette. **C,** Withdraw the pipette and transfer the serum to the sterile eye dropper bottle.

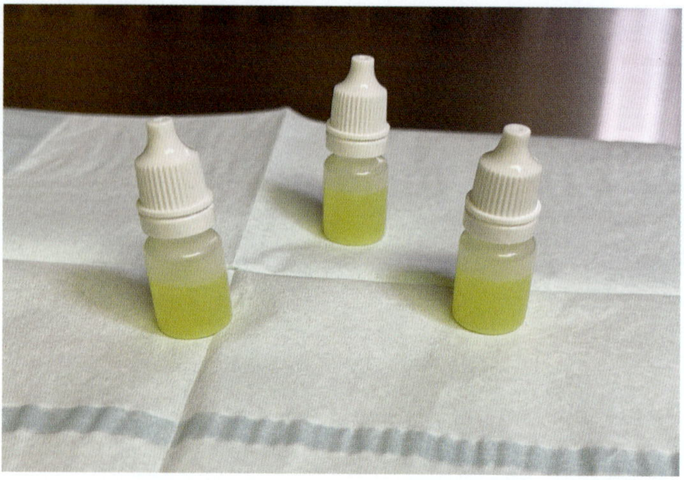

**FIGURE 28-9** Bottled AST. AST should be stored in small bottles. If poor handling practices are noted or the bottle is suspected to be contaminated, the bottle should be discarded. AST, autologous serum tears.

### Use and Storage

Dosing of ASTs can range from twice daily to hourly depending on the severity of the signs and symptoms of the ocular surface disease. Unused bottles can be stored in the freezer for 90 days.[3]

## POSTPROCEDURE CARE/COMANAGEMENT (FOLLOW-UP SCHEDULE)

**Key Postoperative Considerations**

- Apply pressure and a Band-Aid to the venipuncture site.
- Increase fluid intake.
- Avoid strenuous exercise and activity with the arm for 24 hours.
- Return to the clinic 2 to 6 weeks for follow-up.

After blood collection, apply firm pressure to the arm for a few minutes to help facilitate clot formation. Instruct the patient to drink plenty of fluids and to sit or lie down if dizzy. If dizziness remains or becomes severe, they should be instructed to go to the emergency room.[18]

To reduce bruising, the patient can apply a cold compress to the venipuncture site. The patient should be advised to leave the Band-Aid in place for at least 2 hours. Typical phlebotomy protocol and precautions advise avoiding alcohol, caffeine, hot baths, strenuous exercise, and heavy lifting with that arm for the next 24 hours.[19]

The patient should follow up with their eye care professional (ECP) in 2 to 6 weeks to assess the response to the therapy and allow for necessary adjustments in the treatment strategy. Slit-lamp evaluation and staining patterns are useful to determine whether additional treatment with ASTs and/or alternative therapy is needed.[14]

# POTENTIAL COMPLICATIONS AND THEIR TREATMENT

### Key Potential Complications

- Phlebotomy Complications
  - Hematoma/bruising
  - Pain
  - Infection
  - Air embolism (rare)
  - Anemia (rare)
  - Thrombosis (rare)
- AST complications
  - Microbial contamination of the tears during preparation, storage or usage of the ASTs, and possible resultant ocular infection if contamination occurs
  - Immune complex deposition (rare, and only from high-concentration ASTs)

Complications of phlebotomy include hematoma, pain, and infection.[20] Air embolism, anemia, and thrombosis are other more rare but potentially serious side effects of phlebotomy.[21] Bruising after the blood draw is a relatively common side effect. The patient can keep the arm elevated and apply pressure and ice to the area of the needlestick to reduce the probability of hematoma.

Risks of AST use include contamination by bacteria or fungus, which poses an infection risk to the patient. Although the ASTs are prepared utilizing sterile conditions, there are risks for contamination during all phases of preparation.[16]

Due to the lack of preservatives and the high protein content of ASTs, the risk of contamination and growth of microorganisms is higher than when using commercially available preserved treatments. At any time during the preparation, storage, and use of the drops, contamination could occur. The patient must be cautioned not to leave the ASTs unrefrigerated for any length of time. The refrigeration requirement should be considered when patients need to transport the ASTs. Proper handling and storage of the ASTs significantly reduce the risk of contamination or denaturation of the serum proteins.[14]

Patients must also take additional precautions when utilizing the ASTs including not allowing the tip of the dropper to contact the eye, eyelid, or any nonsterile surface.[16] During the informed consent process, the patient should be educated on the risks of bacterial or fungal contamination, how to recognize when a bottle is or may be contaminated, and the potential risks contaminated solutions can pose to the eye.

If a patient presents to the clinic with an infectious corneal infiltrate during AST treatment, it is important to obtain a corneal culture to accurately identify the organism. Timely identification of the causative organism is the key to a favorable outcome.[22] If a corneal culture cannot be obtained within 24 hours, empirical broad-spectrum antimicrobials should be initiated.

There is also a risk of immune complex deposition from frequent dosing (hourly) of high-concentration ASTs (100% serum). Patients who utilize high-concentration ASTs may need more cautious monitoring due to this risk.[23]

## VIDEOS OF PROCEDURES

**Video 28-1**—Serum preparation: collect six vacutainer tubes of blood and allow them to sit at room temperature to clot for at least 2 hours. Then, load the vacutainers into the centrifuge. Before starting the centrifuge, ensure the vacutainers are balanced. A vacutainer tube containing an equal volume of blood (or water used as a balance) should be placed directly across from the first vacutainer. There should always be an even number of tubes. Close the lid of the centrifuge and set the speed and time. The speed dial (on the left side) is set between 2,000 and 4,000 RPM. The timer (on the right) is set for a minimum of 15 minutes. Once the centrifuge stops, remove the vacutainers and observe that the serum is properly spun down from the red blood cells. (Video courtesy of Pamela Theriot and Felicia Croft.)

**Video 28-2**—autologous serum tears (AST) preparation instructions: Set up your sterile field inside the laminar flow hood. Starting with a sterile drape, open the sterile pipettes and eye drop bottles onto the field. Next, dawn your sterile surgical gloves to arrange the field. Prepare the sterile AST drops by placing 1 mL of serum into the sterile eye drop bottle, being careful not to touch the sides of the vacutainer or eye drop bottle. A new pipette should be used each time to reduce the possibility of contamination. Add 1 mL of sterile saline solution to each eye drop bottle containing the serum. This gives 2 mL of 50% solution. Vary the amount of saline solution depending on the concentration of ASTs desired. Once the bottle tips and lids are placed under the sterile hood, the eye drop bottles can be labeled with the patient's name and date. (Video courtesy of Pamela Theriot and Felicia Croft.)

# EFFICACY

ASTs have variable efficacy depending on the concentration of tears used and the severity of the disease being treated. Overall, when compared to artificial tear use or other conventional treatments, ASTs are a great treatment option for many corneal defects.

## Keratoconjunctivitis Sicca/Dry Eye Disease

In a randomized controlled trial (RCT) by Kojima et al, 20 patients with KCS were randomized into treatment (AST) and control groups (artificial tears). AST use was associated with improvement of clinical signs (reduction of fluorescein staining) and symptoms (using a visual analog scale). This study provided evidence that AST use was more effective than artificial tears for KCS treatment.[24]

In a different RCT by Urzua et al, 12 patients with KCS were treated with 20% AST, and Ocular Surface Disease Index (OSDI) symptom scores were taken before and after treatment.

The control group was treated with artificial tears alone. A 50% improvement in the OSDI score was found in the AST treatment group.[25]

In a study by Takamura et al, the efficacy of treatment of PED was 94% in patients receiving ASTs dosed eight times a day. However, only 58% of patients who received ASTs four times a day experienced resolution.[26] The concentration of the ASTs and the dosing must be altered based on the severity of the clinical appearance.

### Graft-versus-Host Disease

The effects of using 20% ASTs to treat 14 patients with GVHD were studied in a case series by Ogawa et al. After 4 weeks of treatment using ASTs 10 times per day, significant improvements were seen in both subjective complaint scores and fluorescein staining. In 50% of participants, the results were maintained for 6 months or more. The other 50% required the use of punctal plugs in order to maintain resolution of the corneal epithelial defects.[27]

### Superior Limbic Keratoconjunctivitis

ASTs as a treatment for SLK were less effective. Although patients had resolution of their fluorescein staining, the symptoms were found to return after discontinuation of the AST therapy. The efficacy of AST therapy varied between 30% and 100% for symptomatic relief and 39% to 61% for reduction of fluorescein. These differences may result from variations in the production and treatment protocol with ASTs.[4]

### Recurrent Corneal Erosions

Patients had an 85% success rate of no recurrence of RCE for 1 to 4 years after treatment with ASTs. The treatment protocol included using ASTs six times daily for 3 months followed by four times daily for another 3 months.[28]

### Sjögren's Syndrome

AST treatment is a safe and effective way to provide essential nutrients to the ocular surface in the treatment of KCS associated with Sjögren's syndrome. In patients with SS who were treated with 20% AST for 4 weeks, 55% of patients saw the resolution of the fluorescein staining.[10]

## CODING/BILLING

### CPT Code

**36415** can be used for all routine venipunctures, not requiring the skill of a physician. However, the production of ASTs is an out-of-pocket product for the patient because there is currently no pharmaceutical coverage for it. The ECP can set the price for the procedure after assessing their costs to produce the product.

Common ICD-10 codes that support the preparation of ASTs:

- **H16.22X**—Keratoconjunctivitis sicca, unspecified eye
- **H04.12X**—Dry eye syndrome, unspecified eye
- **H18.89X**—Persistent epithelial defect, unspecified eye
- **H18.839X**—Persistent epithelial erosion, unspecified eye
- **M35.01**—Sjögren's syndrome with keratoconjunctivitis sicca, unspecified eye
- **H18.83X**—Recurrent corneal erosion, unspecified eye
- **H16.23X**—Neurotrophic keratitis, unspecified eye
- **D89.813**—Graft-versus-host disease

### Important to Note

Production of blood products is regulated by national laws, which may vary significantly between states. It is important to research the exact laws regarding Clinical Laboratory Improvement Amendments (CLIA) and compounding in your state. There are several alternatives to producing AST in your own clinic.

## ALTERNATIVE OPTIONS

There are several alternative ways to prescribe ASTs to your patients if you are unable to make ASTs in your own clinic. There may be a local compounding pharmacy that can make ASTs for your patients. There are also a couple of national companies that will set up your patient to have their blood drawn locally and shipped to their facility to be processed as ASTs. Once the ASTs are produced, they are shipped overnight directly to your patient's home in a refrigerated carton. These companies include:

- Vital Tears—www.vitaltears.com
- Opticyte Tears—www.opticytetears.com
- Arc Point Labs—www.arcpointlabs.com

### Platelet-Rich Plasma Tears

Platelet-rich plasma (PRP) tears are another alternative to ASTs. PRP tears have been reported as a successful treatment for both the signs and symptoms of DED.[29] PRP can contain 2.5 to 8.0 times the concentration of platelets found in whole blood. It is considered to have superior healing effects on the cornea compared to ASTs. This superior healing power is due to both its lower concentration of inflammatory cytokines and its richer concentration of growth factors and other platelet derivatives.[30-32] In addition, PRP tears have a natural analgesic effect to reduce pain.[31]

In a clinical study of over 300 patients with a diagnosis of either aqueous deficient DED or evaporative DED, 87% of patients showed an improvement in symptoms after 6 weeks of therapy using the drops six times per day. Additionally, 76% of patients showed a reduction in fluorescein staining.[30] The use of PRP drops as monotherapy is an effective treatment to improve both the signs and symptoms of moderate to severe DED.[30]

There is a significant difference in the preparation of PRP drops compared to ASTs. The process of preparing the PRP tears maintains the integrity of the platelets and allows the platelets to activate at the site of tissue injury instead of removing them from the serum as is done in AST preparation.[32]

An anticoagulant (Figure 28-10) is added to the syringe prior to the blood being drawn, and the blood is not allowed to clot before it is spun down. Six mL of sodium citrate is used to coat the inside of a 60-mL syringe. The anticoagulant prevents the clotting of the blood and activation of platelets. This keeps the platelets in their native form.

Centrifugation separates the blood components. Unlike serum, PRP is red in color. The PRP is collected with a pipette and put in eye drop bottles.[30] The PRP can be diluted with sterile saline if desired. Fifty percent to 100% concentrations are common for PRP. These drops need to remain refrigerated while not in use. And once refrigerated, they should be discarded after 5 to 7 days.[33] The PRP drops used in Wu's studies were never frozen. Instead, they were prepared fresh each week and kept refrigerated in between.

Several studies have been conducted to determine whether the protein concentrations of PRP differ once it has been frozen and then thawed before use. The results of the studies showed that both the platelet count and growth factor concentrations began to decline after 4 weeks of frozen storage.[34] Once the PRP is frozen, it should be utilized within 1 month.

Again, it is important to note that the production of blood products is regulated by national laws, which may vary significantly between states. It is important to research the exact laws

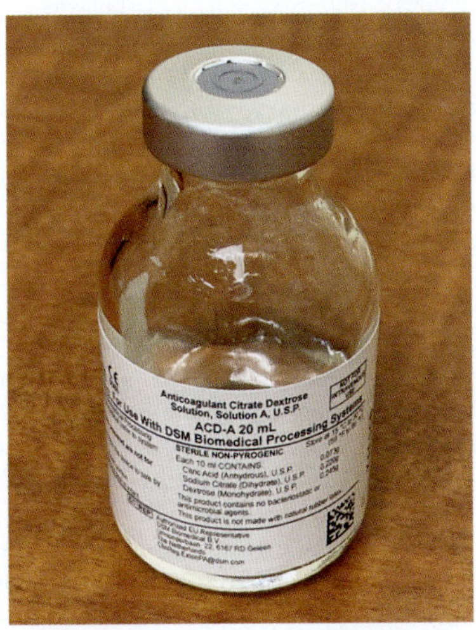


**FIGURE 28-10** Anticoagulant. This is an additive that should be placed in the blood collection container. It prevents platelet activation and clot formation. This allows the platelets to be collected along with the serum and removes the white and red blood cells only.

regarding CLIA and compounding in your state. Some commercially available PRP preparation systems include:

Endoret PRGF—https://bti-biotechnologyinstitute.com/en/solutions/regenerative-medicine/why-endoret-prgf

RegenKit A-PRP—https://www.regenlab.com/products/regenkit-a-prp-2/

# REFERENCES


1. Quinto GG, Campos M, Behrens A. Autologous serum for ocular surface diseases. *Arg Bras Oftalmol.* 2008;71(6 suppl):47-54.
2. Dang V, Hoyle B. Autologous serum tears: an overlooked treatment for dry eye. *Mod Optom.* 2020(July/August):26-28.
3. García-Martín E, Pernía-López S, Romero Jiménez RM, García-Valcárcel B, Martínez-Ortega PA, Sanjurjo-Saez M. The use of autologous serum eye drops for the treatment of ocular surface disorders. *Eur J Hosp Pharm.* 2019;26(6):314-317. doi:10.1136/ejhpharm-2018-001527
4. Geerling G, MacLennan S, Hartwig D. Autologous serum eye drops for ocular surface disorders. *Br J Ophthalmol.* 2004;88(11):1467-1474.
5. Jones L, Downie LE, Korb D, et al. TFOS DEWS II management and therapy report *Ocul Surf.* 2017;15(3):575-628. doi:10.1016/j.jtos.2017.05.006
6. Semeraro F, Forbice E, Braga O, Bova A, Di Salvatore A, Azzolini C. Evaluation of the efficacy of 50% autologous serum eye drops in different ocular surface pathologies. *Biomed Res Int.* 2014;2014:826970. doi:10.1155/2014/826970
7. Gupta A, Monroy D, Ji Z, Yoshino K, Huang A, Pflugfelder SC. Transforming growth factor beta-1 and beta-2 in human tear fluid. *Curr Eye Res.* 1996;15(6):605-614.
8. Jeng BH, Dupps WJ Jr. Autologous serum 50% eyedrops in the treatment of persistent corneal epithelial defects. *Cornea.* 2009;28(10):1104-1108. doi:10.1097/ICO.0b013e3181a2a7f6
9. Craig JP, Nelson JD, Azar DT, et al. TFOS DEWS II report executive summary. *Ocul Surf.* 2017;15(4):802-812. doi:10.1016/j.jtos.2017.08.003
10. Tsubota K, Goto E, Fujita H, et al. Treatment of dry eye by autologous serum application in Sjögren's syndrome. *Br J Ophthalmol.* 1999;83(4):390-395. doi:10.1136/bjo.83.4.390
11. Tsubota K, Goto E, Shimmura S, Shimazaki J. Treatment of persistent corneal epithelial defect by autologous serum application. *Ophthalmology.* 1999;106(10):1984-1989.
12. Young AL, Cheng AC, Ng HK, Cheng LL, Leung GY, Lam DS. The use of autologous serum tears in persistent corneal epithelial defects. *Eye.* 2004;18(6):609-614.
13. Lee GA, Chen SX. Autologous serum in the management of recalcitrant dry eye syndrome. *Clin Experiment Ophthalmol.* 2008;36(2):119-122.
14. Mangan R, Layman S. How (and why) to make autologous serum. *Rev Optom.* Published March 15, 2012. https://www.reviewofoptometry.com/article/how-and-why-to-make-autologous-serum
15. Tahmaz V, Wiesen MHJ, Gehlsen U, et al. Detection of systemic immunosuppressants in autologous serum eye drops (ASED) in patients with severe chronic ocular graft versus host disease. *Graefes Arch Clin Exp Ophthalmol.* 2021;259(1):121-128. doi:10.1007/s00417-020-04865-8
16. Lagnado R, King AJ, Donald F, Dua HS. A protocol for low contamination risk of autologous serum drops in the management of ocular surface disorders. *Br J Ophthalmol.* 2004;88(4):464-465. doi:10.1136/bjo.2003.025528
17. Liu L, Hartwig D, Harloff S, et al. Corneal epitheliotrophic capacity of three different blood-derived preparations. *Invest Ophthalmol Vis Sci.* 2006;47(6):2438-2444. doi:10.1167/iovs.05-0876
18. National Library of Medicine. *WHO Guidelines on Drawing Blood: Best Practices in Phlebotomy.* World Health Organization; 2010. Accessed October 25, 2022. https://www.ncbi.nlm.nih.gov/books/NBK138665/
19. Memorial Sloan Kettering Cancer Center. Instructions after your therapeutic phlebotomy procedure. Accessed October 25, 2022. https://www.mskcc.org/cancer-care/patient-education/instructions-after-your-therapeutic-phlebotomy-procedure
20. Buowari O. Complications of venipuncture. *Adv Biosci Biotechnol.* 2013;4:126-128. doi:10.4236/abb.2013.41A018

21. Ohnishi H Side effects of phlebotomy: pathophysiology, diagnosis, treatment and prophylaxis. *Rinsho Byori.* 2005;53:904-910.
22. Robinson J, Ellen J, Hadel B, Lighthizer N. Collecting a corneal culture: when guesses and hunches won't do, get the facts. *Rev Optom.* Published April 15, 2016. https://www.reviewofoptometry.com/article/collecting-a-corneal-culture
23. McDonnell PJ, Schanzlin DJ, Rao NA. Immunoglobulin deposition in the cornea after application of autologous serum. *Arch Ophthalmol.* 1988;106(10):1423-1425.
24. Kojima T, Ishida R, Goto E, Matsumoto Y, Dogru M, Tsubota K; The efficacy of autologous serum eye drops for Keratoconjunctivitis Sicca A prospective study. *Invest Ophthalmol Vis Sci.* 2004;45(13):3894.
25. Urzua CA, Vasquez DH, Huidobro A, Hernandez H, Alfaro J. Randomized double-blind clinical trial of autologous serum versus artificial tears in dry eye syndrome. *Curr Eye Res.* 2012;37(8):684-688. doi:10.3109/02713683.2012.674609
26. Takamura E, Shiozaki K, Hata H, et al. Efficacy of autologous serum treatment in patients with severe dry eye. In: Sullivan DA, ed. *Lacrimal Gland, Tear Film, and Dry Eye Syndromes 3.* Kluwer Academic/Plenum Publishers; 2002:1247-1250.
27. Ogawa Y, Okamoto S, Mori T, et al. Autologous serum eye drops for the treatment of severe dry eye in patients with chronic graft-versus-host disease. *Bone Marrow Transplant.* 2003;31(7):579-583.
28. Ziakas NG, Boboridis KG, Terzidou C, et al. Long-term follow up of autologous serum treatment for recurrent corneal erosions. *Clin Exp Ophthalmol.* 2010;38(7):683-687. doi:10.1111/j.1442-9071.2010.02304.x
29. López-Plandolit S, Morales MC, Freire V, Grau AE, Durán JA. Efficacy of plasma rich in growth factors for the treatment of dry eye. *Cornea.* 2011;30(12):1312-1317. doi:10.1097/ICO.0b013e31820d86d6
30. Alio JL, Rodriguez AE, Ferreira-Oliveira R, Wróbel-Dudzińska D, Abdelghany AA. Treatment of dry eye disease with autologous platelet-rich plasma: a prospective, interventional, non-randomized study. *Ophthalmol Ther.* 2017;6(2):285-293. doi:10.1007/s40123-017-0100-z
31. Cole BJ, Seroyer ST, Filardo G, Bajaj S, Fortier LA. Platelet-rich plasma: where are we now and where are we going? *Sports Health.* 2010;2(3):203-210. doi:10.1177/1941738110366385
32. Madan M. Platelet-rich plasma eye drops for dry eye disease: separating the myths from the facts. *Mod Optom.* Published November/December 2021. https://modernod.com/articles/2021-nov-dec/platelet-rich-plasma-eye-drops-for-dry-eye-disease
33. Wu TE, Chen CJ, Hu CC, Cheng CK. Easy-to-prepare autologous platelet-rich plasma in the treatment of refractory corneal ulcers. *Taiwan J Ophthalmol.* 2015;5(3):132-135. doi:10.1016/j.tjo.2014.09.001
34. Shiga Y, Kubota G, Orita S, et al. Freeze-dried human platelet-rich plasma retains activation and growth factor expression after an eight-week preservation period. *Asian Spine J.* 2017;11(3):329-336. doi:10.4184/asj.2017.11.3.329

# 29 Conjunctivochalasis Repair

**Edward H. Jaccoma**

## BACKGROUND

Conjunctivochalasis (CCH) is an ocular disorder, which is described as a nonedematous, loose, and redundant conjunctiva, most commonly affecting the inferior bulbar conjunctiva that situates between the lower eyelid and the globe.[1] The condition can affect all parts of the inferior bulbar area, including the nasal, central, or temporal portions. It usually occurs bilaterally, and its prevalence increases with age.[2-4] According to Mimura et al, in their hospital-based study of 1,416 patients, the prevalence of CCH increased dramatically with age:

- 1 to 10 years = 6.8%
- 11 to 20 years = 36.2%
- 21 to 30 years = 61.5%
- 31 to 40 years = 71.4%
- 41 to 50 years = 90.2%
- 51 to 60 years = 94.2%
- 61 to 70 years = 98.0%
- 71 to 80 years = 99.0%
- 81 to 90 years = 98.5%
- 91 to 100 years = 100.0%[4]

The pathogenesis of CCH, though there is no consensus, roots in the loss of conjunctival epithelial cohesiveness and increased collagenolytic activity due to an inflammatory pathway that may, at least in part, relate to increased friction from poor tear lubrication.[2,3] It relates to other ophthalmic conditions such as ocular irritation, pterygium, dryness, subconjunctival hemorrhage (SCH), and blurred vision.[5,6] A recent study has shown a decrease in tear break-up time (TBUT) and delayed tear clearance in patients with significant CCH.[2,7] The redundant conjunctiva can impact the normal function of the tear meniscus along the lid margin, leading to a reduction in tear volume of the inferior fornix, which serves as a reservoir. This affects the even delivery of tears to the ocular surface. The disruption of structure results in the impairment of conjunctival function, leading to tear film thinning and instability.[8-10] A recent report by Pflugfelder et al noted that tear meniscus height was elevated in eyes with CCH due to redundant conjunctiva protruding into the inferior fornix. This has the effect of pushing the tear meniscus anteriorly over the lid margin, while diminishing the reservoir capacity of the inferior fornix. Tear anterior migration, coupled with the elevated osmolarity and inflammatory mediators that are common to CCH and dry eye disease (DED), can lead to changes in the lid margin and Meibomian gland (MG) orifices observed as increased degrees of Marx's line, which is associated with worsening of DED. They also pointed to the importance of identifying and treating CCH before these structural changes occur.[11]

Meibomian gland dysfunction (MGD) is one major cause of DED.[12] MGs are holocrine, sebaceous glands that secrete meibum, which is a lipid that consists of cholesterol, triacylglycerol, free fatty acids, wax ester, and phospholipids. This secretion serves as a coat to stabilize the tear film by retarding evaporation. Therefore, dysfunction of these glands leads to a decrease in TBUT, causing the typical symptoms of dry eye, including redness, irritation, and sandy sensations that patients with DED experience and frequently report.[13,14]

Thermal pulsation treatment is the leading predicate treatment for reducing obstructions shown to result in the majority of MGD cases. A recent study has shown the benefits of utilizing radiofrequency (RF) to melt and express these obstructions and improve dry eye signs and symptoms associated with obstructive MGD.[15] It seems apparent that obstructive MGD would be a leading cause of CCH as the lack of lubrication from these oil glands leads to an increase in friction from each blink, thus exacerbating the condition. Lack of oil also increases evaporation, which subsequently increases tear osmolarity and inflammation, leading to additional CCH through breakdown of more collagen. The worsening of CCH will lead to negative effects on the tear film and tear distribution, which will worsen DED and result in more severe and refractory dry eye symptoms. Treatment of CCH should improve DED by recovering the tear meniscus function and reestablishing the volume and reservoir functionality of the inferior fornix. At the same time, treating MGD could help fix the root cause of CCH.

## INDICATIONS FOR TREATMENT

### Key Indications

- Symptoms and signs consistent with CCH
- Sufficient CCH to account for the signs and symptoms (generally Lid-Parallel Conjunctival Folds [LIPCOF] grade 2 or more, with evidence of tear film dysfunction) (Figures 29-1A,B to 29-3)
- Obstructive MGD signs and symptoms (usually coexistent with CCH)
- Sufficient clinical evidence to exclude other primary or significant co-contributors that should be dealt with before instituting a surgical approach to the CCH

In the author's experience, the most common indications for CCH plication (CCHP) and (off-label) RF thermal expression of obstructed MGs (ThermaLid) are any combination of the following:

- A rapid TBUT (ideally <10 and commonly <5 seconds)
- Tear film obstruction or obliteration by the CCH that inhibits a rapid return of tear volume from a dried inferior fornix with slit-lamp monitoring of a return of the fluorescein-stained tear film meniscus (generally >2 seconds or 1 blink to restore the meniscus)
  - Staining of the conjunctival folds with Rose Bengal or Lissamine Green
- Frequent SCHs
- Evidence of obstructive MGD (waxy plugging or poor MG expression)

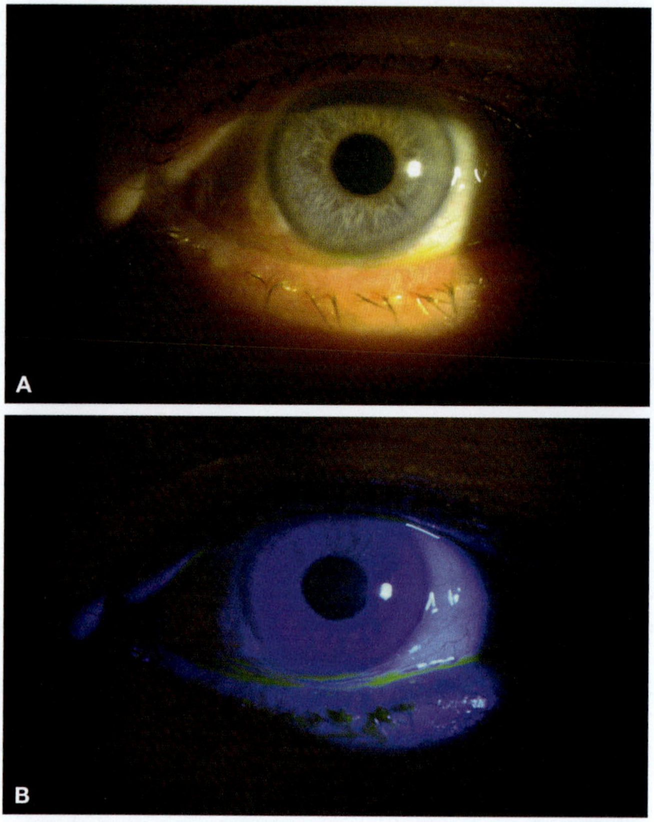


**FIGURE 29-1** **A,** Grade 3 CCH. **B,** Grade 3 CCH as seen with sodium fluorescein stain. CCH, conjunctivochalasis.

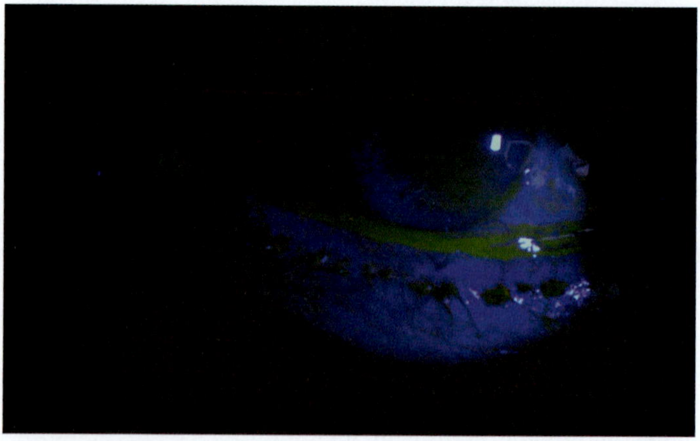

**FIGURE 29-2** Another Grade 3 CCH case as seen with sodium fluorescein stain. CCH, conjunctivochalasis.

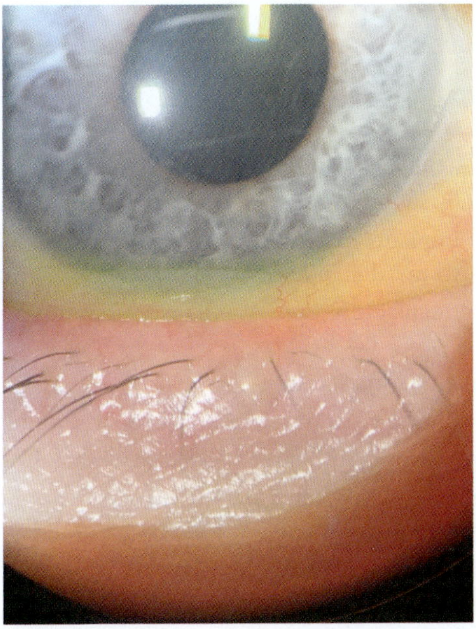

FIGURE 29-3 Grade 4 CCH. CCH, conjunctivochalasis.

There are many nonsurgical methods, including topical lubricants in the form of eye drops, ointments, and topical corticosteroids, to manage CCH. Each of these treatments can serve to improve tear film stability and lessen the mechanical friction from each blink that could worsen the redundant conjunctiva. However, such benefits are typically transient, while surgical treatments, such as conjunctival cauterization or conjunctival excision with or without graft or scleral fixation of the conjunctiva, can each provide a definitive treatment for CCH.[16]

Electrosurgical RF systems, which made their debut in 1928, are now widely utilized to treat CCH by providing a definitive cauterization of the redundant conjunctival folds. This treatment has been shown to improve symptoms of CCH by causing physical damage to the tissue, leading to subsequent shrinkage and flattening of the redundant conjunctiva.[17-20] However, its effectiveness in a combination treatment to target DED caused by MGD has not received much attention.

Initial grading of CCH utilizes the LIPCOF system described by Hoh but modified according to the following:

- LIPCOF grade 0 indicates the lack of the conjunctival folds.
- LIPCOF grade 1 means there was only one conjunctival fold upon examination.
- LIPCOF grade 2 illustrates multiple conjunctival folds that do not extend the tear meniscus upon examination.
- LIPCOF grade 3 represents multiple conjunctival folds that extend the tear meniscus upon examination.
- LIPCOF grade 4, which signifies a fold hanging over the margin of the lid upon examination, was added to the grading system as these patients are blinking on their conjunctiva, so that stronger blinking results in additional trauma and discomfort.

The LIPCOF grading has been shown to correlate with the dry eye symptoms reported subjectively by patients.[21,22]

# CONTRAINDICATIONS

## Key Contraindications

- Presence of an implanted electrical device that cannot be safely turned off and could be interfered with by subjecting the patient to RF energy (i.e., cardiac pacemakers)
- Presence of metal implants in or near to the treatment area (i.e., metallic implants, shrapnel, or tattooed metallic ink in the eyelid or immediate orbital area)
- Active ocular or periocular infections or inflammations (i.e., infectious conjunctivitis, keratitis, uveitis)
- Presence of a glaucoma filtration bleb
- Active thyroid eye disease (TED) or ocular cicatricial pemphigoid (OCP)
- Patient with recent eye or eyelid surgery (typically within 1 month)
- Pregnant patients (use of this combination treatment has not been investigated in pregnancy, and though it seems unlikely to cause harm, it is not recommended)
- Patients with unrealistic expectations, are uncooperative, or unable to hold still

Using radio frequency over metal implants risks excessive heating and arcing (akin to putting a metal spoon in a microwave oven). Significant intra- or periocular inflammation would also preclude the use of a cauterizing surgery, as it could aggravate the already active inflammation and potentially adversely influence the outcome of the surgery. Use in eyes with existing glaucoma filtration blebs would also add high risk of fibrosing the filtration area and possibly losing the efficacy of the bleb. Intraocular surgeries such as cataract, corneal transplant, glaucoma, and retinal operations require clinical judgment, as undue manipulation of the eye might result in opening a less fully healed corneal or scleral incision and result in an open globe. Consideration should be made for generally waiting a month or more for most ocular and eyelid surgeries and perhaps a year or more for penetrating keratoplasty to heal.

Relative contraindications include active co-contributors such as active allergic conjunctivitis, frequent recurrent corneal infections like herpes simplex virus (HSV) keratitis, or recurrent inflammations like noninfectious iritis, as the healing from cauterizing the conjunctiva may allow an overabundant edematous reaction (stretching the conjunctiva while it is healing, so as to reduce the efficacy of otherwise shrinking and reattaching the redundant folds of CCH) or reactivation of the infection or inflammation. Patients with glaucoma who are steroid responders should be monitored closely for excessive pressure spikes with the steroids required to heal sufficiently after the plication. Patients who expose their eyes routinely to airborne dirty or chemical fumes should avoid that environment during the acute healing phase postoperatively (generally a minimum of 3–5 days) to avoid infecting or excessively irritating their healing conjunctiva. Patients with a history of keloid formation are a special consideration (though this tends to be a dermal reaction and not as likely with moist mucous membranes). The author has treated a few keloid formers and has monitored their healing more closely and generally extend their postoperative topical steroid treatment to limit the risk of excessive scarring.

# INFORMED CONSENT CONSIDERATIONS

## Key Informed Consent Adverse Events Listed

- IOP spike (from the steroid treatment postop)
- Inflammation (normal to excessive) which may result in unwanted scarring
- Symblepharon, possibly with restriction to extraocular motility
- Infection
- Transient blurring of vision
- Under- or overtreatment, possibly requiring additional surgery
- Bleeding/SCH
- Conjunctival inclusion cyst (usually minor, but can be treated with further cautery or removal if needed)
- Partial or incomplete expression of clogged MGs

Informed consent should include a description of the procedure in plain language. For example, "After numbing your eye, a cauterizing device will be used to lightly burn the redundant conjunctiva, allowing the membrane to heal smoothly and tightly to the underlying eye tissue. This can help mobilize tears residing under the lower eyelid area so they can easily replace the used-up tears on the exposed surface of your eye. The heat from the same device can be reduced to levels adequate to melt the waxy obstructions in your eyelid's oil glands without burning you and allow these liquid oils to be expressed from these glands to unclog them. This is considered an off-label application of this heating device, in that the Food and Drug Administration (FDA) has not evaluated it specifically for this application, but several studies support the safety and efficacy of this technique and the FDA has approved this for cosmetic applications that use a similar skin-heating technique to reduce the fine lines and wrinkles in facial skin."

"Potential alternative treatments include use of lubricating or anti-inflammatory eye drops, monitoring, or a more invasive surgery such as removing the loose conjunctival membrane and either allowing it to heal over the raw, exposed white area of your lower eyeball directly, or grafting a membrane such as amnion with glue or stitches to facilitate the healing.

Risks and complications inherent to any conjunctival cautery procedure include but are not limited to the following:

- Increased eye pressure
- Eye inflammation
- Irritation
- Temporary blurring of vision

Complications more specific to CCHP include the following:

- Subconjunctival hemorrhage (common, but transient bruising under the clear membrane, leaving a days-to-weeks-long, bright red area on the white of the eye)

- The need for a repeat CCHP procedure (uncommon in the first 3–5 years)
- Risk of perforation of the eyeball from the anesthetic injection potentially resulting in permanent vision loss (not yet reported for this procedure but theoretically possible)
- Burning the cornea or eyelid, which can cause an injury that can be painful and take days to heal (unlikely with adequate patient cooperation)."

A note from the counseling physician should be included and phrased similar to: "I have counseled this patient as to the nature of the proposed procedure, the attendant risks involved, and the expected results." The patient's and doctor's names should be printed and signed with the date as well as a witness (typically a staff member).

## PREOPERATIVE CARE

### Key Preoperative Considerations

- Adequate clinical examination and review of treatments already tried to ameliorate signs and symptoms. Examination typically involves the following:
  - An anesthetic Schirmer's test to determine the degree of aqueous tear deficiency
  - MG expression
  - Infrared (IR) meibography
  - TBUT to determine the degree of MGD
  - The assessment of CCH by grade and by clinical signs of friction and tear film disruption
- Determination of lid wiper epitheliopathy (another co-contributor and related to friction from MGD), lid position, presence of floppy lids, nocturnal lagophthalmos, papillary conjunctivitis, and SPK
- Superior limbal keratoconjunctivitis (SLK) is likely a covariant of inferior CCH, with related mechanisms of etiology and in the author's experience, can be treated in similar fashion as is common CCH, as long as other obvious potential etiologies such as TED, contact lens–related irritation, and graft-versus-host reactions are either excluded or concomitantly dealt with.

## PREOPERATIVE PREPARATION

- Preoperative drops: alpha-agonist (a vasoconstrictor such as brimonidine) and proparacaine
- Lid cleaning/prepping (minimum of a hypochlorous acid spray over the closed lids. Consider debridement of the lid margin to remove surface biofilm and waxy debris that can additionally clog the MGs and a ZEST or BlephEx lid hygiene treatment if lid hygiene is not optimal)
- Study patients underwent a combination treatment that includes cauterization and thermal lid expression (ThermaLid) therapy by utilizing the single 4 MHz Monopolar RF Pellevé S5 generator system to target both MGD and CCH.[16-19] The author currently commonly

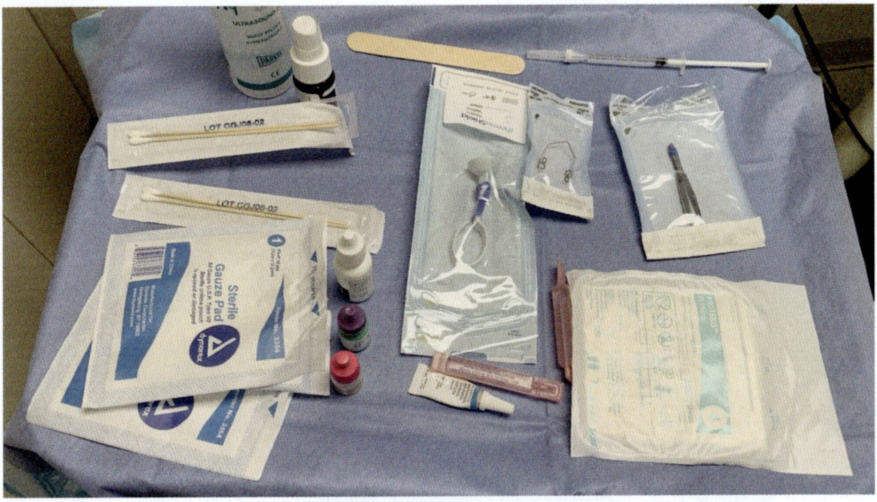


**FIGURE 29-4** Instrument tray set up for CCH repair. CCH, conjunctivochalasis.

uses a Cynosure TempSure Envi system with the Cynosure EyeEnvi (also referred to as the miniEnvi) handpiece for the plication and ThermaLid treatment, though an appropriate high-end IR camera may be used to monitor lid temperatures with an older, Pelleve 10-mm handpiece, as the initial study did.

- A sterile or aseptic setup is recommended on a Mayo stand, and sterile gloves are recommended. Extra 4 × 4 gauze, cotton-tipped applicators, the smooth angled MacPherson forceps (no teeth), the 1 mL syringe of anesthetic with a 33-gauge needle, and a wire eyelid speculum (which can be used in cases where patients have difficulty in keeping lids open) can be placed on the covered Mayo stand in preparation (Figure 29-4). An eye shield (ThermaShield) can also be placed if doing a ThermaLid heat treatment.

## PROCEDURE AND SETTINGS

- Administration of topical anesthetic is followed by a sterile, wooden, cotton-tipped applicator soaked in proparacaine and left in the nasal inferior fornix for 1 minute (Figure 29-5). A 33-gauge needle on a 1-mL tuberculin-style syringe is used for local, inferior bulbar subconjunctival total injection of approximately 0.2 to 0.3 mL 1% lidocaine with 1:100,000 epinephrine to the treatment eye (Figure 29-6). Injecting first in the cotton-tipped applicator medial area ensures minimal discomfort, and 10 to 20 seconds of light pressure of a 4 × 4 sterile gauze pad over the closed lids allows the dispersal of the anesthetic under the conjunctiva. A series of three such 0.05 to 0.1 mL injections—starting with the medial, followed by a central and then temporal bulbar injection, affords optimal anesthesia.
- Placement of a neutral plate on the patient's back, between the shoulders, ensures full contact of the plate with the patient's skin. The physician then instructs the patient to upgaze

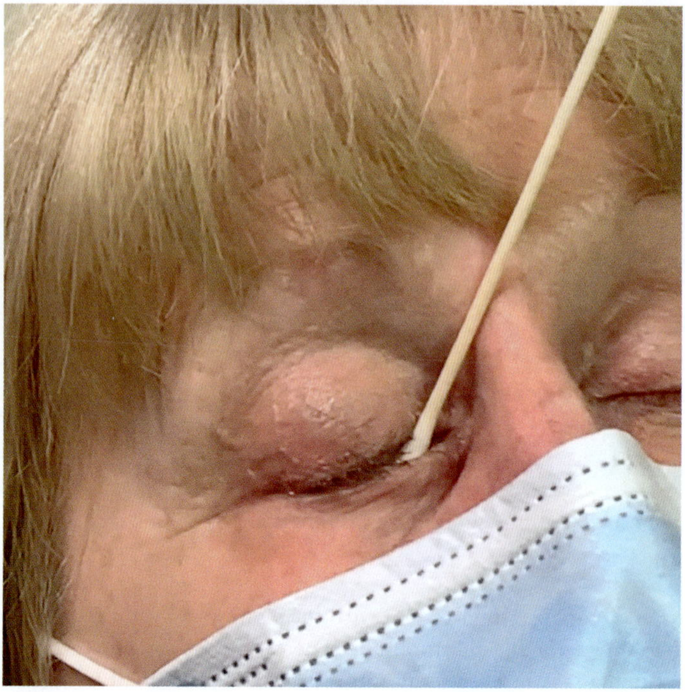

**FIGURE 29-5** This is the preoperative photo prior to injecting the lidocaine with epinephrine subconjunctivally. The eye has received two drops of proparacaine, a drop of brimonidine, and had a cotton-tipped applicator soaked in proparacaine in the medial inferior fornix for 1 minute prior to injecting the anesthetic. This allows for vasoconstriction and provides topical anesthesia, so the patient usually feels no discomfort from the few small injections using a 33-gauge needle along the inferior bulbar conjunctival area.

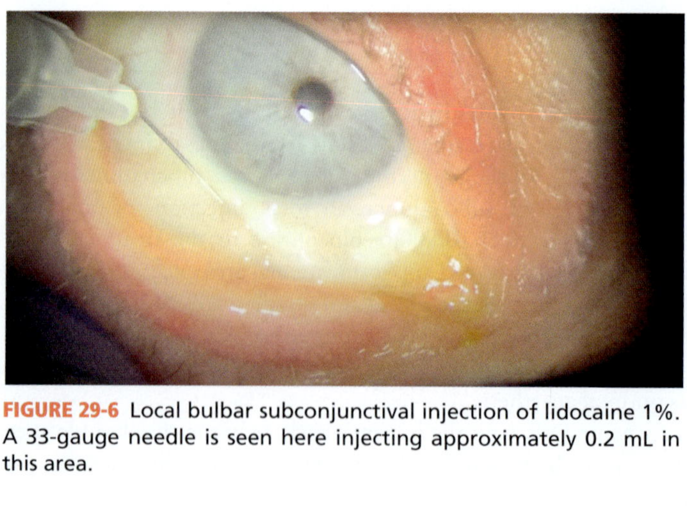

**FIGURE 29-6** Local bulbar subconjunctival injection of lidocaine 1%. A 33-gauge needle is seen here injecting approximately 0.2 mL in this area.

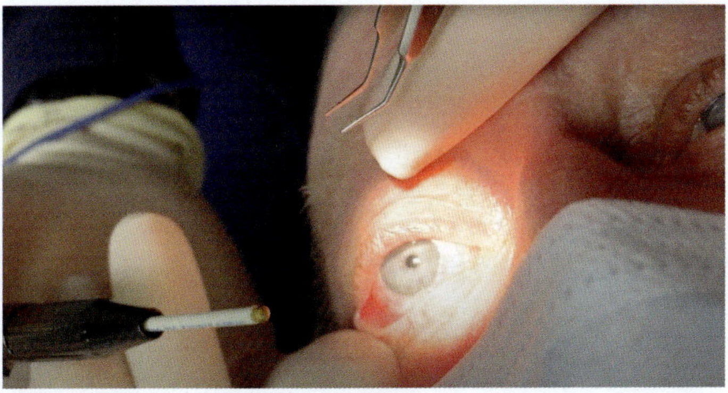

**FIGURE 29-7** The lax right lower lid allows substantial distraction and eversion to expose the redundant conjunctiva for treatment. If there is significant ectropion, the concomitant ignipuncture can be done to tighten and "turn" the lid back into apposition, by serially deeply burning 1 to 2 mm trans-tarsally along the inferior border of the tarsus (approximately 3–5 such burns can be used depending on the amount of malposition to be treated).

at the slit lamp while the lower lid is manually retracted to expose the lower bulbar CCH. Alternatively, this can be done with the patient lying flat on an operating table and an operating microscope used in place of the slit lamp.

- Treating CCH utilizes the surgical handpiece in the CUT mode with usage of a smooth, angled MacPherson forceps to grasp the redundant tissue and a 2-mm ball tip electrode to apply energy to the inferior fornix folds on a power setting of 4 on the 4 MHz Monopolar RF Pellevé S5 generator system or TempSure Envi surgical RF device (Figures 29-7 to 29-13). In the author's experience, the waveform of the "cut" mode seems to work best for lightly "searing" the conjunctiva with the 2-mm ball tip (Figures 29-7 to 29-13).
- Avoid treating within 2 mm of the limbus (to avoid corneal burns or potentially disturbing the limbal stem cells). The deepest fornix folds are treated first in a circumferential, near contiguous line, with subsequent, less peripheral zones of CCH treated serially until there is a sense of adequate tightening of the conjunctiva (few if any residual folds and a flat forceps stroking or "strumming" of the membrane from limbus to fornix suggests a smooth contour. A coagulum of conjunctival cells and mucous is commonly brushed loose with this stroking and may be wiped free with a cotton-tipped applicator).
- The amount of time locally injected anesthesia is applied until the time the CCH is fully plicated generally ranges from 3 to 5 minutes depending on patient cooperation and the amount of CCH to plicate.

After CCHP, a ThermaLid treatment of obstructive MGD, which was described in detail and referred to as the "ThermaLid treatment," in the previous publication, "MGD-Related Dry Eye Treatment Study: the ThermaLid™ Procedure," can then be performed.[17] The sole deviation from that protocol is using a flexible handled, hard plastic corneal eye shield to cover the cornea (a ThermaShield), though any appropriate, plastic, scleral eye shield can be used

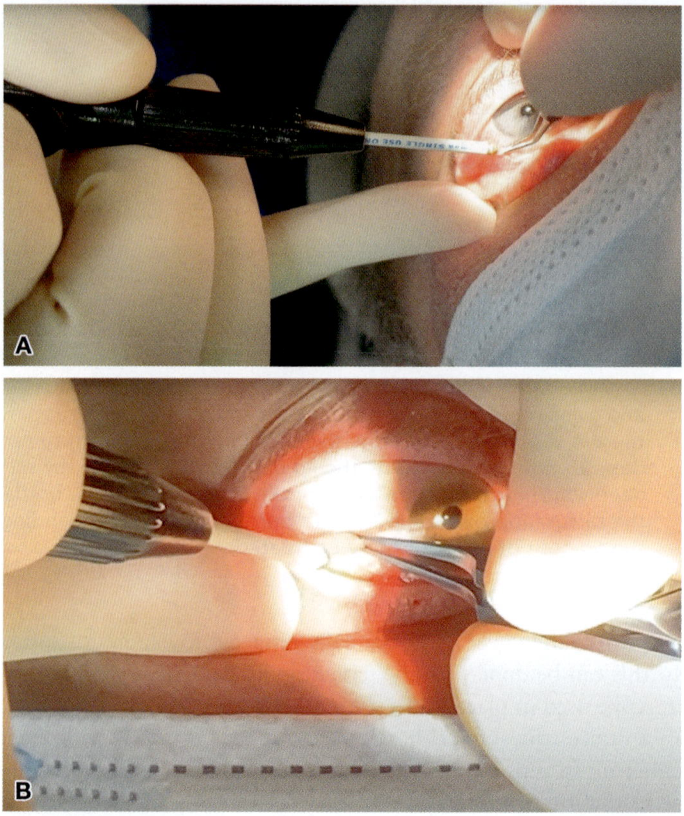


**FIGURE 29-8** **A,** Using the angled McPherson forceps to grasp the redundant, parallel conjunctival folds, the 2-mm ball tip is used with a power of 4 on the "cut" mode of the TempSure to lightly "sear" the conjunctiva serially along the inferior fornix. **B,** The plications extend upward over the lateral bulbar conjunctiva as needed to smooth and tighten the conjunctiva within the "blink area."

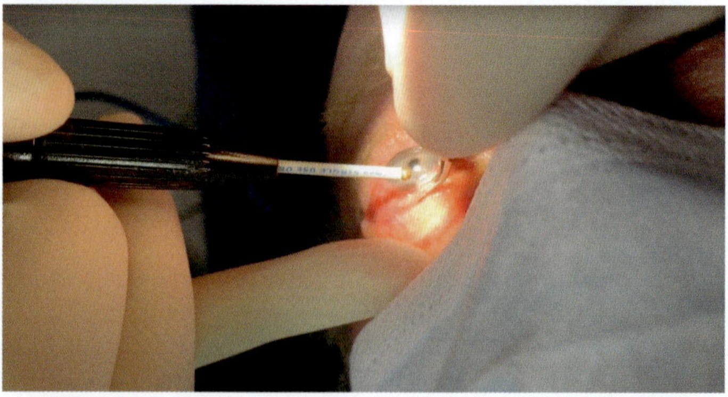

**FIGURE 29-9** Further serial plication extending along the inferior fornix and turning upward to treat the medial bulbar redundant conjunctiva within the "blink area."

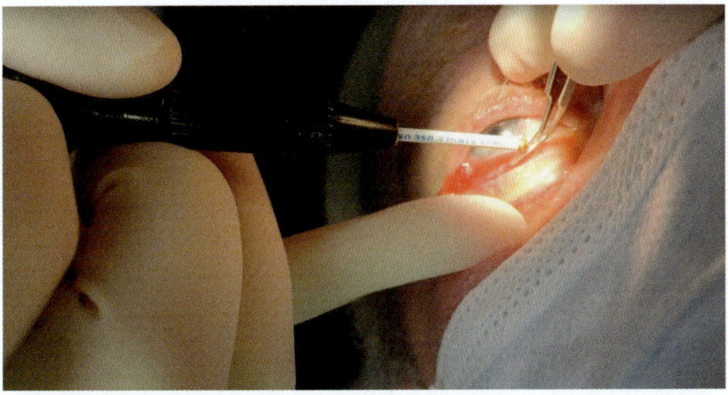

**FIGURE 29-10** Further serial plication extending along the inferior fornix and turning upward to treat the medial bulbar redundant conjunctiva within the "blink area."

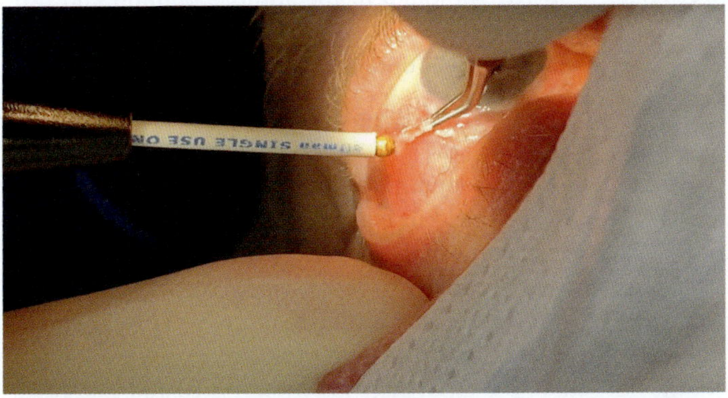

**FIGURE 29-11** Serial folds may mean extending the rows of plication from the most inferior to sequentially more mid-bulbar (avoiding the 2-mm perilimbal area to avoid damaging limbal stem cells).

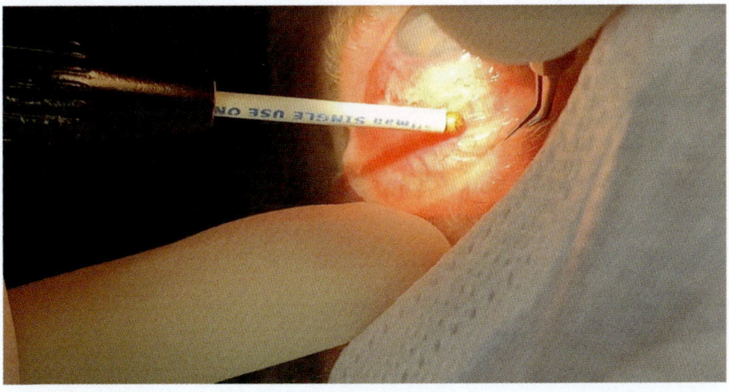

**FIGURE 29-12** It is possible to tap the tip and burn focal "spots" along the redundant conjunctiva as needed, though lifting the conjunctiva off the sclera allows for less discomfort and a broader "searing" effect. It also can help gauge the amount of redundancy to be treated.

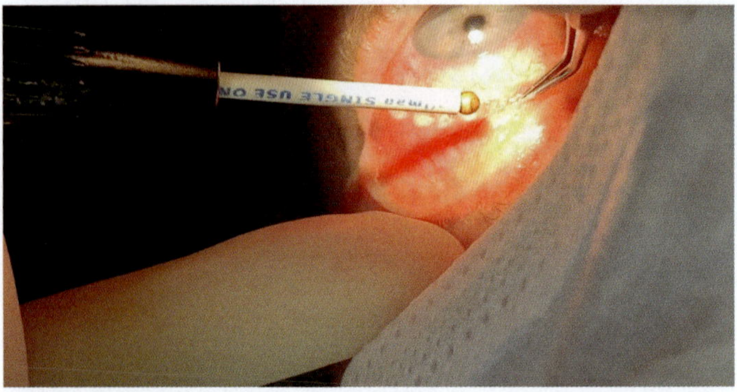

**FIGURE 29-13** This photo demonstrates the "whitening" common to the plicating burns.

as plastic is nonconductive to RF. Although in the author's opinion and experience, during heated expression, loose scleral shields tend to migrate under the counterpressure and may not provide adequate "backpressure" to effect optimal expression of molten oils.

- When using the TempSure Envi, it is possible to set the power to 8 and the temperature to 41 or 42°C for the ThermaLid treatment (Video 29-1). A fresh ½ teaspoon-sized dollop of ultrasound gel is applied to the upper and lower eyelid with a wooden tongue blade with the shield in place over the cornea and under the lids. The RF 10 mm handpiece is used to gently apply RF energy per the above settings, back and forth over the upper and then lower eyelid, with the endpoint of at least 1 minute at the intended temperature of 41 to 42°C and a frequent feeling that the "waxy ridge" of the lid margin has been "melted," so that it passes over the margin of the lid, encountering no "ski-jump-like" resistance and the full area of the tarsal plate has been heated and expressed.

# POSTOPERATIVE CARE/COMANAGEMENT (FOLLOW-UP SCHEDULE)

## Key Postoperative Considerations

Following the ThermaLid heated expression, the ThermaShield (or other appropriate plastic, nonconductive eye shield) is removed; fresh, sterile saline is used to rinse the eye and eyelid area; and 4 × 4 gauze is used to absorb the saline (approximately 2–3 mL is generally required).

- Postoperative drops: A drop of a tobramycin and dexamethasone solution is applied.
- Erythromycin, gentamycin, or other appropriate antibiotic eye ointment is applied to the operated eye.
- IOP check and assessment of conjunctival healing (generally 3–5 weeks postprocedure, though clinical judgment is required to determine optimal intervals, depending on the patient's history and preoperative exam)

After treatments, a typical patient is prescribed a tapered course of a combination of tobramycin and dexamethasone ophthalmic drops with a scheduled follow-up within 1 month (sooner in cases of severe ocular surface disease or advanced glaucoma where steroid response might be an issue) with instructions to the patient to return if any increased redness, increased pain, or decreased vision is noted. If needed, treatment of the fellow eye can be scheduled 4 to 6 weeks after the first eye and may coincide with the follow-up of the first eye, allowing a full recovery from the initial treatment. The final follow-up is typically 4 to 6 weeks after completion of treatment of one or both eyes, at which time symptoms are evaluated and a dry eye exam performed.

# POTENTIAL COMPLICATIONS AND THEIR TREATMENT

## Key Potential Complications to Look For

- IOP spike (from the steroid treatment postoperatively)
- Inflammation (normal to excessive) which may result in unwanted scarring
- Symblepharon, possibly with restriction to extraocular motility
- Poor healing may be a sign of an unrecognized autoimmune disease, and consideration of a conjunctival biopsy and/or autoimmune workup can be made if an extended taper of 1% prednisolone acetate suspension is inadequate at reducing conjunctival inflammation after 1 month.
- Infection
- Transient blurring of vision
- Under- or overtreatment, possibly requiring additional surgery
- Bleeding/SCH
- Conjunctival inclusion cyst (usually minor, but can be treated with further cautery or removal if needed)
- Partial or incomplete expression of clogged MGs

As with any conjunctival operative procedure in a dry eye patient, one possible complication is poor healing. Typically, the expression of oils during the ThermaLid will leave the tears depleted of tear oils for 3 to 5 days, and it may take several weeks to see more normal amounts of oils being expressed. In eyes with advanced ocular surface disease, consideration for application of a Prokera amniotic membrane at a 1-day postoperative visit can be made if the ocular surface appears to be at risk of further embarrassment. The membrane and its plastic ring can act as a conformer that dissolves and releases biologically active pro-healing and anti-inflammatory products that can help avoid symblepharon or other results of poor healing.

## VIDEO OF PROCEDURE

**Video 29-1**—Conjunctivochalasis (CCH) plication along with a ThermaLid treatment is seen in this video and explained by the author throughout the video.

## EFFICACY

Efficacy is best summarized by the results from the study Liem Nguyen and Edward Jaccoma published:

- All patients in the patient population completed a bilateral treatment regimen.
- Evaluation of photographs showed marked improvement in CCH (Table 29-1, Figures 29-14 to 29-17A-F).

**TABLE 29-1** COMPARISON BETWEEN AVERAGE PRE- AND POSTTREATMENT LIPCOF CCH GRADING

| | CCH GRADING BASELINE | | CCH GRADING FOLLOW-UP | |
|---|---|---|---|---|
| SUBJECT | OD (R) | OS (L) | OD (R) | OS (L) |
| 1 | 2.5 | 2.5 | 0.5 | 0.5 |
| 2 | 2 | 2 | 0 | 0 |
| 3 | 3 | 3 | 0 | 0 |
| 4 | 2.5 | 2.5 | 0.5 | 0.5 |
| 5 | 2.5 | 2.5 | 1.5 | 0 |
| 6 | 3.5 | 3.5 | 0.5 | 0.5 |
| 7 | 3 | 3 | 1 | 0 |
| 8 | 2 | 2 | 0 | 0 |
| 9 | 2.5 | 2.5 | 0 | 0 |
| 10 | NA | 2.5 | NA | 0 |
| 11 | 2.5 | 2.5 | 0 | 0 |
| 12 | 3 | 3 | 0.5 | 0 |
| 13 | 2.5 | 2.5 | 0 | 0 |
| 14 | 2 | 2 | 1.5 | 1.5 |
| 15 | 1.5 | 1.5 | 0 | 0 |
| 16 | 1.5 | 1.5 | 0 | 0 |
| 17 | 1.5 | 1.5 | 0 | 0 |
| 18 | 2.5 | 2.5 | 2 | 2 |
| 19 | 2 | 2.5 | 0 | 0 |
| 20 | 2 | 2 | 1 | NA |
| 21 | 1.5 | 1.5 | 0 | 0 |
| 22 | 3 | 2 | 0 | 0 |
| 23 | 2 | 1.5 | 0 | 0 |
| 24 | 2 | 2 | 0 | 0 |
| 25 | 1.5 | 1.5 | 0 | 0 |
| Average | 2.27 | 2.24 | 0.38 | 0.21 |

CCH, conjunctivochalasis; LIPCOF, lid-parallel conjunctival folds.

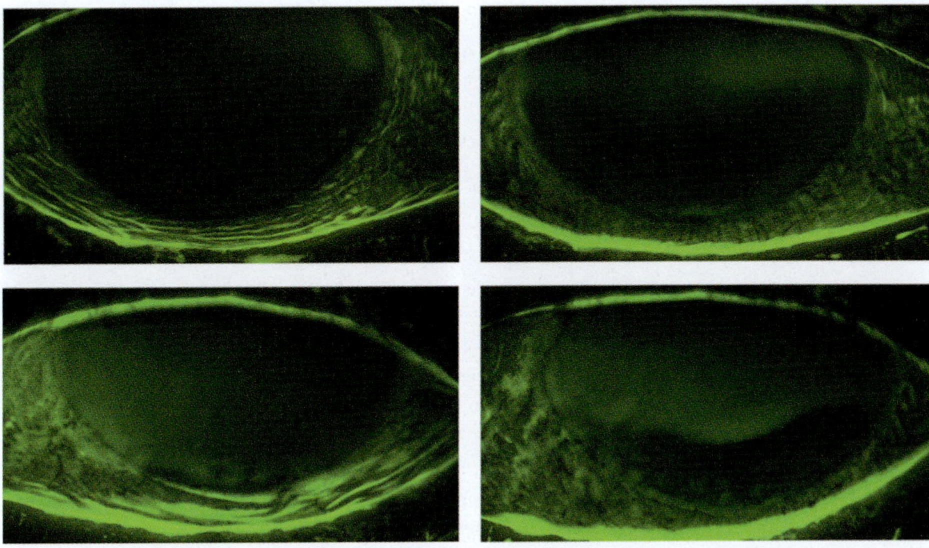

FIGURE 29-14 Fluorescent stain imaging. Fluorescent stain of before (OD [top left], OS [bottom left]) and after (OD [top right] and OS [bottom right]) conjunctival plication treatment. Conjunctivochalasis is bilaterally improved with decrease in inferior bulbar conjunctival folds.

A

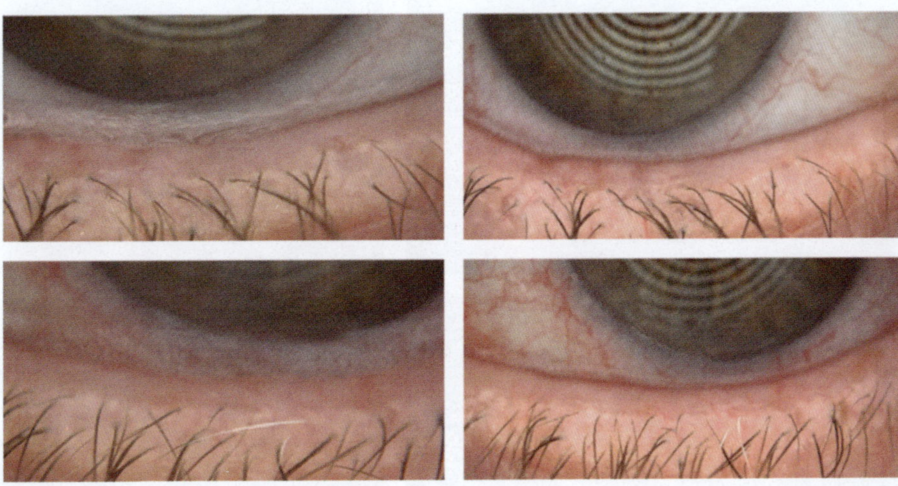

FIGURE 29-15 A, Tear distribution imaging. Imaging of the eyes before (OD [top left], OS [bottom left]) and after (OD [top right] and OS [bottom right]) conjunctival plication treatment. Tear distribution improved bilaterally with better distribution across both eyes with a significant decrease in tear film volume along the lower eyelid.

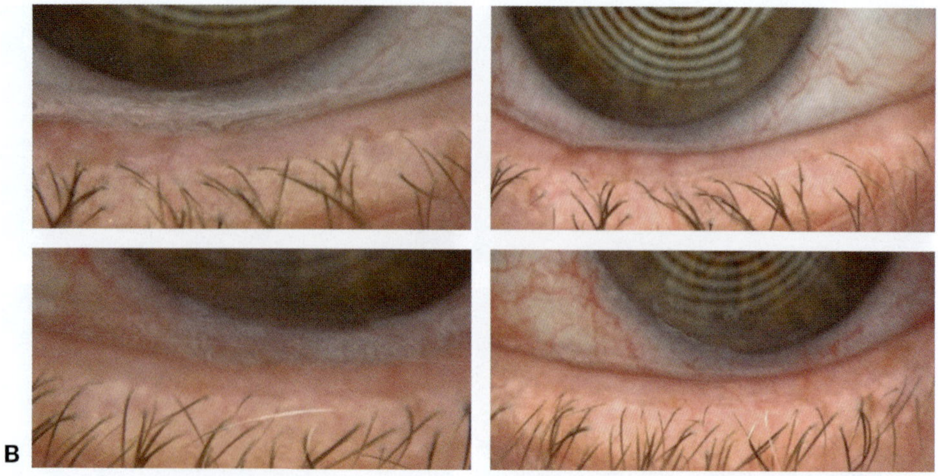

**FIGURE 29-15** (*continued*) **B,** More magnified image showing similar marked improvement of CCH after plication treatment (two right images). CCH, conjunctivochalasis.

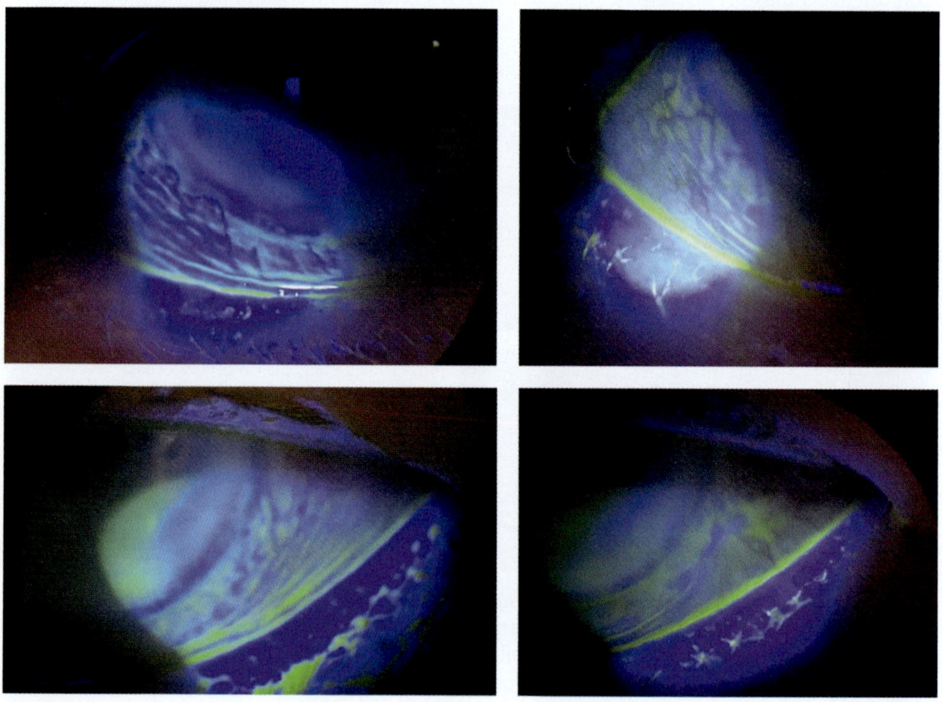

**FIGURE 29-16** Two photos on the left are showing the preoperative appearance of the CCH. The two photos on the right are after CCHP treatment. CCH, conjunctivochalasis; CCHP, CCH plication.

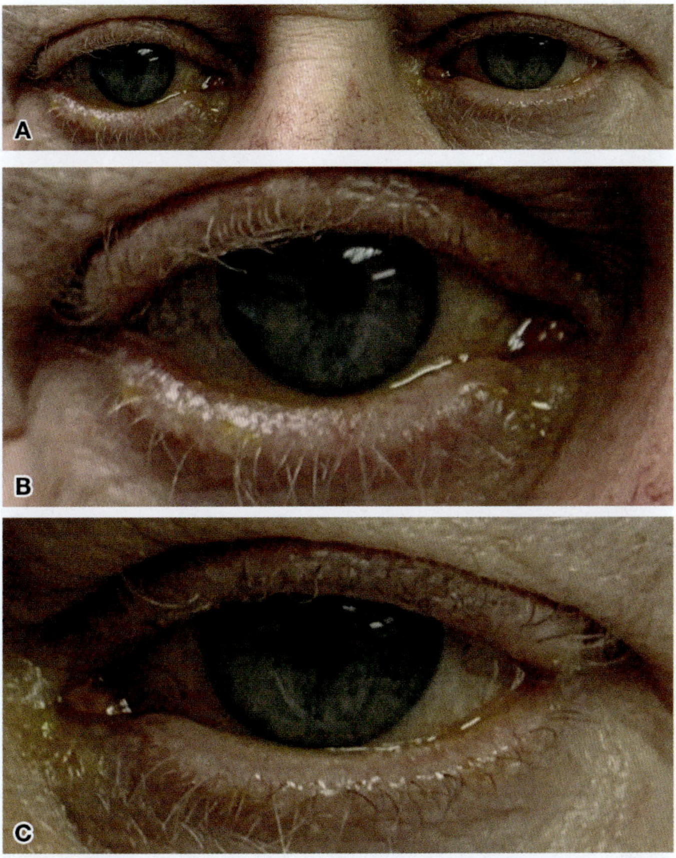


**FIGURE 29-17** **A,** This patient had CCH plication (CCHP) and a ThermaLid procedure for the more affected left eye approximately 1 month prior to this photo and is preparing for the same treatment for the right eye. The lax right lower lid is likely to have some lid tightening from the radiofrequency (RF) over the lid skin. **B,** Preoperative photo of the right lower lid and CCH. **C,** One-month postoperative photo of the left eye following CCHP and ThermaLid treatment. **D,** Preoperative photo of the untreated right eye CCH. **E,** Preoperative photo of the right eye using less light to reveal the greater degree of CCH. The conjunctiva lies over the lid margin, functioning as a "gasket" that seals the tears of the inferior fornix from exchanging with the "old tear" covering the cornea. Blinking brings the lids together over this fold, effectively "blinking on the conjunctiva," which potentially can cause trauma to conjunctival vessels, resulting in subconjunctival hemorrhages and inflammation. **F,** This is the 1-month postoperative photo of the left eye following the CCHP and ThermaLid treatment. The tear film rests evenly along the lower lid, and the conjunctival folds have been smoothed out from the plications. CCH, conjunctivochalasis. (From: TempSure Conjunctival Chalasis (CCH) plication with ThermaLid heated expression of obstructive MGD. https://www.youtube.com/watch?v=6ULZrYOEBmM)

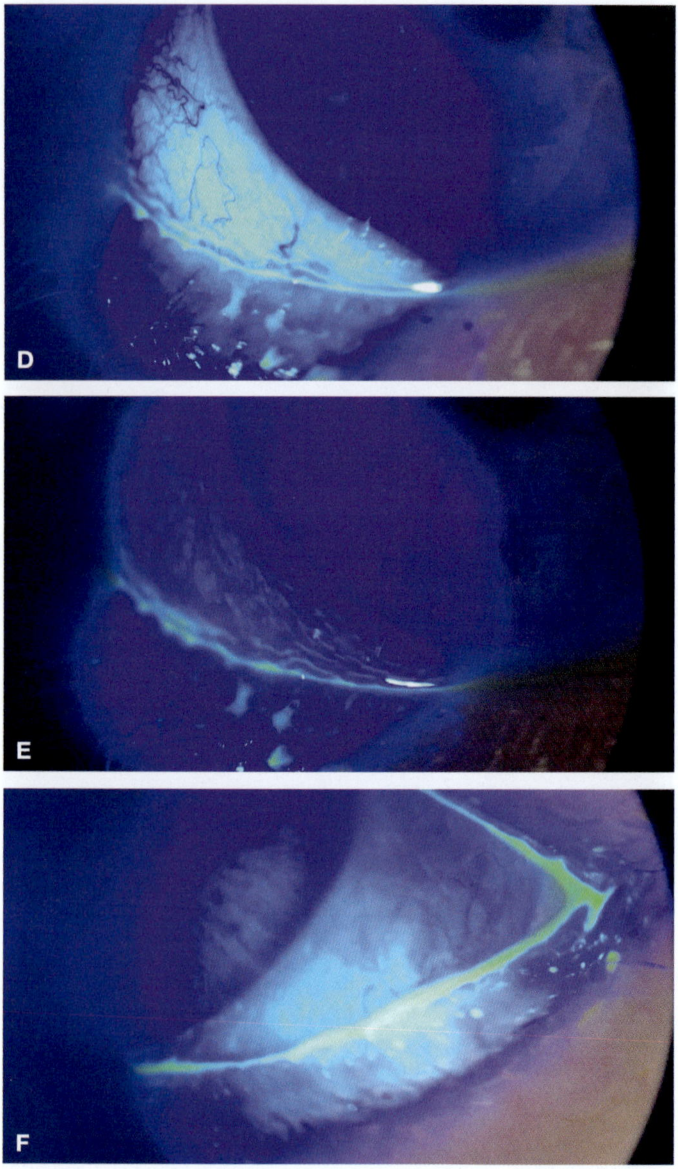


**FIGURE 29-17** *(continued)*

- Standard Patient Evaluation of Eye Dryness (SPEED) total decreased by 33.5% ($p = 0.001$), and subject responses indicated that 80% of the subjects noted improvement (Table 29-2).
- The average total number of Meibomian glands yielding liquid secretion (MGYLS) increased by 12.4% posttreatment ($p = 0.177$).

**TABLE 29-2** CHANGE OF SPEED SCORE FOR EACH SUBJECT WHEN COMPARED BETWEEN PRETREATMENT AND POSTTREATMENT DATA

| SUBJECT | SPEED CHANGE |
|---|---|
| 1 | −1 |
| 2 | −1 |
| 3 | −20 |
| 4 | 2 |
| 5 | 8 |
| 6 | −5 |
| 7 | −3 |
| 8 | 1 |
| 9 | −6 |
| 10 | −4 |
| 11 | 3 |
| 12 | −4 |
| 13 | −3 |
| 14 | −4 |
| 15 | −16 |
| 16 | −16 |
| 17 | −13 |
| 18 | −8 |
| 19 | −4 |
| 20 | −13 |
| 21 | −4 |
| 22 | −1.5[a] |
| 23 | −11 |
| 24 | NA |
| 25 | −2 |

[a]Patient response was in between two numbers during posttreatment evaluation.

**TABLE 29-3 RECORDED MEASUREMENTS DURING THE STUDY**

| MEASUREMENT | BASELINE | FOLLOW-UP | IMPROVEMENT | *p*-VALUE |
|---|---|---|---|---|
| **SPEED** | 15.6 ± 7.0 | 10.3 ± 7.1 | 5.2 ± 6.7 | 0.001 |
| **NTBUT** | 10.1 ± 5.7 | 11.3 ± 5.8 | 1.3 ± 5.6 | 0.177 |
| **Schirmer** | 11.3 ± 7.9 | 12.7 ± 6.3 | 1.4 ± 6.9 | 0.178 |
| **MGYLS**[a] | 23.6% | 46.8% | 23.2% | <0.001 |
| **Tear Meniscus Height** | 0.4 ± 0.2 | 0.3 ± 0.1 | 0.2 ± 0.2 | <0.001 |

MGYLS, Meibomian glands yielding liquid secretion; NTBUT, non-invasive tear break up time; SPEED, Standard Patient Evaluation of Eye Dryness.

[a]MGYLS reported as percentage of subjects with moderate or copious secretion.

- Schirmer's test results also increased by 12.2% ($p = 0.178$) (Table 29-3).
- Common side effects were tenderness and ocular irritation, which subsided within 2 to 5 days, and redness, which receded within 2 to 4 weeks. This is consistent with other studies that utilize a similar RF plication method on other patient populations.[16-19,23,24]

## CODING/BILLING

**CPT code: 68330**—Repair of symblepharon; conjunctivoplasty, without graft. The code 68330 carries a 90-day global period. If both eyes are treated on the same day, payers will usually reimburse 100% for the first eye and 50% for the second eye.

Common ICD-10 codes that support this procedure include the following:

- **H11.821**—Conjunctivochalasis, right eye
- **H11.822**— Conjunctivochalasis, left eye
- **H11.823**— Conjunctivochalasis, bilateral

## REFERENCES


1. Hughes WL. Conjunctivochalasis. *Am J Ophthalmol.* 1942;25:48-51.
2. Wang Y, Dogru M, Matsumoto Y, et al. The impact of nasal conjunctivochalasis on tear functions and ocular surface findings. *Am J Ophthalmol.* 2007;144:930-937.
3. Murube J. Characteristics and etiology of conjunctivochalasis: historical perspective. *Ocul Surf.* 2005;3:7-14.
4. Mimura T, Yamagami S, Usui T, et al. Changes of conjunctivochalasis with age in a hospital-based study. *Am J Ophthalmol.* 2009;147:171-177.
5. Di Pascuale MA, Espana EM, Kawakita T, Tseng SC. Clinical characteristics of conjunctivochalasis with or without aqueous tear deficiency. *Br J Ophthalmol.* 2004;88:388-392.
6. Meller D, Li DQ, Tseng SC. Regulation of collagenase, stromelysin, and gelatinase B in human conjunctival and conjunctivochalasis fibroblasts by interleukin-1beta and tumor necrosis factor-alpha. *Invest Ophthalmol Vis Sci.* 2000;41:2922-2929.
7. Le Q, Cui X, Xiang J, et al. Impact of conjunctivochalasis on visual quality of life: a community population survey. *PLoS One.*2014;9:e110821.
8. McDonald JE, Brubaker S. Meniscus-induced thinning of tear films. *Am J Ophthalmol.* 1971;72:139-146.
9. Doane MG. Blinking and the mechanics of the lacrimal drainage system. *Ophthalmology.* 1981;88:844-851.

10. Yokoi N, Komuro A, Nishii M, Inagaki K, Tanioka H, et al. Clinical impact of conjunctivochalasis on the ocular surface. *Cornea.* 2005;24:S24-S31.
11. Pflugfelder SC, Gumus K, Feuerman J, Alex A. Tear volume-based diagnostic classification for tear dysfunction. *Int Ophthalmol Clin.* 2017;57(2):1-12. doi:10.1097/IIO.0000000000000162
12. Lemp MA, Crews LA, Bron AJ, Foulks GN, Sullivan BD. Distribution of aqueous-deficient and evaporative dry eye in a clinic-based patient cohort: a retrospective study. *Cornea.* 2012;31(5):472-478.
13. Heiligenhaus A, Koch JM, Kemper D, Kruse FE, Waubke TN. [Therapy in tear film deficiencies]. Therapie von Benetzungsstorungen. *Klin Monatsbl Augenheilkd.* 1994;204:162-168.
14. Bron AJ, Tiffany JM. The contribution of meibomian disease to dry eye. *Ocul Surf.* 2004;2:149-165.
15. Jaccoma E, Litherland C, Jaccoma A, Ahmed A. Pellevé™ vs Lipiflow™ MGD-related Dry Eye Treatment Study: the ThermaLid™ procedure. *J Dry Eye Dis.* 2018;1:11-21. doi:10.22374/jded.v1i1.2
16. Marmalidou A, Kheirkhah A, Dana R. Conjunctivochalasis: a systematic review. *Surv Ophthalmol.* 2017;63:554-564.
17. Haefliger IO, Vysniauskiene I, Figueiredo AR, Piffaretti JM. Superficial conjunctiva cauterization to reduce moderate conjunctivochalasis. *Klin Monatsblätter Augenheilkd.* 2007;224:237-239.
18. Gumus K, Crockett CH, Pflugfelder CH. Anterior segment optical coherence tomography: a diagnostic instrument for conjunctivochalasis. *Am J Ophthalmol.* 2010;150:798-806.
19. Arenas E, Munoz D. A new surgical approach for the treatment of conjunctivochalasis: reduction of the conjunctival fold with bipolar electrocautery forceps. *Sci World J.* 2016;2016:6589751
20. Trivli A, Dalianis G, Terzidou C. A quick surgical treatment of conjunctivochalasis using radiofrequencies. *Healthcare (Basel).* 2018;6(1):14. doi:10.3390/healthcare6010014
21. Na KS, Mok JW, Kim JY, Rho CR, Joo CK. Correlations between tear cytokines, chemokines, and soluble receptors and clinical severity of dry eye disease. *Invest Ophthalmol Vis Sci.* 2012;53(9):5443-5450.
22. Lemp MA, Foulks GN. The definition and classification of dry eye disease: report of the Definition and Classification Subcommittee of the International Dry Eye WorkShop. *Ocul Surf.* 2007;5(2):75-92.
23. Caglayan M, Kosekahya P. Comparison of electrocoagulation and conventional medical drops for treatment of conjunctivochalasis: short-term results. *Turk J Ophthalmol.* 2018;48:61-65.
24. Kashima T, Akiyama H, Miura F, Kishi S. Improved subjective symptoms of conjunctivochalasis using bipolar diathermy method for conjunctival shrinkage. *Clin Ophthalmol.* 2011;5:1391-1396.

# 30 Concretion Removal

**Jeff M. Miller • Leonid Skorin, Jr**

Conjunctival concretions are small yellowish-white deposits that are usually less than 1 mm in size and commonly found within the palpebral conjunctiva[1] (Figure 30-1). They are especially common in the older adult population and typically located in the inferior palpebral conjunctiva although they can occur superiorly.[2,3] These lesions are comprised of degenerated epithelial cells, proteins secreted by the conjunctival tissue, as well as some calcium deposits.[4,5]

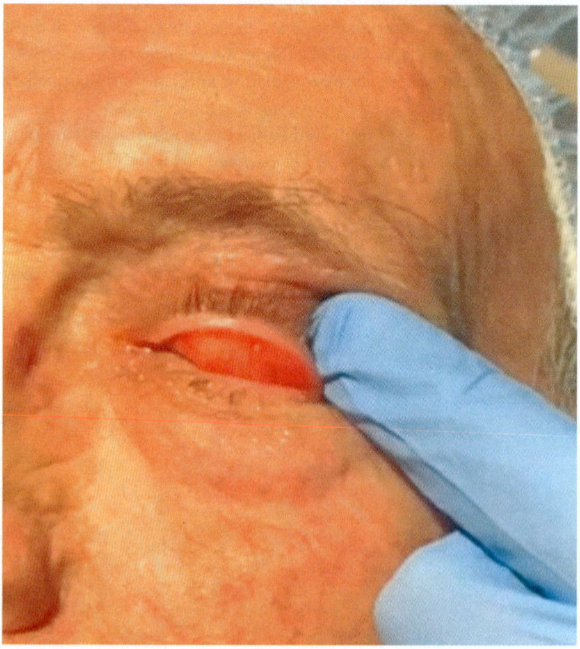

**FIGURE 30-1** Concretion located along the superior palpebral conjunctiva.

# INDICATIONS

## Key Indications

- Chronic conjunctivitis
- Blepharitis
- Atopic conjunctivitis
- Vernal conjunctivitis
- Post-trachomatous degeneration
- History of sulphadiazine eye drop use

Conjunctival concretions have been associated with inflammatory conditions such as chronic conjunctivitis and blepharitis,[1,6] atopic conjunctivitis,[4,7] vernal conjunctivitis,[7] post-trachomatous degeneration,[5,7] and sulphadiazine eye drop administration.[8]

Concretions are often asymptomatic and noticed incidentally by the clinician on a slit-lamp exam. These typically do not require any intervention or may only require observation. Their gelatinous, paste-like consistency has been put forward as a reason why many patients experience no symptoms.[5] Occasionally, a concretion can cause irritation and a foreign-body sensation as the deposit erodes through the conjunctival epithelial layer.[1,3] If the eroded concretion is located on the superior eyelid, it is more likely to rub the bulbar conjunctiva or cornea during the blinking process. This may lead to a corneal abrasion.[3]

In one study of 100 patients at a single eye clinic, concretions were found in 42% of patients seen. Concretions were found in 45% of male subjects and in 29% of females studied. There was no significant difference between the number of concretions found between the upper and lower eyelids of either eye. Superficial concretions were 3½ times as common as deep concretions. Only 7% of patients with concretions were found to have symptoms of irritation that could be attributed to the presence of the concretions.[3]

Conservative treatment options for minimally symptomatic concretions include viscous artificial tears. More symptomatic concretions can usually be removed at the slit lamp by the clinician although larger deposits may require surgical excision.

# CONTRAINDICATIONS

## Key Contraindications

- The patient is unable to remain stable in the slit lamp.
- The patient is unable to maintain fixation.
- Poor patient cooperation in general.
- The patient is using an anticoagulation medication (relative contraindication).

There are few contraindications to the removal of bothersome concretions. For superficial concretion removal, the patient needs to be cooperative, be able to remain stable behind the slit lamp, and be able to maintain fixation.

A relative contraindication would be the use of an anticoagulation medication. Special attention may be needed for those patients who are on an anticoagulation agent such as heparin, warfarin, or one of the direct oral anticoagulant medications such as rivaroxaban or apixaban.[9]

# PREOPERATIVE PREPARATION

## Necessary Instrumentation for Superficial Concretion Removal

1. Ophthalmic topical anesthetic (e.g., tetracaine 0.5%, proparacaine 0.5%)
2. Slit lamp
3. 30 gauge × ½ inch needle and/or needlepoint forceps

Necessary instrumentation for deep concretion removal:

1. Lidocaine hydrochloride 3.5% ophthalmic gel
2. Lidocaine 1% or 2% with 1:100,000 epinephrine injectable anesthetic
3. Povidone–iodine 5% ophthalmic solution
4. 30 gauge × ½ inch needle with 3-mL syringe for anesthetic
5. Sterile fenestrated drape
6. Number 11 surgical blade
7. 2-mm curette
8. Sterile cotton-tipped applicators
9. Ophthalmic antibiotic ointment

# PROCEDURE

## Key Procedural Steps

### *Superficial Concretions*

- Patient is comfortably and securely positioned.
- Fixation target is established.
- 30-gauge needle and cotton-tipped applicator are accessible on the slit-lamp stand.
- 30-gauge needle is positioned bevel up for the procedure.

### *Deep Concretions*

- Patient placed in supine position.
- Combination of topical ophthalmic and injectable anesthesia is performed.

- The eye is sterilely prepped and draped.
- A horizontal incision with a number 11 surgical blade is performed through the palpebral conjunctiva above the concretion.
- Curette used to scrape and remove concretion.
- Local pressure is applied for hemostasis.
- Topical ophthalmic antibiotic is applied.

### *Excision of Superficial Concretions*

After initial slit lamp evaluation of the palpebral conjunctiva, proparacaine or other ophthalmic anesthetic can be instilled in both eyes to minimize the blink reflex. While viewing through the slit lamp, a 30 gauge × ½ inch needle (without syringe) can be placed, bevel up, underneath the concretion and used to dislodge the deposit.[6] Alternatively, fine needlepoint forceps can be used in place of the 30 gauge × ½ inch needle to remove the concretion. Mild bleeding may be encountered and can be stopped by applying gentle pressure to the outer lid in the area that was treated or by applying pressure with a sterile cotton-tipped applicator directly to the area. If there is significant conjunctival disruption, consider an ophthalmic antibiotic solution such as trimethoprim–polymyxin B or tobramycin.

### *Excision of Deep Concretions*

Removal of deep concretions is performed under local anesthesia using no sedation. The patient is placed in a supine position, and lidocaine hydrochloride 3.5% ophthalmic gel is placed on the globe. Lidocaine 1% or 2% with 1:100,000 epinephrine is injected adjacent to the concretion using a 30 gauge × ½ inch needle on a 3-mL syringe (Figure 30-2). This is done for local anesthesia and vasoconstriction to reduce bleeding during the procedure. The eye is prepped with one drop of povidone–iodine 5% ophthalmic solution, and the face is covered with a sterile fenestrated drape. Prior to surgery, the site is tested to ensure anesthesia has taken effect. Once this is confirmed, the clinician makes a horizontal incision with a number 11 surgical blade through the palpebral conjunctiva above the concretion (Figure 30-3). Using a 2-mm curette, the clinician then scrapes and removes the concretion (Figure 30-4). Pressure is applied over the incision with a sterile cotton-tipped applicator for hemostasis. After hemostasis is achieved, topical antibiotic ointment is applied for prophylaxis. Cauterization and suturing of the surgical site are not usually necessary. These incisions are small and will stop bleeding with applied pressure and heal rapidly by secondary intention (deliberately leaving the surgical wound open, allowing the body to heal on its own).[10] Figure 30-5 shows the eyelid postprocedure.

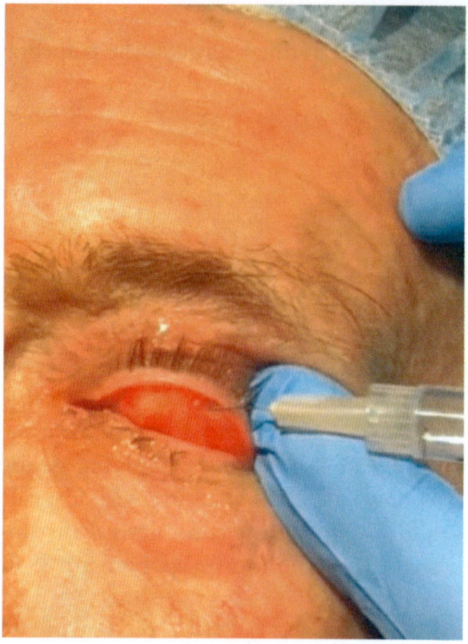

**FIGURE 30-2** Local injection of lidocaine with epinephrine being performed to provide proper anesthesia.

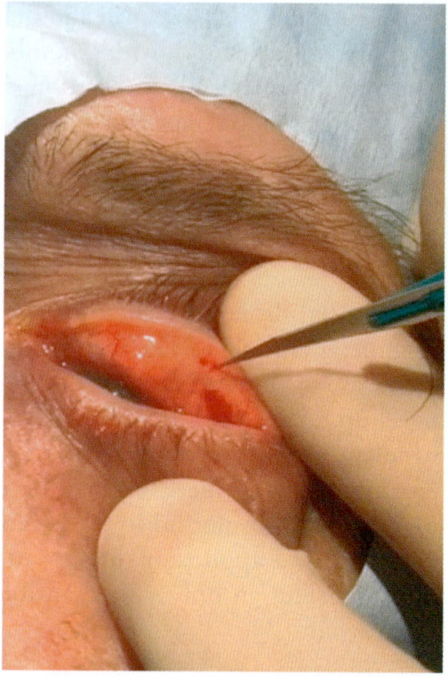

**FIGURE 30-3** Incision with a number 11 blade through the palpebral conjunctiva directly above the concretion.

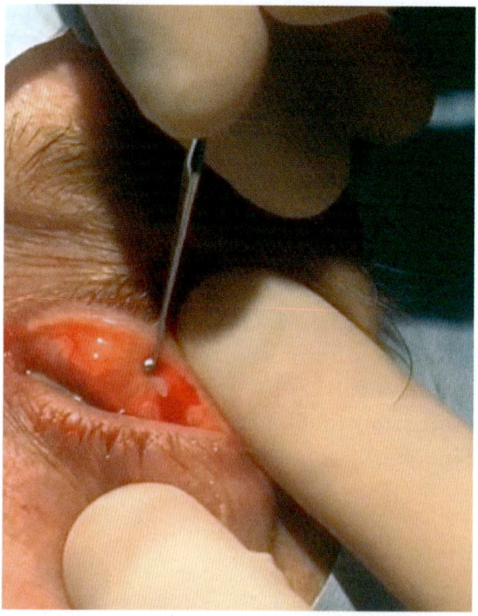

**FIGURE 30-4** Curette being used to scoop out the concretion.

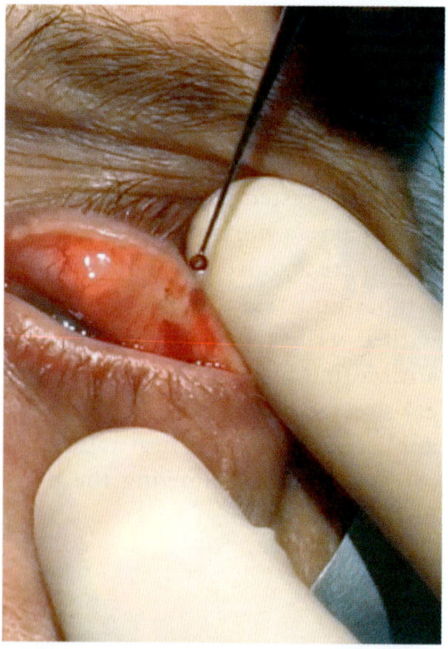

**FIGURE 30-5** The concretion has been completely removed. Note the concretion within the curette, and the area where the concretion was located showing no residual concretion material remaining.

# POSTOPERATIVE CARE/COMANAGEMENT (FOLLOW-UP SCHEDULE)

**Key Postoperative Considerations**

- Ophthalmic antibiotic ointment twice a day (BID) for 5 to 7 days
- Over-the-counter pain medication as necessary
- Recheck in 1 week

The patient is usually seen 1 week after concretion removal although they can also be instructed to only return to the clinic if they notice any persistent discharge, pain, redness, swelling, or other signs of infection. The patient should continue their ophthalmic antibiotic eye drop four times a day (QID) or ophthalmic antibiotic ointment BID for 5 to 7 days. Over-the-counter pain medications can be used by the patient as necessary. Usually, minimal postoperative pain is experienced by the patient.

# POTENTIAL COMPLICATIONS AND THEIR TREATMENT

**Key Potential Complications**

- Postoperative infection
- Persistent bleeding, especially if the patient is on anticoagulation medication
- Recurrence of concretion

Using a sterile technique during the concretion removal and treating the patient with an ophthalmic antibiotic eye drop or ointment after the removal minimizes the risk of postoperative infection. Persistent bleeding is rare because the incisions are very small. Persistent bleeding can occur if the patient is on anticoagulant medication.[9] Recurrence of concretions is common, but most will remain asymptomatic. The patient should be advised of a possible recurrence.

## VIDEO OF PROCEDURE

**Video 30-1**—Excision of deep concretion located within the palpebral conjunctiva of the upper eyelid. Local anesthesia with no sedation. A number 11 surgical blade is used to make a horizontal incision over the symptomatic deep concretion. The concretion is removed using a curette. After hemostasis is attained, the incision is left to heal by secondary intention. (Video courtesy of Leonid Skorin Jr and Kynndyl Giannonatti.)

## EFFICACY

There are no major studies regarding the efficacy of concretion removal. Kulshrestha and Thaller found that out of 100 patients evaluated, 42% were found to have concretions and only 3 patients (7% of those with concretions) were symptomatic and needed their concretions excised.[3] All these concretions were graded as being superficial, and the clinicians used "a needle after instillation of topical anesthetic" to remove the concretions.[3] At a 1-week follow-up, all 3 patients were asymptomatic.[3]

## CODING/BILLING

**CPT code: 65210**—Removal of foreign body, external eye; conjunctival embedded (includes concretions), subconjunctival, or scleral nonperforating

Common ICD-10 codes that support this procedure include the following:

- **H11.121**—Conjunctival concretions, right eye
- **H11.122**—Conjunctival concretions, left eye
- **H11.123**—Conjunctival concretions, bilateral

## REFERENCES

1. Boruchoff SA. *Anterior Segment Disease: A Diagnostic Color Atlas*. Butterworth Heinemann; 2001:145.
2. Haicl P, Jankova H. [Prevalence of conjunctival concretions]. *Cesk Slov Oftalmol.* 2005;61(4):260-264.
3. Kulshrestha MK, Thaller VT. Prevalence of conjunctival concretions. *Eye.* 1995;(9):797-798.
4. Chin GN, Chi EY, Bunt AH. Ultrastructural and histochemical studies of conjunctival concretions. *Arch Ophthalmol.* 1980;98(4):720-724.
5. Chang SW, Hou PK, Chen MS. Conjunctival concretions. Polarized microscopic, histopathologic, and ultrastructural studies. *Arch Ophthalmol.* 1990;108(3):405-407.
6. Simon-Castellevi G, Simon-Castellevi S, Simon-Castellevi JM, Simon-Castellevi C, Simon-Tor JM, Pita-Salorio D. Conjunctiva. In: Agarwal A, ed. *Handbook of Ophthalmology*. SLACK Incorp; 2006:191-228.
7. Roy FH. *Ocular Differential Diagnosis*. 5th ed. Lea & Febiger; 1993:253-254.
8. Boettner EA, Fralick FB, Wolter JR. Conjunctival concretions of sulfadiazine. *Arch Ophthalmol.* 1974;92(5):446-448.
9. Christenson G, Skorin L. Black and blue and red all over. *Rev Optom.* 2021;158(7): 82-83.
10. Skorin L, Genereux L. Secondary intention healing of graft donor site wound dehiscence following ectropion repair with autologous graft. *Clin Surg Ophthalmol.* 2014;32(4):101-102.

## SUPPLEMENTAL READING

1. Giannonatti K, Skorin L. Cutting out calcifications. *Rev Optom.* Published February 15, 2019. https://www.reviewofoptometry.com/article/cutting-out-calcifications

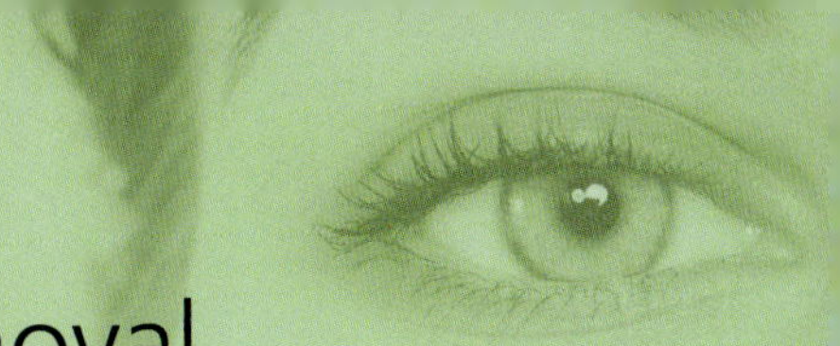

# 31 Pterygium Removal

Karl Stonecipher • Arun C. Gulani • Aaishwariya A. Gulani

Pterygium originates from the Greek words "pteryx" and "pterygion," which mean "wing" and "fin." Its new Latin origins date from approximately 1650 to 1660. However, pterygium, a disease of the eye, has origins as far back as 1000 BC, first described by Sushruta. It is a raised, triangular-shaped growth of the conjunctiva that has grown on to the surface of the cornea. This pathology is distinguished from a pinguecula, which is a raised, yellow-colored growth next to or abutting the cornea. A pterygium can spread across the surface of the cornea.[1,2] Multiple population studies exist regarding pterygium. These vary with race and risk factors, but the prevalence range is from 1% to 30%. The pooled prevalence is around 10%.[3-7]

## DIFFERENTIAL DIAGNOSIS

- Pinguecula
- Phlyctenule
- Limbal dermoid
- Papilloma
- Nodular scleritis
- Limbal squamous cell carcinoma
- Ocular surface squamous neoplasia

The most important diagnosis to distinguish is pathologic neoplasia.[8]

**Risk Factors**

- Age
- Male gender
- Outdoor job
- Low education
- Rural residence
- Low income
- Darker skin complexion
- Smoking
- Geographic latitude 40° around the equator (10 times higher rate)
- Ultraviolet light exposure (time and amount)[3-16]

Despite numerous studies performed on the pathophysiology of pterygium, the exact etiology of pterygium formation is not fully known. Genetics, immune mechanisms, inflammation, and environmental irritation are potential risk factors. The link between increased time of exposure to ultraviolet light and chronic irritation of the ocular surface related to dry, hot, windy, and dusty conditions is well known.[16] Secondary to changes in the local ocular surface homeostasis, the main items seen in a pterygium include clusters of proliferating limbal stem cells, disruption of Bowman's layer along the apex of the pterygium itself, and epithelial metaplasia.[17] Di Girolamo et al reported that experimental models in animals have failed and that pterygium appears to be an ocular disease only seen in humans.[18]

## INDICATIONS

### Key Indications

- Involvement of, or threat to, the visual axis
- Loss of vision from astigmatism
- Restriction of eye movement
- Atypical appearance suggesting dysplasia
- Increasing size (easily documented with computed topography)
- Symptoms of irritation and complaints of redness
- Cosmetic issues

Early intervention will reduce the risk of vision loss secondary to corneal scarring. If a pterygium is left alone, eye movement and increased astigmatism can result in visual compromise. If there is any suspicion of neoplasia, removal and pathologic evaluation is important to aid in the diagnosis, with additional treatment administered if indicated. Many patients may present with cosmetic complaints secondary to their pterygium. The persistent redness in their eyes can cause patients to seek out treatment. As with all surgeries, a thorough discussion of the surgery's risks and benefits is indicated.[19,20]

## CONTRAINDICATIONS

### Key Contraindications

- Patient responds well to conservative therapy.
- No visual compromise
- Patient is at high risk for postoperative pterygium recurrence.

Pterygium removal is not an urgent or emergent issue, and not all pterygia have to be removed. Conservative treatments such as topical lubrication or topical pulsed steroids are options. Preventive measures such as hats or sunglasses can be discussed, and the risk of surgery and recurrence should be discussed with each patient. Although surgical intervention is relatively straightforward, it is still not without risks and systemic health risks should be addressed prior to surgical intervention.[19,20]

# PREOPERATIVE PREPARATION

## Instrumentation

- Proparacaine ophthalmic 0.5% or tetracaine ophthalmic 0.5% supplemented with subconjunctival lidocaine 0.5% to 1% with or without epinephrine 1:100,000
- 50:50 dilute povidone–iodine 5% solution
- Toothed and nontoothed forceps
- Wescott and Vannas scissors
- Eyelid speculum
- Surgical spear sponges
- 4 × 4 gauze sponges/pads
- Bandage soft contact lens (optional)

Instruments will vary from surgeon to surgeon. A simple setup is seen in Figure 31-1.

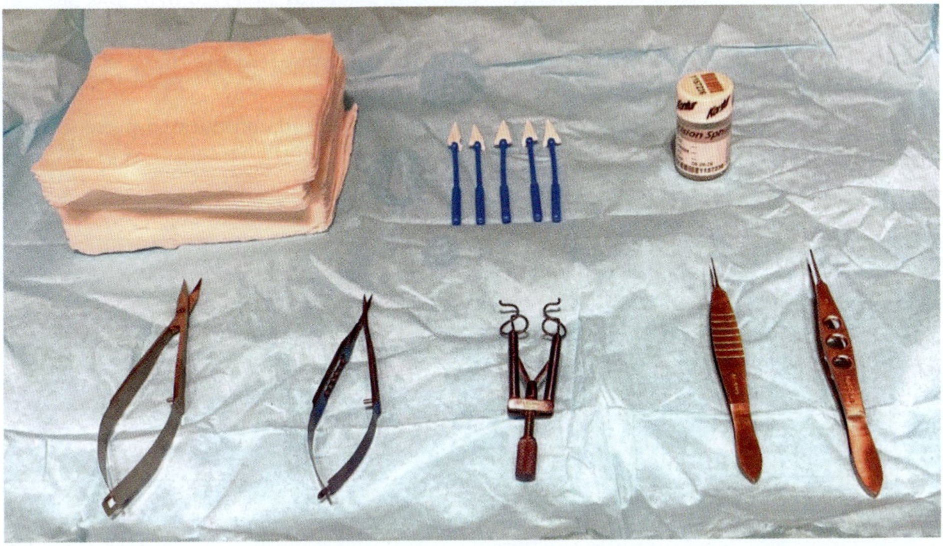

**FIGURE 31-1** A typical setup for pterygium surgery. Included are forceps, scissors, lid speculum, surgical spear sponges, and 4 × 4 gauze sponges/pads. A bandage contact lens of choice may be required postoperatively. Some surgeons elect not to use a bandage contact lens postoperatively.

A simple preparation prior to the procedure using a 50:50 dilute povidone–iodine 5% solution has been described and shown to reduce bacterial colonies in patients prior to ophthalmic surgery. Adding a topical wide-spectrum antibiotic for 3 days prior to the procedure and after the procedure is even more effective.[21,22]

# PROCEDURE

Staging and surgery assessment scales

Maheshwari published the following simple grading scale using computed topography, which is a simple way to follow progression with pterygia:

Grade 1—between limbus and a point midway between limbus and pupillary margin
Grade 2—head of the pterygium present between a point midway between limbus and pupillary margin (nasal pupillary margin in case of nasal pterygium and temporal margin in case of temporal pterygium)
Grade 3—crossing pupillary margin[23]

Prabhasawat et al published the following grading scale for recurrent pterygium:

Grade 1—consists of cases with a normal operative site
Grade 2—indicates the presence of fine episcleral vessels without fibrous tissue
Grade 3—represents cases with fibrous tissue not invading the cornea
Grade 4—indicates true recurrent pterygia with fibrovascular tissue invading the cornea[24]

Johnston et al published a comprehensive staging scale for pterygium (Table 31-1 and Figure 31-2).[25]

Reliable pterygium surgery assessment scales have been presented by Zhang et al and will not be covered in detail.[26]

Figures 31-3 to 31-8 show both typical early presentation and complicated presentation of pterygia.

| TABLE 31-1 A COMPREHENSIVE STAGING SCALE FOR PTERYGIUM |
| --- |
| Stage 0 represents pingueculum, posterior to the limbus. |
| Stage 1 is tissue involvement in the limbus. |
| Stage 2 is tissue just onto the limbus. |
| Stage 3 is tissue between the limbus and pupillary margin. |
| Stage 4 is tissue central to the pupillary margin. |

Used with permission of Association for Research in Vision and Ophthalmology, from Johnston SC, Williams PB, Sheppard JD, Jr. A comprehensive system for pterygium classification. *Invest Ophthalmol Vis Sci.* 2004;45(13):2940. Date of download 11.25.22; permission conveyed through Copyright Clearance Center, Inc.

| Conjunctival and Corneal Tissue Surface Vascularity (V) | Conjunctival Tissue Thickness (C) | Corneal Tissue Thickness (K) | Corneal Leading Edge Pigmentation or Ferry Line (P) |
|---|---|---|---|
| V0—No discernable vascularity | C0—Conjunctival ectasia or thinning | K0—Corneal ectasia or thinning with flat overlying tissue | P0—No discernable pigment line |
| V1—Minimal papillary response without visible intact vessels | C1—Flat tissue | K1—Flat tissue | P1—Faint interrupted pigment line |
| V2—Normal Vascularity | C2—Minimally elevated tissue | K2—Minimally elevated tissue | P2—Minimal pigment line similar to ipsilateral Hudson–Staheli line |
| V3—Moderate vascularity and vessel congestion, more dense than conjunctiva | C3—Tissue elevation up to 1 mm with minimal or no epithelial staining | K3—Tissue elevation up to 1 mm with minimal or no epithelial staining | P3—Moderate, intensely colored pigment line |
| V4—Severe vascularity with vessel congestion and dilation | C4—Tissue elevation over 1 mm with epithelial staining or erosion | K4—Tissue elevation over 1 mm with epithelial staining or erosion | P4—Dense, deeply colored or elevated pigment line |

**FIGURE 31-2** Subclassification of the conjunctival and corneal tissue surface vascularity; conjunctival tissue thickness; corneal tissue thickness and corneal leading-edge pigmentation or ferry line. (Used with permission of Association for Research in Vision and Ophthalmology, from Johnston SC, Williams PB, Sheppard JD, Jr. A comprehensive system for pterygium classification. *Invest Ophthalmol Vis Sci*. 2004;45(13):2940. Date of download 11.25.22; permission conveyed through Copyright Clearance Center, Inc.)

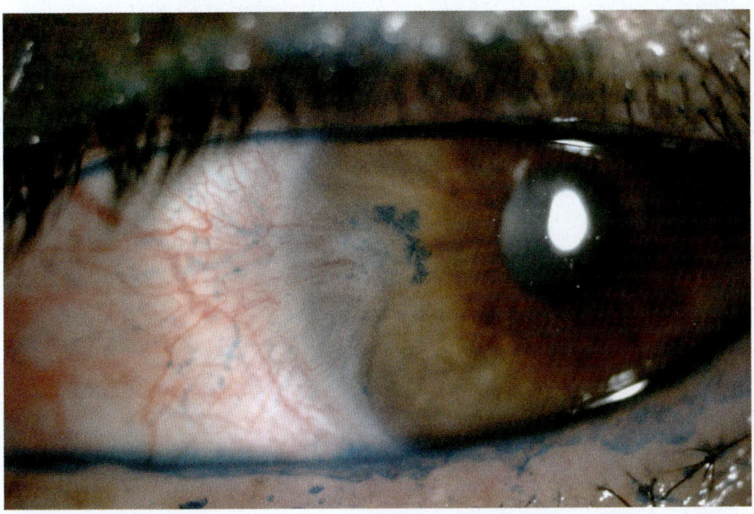

**FIGURE 31-3** Pterygium between limbus and a point midway between limbus and pupillary margin. (Courtesy of Alanna Nattis, DO.)

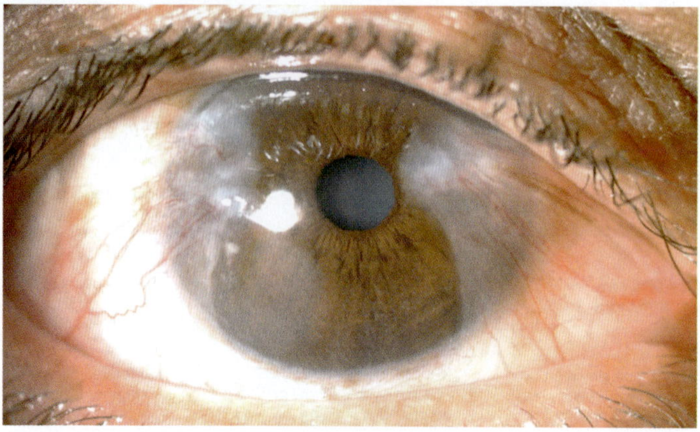

**FIGURE 31-4** Double-headed (nasal and temporal) pterygia. (Courtesy of Alanna Nattis, DO.)

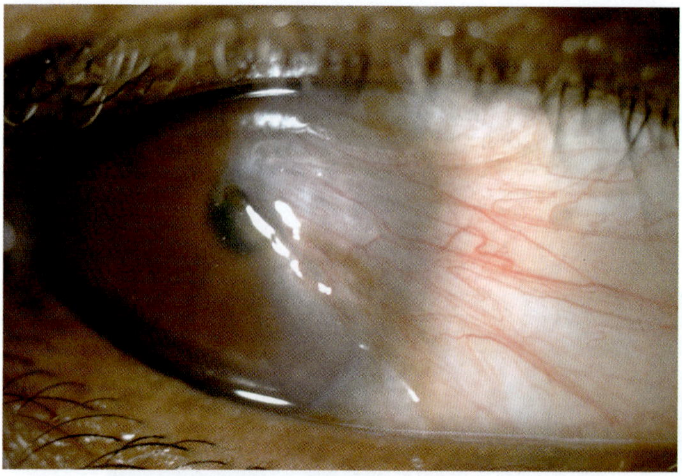

**FIGURE 31-5** Pterygium encroaching on to visual axis. (Courtesy of Alanna Nattis, DO.)

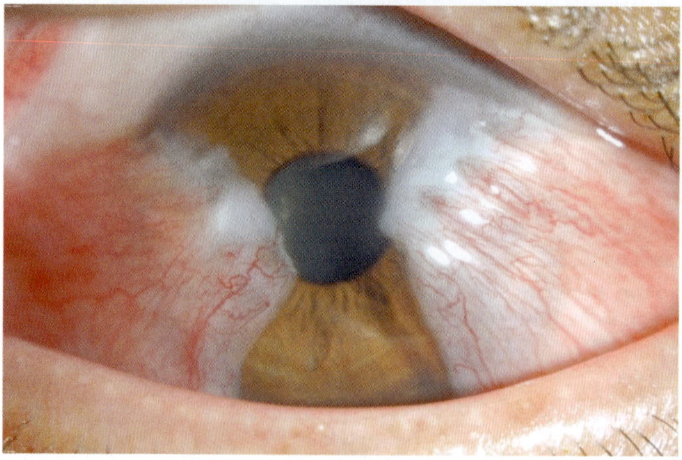

**FIGURE 31-6** Double-headed (nasal and temporal) pterygia encroaching beyond the pupillary margins. (Courtesy of Brandon D Ayres, MD.)

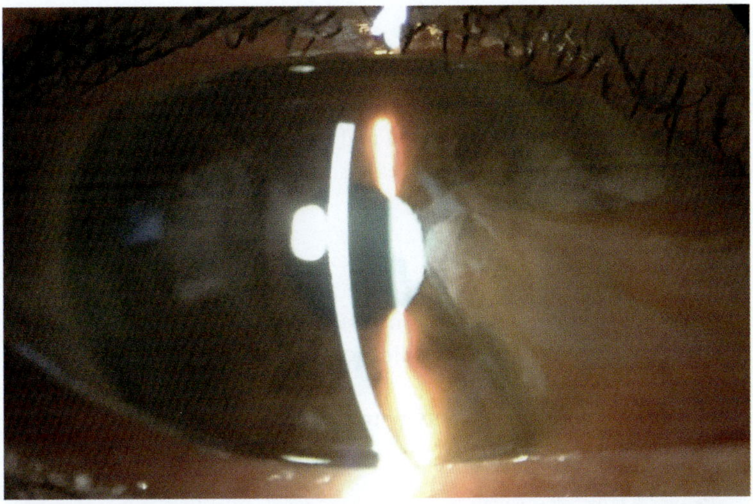

**FIGURE 31-7** Pterygium at the pupillary margin. (Courtesy of Karl Stonecipher, MD.)

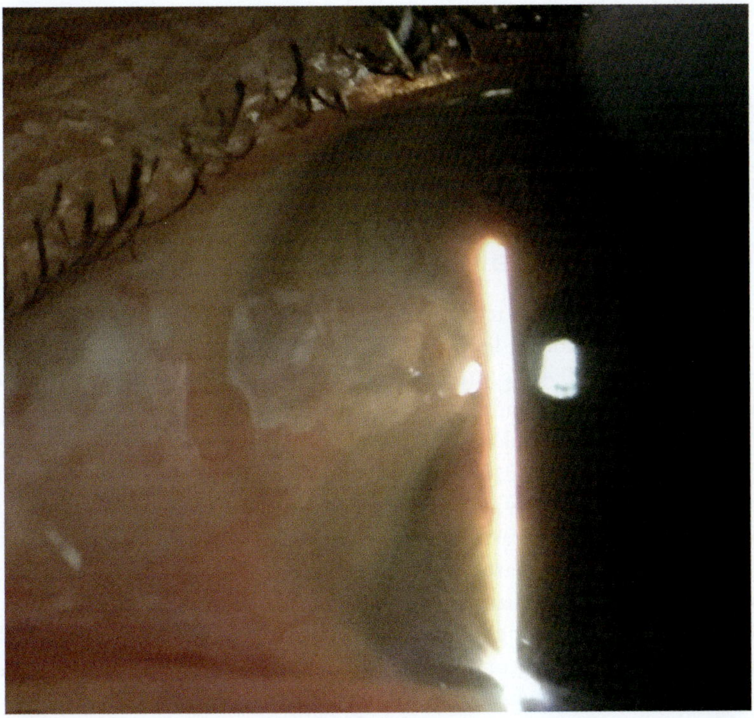

**FIGURE 31-8** Atrophic appearing pterygium. (Courtesy of Karl Stonecipher, MD.)

## Anesthesia

Anesthesia varies from patient to patient and surgeon to surgeon. Most patients can have topical anesthesia with proparacaine ophthalmic 0.5% or tetracaine ophthalmic 0.5% supplemented with subconjunctival lidocaine 0.5% to 1% with or without epinephrine 1:100,000. Rarely, a retrobulbar block or general anesthesia is indicated.

## Treatments

When an ocular surgical problem presents such an array of potential treatment options, it usually means that there is more than one successful option. This chapter will only cover the top options that are used at the time of publication with the best options to reduce recurrence and complications.

Sarkar and Tripathy describe the variety of techniques with and without adjuvants.[27]

**Techniques with or without Adjuvants**

- Avulsion technique[28,29]
- Simple excision technique[30,31]
- Bare sclera technique[32-37]
- Primary closure[38]
- Transplantation of the head of the pterygium[39,40]
- Conjunctival autograft technique[41-44]
- Conjunctival rotational autograft[45-47]
- Limbal conjunctival autotransplant[48-53]
- Amniotic membrane grafting[54,55]
- Lamellar or penetrating keratoplasty[56]

The author has chosen to focus on the techniques that are commonly used.

## Bare Scleral Technique with Adjuvants

Since ancient times, a bare scleral technique was utilized, but recurrence rates of 29% to 89% have been recorded.[16] The author looked at 248 consecutive cases with bare scleral technique and topical mitomycin C (0.4 mg/mL) postoperatively twice per day for 5 days. Recurrence was seen in only 1 (0.4%) patient that presented with nasal and temporal pterygium in the same eye compromising the visual axis. Both pterygia were treated at the same surgery.

Prior to anesthesia and removal, marking of the boundaries of the pterygium with a surgical marking pen or handheld cautery will help the surgeon to distinguish normal and abnormal tissue boundaries. The bare sclera technique simply involves excising the head and body of the pterygium with blunt and sharp dissection using forceps and scissors. After removing the pterygium, a diamond burr is utilized to smooth the limbal edges and irregular corneal surface. Next, dissect the conjunctiva using blunt and sharp dissection to remove abnormal tissue and Tenon's capsule. Originally, surgeons left bare sclera behind and allowed re-epithelialization; however, today most surgeons who utilize this technique will use mitomycin C. However, the following adjuvants have also been used in the past: beta irradiation, thiotepa, 5-fluorouracil, cyclosporine, or bevacizumab.

## Pterygium Excision With Preservation of Conjunctiva With Injection of Adjuvant

When looking for a simple technique with primary pterygium surgery, a modification of the Anduze technique with the addition of an adjuvant such as mitomycin C is quick and simple. It consists of a scleral conjunctival flap technique with the single application of 0.1 mL of 0.4 mg/mL of mitomycin C to the subconjunctival space. The recurrence rate in a large series was 0.35%.[38,57,58]

## Amniotic Membrane Grafting

The amniotic membrane grafting technique reports recurrence rates from 2% to 10% for primary pterygium and as high as 42% in recurrent pterygium without adjunctive intraoperative or postoperative therapy. It is thought that with amniotic membrane utilization, there is a reduction of inflammation and fibrosis promoting more normal re-epithelialization. After excision of the pterygium, the bare sclera is covered with an amniotic membrane, with the basement membrane facing up and the stroma facing down. Fibrin glue is applied to help the graft adhere to the scleral bed. Amniotic membranes that are bidirectional exist as well. An advantage of this technique over the autograft technique is preservation of the patient's normal anatomy and conjunctiva (e.g., preservation of conjunctiva for potential future glaucoma surgery).

## Conjunctival Autograft or Rotational Autograft Technique

The conjunctival autograft technique has recurrence rates as low as 1% to as high as 40% without adjunctive therapy.[16] After the dissection of the pterygium as described earlier, a previously harvested autograft usually obtained from the superior temporal bulbar conjunctiva or rotated into position is utilized to cover the exposed scleral bed. Sizing of the graft is determined based on the defect needed to cover prior to harvesting of the tissue. Of note, the graft needs to be dissected free of Tenon's tissue to ensure the best outcomes cosmetically and reduce the risk of recurrence. The graft can either be sutured using an 8-0 Vicryl suture or glued into position using fibrin glue.

When you look at the above four options, most surgeons choose one of the latter two. However, the recurrence rates for the first two are 0.39% and 0.4%, respectively. Clearfield et al did a Cochrane meta-analysis of 1,947 eyes of 1,866 patients showing superiority of the conjunctival autograft over amniotic membrane with a risk ratio for recurrence of pterygium (primary and recurrent) of 0.53% (95% confidence interval: 0.33–0.85; $p = 0.009$) at 6-month follow-up and recurrence rates from 3.33% to 16.7% in the conjunctival autograft group and 2.6% to 42.3% in the amniotic membrane group. The authors of this study concluded that a thorough pterygium and Tenon's tissue removal combined with a conjunctival autograft transplantation is considered a superior alternative to reduce recurrence and complications.[59] Gulani et al, however, feel the most effective, least complicated and best cosmetic option involves extensive tenonectomy, adjunctive fibrin-glued amniotic membrane transplantation, and adjunctive mitomycin C.[60]

# POSTOPERATIVE CARE/COMANAGEMENT (FOLLOW-UP SCHEDULE)

## Key Postoperative Considerations

- Topical antibiotic for 7 to 10 days
- Topical or depot corticosteroid until all signs of inflammation and vascularity are controlled
- Therapeutic bandage soft contact lenses to promote re-epithelialization and reduce postoperative pain
- Short-term oral narcotics can be used as needed for pain.
- Topical lubricating drops or punctal occlusion for accompanying dry eye symptoms
- Sunglasses with ultraviolet light protection, hats, and so on, as nutritional or environmental intervention
- Oral doxycycline (in combination with or alone) with topical azithromycin
- Mitomycin C must be managed and followed closely if used postoperatively.

Postoperatively, surgeons vary on their topical corticosteroid (prednisolone acetate, fluorometholone, or loteprednol) use and their taper of the corticosteroid.[61] The most commonly prescribed antibiotic is fluoroquinolone, which is used three to four times per day for 1 week.

## Adjuvants

Multiple adjuvants have been used with varying results as listed in Table 31-2.[16] The following are the adjuvants used intraoperatively and/or postoperatively:

- Beta irradiation
- Thiotepa
- 5-Fluorouracil
- Mitomycin C
- Bevacizumab
- Cyclosporine

## Comanagement

Comanagement of patients really varies from surgeon to surgeon, referral source to referral source, and state to state regarding the standard of care. With that said, the surgeon is responsible for any complications that arise from the intervention. Comanagement also varies based on the original intervention and whether adjunctive therapies are used (i.e., postoperative bandage contact lens, amniotic membrane, adjuvants, etc.). Topical drops have been discussed, but one note to mention is that topical nonsteroidal anti-inflammatory agents and topical anesthesia can create complications of their own accord and are not recommended by most sources. Therapeutic bandage soft contact lenses are used because they promote re-epithelialization and reduce postoperative pain. Topical mydriatics such as homatropine 5%, Mydriacyl 1% (Alcon

### TABLE 31-2 SUMMARY OF SURGICAL TECHNIQUES AND ADJUVANT OPTIONS FOR THE TREATMENT OF PTERYGIUM

| THE BASIC SURGICAL TECHNIQUE | ADJUVANT OPTION | RECURRENCE RATE ACCORDING TO PROSPECTIVE COMPARATIVE OR NONCOMPARATIVE STUDIES (%) |
|---|---|---|
| Bare sclera | None | 24–89 |
| | Beta irradiation | 0.5–52 |
| | Topical postoperative thiotepa | 3–45 |
| | Intraoperative 5-FU | 11–36 |
| | Preoperative MMC injection | 4–6 |
| | Intraoperative MMC application | 3–38 |
| | Postoperative topical MMC | 0–38 |
| | Intraoperative subconjunctival bevacizumab injection | 57.6 |
| | Postoperative topical bevacizumab | 0–41.7 |
| | Postoperative topical cyclosporine 0.05% | 12–22.2 |
| Conjunctival or conjunctival–limbal autografting | None | 1–40 |
| | Intraoperative 5-FU | 3.7–12 |
| | Intraoperative MMC | 0–9 |
| | Postoperative topical MMC | 6.5–21 |
| | Subconjunctival bevacizumab injection | 0–18.8 |
| | Postoperative topical cyclosporine 0.05% | 3.4–7.5 |
| Amniotic membrane transplantation | None | 2.6–42.3 |
| | Intraoperative MMC | 16–21 |

FU, fluorouracil; MMC, mitomycin C.

From Shahraki T, Arabi A, Feizi S. Pterygium: an update on pathophysiology, clinical features, and management. *Ther Adv Ophthalmol.* 2021;13. doi:10.1177/25158414211020152. Table 1.

Laboratories, Inc.), or Cyclogyl 1% (Alcon Laboratories, Inc.) can be used if indicated but may cause irritation. Short-term oral narcotics can be used as needed for pain.

Coexisting dry eye disease must be managed aggressively whether that be topical drops or intervention such as punctal occlusion (temporary collagen, silicone, or cauterization). Nutritional or environmental interventions (sunglasses with ultraviolet light protection, hats, etc.) are always good options.

Topical antibiotics are typically used during the first 7 to 10 days based on re-epithelialization. Topical or depot steroids are indicated until all signs of inflammation and vascularity are controlled. Oral doxycycline (in combination with or alone) with topical azithromycin has beneficial nonantimicrobial effects, including anti-inflammatory, anticollagenase, meibomian lipid viscosity reduction, vascular stabilization, and anti-matrix metallopeptidase 9 activities.

Mitomycin C, either intraoperative or used postoperatively, must be managed and followed closely. Intraocular pressure with prolonged steroid use must be monitored appropriately.

## POTENTIAL COMPLICATIONS AND THEIR TREATMENT

Patients need to be fully informed about possible complications before the surgery. Complications can occur during the operation or may present later. The discussion of recurrence diagnosis and management cannot be adequately covered in this book chapter.[19] There is a current review by Ghiasian et al on this topic.[62]

Intraoperative complications include:

- Perforation of the globe
  This is a surgical emergency and requires appropriate techniques with globe closure.
- Thinning of sclera or cornea from dissection
  Observation can be employed, but when globe perforation is apparent, amniotic membrane supplementation can be tried but patch grafting with sclera may be needed.
- Intraoperative bleeding
  As always quoted, "all bleeding eventually stops." However, simple techniques such as pressure, topical phenylephrine or phenylephrine placed on a sponge, and cauterization are the standard options.
- Excessive cautery
  If excessive cauterization is undertaken, then scleral necrosis and other complications can occur.
- Muscle damage
  Identification of all anatomic structures is imperative, especially in advanced cases. First identify the anatomic structures before proceeding with excision of the pterygium, Tenon's capsule, or conjunctiva.
- Reversing the conjunctival autograft (placing its epithelial surface down)
  Simple marking of the conjunctival autograft is a wise technique. Anatomy can get confusing, especially when excessive bleeding occurs.

Early postoperative complications include:

- Persistent epithelial defects
  As with any surgery involving the corneal epithelium, re-epithelialization is of utmost importance. Many surgeons choose to prophylactically place bandage soft contact lenses and use temporary or permanent reversible punctal occlusion as a preventative measure. Amniotic membrane placement at the time of surgery or after surgery are options for management. Of course, aggressive lubrication is encouraged, and autologous serum or topical albumin are postoperative options.
- Dellen formation (an area of corneal thinning adjacent to limbal swelling that prevents normal wetting of the corneal surface)
  Many of the options listed previously will also be utilized for Dellen formation. In some cases, the addition of eye patching or closure may be necessary for resolution.
- Hematoma beneath the graft
  Observation is prudent, but if excessive, reoperation may be necessary.
- Loss of graft
  Again, observation is an option. Depending on where the graft was obtained, another location for harvesting a replacement graft or using the other eye for donation is an option for repair.

- Pyogenic granuloma
  These benign lesions can occur after surgery or with the use of adjuvants. Despite their name, they are really a proliferative vascular response that consists of immature capillary channels within a myxoid stroma of lymphocytes, leukocytes, fibroblasts, and plasma cells. Treatment with topical corticosteroids initially is an option, but ultimately excision with cauterization is usually indicated.

Late complications include:

- Recurrence
  Recurrent pterygium treatment has been reviewed by Ghiasian et al[62]
- Corneal scleral necrosis and scleritis
  Late corneal scleral necrosis and scleritis are rare ocular complications. Surgical intervention with patch grafting may be indicated, and in addition to topical treatments, systemic intervention is necessary. Referral to surgeons who routinely deal with this patient population is prudent.[63]
- Endophthalmitis
  This book chapter cannot adequately cover the treatment of endophthalmitis. Emergent referral to a specialist who treats this patient population is indicated.

## VIDEOS OF PROCEDURES

**Video 31-1**—Dr. William Trattler shows us a modification of the Anduze technique using 0.1 mL of mitomycin C 0.4 mg/mL to the subconjunctival space after superficial dissection of the head of the pterygium and removal of tenons. It is a one-time application of mitomycin C intraoperatively, and the reported 10-year series by Dr. Anduze showed a recurrence rate of 0.35% without vision-threatening complications.

**Video 31-2**—Pearls for immediate and long-term success for cosmetic pterygium surgery: Gulani SPARKLE Technique. In this video, you can see the Gulani iceberg concept where the entire pterygium is traced down to its roots (tentacles) and dissected right up to the medial rectus, following which the anatomy is clearly defined, so the tenons and conjunctival layer are easily identifiable. The corneal scar is always addressed without any blades or sharp dissection by using centripetal movements. Mitomycin C Weck-Cel pieces are placed between the tenons and conjunctival pocket, which is further sealed with Tisseel fibrin glue to prevent recurrence as well as avoid exposure to the sclera. Tisseel fibrin glue is also used to adhere an amniotic graft to the underlying sclera. The amniotic graft is gently placed within the fornix as well as on the sclera. Finally, a single, superficial and precise peri-limbal cut of the excess amniotic tissue without impacting the underlying cornea so these patients not only have a great looking eye starting day one, but they are also ready for vision corrective surgery within a week. The final appearance of the eye so patients can actually go up to a mirror immediately after surgery and day one post surgery as part of our protocol.

# EFFICACY

There are many ways to evaluate the effectiveness of an intervention. With pterygium surgery and the plethora of options available, we will only recommend the reader to Table 31-2 from Shahraki et al, which outlines the recurrence rates with a variety of interventions over time.[16]

## CODING/BILLING

The most common ways to code for cases of pterygium excision without a conjunctival autograft and with an:

- Amniotic membrane, single layer or multilayer, sutured: Use Current Procedural Terminology (CPT) code 65426.
  - Avoid combination use of CPT codes 65779 and 65426, which is not considered appropriate because 65426 does not specify the type of graft and because the amniotic membrane is the graft. It is not appropriate to bill CPT code 65420 for excision or transposition of pterygium, without graft.
- Amniotic membrane, single layer or multilayer, glued: Use CPT code 65426.
  - Avoid combination use of CPT codes 66999 and 65425, which is no longer considered appropriate because 65426 does not specify the type of graft. As explained previously, it is not appropriate to bill CPT code 65420.

The most common ways to code for cases of pterygium excision with a conjunctival autograft and with an:

Amniotic membrane, single layer, or multilayered, sutured: Use CPT codes 65426 and 65779.
Amniotic membrane, single layer or multilayer, glued: Use CPT codes 65426 and 66999.
For placement of an amniotic membrane using tissue glue: Use 66999.

## REFERENCES


1. Rosenthal JW. Chronology of pterygium therapy. *Am J Ophthalmol.* 1953;36(11):1601-1616.
2. Singh V. Sushruta: the father of surgery. *Natl J Maxillofac Surg.* 2017;8(1):1-3. doi:10.4103/njms.NJMS_33_17
3. Luthra R, Nemesure BB, Wu SY, et al. Frequency and risk factors for pterygium in the Barbados Eye Study. *Arch Ophthalmol.* 2001;119:1827-1832.
4. Cajucom-Uy H, Tong L, Wong TY, et al. The prevalence of and risk factors for pterygium in an urban Malay population: the Singapore Malay Eye Study (SiMES). *Br J Ophthalmol.* 2010;94:977-981.
5. West S, Muñoz B. Prevalence of pterygium in Latinos: proyecto VER. *Br J Ophthalmol.* 2009;93:1287-1290.
6. Fotouhi A, Hashemi H, Khabazkhoob M, et al. Prevalence and risk factors of pterygium and pinguecula: the Tehran Eye Study. *Eye.* 2009;23:1125-1129.
7. Ma K, Xu L, Jie Y, et al. Prevalence of and factors associated with pterygium in adult Chinese: the Beijing Eye Study. *Cornea.* 2007;26:1184-1186.
8. Liu L, Wu J, Geng J, et al. Geographical prevalence and risk factors for pterygium: a systematic review and meta-analysis. *BMJ Open.* 2013;3:e003787.
9. Wu K, He M, Xu J, et al. Pterygium in aged population in Doumen County, China. *Yan Ke Xue Bao.* 2002;18:181-184.
10. Moran DJ, Hollows FC. Pterygium and ultraviolet radiation: a positive correlation. *Br J Ophthalmol.* 1984;68(5):343-346.
11. Tan CS, Lim TH, Koh WP, et al. Epidemiology of pterygium on a tropical island in the Riau Archipelago. *Eye.* 2006;20:908-912.
12. McCarty CA, Fu CL, Taylor HR. Epidemiology of pterygium in Victoria, Australia. *Br J Ophthalmol.* 2000;84:289-292.
13. Viso E, Gude F, Rodríguez-Ares MT. Prevalence of pinguecula and pterygium in a general population in Spain. *Eye.* 2011;25:350-357.

14. Coroneo MT. Pterygium as an early indicator of ultraviolet insolation: a hypothesis. *Br J Ophthalmol.* 1993;77:734-739.
15. Mackenzie FD, Hirst LW, Battistutta D, et al. Risk analysis in the development of pterygia. *Ophthalmology.* 1992;99:1056-1061.
16. Shahraki T, Arabi A, Feizi S. Pterygium: an update on pathophysiology, clinical features, and management. *Ther Adv Ophthalmol.* 2021;13. doi:10.1177/25158414211020152
17. Chui J, Di Girolamo N, Wakefield D, et al. The pathogenesis of pterygium: current concepts and their therapeutic implications. *Ocul Surf.* 2008;6:24-43.
18. Di Girolamo N, Chui J, Coroneo MT, et al. Pathogenesis of pterygia: role of cytokines, growth factors, and matrix metalloproteinases. *Prog Retin Eye Res.* 2004;23:195-228.
19. Hall AB. Understanding and managing pterygium. *Community Eye Health.* 2016;29(95):54-56.
20. Hirst LW. The treatment of pterygium. *Surv Ophthalmol.* 2003;48:145-180.
21. Apt L, Isenberg S, Yoshimori R, Paez JH. Chemical preparation of the eye in ophthalmic surgery. III. Effect of povidone-iodine on the conjunctiva. *Arch Ophthalmol.* 1984;102(5):728-729. doi:10.1001/archopht.1984.01040030584025
22. Isenberg SJ, Apt L, Yoshimori R, Khwarg S. Chemical preparation of the eye in ophthalmic surgery. IV. Comparison of povidone-iodine on the conjunctiva with a prophylactic antibiotic. *Arch Ophthalmol.* 1985;103(9):1340-1342. doi:10.1001/archopht.1985.01050090092039
23. Maheshwari S. Pterygium-induced corneal refractive changes. *Indian J Ophthalmol.* 2007;55(5):383-386. doi:10.4103/0301-4738.33829
24. Prabhasawat P, Barton K, Burkett G, Tseng SC. Comparison of conjunctival autografts, amniotic membrane grafts, and primary closure for pterygium excision. *Ophthalmology.* 1997;104(6):974-985. doi:10.1016/s0161-6420(97)30197-3
25. Johnston SC, Williams PB, Sheppard JD Jr. A comprehensive system for pterygium classification. *Invest Ophthalmol Vis Sci.* 2004;45(13):2940.
26. Zhang Z, Qian T, Zhu B, Liu H, Sun X, Xu X. Development of a valid and reliable pterygium surgery assessment scale for ophthalmology residents. *BMC Med Educ.* 2021;21(1):511. doi:10.1186/s12909-021-02934-y
27. Sarkar P, Tripathy K. Pterygium. In: *StatPearls [Internet].* StatPearls Publishing; 2022. Updated August 22, 2022. https://www.ncbi.nlm.nih.gov/books/NBK558907/
28. Zolli CL. Experience with the avulsion technique in pterygium surgery. *Ann Ophthalmol.* 1979;11(10):1569-1576.
29. Gibson JB. Brisbane survey of pterygium. *Trans Ophthalmol Soc Aust.* 1956;16:125-134.
30. Youngson RM. Recurrence of pterygium after excision. *Br J Ophthalmol.* 1972;56(2):120-125. doi:10.1136/bjo.56.2.120
31. Krag S, Ehlers N. Excimer laser treatment of pterygium. *Acta Ophthalmol (Copenh).* 1992;70(4):530-533. doi:10.1111/j.1755-3768.1992.tb02127.x
32. D'Ombrain A. The surgical treatment of pterygium. *Br J Ophthalmol.* 1948;32(2):65-71. doi:10.1136/bjo.32.2.65
33. Alpay A, Uğurbaş SH, Erdoğan B. Comparing techniques for pterygium surgery. *Clin Ophthalmol.* 2009;3:69-74.
34. Kareem AA, Farhood QK, Alhammami HA. The use of antimetabolites as adjunctive therapy in the surgical treatment of pterygium. *Clin Ophthalmol.* 2012;6:1849-1854. doi:10.2147/OPTH.S38388
35. Verma N, Garap JA, Maris R, Kerek A. Intraoperative use of mitomycin C in the treatment of recurrent pterygium. *P N G Med J.* 1998;41(1):37-42.
36. Yanyali AC, Talu H, Alp BN, Karabas L, Ay GM, Caglar Y. Intraoperative mitomycin C in the treatment of pterygium. *Cornea.* 2000;19(4):471-473. doi:10.1097/00003226-200007000-00013
37. Demirok A, Simsek S, Cinal A, Yasar T. Intraoperative application of mitomycin C in the surgical treatment of pterygium. *Eur J Ophthalmol.* 1998;8(3):153-156. doi:10.1177/112067219800800306
38. Anduze AL. Merest sclera technique for primary pterygium surgery. *Ophthalmic Surg.* 1989;20(12):892-894.
39. Staz L. A modification and extension of the McReynolds' operation for pterygium. *Br J Ophthalmol.* 1945;29(4):193-196. doi:10.1136/bjo.29.4.193
40. Wilson SE, Bourne WM. Conjunctival Z-plasty in the treatment of pterygium. *Am J Ophthalmol.* 1988;106(3):355-357. doi:10.1016/0002-9394(88)90377-7
41. Lewallen S. A randomized trial of conjunctival autografting for pterygium in the tropics. *Ophthalmology.* 1989;96(11):1612-1614. doi:10.1016/s0161-6420(89)32667-4

42. Ti SE, Chee SP, Dear KB, Tan DT. Analysis of variation in success rates in conjunctival autografting for primary and recurrent pterygium. *Br J Ophthalmol.* 2000;84(4):385-389. doi:10.1136/bjo.84.4.385
43. Kenyon KR, Wagoner MD, Hettinger ME. Conjunctival autograft transplantation for advanced and recurrent pterygium. *Ophthalmology.* 1985;92(11):1461-1470. doi:10.1016/s0161-6420(85)33831-9
44. Cohen RA, McDonald MB. Fixation of conjunctival autografts with an organic tissue adhesive. *Arch Ophthalmol.* 1993;111(9):1167-1168. doi:10.1001/archopht.1993.01090090017006
45. Kumar S, Singh R. Pterygium excision and conjunctival autograft: a comparative study of techniques. *Oman J Ophthalmol.* 2018;11(2):124-128. doi:10.4103/ojo.OJO_6_2017
46. Haider TA, Al-Amin LM, Bamashmus MA, Ali SF. Ninety-degree conjunctival rotation autograft versus zero- and 180-degree rotation autograft for pterygium surgery. *Saudi Med J.* 2009;30(4):519-523.
47. Alp BN, Yanyali A, Ay GM, Keskin O. Conjunctival rotation autograft for primary pterygium. *Ophthalmologica.* 2002;216(5):333-336. doi:10.1159/000066188
48. Gris O, Güell JL, del Campo Z. Limbal-conjunctival autograft transplantation for the treatment of recurrent pterygium. *Ophthalmology.* 2000;107(2):270-273. doi:10.1016/s0161-6420(99)00041-x
49. Malik KP, Goel R, Gutpa A, et al. Efficacy of sutureless and glue free limbal conjunctival autograft for primary pterygium surgery. *Nepal J Ophthalmol.* 2012;4(2):230-235. doi:10.3126/nepjoph.v4i2.6537
50. Al Fayez MF. Limbal versus conjunctival autograft transplantation for advanced and recurrent pterygium. *Ophthalmology.* 2002;109(9):1752-1755. doi:10.1016/s0161-6420(02)01160-0
51. Masters JS, Harris DJ Jr. Low recurrence rate of pterygium after excision with conjunctival limbal autograft: a retrospective study with long-term follow-up. *Cornea.* 2015;34(12):1569-1572. doi:10.1097/ICO.0000000000000597
52. Fernandes M, Sangwan VS, Bansal AK, et al. Outcome of pterygium surgery: analysis over 14 years. *Eye (Lond).* 2005;19(11):1182-1190. doi:10.1038/sj.eye.6701728
53. Syam PP, Eleftheriadis H, Liu CS. Inferior conjunctival autograft for primary pterygia. *Ophthalmology.* 2003;110(4):806-810. doi:10.1016/S0161-6420(02)01970-X
54. Essex RW, Snibson GR, Daniell M, Tole DM. Amniotic membrane grafting in the surgical management of primary pterygium. *Clin Exp Ophthalmol.* 2004;32(5):501-504. doi:10.1111/j.1442-9071.2004.00884.x
55. Ma DH, See LC, Liau SB, Tsai RJ. Amniotic membrane graft for primary pterygium: comparison with conjunctival autograft and topical mitomycin C treatment. *Br J Ophthalmol.* 2000;84(9):973-978. doi:10.1136/bjo.84.9.973
56. Laughrea PA, Arentsen JJ. Lamellar keratoplasty in the management of recurrent pterygium. *Ophthalmic Surg.* 1986;17(2):106-108.
57. Gupta VP, Sanghi S, Rohatgi J, Dhaliwal U. Outcomes of preoperative intrapterygial injection of mitomycin C for pterygium excision with and without inferior conjunctival flap. *Oman J Ophthalmol.* 2019;12(3):171-176. doi:10.4103/ojo.OJO_129_2018.
58. Anduze AL. Pterygium surgery with mitomycin-C: ten-year results. *Ophthalmic Surg Lasers.* 2001;32(4):341-345.
59. Clearfield E, Hawkins BS, Kuo IC. Conjunctival autograft versus amniotic membrane transplantation for treatment of pterygium: findings from a Cochrane Systematic Review. *Am J Ophthalmol.* 2017;182:8-17. doi:10.1016/j.ajo.2017.07.004
60. Gulani AC, Gulani AA. Cosmetic pterygium surgery: techniques and long-term outcomes. *Clin Ophthalmol.* 2020;14:1681-1687. doi:10.2147/OPTH.S251555
61. Sheppard JD, Mansur A, Comstock TL, Hovanesian JA. An update on the surgical management of pterygium and the role of loteprednol etabonate ointment. *Clin Ophthalmol.* 2014;8:1105-1118. doi:10.2147/OPTH.S55259
62. Ghiasian L, Samavat B, Hadi Y, Arbab M, Abolfathzadeh N. Recurrent pterygium: a review. *J Curr Ophthalmol.* 2022;33(4):367-378. doi:10.4103/joco.joco_153_20
63. Doshi RR, Harocopos GJ, Schwab IR, Cunningham ET Jr. The spectrum of postoperative scleral necrosis. *Surv Ophthalmol.* 2013;58(6):620-633. doi:10.1016/j.survophthal.2012.11.002

## SUPPLEMENTAL READING

1. Dr. Arun Gulani's PowerPoint presentation on ART of Pterygium Surgery: Cosmetic Outcomes & 21 Years Follow up.

# 32 Subconjunctival and Sub-Tenon's Injections

John Berdahl • Justin Schweitzer • Kristin Mohr

Medication to the eye is administered via topical administration or in the form of intravitreal, subconjunctival, or sub-Tenon's injection. This chapter explores the various pros and cons of subconjunctival and sub-Tenon's injection. Poor patient compliance and poor ocular drug penetration is the main benefit of injection as a vehicle for medication delivery. Both types of injections are used in surgical settings according to surgeon preference.

## INDICATIONS

### Subconjunctival Injection Indications

**Key Subconjunctival Injection Indications**

- Inflammatory etiologies
  - Anterior, noninfectious, non-necrotizing scleritis
  - Intermediate uveitis
- Severe infection
- Perioperatively for anesthesia
- Anti-fibrotic agents
  - Pre- and postsurgical 5-fluorouracil (5-FU) or mitomycin C (MMC)

Subconjunctival injections are simple procedures utilized in a variety of clinical and surgical circumstances to deliver localized medication. The use of subconjunctival medication injections has declined over the years, but it remains an important tool to be cognizant of in certain situations. Poor patient compliance and poor ocular drug penetration are two clinical indications where a subconjunctival injection is an excellent alternative. Consider a subconjunctival injection in scenarios where topical drugs are not eliciting the desired response in treatment.

From a clinical standpoint, a subconjunctival steroid injection is indicated in patients with anterior non-necrotizing scleritis who cannot tolerate systemic therapy.[1] Noninfectious anterior scleritis is a potentially sight-threatening condition characterized by inflammation of the sclera and is the most common form of scleritis.[1] Categorically, anterior scleritis falls into either necrotizing or non-necrotizing. Subconjunctival steroid injections for necrotizing scleritis are controversial at this time due to extensive scleral thinning and the risk of perforation. Therefore, these injections should only be used in patients without uveoscleral thinning. First-line treatments involve a combination of oral nonsteroidal anti-inflammatory drugs (NSAIDs) or corticosteroids. Difficulty during a steroid taper with recalcitrant scleritis or encounters with undesirable oral steroid side effects such as osteoporosis, liver toxicity, cushingoid features, insomnia, gastritis, anxiety, headaches, diabetes mellitus, or alopecia are all reasons to proceed with subconjunctival steroid injection.[2]

Scleritis with infectious etiologies poses a difficult treatment challenge due to the presence of an infection with a concurrent risk of scleral perforation. Moreover, symptoms for infectious scleritis mimic scleritis from an underlying autoimmune or idiopathic etiology.[3] It is important to differentiate infectious versus noninfectious through a careful case history. Infectious scleritis is often secondary to previous ocular surgery, pterygium excision, endophthalmitis, post anti-neoplastic agents, eye injury, or radiation.[3] The most common infectious organisms include *Pseudomonas aeruginosa, Nocardia, Streptococcus, Haemophilus, Candida,* and *Aspergillus.*[3] First-line treatment includes broad-spectrum or topical fortified antibiotics. Patients who are not responding to these therapies may be treated with either subconjunctival or intravenous (IV) vancomycin in culture-positive methicillin-resistant *Staphylococcus aureus.*[4]

From a surgical standpoint, subconjunctival injections are indicated before a vitreoretinal surgery or cataract extraction surgery for the purpose of anesthesia. This may be preferred over topical anesthesia depending on the preferred surgical technique.

Antimetabolites are used as antifibrotic agents in glaucoma filtering procedures as an off-label use to limit the degree of scarring. Antimetabolites are most commonly used at the time of surgery and during surgical revision of filtration procedures to manage appropriate bleb formation. The use of 5-FU postfiltration surgery has proven to improve the success rate of trabeculotomy surgery.[5] Subconjunctival use of 5-FU increases maintenance of intraocular pressure (IOP) control and lowers the risk of reoperation. In the Fluorouracil Filtering Surgery Study, 0.5 mL of 10 mg/mL of 5-FU was injected twice daily on postoperative days 1 to 7 and once daily on postoperative days 8 to 14. 5-FU is administered as an adjunct after a needling procedure to revive blebs. Risks with the use of 5-FU include corneal epithelial toxicity, endophthalmitis, and ocular pain. Recent studies have shown MMC offers several advantages for bleb revisions.[6] MMC lowers the risk of bleb encapsulation and offers better IOP control.[6] Subconjunctival injection of 5-FU or MMC may also be indicated before pterygium removal.

## Sub-Tenon's Injection Indications

### Key Sub-Tenon's Injection Indications

- Surgical
  - Cataract
  - Strabismus
  - Vitreoretinal
  - Optic nerve fenestration

- Intermediate uveitis/pars planitis
- Infectious posterior uveitis
    - Toxocariasis
- Birdshot choroidopathy (vitiliginous chorioretinitis)
- Behcet's disease
- Cystoid macular edema (CME)
- Posterior scleritis

Sub-Tenon's injections are indicated from a surgical standpoint in cataract extraction, strabismus surgery, vitreoretinal surgery, and optic nerve fenestration surgery. It is at the surgeon's discretion on indication and methodology.

CME is the accumulation of fluid within the macula and is identified by optical coherence tomography through the presence of cystic spaces in the outer plexiform layer of the retina. Cataract extraction, post-laser treatment, uveitis, diabetic retinopathy, macular telangiectasia, vein occlusions, vasculitis, epiretinal membranes, hypertensive retinopathy, exudative age-related macular degeneration, occult rhegmatogenous retinal detachments, intraocular tumors, collagen vascular diseases, hypotony, and chronic inflammation are all causes of CME.[7] Fluorescein angiography is another imaging technique used to identify early leakage of the macula, often in a petaloid pattern. A sub-Tenon's steroid injection (triamcinolone acetonide 40 mg/mL) is indicated in cases where topical steroid and NSAIDs medication are ineffective.

Intermediate uveitis is characterized by inflammation of the ciliary body, pars plana, and vitreous. Similarly, pars planitis presents with the same characteristics but with a vitritis, exudates, and retinal vasculitis.[8] Both intermediate uveitis and pars planitis are often idiopathic in nature. An appropriate laboratory workup that includes human leukocyte antigen-DR2, angiotensin converting enzyme, chest radiographs, serum lysozyme, complete blood count, Venereal Disease Research Laboratory, fluorescent treponemal antibody-absorbed, Lyme titers, toxocariasis, toxoplasmosis, and immunoglobulin G (IgG) and IgM serology is conducive to rule out inflammatory systemic conditions.[8] Management includes a posterior sub-Tenon's steroid injection (triamcinolone acetonide 40 mg/mL) if vision is affected by CME or inflammation in conjunction with oral steroids.

Posterior uveitis caused by toxocariasis presents as unilateral, multifocal yellow granulomas caused by the roundworm *Toxocara canis*. When *T. canis* is suspected, ELISA testing for antibody titers is useful for confirmation. In cases of severe posterior inflammation, a sub-Tenon's injection (triamcinolone acetonide 40 mg/mL) along with oral prednisolone is indicated.

Birdshot choroidopathy (vitiliginous chorioretinitis) falls into a category of White Dot syndromes characterized by posterior uveitis. Treatment is observation unless there is significant visual involvement including CME or significant inflammation. In these cases of visual impairment, sub-Tenon's injection (triamcinolone acetonide 40 mg/mL) is administered.[9]

Behcet's disease is accompanied by aphthous oral ulcers, genital ulcers, and bilateral nongranulomatous uveitis.[10] Positive lab tests for antinuclear antibody, erythrocyte sedimentation rate, C-reactive protein, and serum proteins are common but not exclusive. Topical and oral steroids are indicated in mild–moderate cases. In severe cases, a sub-Tenon's injection (triamcinolone acetonide 40 mg/mL) is indicated.

Posterior scleritis can produce elevations of the choroid that lead to choroidal folds, retinal detachment, vitritis, optic disc edema, scleral thickening, proptosis, limited extraocular motility, and angle closure glaucoma.[10] Oral and even high-dose IV steroids are a primary treatment, but a sub-Tenon's injection may be required (triamcinolone acetonide 40 mg/mL).

## CONTRAINDICATIONS

### Subconjunctival injection

- Contraindications
  - Injection of steroids over thinned sclera can cause a rupture at the site of the injection.

### Sub-Tenon's injection

- Limitations
  - Previous sub-Tenon's block in the same quadrant
  - Previous extensive vitreoretinal surgery
  - Previous repeated strabismus surgery
  - Eye trauma
  - Infection to the orbit
- Relative contraindications
  - Severe ocular pemphigoid
  - Surgery requiring complete akinesia
  - Surgeries where subsequent chemosis and subconjunctival hemorrhaging may alter the outcome of the procedure
    - Example: glaucoma filtering surgery

## PREOPERATIVE PREPARATION

### Materials and instrumentation

- Proper medication to be injected
- Topical ophthalmic anesthetic (proparacaine 0.5% or tetracaine 0.5%)
- 1-, 3-, or 5-mL tuberculin syringe
- Sterile 27- or 30-gauge ½ inch needle to draw up medication for subconjunctival injection
- Sterile 18- or 20-gauge ½ inch needle to draw up medication for sub-Tenon's injection
- Curved cannula
- Jeweler's forceps or Colibri forceps
- Alcohol swab
- Lid speculum
- Gloves
- 4 × 4 inch multipurpose gauze pads
- Dissecting scissors (for sub-Tenon's injection)

# PROCEDURE

## Subconjunctival Injection

- Obtain informed consent and discuss all risks/benefits/alternatives of the procedure.
- Position the patient to lie back comfortably with proper neck support.
- Wash hands and put on appropriately sized sterile gloves.
- Instill one drop of topical proparacaine 0.5% or tetracaine 0.5%.
- Instill topical phenylephrine 2.5% to constrict blood vessels and reduce the risk of subconjunctival hemorrhage.
- Disinfect the vial top of medication with the alcohol swab and withdraw the necessary amount of medication with a sterile 27- or 30-gauge needle.
- Withdraw the needle from the vial. Expel any air bubbles and measure to the appropriate volume (mL) amount of desired medication.
- Insert the lid speculum or alternatively instruct the patient to look in the opposite direction of the location of the injection.
  - The superior-temporal quadrant of the conjunctiva is most commonly used for injection location as this allows most space between recti muscle insertions.
    - Instruct the patient to look down.
  - In the event of inferior subconjunctival injections, instruct the patient to look up.
- "Tent" up the conjunctiva with Jeweler's or Colibri forceps with the nondominant hand.
- Position the needle tangentially to the elevated conjunctival tent, with the bevel of the needle facing down ("bevel down").
  - The needle should be pointed away from the cornea.
- Inject the desired amount of medication—typically 0.25 to 1 mL of medication—while ensuring the bevel remains down as the medication is injected (Figures 32-1 to 32-3).

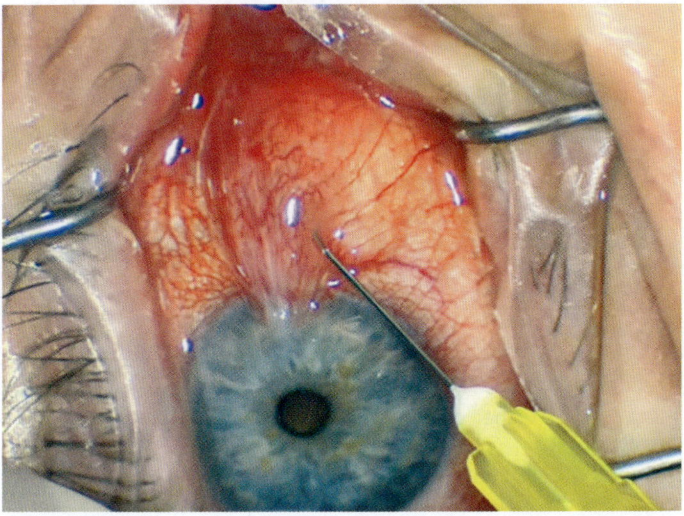

**FIGURE 32-1** Subconjunctival injection during a pterygium removal.

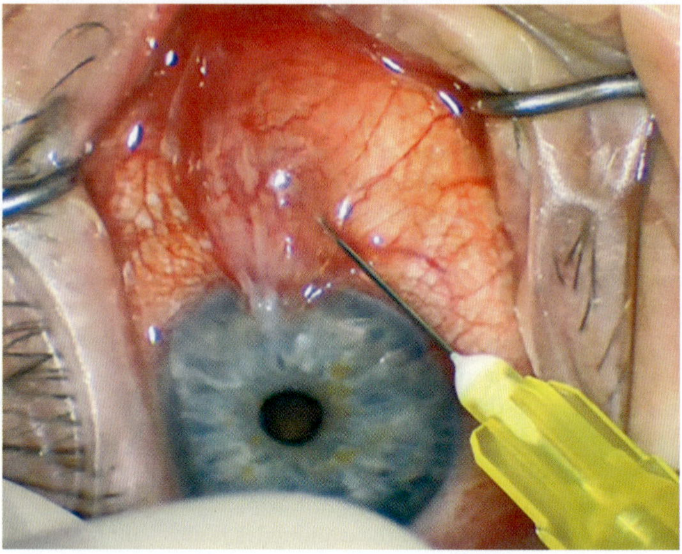

**FIGURE 32-2** Subconjunctival injection with "ballooning" of the conjunctiva as the medication is injected.

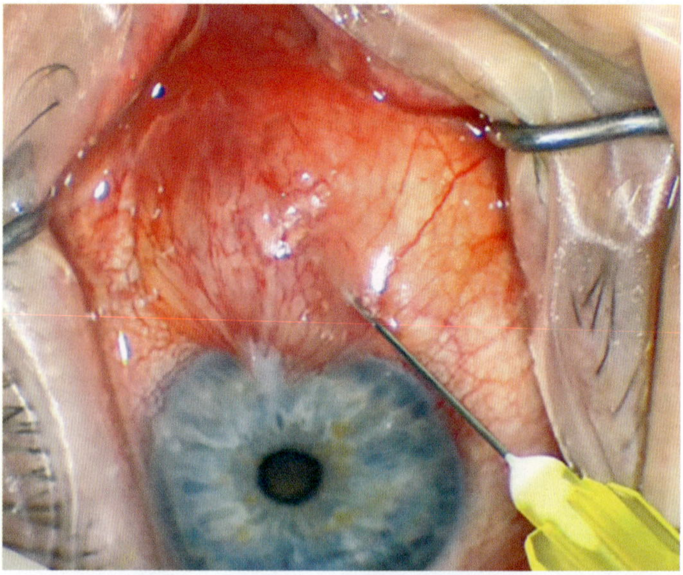

**FIGURE 32-3** Further conjunctiva "ballooning" before the needle is retracted.

- Avoid instilling medication on the ocular surface.
  - 5-FU is toxic to the cornea and may cause an abrasion or subsequential haze.
- Retract the needle and dispose in an appropriate sharps disposal container.
- Ask the patient to close their eyes to ensure eyelids are able to properly close.
- Apply a gauze pad against the closed eye to allow injected medication to distribute across the subconjunctival surface for approximately 30 seconds.
- Educate the patient on possible side effects, most often including subconjunctival hemorrhaging.
- Instruct patient on when to return to the clinic for follow-up.

## Sub-Tenon's Injection

- Obtain informed consent.
- Place the patient in a supine position. Wash hands and put on appropriately sized sterile gloves.
- Instill one drop of topical proparacaine 0.5% or tetracaine 0.5%.
- Instill one drop of topical phenylephrine 2.5% to constrict blood vessels and reduce the risk of subconjunctival hemorrhage.
- Disinfect the vial top of medication with the alcohol swab, and withdraw the necessary amount of medication with a sterile 27- or 30-gauge needle.
- Withdraw the needle from the vial. Expel any air bubbles and measure to the appropriate mL amount of desired medication.
- Perform a needle exchange to a curved cannula.
- Insert lid speculum on the upper and lower lid.
- Instruct the patient to look up.
- "Tent" up both the subconjunctival tissue and Tenon's capsule with forceps.
  - Tenon's capsule will not tent up as high and will create more resistance.
- Dissect toward the sclera with scissors to enlarge sub-Tenon's space.
- Point the cannula away from the cornea and position the syringe and needle tangentially to the elevated sub-Tenon's tent.
- Once in proper position, the cannula should be nearly perpendicular to the surface of the eye with a nearly vertical orientation.
- If resistance is met while positioning the cannula, withdraw and reposition.
- Inject the desired amount of medication into sub-Tenon's space.
- Retract cannula and dispose in appropriate sharps disposal container.

# POSTOPERATIVE CARE/COMANAGEMENT (FOLLOW-UP SCHEDULE)

## Subconjunctival Injection Postoperative and Comanagement Care

- Subconjunctival hemorrhages are relatively common; patient should be well educated about appearance.
- Place a cool pack over the eyes TID–QID over the next 24 hours.
- Do not rub the eyes.

- Advise the patient to return to the clinic if pain, changes or loss of vision, or ocular discharge occurs.
- Follow up as appropriately indicated for monitoring the underlying condition.

### Sub-Tenon's Injection Postoperative and Comanagement Care

- Eye shields are indicated especially after surgery.
- Do not rub the eyes.
- Advise the patient to return to the clinic if pain, changes or loss of vision, or ocular discharge occurs.
- Follow up as appropriately indicated for monitoring the underlying condition.

## POTENTIAL COMPLICATIONS AND THEIR TREATMENT

### Subconjunctival Injections

- Subconjunctival hemorrhage:
  Self-limiting in nature. There is no treatment, but it is optional to add artificial tears as lubricant.
- Ocular hypertension:
  Treatment consists of topical antihypertension drops. In the event of a steroid response, continue monitoring IOP over the course of several weeks.
- Episcleritis/Scleritis:
  Treat with topical steroid and topical/oral NSAIDs.
- Cataract formation:
  Debate on causation versus correlation remains controversial. Commonly, patients are using systemic steroids to battle scleritis. Treatment: cataract extraction
- Scleral necrosis/melt:
  Debate on causation versus correlation remains controversial. Strongly associated with scleritis. Treatment involves either systemic immunosuppressant drugs or a Tenon's membrane flap with amniotic membrane coverage. An amniotic membrane coverage is most commonly used in scenarios of postoperative scleral necrosis following pterygium excision. A corneoscleral patch graft with amniotic membrane coverage is also an option.

### Sub-Tenon's Injections

**Minor complications**

- Pain
  - Pain from the local anesthetic solution is due to the widening and stretching of the sub-Tenon's space during the injection.
  - Treatment: Minimize through adequate surface anesthesia, slow insertion of the cannula, and slow injection.
- Chemosis
  - A result of an anterior spread from sub-Tenon's space into the conjunctiva

- Can also result from incorrect injection into the subconjunctival space rather than sub-Tenon's space
- May occur if the dissection from the conjunctiva from Tenon's capsule is insufficient or if there is excess volume of injected anesthesia
- Treatment: To minimize this, ensure adequate cannula length, be sure to dissect carefully, and apply gentle pressure to the globe after injection.

- Subconjunctival hemorrhage
  - A result due to tearing of blood vessels during dissection of the conjunctiva from Tenon's capsule
  - The hemorrhaging may remain localized or spread.
  - To differentiate this from conjunctival vasodilation, anterior segment evaluation of the conjunctiva is necessary to compare preinjection and postinjection appearance.
  - Patients on antiplatelet agents experience subconjunctival hemorrhaging at a higher incidence.
  - Patients should not discontinue antiplatelet therapy, as discontinuing medication has no effect on intraoperative course or postoperative outcome.
  - Treatment: none, may add topical lubrication through artificial tears
  - To minimize, carefully dissect to prevent shearing of blood vessels.
  - Apply gentle pressure to the globe with vasoconstrictor-soaked cotton buds.
  - Localized cautery can reduce the frequency of subconjunctival hemorrhage.

**Major complications**

- Brain stem anesthesia[11]
  - Due to the spread of local anesthesia to the central nervous system (CNS) through the subarachnoid space. This can occur from accidental injection into the posterior sub-Tenon's space, which enters the subarachnoid space through the optic nerve sheath.
  - Can also occur from unintentional perforation of the Tenon's capsule, which can cause subsequent local anesthesia deposition into the intraconal space and spread to the CNS through an orbital foramen
  - Symptoms: drowsiness, confusion, loss of verbal contact, cranial nerve palsies, convulsions, cardiac arrest, respiratory depression
  - Treatment: Maintain airway, provide oxygenation, IV therapy, and vasopressor agents.
- Globe perforation[11]
  - Reported in cases of scleral scarring from previous retinal detachment surgery
  - Prevention: case reports of pain when not waiting long enough for anesthesia to kick in
  - Higher chance of this if the patient is squeezing their eyes shut
  - Treatment: immediate surgery to close the open globe wound
- Orbital and/or retrobulbar hemorrhage[11]
  - Unknown etiology; may be caused by excessive digital massage
  - Direct trauma to blood vessels from the cannula is a possibility.
  - Suspect this if the globe becomes proptosed over a period of a few minutes.
  - Lid swelling and conjunctival blood vessel engorgement can occur.
  - Treatment: Check IOP and retinal circulation. Reduce the compartment pressure and IOP through topical antihypertensive drops. Immediate oculocompression may be necessary.
- Retinal ischemia[11]
  - Closure of central retinal vessels

    - Cause is unknown, may be from an increase in IOP exceeding the mean arterial pressure in the ophthalmic or central artery.
    - May be caused by anesthetic blockade of the vasodilator nerves
    - Significant and consider in patients with compromised ocular circulation or significant glaucomatous optic neuropathy
    - Retinal artery occlusions treatment:
        - Digital massage, IV acetazolamide, methylprednisolone
        - Paracentesis of aqueous humor to decrease IOP acutely
- Optic nerve damage
- Rectus muscle dysfunction
    - Diplopia is mostly caused by inferior rectus damage caused by the sub-Tenon's block. Direct trauma to the muscle with hematoma formation.
        - Concurrent orbital bruising
        - Can occur from direct trauma to the muscle with either the scissors or trauma by the rigid metal cannula
- Orbital swelling
    - Proptosis
    - Possible causes: infection, inflammation, or reaction to the anesthetic agent
    - Treatment: oral and systemic antibiotics with or without steroids
    - Oral antihistamines may also resolve the orbital swelling.
    - Chance of endophthalmitis and orbital cellulitis

## VIDEOS OF PROCEDURES

**Video 32-1**—Subconjunctival injection. A 30-gauge needle is injected into the conjunctiva (as seen before a surgical pterygium removal). The conjunctiva "balloons" upward as lidocaine is injected. The needle is then retracted from the subconjunctival space.

**Video 32-2**—Sub-Tenon's injection. A sub-Tenon's block is performed during an aqueous tube shunt surgery. Westcott scissors are used to dissect the subconjunctiva from Tenon's capsule. A 19-gauge cannula is inserted between the created space, and anesthesia is injected behind the globe posteriorly.

# EFFICACY

Subconjunctival injections of steroid for non-necrotizing scleritis may take several days to take effect, and these patients should still have daily or close to daily monitoring. Likewise, subconjunctival injections for antibiotic use warrant daily monitoring of the patient's condition. Surgical effects of analgesia, akinesia, or antimetabolite use will be achieved within 1 to 10 minutes for both subconjunctival and sub-Tenon's injections. In cases of posterior scleritis, patients should also be monitored daily or close to daily until resolution of the condition. Posterior segment pathology may take an undermined amount of time until resolution due to the severity of the disease being treated and close monitoring is expected.

# CODING/BILLING AND MODIFIERS

For sub-Tenon's injections, Current Procedural Terminology (CPT) code 67515 is used: "Injection of medication or other substance into Tenon's capsule."

For subconjunctival injections, CPT code 68200 is used: "Subconjunctival injection."

Report the appropriate laterality modifier (i.e., LT for left side, RT for right side, 50 for bilateral). Neither procedural codes have a global period.

According to CMS-established guidelines, there are several instances to not report either CPT code separately.[12] These include:

- If a medically necessary anti-sclerosing agent at the same patient encounter as surgery to correct glaucoma is necessary
- If the injected substance is an anesthetic agent used by the physician in order to perform an operative procedure
- If the injected substance is an anesthetic agent used by the physician for the use of post-operative pain management and the same physician is responsible for the original surgical procedure
- In the instance of injection of antibiotic, steroid, or NSAID during a cataract extraction or other ophthalmic procedure
- In the instance of a procedural paracentesis because the injections are inherent and an integral component of the paracentesis procedure

Common ICD-10 codes that are billable for this procedure include:

**Subconjunctival injection ICD-10 Codes**

- **H15.0 to H15.009**—Unspecified scleritis
- **H15.01 to H15.019**—Anterior scleritis
- **H15.02 to H15.029**—Brawny scleritis
- **Z98.83**—Filtering (vitreous) bleb after glaucoma surgery status
- **T81.89XA**—Other complication of procedures not elsewhere classified, initial encounter
- **Z98.89**—Other specified postprocedural states

**25 Modifier**

- CPT states that the two above CPT codes only cover the procedure itself. A -25 modifier indicates a separate evaluation and management by the same physician on the exact same encounter date of the other injection service. This is indicated and appropriate where the injection serves as a separate evaluation and management that was performed on the same date of service. The -25 modifier should be added to the appropriately leveled examination CPT code.

**Sub-Tenon's injection ICD-10 codes**

- **H30.00 to H30.133**—Chorioretinal inflammation
- **M35.2**—Behcet's disease
- **H15.0 to H15.009**—Unspecified scleritis

- **B83.0**—Visceral larva migrans
- **H30.20 to H30.23**—Posterior cyclitis
- **H20.9**—Unspecified iridocyclitis
- **H59.031 to H59.033**—CME following cataract surgery
- **H35.351 to H35.353**—CME

**J codes—Both subconjunctival and sub-Tenon's injection**

- **J3300**—Injection, triamcinolone preservative free 1 mg
- **J3301**—Injection, triamcinolone acetonide, 40 mg/1 mL per 10 mg vial
  - Kenalog-10
  - Kenalog-40
  - Tri-Kort
  - Kenaject-40
  - Kenacort A-40
  - Triam-A
  - Trilog
- **J3304**—Injection, triamcinolone acetonide, preservative-free, extended-release, microsphere formulation 1 mg
- **J1020**—Methylprednisolone 20 mg
- **J1030**—Methylprednisolone 40 mg
- **J1040**—Methylprednisolone 80 mg
- **J0696**—Ceftriaxone sodium injection 250 mg
- **J0713**—Ceftazidime injection 500 mg
- **J0714**—Ceftazidime and avibactam 0.625 g
- **J1580**—Garamycin, gentamicin up to 80 mg
- **J3370**—Vancomycin HCl injection 500 mg
- **J3260**—Tobramycin sulfate 80 mg
- **J7682**—Tobramycin non-comp unit 300 mg
- **J0285**—Amphotericin B 50 mg
- **J0287**—Amphotericin B lipid complex 10 mg
- **J0289**—Amphotericin B liposome injection 10 mg
- **J9280**—Mitomycin injection 5 mg
- **J9190**—Fluorouracil injection 500 mg
- **J2001**—Lidocaine injection 10 mg
- **J7999**—Compounded drug, not otherwise classified
- **NOC code**—Use only if there is no valid Healthcare Common Procedure Coding System code that describes the drug.

**Procedure note documentation requirements according to the American Academy of Ophthalmology[13]**

- Diagnosis or indication for injection
- Site of injection, eye(s) treated
- Medication name, how much was injected (in milligrams and volume in milliliters), and lot number

- How much of a drug is wasted
  - If less than 1 unit, document with verbiage "residual medication less than 1 unit discarded."
  - Multidose versus single dose
    - In the event of a multidose vial, you are paid only for the amount administered to the patient and not any amount that is discarded.
- Route of administration
- Physician signature, legible or secure if electronic
- Usage of a covered diagnosis by the payer. If the diagnosis is not included in the payer policy, the patient is responsible for the injection and drug costs.
- Documentation that the patient desires treatment
- Informed consent on the file of first injection and/or change in medication or eye
- Maintenance of legible medication administration records

## REFERENCES


1. Bagheri N, Wajda BN. Scleritis. In: Bagheri N, Wajda BN, eds. *The Wills Eye Manual: Office and Emergency Room Diagnosis and Treatment of Eye Disease*. 7th ed. Lippincott Williams and Wilkins; 2017:117-119.
2. Sohn W R, Read R, Roufas A, et al. Long-term, multicenter evaluation of subconjunctival injection of triamcinolone for non-necrotizing, noninfectious anterior scleritis. *Ophthalmol.* 2011;118(10): 1932-1937. doi:10.1016/j.ophtha.2011.02.043
3. Hodson GA, Karp CL, Davis JL, et al. Epidemiology and visual outcomes in patients with infectious scleritis. *Cornea.* 2013;32(4):466-472. doi:10.1097/ICO.0b013e318259c952
4. Kumar S, Das S, Sharma S, Sahu K. Clinico-microbiological profile and treatment outcome of infectious scleritis: experience from a tertiary eye care center of India. *Intl J Inflamm.* 2012;753560-753568. doi:10.1155/2012/753560
5. Fluorouracil filtering surgery study one-year follow-up. *Am J Ophthalmol.* 1989;108(6):625-635. doi:10.1016/0002-9394(89)90853-2
6. Amini E, Esmaili A, Zarei R, Amini N, Daneshvar R. Office-based slit-lamp needle revision with adjunctive mitomycin-C for late failed or encapsulated filtering blebs. *Middle East Afr J Ophthalmol.* 2012:19(2):216-221. doi:10.4103/0974-9233.95255
7. Friedman NJ, Kaiser PK, Pinedo R. Cystoid macular edema. In: Friedman PR, Kaiser PK, Pinedo R, eds. *The Massachusetts Eye and Ear Infirmary illustrated Manual of Ophthalmology*. 3rd ed. Saunders/Elsevier; 2014:383-385.
8. Friedman NJ, Kaiser PK, Pinedo R. Intermediate uveitis/pars planitis. In: Friedman PR, Kaiser PK, Pinedo R, eds. *The Massachusetts Eye and Ear Infirmary illustrated Manual of Ophthalmology*. 3rd ed. Saunders/Elsevier; 2014:412-413.
9. Friedman NJ, Kaiser PK, Pinedo R. Birdshot choroidopathy vitiliginous chorioretinitis. In: Friedman PR, Kaiser PK, Pinedo R, eds. *The Massachusetts Eye and Ear Infirmary Illustrated Manual of Ophthalmology*. 3rd ed. Saunders/Elsevier; 2014:430-431.
10. Friedman NJ, Kaiser PK, Pinedo R. posterior uveitis: other inflammatory disorders. In: Friedman PR, Kaiser PK, Pinedo R, eds. *The Massachusetts Eye and Ear Infirmary Illustrated Manual of Ophthalmology*. 3rd ed. Saunders/Elsevier; 2014:433-438.
11. Kumar EH, Dodds C. Sub-Tenon's anaesthesia: complications and their prevention. *Eye. (Lond)* 2011;25(6):694-703. doi:10.1038/eye.2011.69
12. Centers for Medicare & Medicaid Services. Chapter VIII. Accessed January 1, 2022. https://www.cms.gov/files/document/chapter8cptcodes60000-69999final11.pdf
13. Edgar JS, Woodke, J. How to ensure your recordkeeping for injections is complete. *Am Acad Ophthalmol.* Accessed March 2, 2020. www.aao.org/young-ophthalmologists/yo-info/article/ensure-recordkeeping-for-injections-is-complete

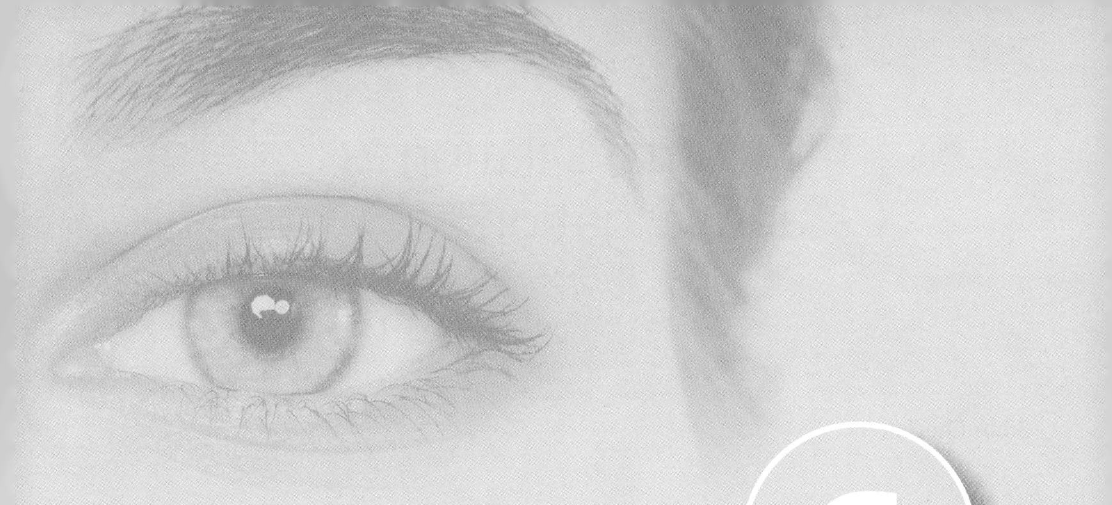

# SECTION 6

# Lacrimal Procedures

# 33 Lacrimal Dilation and Irrigation

**Bibin Cherian**

Epiphora, excessive tearing caused by overproduction of tears or secondary to poor drainage, is a common complaint that can cause a negative impact on the quality of life for patients. Ocular surface diseases (blepharitis, dry eye, etc.), eyelid abnormalities (ectropion, trichiasis, etc.), or lacrimal system issues (punctal stenosis, dacryocystitis, etc.) can all play a part in excessive tearing for patients.[1] In most instances of unilateral epiphora secondary to lacrimal system disorders, nasolacrimal duct obstruction (NLDO) tends to be the culprit.[2]

Dilation and irrigation (D&I) is a straightforward procedure that can be used to open up an NLDO and confirm patency. The punctum is dilated, and balanced salt solution (BSS) is flushed through. If successful, the patient will taste the BSS as it drains through the nasopharynx.[3] For unresolving cases, a referral for dacryocystorhinostomy (DCR) may be warranted.[4,5]

## INDICATIONS

### Key Indications

- Punctal stenosis
- Canalicular obstruction
- Intracanalicular plug

NLDO can be congenital or acquired later in life.[1] The lower end of the nasolacrimal duct (NLD) near the valve of Hasner is the last part to canalize with patency usually occurring soon after birth. In cases of congenital NLDO, spontaneous resolution occurs in around 85% of infants within the first year of life. Oftentimes, the parents of infants with NLDO are advised to massage the lacrimal sac (Crigler maneuver) to relieve the obstruction.[3,4] The most common reasons for acquired NLDO or punctal stenosis tend to be from either idiopathic causes or chronic blepharitis. Involutional changes are a supposed pathogenesis that leads to narrowing or occlusion of the puncta with age, whereas chronic inflammation can lead to fibrosis in the lacrimal system. Accounting for around 20% in some studies, chronic dacryocystitis is another common etiology for acquired NLDO.[1] Foreign bodies such as eyelashes, dacryoliths, or retained punctal plugs can also lead to mechanical obstructions. Other less common causes include topical drugs, eye or eyelid infections, or rarely tumors.[5-7]

D&I can be warranted for instances of stenosis or blockage of the nasolacrimal apparatus. Either the fluorescein dye disappearance test or the Jones 1 test can be used to assess if either is present or if there is another underlying etiology.[6,8] It is also important to understand the anatomy of the lacrimal system to properly evaluate where the blockage is suspected to be.

The nasolacrimal drainage system drains in the following order: puncta, canaliculi, lacrimal sac, and then the NLD that empties into the nasal cavity. Both upper and lower lids have a punctum that can be visualized when slightly everting the medial edge of the eyelid. Tears drain from the puncta into the canaliculi, which pass vertically about 2 mm before turning medially and running 8 mm horizontally to reach the lacrimal sac. The superior and inferior canaliculi typically unite to form the common canaliculus before entering the lateral wall of the lacrimal sac. The angle at which the canaliculus enters the sac and a small flap of mucosa (Rosenmüller valve) prevents the reflux of tears. The lacrimal sac is around 10 to 12 mm long and empties into the NLD, which runs between 12 and 18 mm in length. This duct terminates in the inferior meatus of the nose where the valve of Hasner lies. This mucosal fold prevents retrograde movement of fluid from the nasal cavity into the duct.[2,3,9]

Tears secreted by the lacrimal gland pass along the ocular surface. Although some tear fluid is lost via evaporation or conjunctival reabsorption, the vast majority passes through the nasolacrimal drainage system. Most of the drainage occurs through the lower puncta because of gravitational forces. With eyelid closure, the orbicularis oculi muscle creates positive pressure that forces tears down the NLD and into the nasopharynx. When the eyes open, the canaliculi and lacrimal sac expand, which creates a negative pressure that draws tears into the sac from the canaliculi. Normal tear meniscus height is 0.2 to 0.4 mm versus 0.6 mm or greater in patients with epiphora.[2,3,9]

The dye disappearance test can be performed to determine if the tears are draining at a proper rate. Abnormal drainage can be indicative of an NLDO. Equal amounts of fluorescein dye are instilled in each eye onto the conjunctiva. The patient should be instructed to blink normally and not excessively squeeze their eyes. Any excess dye that has spilled onto the cheeks can be wiped away, but do not allow the patient to blot the eyelids as it can draw the fluorescein and tears out of the conjunctival sac. After 5 minutes, no retained fluorescein or a very thin meniscus should be noted with normal results. If tear heights are unequal, it implies the eye with the larger meniscus likely has an impaired tear drainage. It is unlikely for there to be unilateral poor meniscus secondary to dry eye or unilateral pseudo-epiphora from reflex tearing.[2,6,8] Often the tears will overflow medially if there is an outflow obstruction versus laterally over the outer cheek when it is an eyelid cause.[5]

Jones 1 is another test that is performed by moistening one to two fluorescein strips and touching it to the inferior palpebral conjunctiva of each eye. It is important that sufficient dye is instilled to minimize the possibility of a false test result. The patient should be allowed to sit and blink normally for 5 minutes. Afterward, the patient can occlude a nostril on the unaffected side (or one nostril at a time if bilateral) and blow their nose into a white tissue.[6,8] Another option is to roll a sterile cotton swab inside the nostril. If the system is patent, there should be fluorescein evident with a cobalt blue filter on either the tissue or swab.

With Jones 1 testing, if fluorescein *is recovered* on the affected side, no further testing is required. Reflex tearing or other dry eye etiologies should be considered. D&I can still be considered if there is thought to be a partial obstruction that can be relieved. If *no dye is recovered*, it is because of some degree of blockage, failure of the lacrimal pump system, or a false test secondary to insufficient fluorescein instillation. The punctum on the affected side can be dilated and the test is repeated to see if the source is punctal stenosis; however, this can usually be observed during clinical evaluation.[6]

## CONTRAINDICATION

**Key Contraindications**

- Acute dacryocystitis
- Canaliculitis
- Dacryocystocele

D&I is contraindicated in any cases of acute infection of the lacrimal drainage system. The most serious one a practitioner should be aware of is acute dacryocystitis. This involves an infection, typically streptococcal or staphylococcal, of the lacrimal sac usually secondary to NLDO. D&I can potentially cause the infection to spread, leading to an orbital cellulitis and should thus be avoided. Patients will present with pain in the medial canthus with associated swelling and erythema. Lacrimal sac palpation will be painful. Treatment in these cases consists of oral antibiotics such as amoxicillin. Referral for DCR may be required after the infection has resolved to minimize recurrent infection or if epiphora persists. External DCR has a success rate of 70% to 90% to resolve subsequent epiphora in chronic cases.[1,3,5]

Canaliculitis is a relative contraindication with varying treatment among clinicians. Presentation will typically include mild tenderness near the medial canthus and a "pouting" of the puncta that is pathognomonic for the condition. Expression of mucopurulent discharge or concretions from the puncta can be noted. Although this indicates an active infection, there is no involvement with the lacrimal sac. The patient can be placed on a topical antibiotic or carefully irrigated with an antibiotic solution. If unsure of the etiology, refrain from performing D&I.[3,6,10]

Dacryocystoceles are mild enlargements of the lacrimal sac in an infant that appear as a bluish mass. These can be present at birth but only detected later as tear production increases. It is caused by an accumulation of mucus or amniotic fluid in the lacrimal sac and should be monitored to rule out nasal obstruction or further development into dacryocystitis. Initial treatment involves warm compresses, digital massage, and topical antibiotics. Referral to a pediatric ophthalmologist would be warranted if additional treatment is needed because of the need for general anesthesia.[3,4,10]

## INFORMED CONSENT

Although D&I is straightforward, it is important to obtain an informed consent. Simple language should be used to describe the process: "Anesthetic eye drops will be used to numb the eyes and lessen the discomfort. A small metal tool will be used to widen the puncta (small openings on the eyelids) where the tears drain. A thin metal tool will then be placed through the opening and a sterile salt solution will be injected to try and loosen up any blockages. You may taste the salt solution as it drains."

Alternative treatments such as monitoring or invasive surgery should be listed. Common or possible risks that should be disclosed include pain, discomfort, bleeding, swelling, infection, or need for referral for another type of procedure. They should also be aware that D&I may need to be repeated in the future.

The patient's and doctor's name should be both printed and signed on the informed consent alongside a witness, for example, staff member. The consent form should be dated and stored in the patient's records.

## PREOPERATIVE CARE

Patients with an outflow obstruction tend to be more symptomatic in the mornings or when in windy or cold environments. Complaints of overflowing tears on the cheek, especially medially, tend to also be an indication of a lacrimal obstruction issue rather than hypersecretion.[3,5] Confirm the etiology of the epiphora with either the dye disappearance test or the Jones 1 test. If the lacrimal system is determined to have an obstruction, then proceed with D&I. Behind the slit lamp, the puncta can be evaluated to determine the size of dilator if necessary and cannula (if multiple available).

Prepare the necessary instruments for the procedure with appropriate sterile techniques. The tools needed are a topical anesthetic (e.g., proparacaine 0.5% or tetracaine 0.5%), punctum dilator, irrigation cannula, sterile BSS, and a syringe (3, 5, and 10 mL) (Figure 33-1). Use

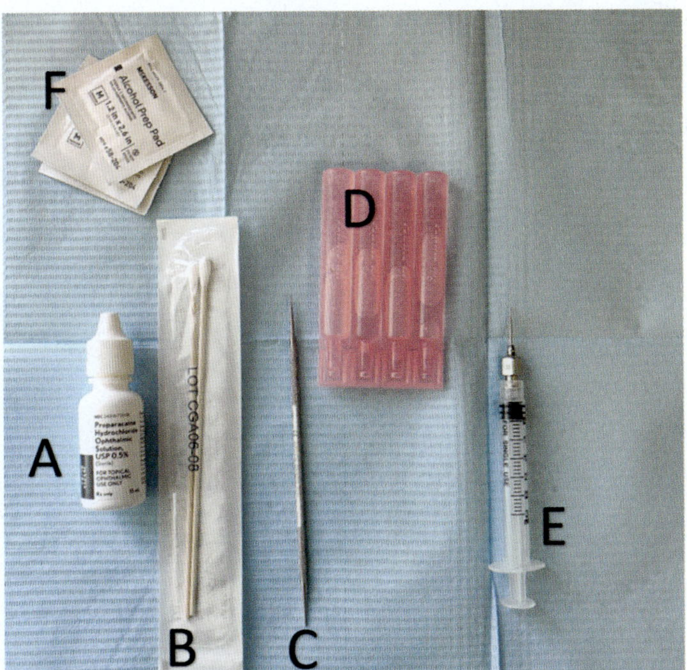


**FIGURE 33-1** Instrumentation preoperative setup. **A,** Proparacaine 0.5% bottle. **B,** Cotton-tipped applicators. **C,** Punctum dilator. **D,** Sterile saline. **E,** Syringe with cannula attached. **F,** Alcohol prep pads.

the largest cannula that can comfortably fit in the punctum, with sizes ranging from 27 gauge to 19 gauge.[11] Fill the syringe with 3 to 5 mL of the saline and push through all but 1 mL to thoroughly rinse any disinfectant in the cannula.[3,6]

## PROCEDURE

1. Topical anesthetic is not required but based on patient and practitioner comfort. Instill a drop of anesthetic on to the eye. For additional comfort, consider holding an anesthetic-soaked cotton tip applicator (CTA) directly on to the puncta. Mildly evert the lid, and firmly place CTA on the inferior punctum (Figure 33-2). Have the patient close their eyes for several minutes to ensure the soaked CTA contacts both puncta.
2. Although this procedure can be done in the slit lamp, it is often easier to perform outside of it if the punctum can be visualized.[12] Recline the patient in the chair or confirm the patient is in a comfortable position. Have the patient direct their gaze out and away from the puncta that is being irrigated. For instance, have the patient look superior temporally when irrigating the inferior punctum. Provide "verbal valium"—talking the patient through the procedure to ensure they remain still.
3. Pull the eyelid away from the globe and insert the dilator vertically into the punctum opening for about 2 mm (Figures 33-3 to 33-5).

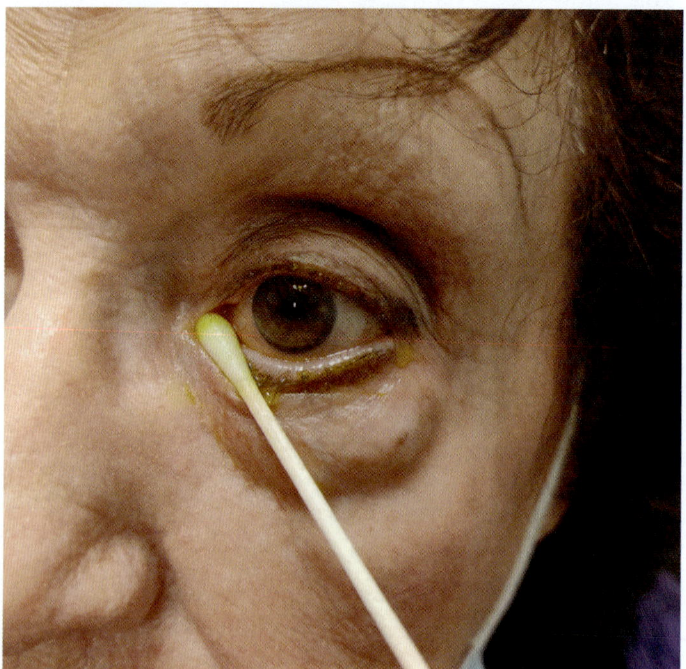

**FIGURE 33-2** Holding proparacaine 0.5% soaked cotton-tipped applicator directly on the puncta.

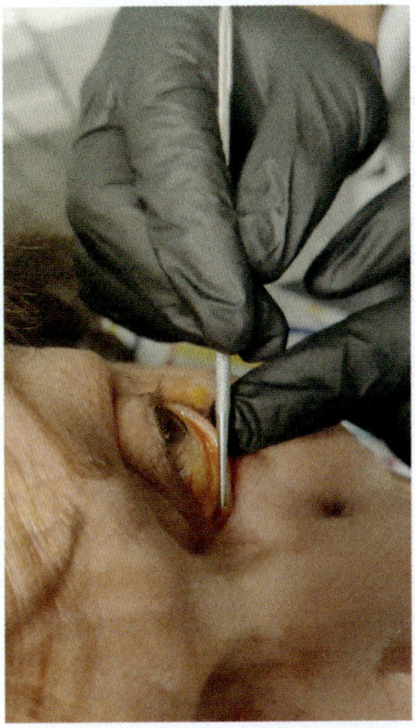

**FIGURE 33-3** When dilating, start advancing 2 mm vertically. Have the patient look up and away.

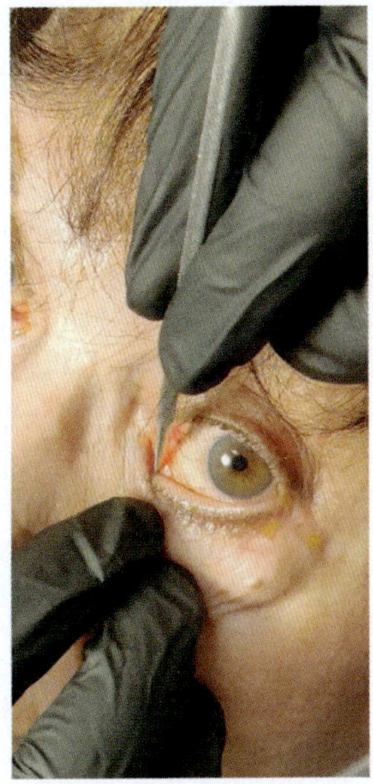

**FIGURE 33-4** Another angle of initial dilation with vertical motion.

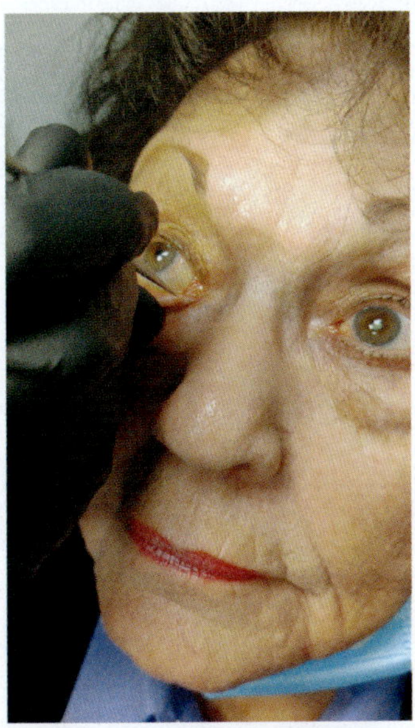

**FIGURE 33-5** Angle of dilation with opposite eye. Keep fulcrum point (such as finger) on patient's lower lid or cheek for stability.

4. If it appears to be tight, gently roll the dilator back and forth to advance into the opening.[11]
5. Once the dilator is inserted about 1 to 2 mm, pull the eyelid laterally to straighten out the canaliculus. Rotate the dilator 90° to assume a horizontal orientation. Continue slowly advancing the dilator (Figures 33-6 and 33-7). Whitening around the punctum opening indicates expansion. Do not force the dilator too deep and retract if the patient notes discomfort or a sharp pain.[6,10]
6. Immediately insert the cannula after dilating the punctum (Figures 33-8 to 33-11). If the punctum isn't opened sufficiently or closes back quickly, consider a smaller gauge cannula, repeating with a larger dilator, or further advancement of the dilator.
7. Using a similar technique, insert the cannula 1 to 2 mm vertically and then pull the eyelid taut laterally before advancing it horizontally another 2 to 4 mm into the horizontal canaliculus (Figures 33-12 to 33-14). Respect the eyelid anatomy as appreciated with the dilator.
8. Upon advancement, a small pop can be felt if there is a membranous obstruction from the common canaliculus into the lacrimal sac. If there is a complete block in the canaliculus, a soft stop can be felt as the cannula does not reach the bone. A hard stop, noticed when it does reach bone, indicates the obstruction is likely further down the lacrimal sac or in the NLD. The cannula should not be advanced when either a soft or hard stop is felt.[3,5,6]

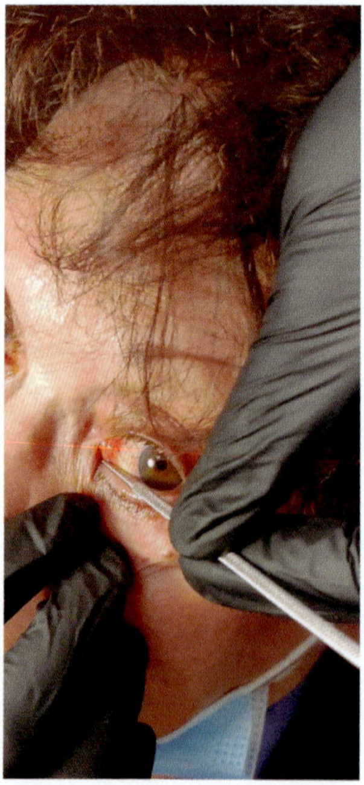

**FIGURE 33-6** Rotate the dilator 90° to the horizontal orientation and then advance another 4 to 6 mm.

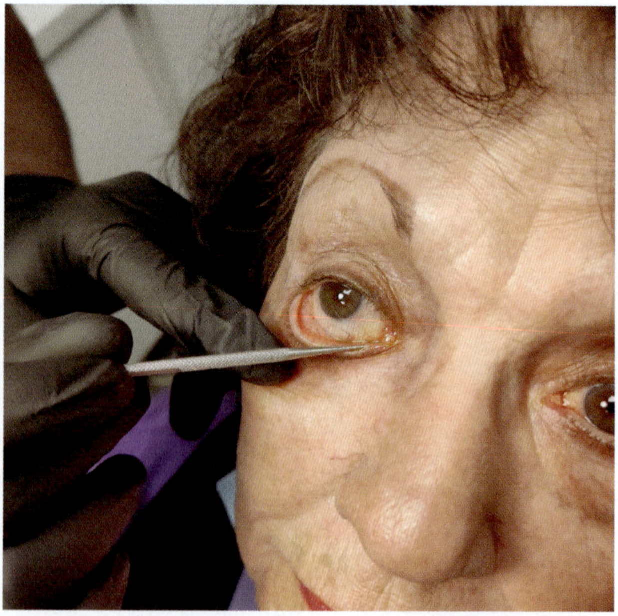

**FIGURE 33-7** When advancing the dilator, try not to come to a hard stop to minimize patient discomfort.

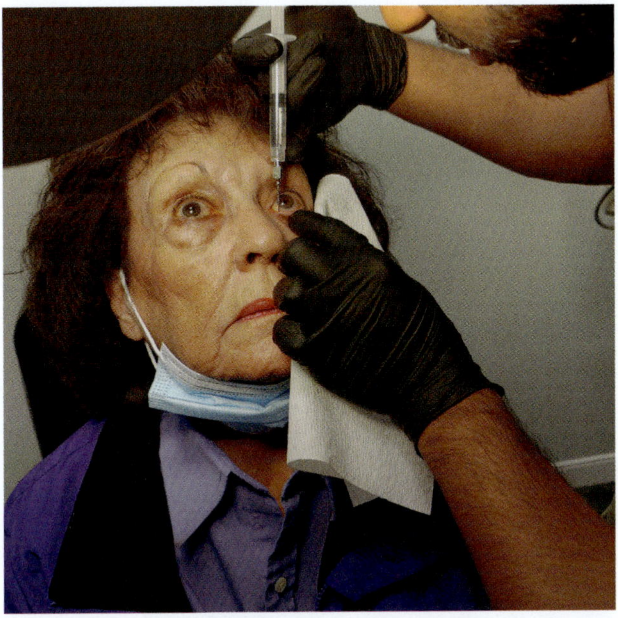

**FIGURE 33-8** Quickly switch to saline syringe/cannula with vertical orientation.

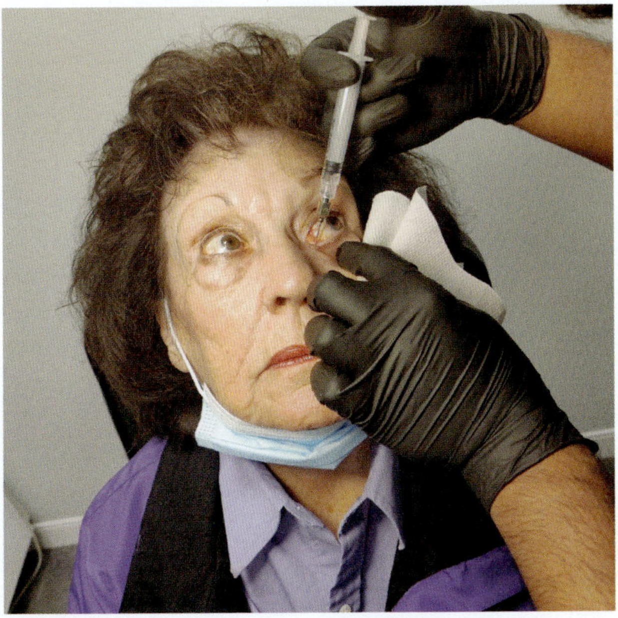

**FIGURE 33-9** Advance 2 mm vertically as before with patient looking away.

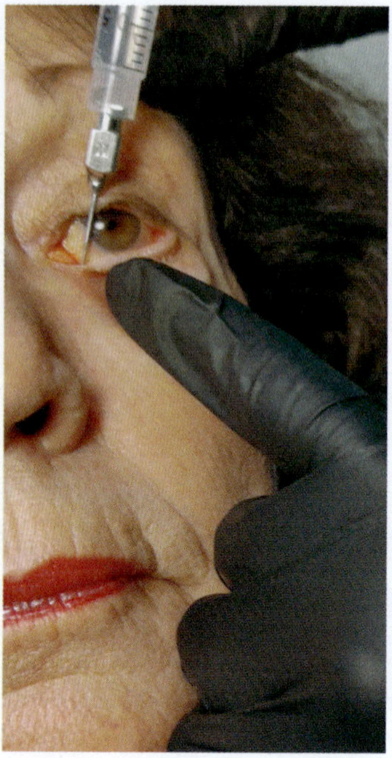

FIGURE 33-10 Another angle of vertical orientation.

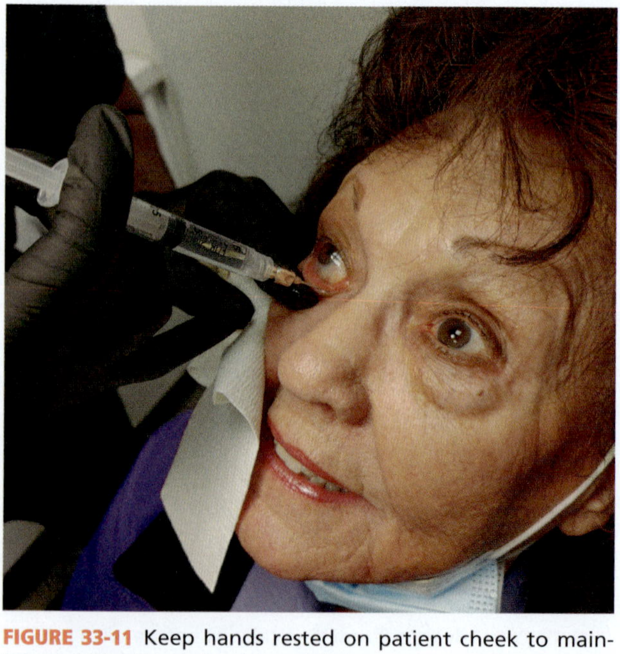

FIGURE 33-11 Keep hands rested on patient cheek to maintain stability throughout procedure.

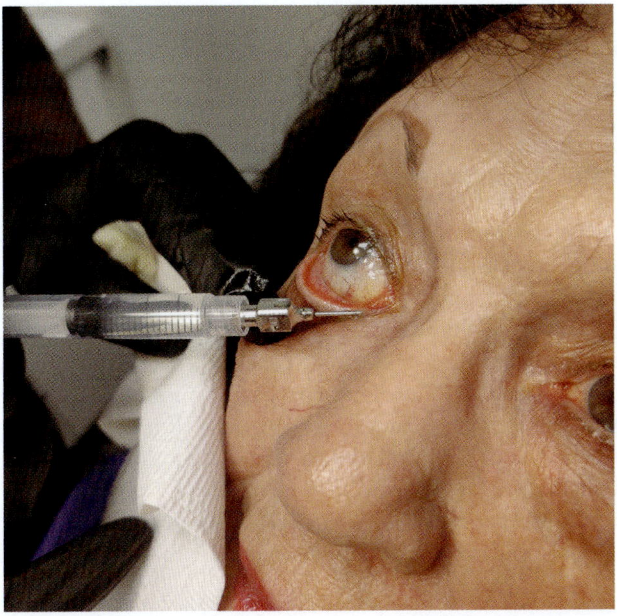

**FIGURE 33-12** Switch to the horizontal orientation to continue advancing cannula and syringe.

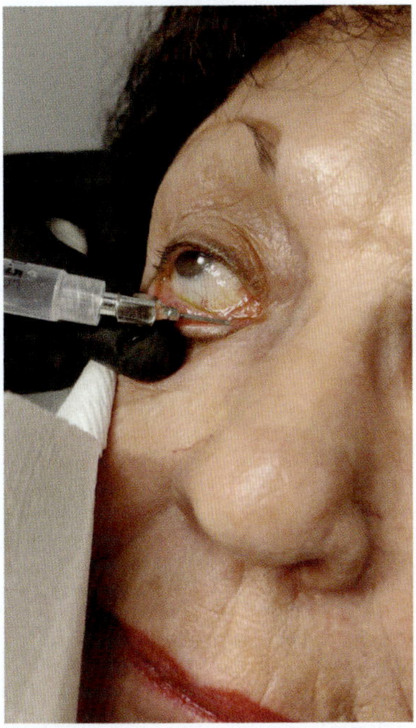

**FIGURE 33-13** Advance 4 to 6 mm before injecting saline solution.

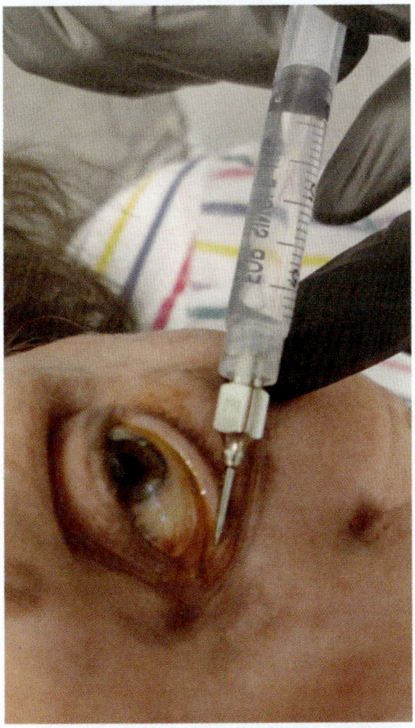

**FIGURE 33-14** Another angle of horizontal orientation while holding the eyelid taut.

9. While maintaining the position of the cannula, gently apply pressure to the plunger to introduce 2 to 3 mL of saline into the canaliculus (Figure 33-15).[10] Don't force the fluid if significant resistance is encountered. Withdraw and then reintroduce the cannula as necessary if resistance occurs.
10. Once saline is introduced, the patient should report detecting it in their throat or nose if the D&I is successful. At this point, the cannula can be slowly withdrawn.

If saline is noted to reflux from the canaliculus during irrigation, it is likely that there is a proximal obstruction or stenosis. If the saline refluxes from the opposite punctum, there is a blockage in the common canaliculus, lacrimal sac, or NLD (Figure 33-16). A CTA can be placed on the opposite punctum while attempting to irrigate again.

If irrigation is performed during a concurrent canaliculitis or other purulent discharge, patients may notice more tenderness. The discomfort can be minimized by adding a few drops of proparacaine 0.5% in the syringe when initially irrigating. It is important to complete the procedure with 0.1 to 0.2 mL of an ophthalmic antibiotic solution within the syringe, after good lacrimal flow is established.[11-13]

*When cleaning and disinfecting the cannula after completion of the procedure, a 3- to 5-mL syringe and rolled alcohol prep pad can be used to prevent future blockage of the cannula lumen from*

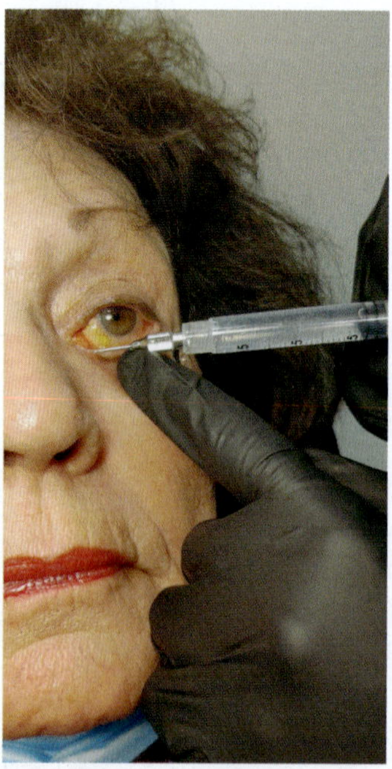

**FIGURE 33-15** Depress plunger and inject saline through the lacrimal system.

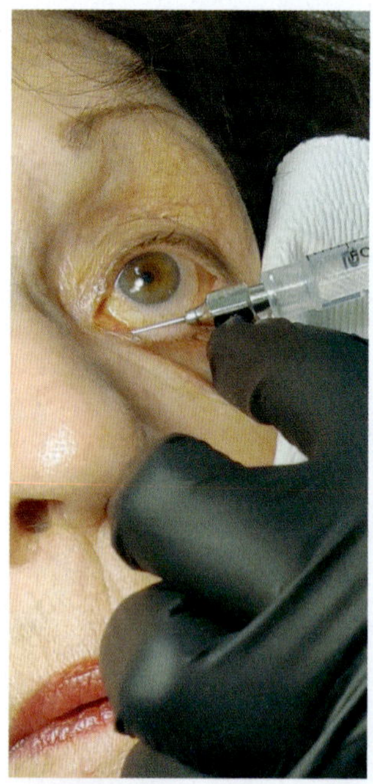

**FIGURE 33-16** Note the fluid regurgitation from the superior puncta, which can be indicative of a proximal blockage.

*any residual evaporated BSS. Roll the pad and place it into the syringe with the cannula attached. Attach the plunger and forcefully push out all alcohol from the pad through the cannula. The cannula can be left to air-dry afterward or autoclaved, if an autoclave is available.*

## POSTOPERATIVE CARE (FOLLOW-UP SCHEDULE)

If the procedure is successful and the system is determined to be patent, no follow-up is usually necessary. However, if no fluid is tasted in the nasopharynx by the patient, the patient should be referred for a lacrimal consult.[5]

The procedure should be detailed in the chart along with the results—whether there was regurgitation from the puncta, blockage that could not be opened, or the system was patent. A comment should be included to acknowledge that the patient tolerated the procedure well and left in no discomfort.

Patients should note improvement in epiphora soon after having a successful irrigation. Prior to leaving, they should be instructed to return to the clinic if swelling, pain, or other symptoms arise. Although not required, some practitioners may consider having the patient return in 1 to 2 weeks after the procedure to confirm that the lacrimal system has remained patent.

## POTENTIAL COMPLICATIONS AND THEIR TREATMENT

### Key Complications

- Discomfort
- Swelling
- Redness
- Pain
- Infection
- Bleeding

As with any procedure, it is possible for the procedure to be ineffective. As described, an NLDO can be significant enough that D&I cannot create patency. In these cases, an oculoplastic referral is warranted.

The most common complication will be discomfort if the anatomy of the lacrimal system isn't respected.[6] If the dilator or cannula is forced forward, the patient may note pain. If any inflammation is present prior to the procedure, the area will already be tender to begin with.[5] The procedure should be performed gently to minimize risks of discomfort or even bleeding secondary to piercing of tissue from the dilator or cannula.

At the end of the procedure, an ophthalmic antibiotic can be used in the syringe to flush the NLD once good flow is established. If swelling or pain become present postprocedure, consider placing the patient on an oral antibiotic and using cool compresses for any accompanying inflammation.

## VIDEOS OF PROCEDURES

**Video 33-1**—Lacrimal dilation and irrigation. Proparacaine 0.5% soaked cotton-tipped applicator held to puncta for local tissue anesthesia. Dilator advanced into puncta 2 mm vertically before rotating to horizontal orientation for another 4 to 6 mm. Quickly switch to syringe/cannula and follow same pathway to respect lacrimal system anatomy. Inject saline into the system to remove blockages. (Video courtesy of Bibin Cherian.)

**Video 33-2**—Lacrimal dilation and irrigation. Different technique using 4% lidocaine soaked soft cell surgical sponge to anesthetize puncta. Lacrimal dilator used to aggressively dilate. Note whitening of tissue around puncta indicating expansion. Curved lacrimal cannula on syringe used to irrigate puncta. Observe mucus plug that regurgitates. (Video courtesy of Richard Castillo.)

**Video 33-3**—Lacrimal dilation and irrigation. Epiphora differential diagnoses reviewed. Proparacaine 0.5% soaked cotton-tipped applicator held to puncta for local tissue anesthesia. Dilator advanced into puncta. Note gentle rotation while advancing dilator. Immediately introduce cannula/syringe after proper puncta dilation. Inject saline into the system to remove blockages. (Video courtesy of Nathan Lighthizer.)

# EFFICACY

Only a few studies in the literature have investigated the etiology of epiphora. One of the first studies was by Mainville and Jordan, which showed NLDO was the culprit in close to 50% of patients with epiphora. Dry eye reflex tearing came in second at 40%.[14] Other studies showed similar findings with stenosis, NLDO, or ocular surface disease being the leading contributors.[1] Effectiveness of D&I can vary depending on whether the etiology was correctly determined to be because of an NLDO and the size of the obstruction.

# BILLING/CODING AND MODIFIERS

To be reimbursed for the procedure, it is important to include the patient's symptoms, reasoning for D&I, how it was performed, and the result in the chart. Also, document how the patient tolerated the procedure and if or when a follow-up can be expected.[12]

- **CPT code: 68801**—Dilation of lacrimal punctum, with or without irrigation
- **CPT code: 68840**—Probing of lacrimal canaliculi, with or without irrigation

Other related CPT codes include:

- ***CPT code: 68810***—*Probing of NLD, with or without irrigation*
- ***CPT code: 68811***—*Probing of NLD, with or without irrigation; requiring general anesthesia*
- **CPT 68810/68811** are primarily pediatric procedures and rarely necessary for adults. CPT 68840 is more commonly performed in an adult population. Unusually frequent billing of 68810 may trigger a review as per the Centers for Medicare and Medicaid Services.

*Reimbursement will only be made for one of these CPT codes performed on the same day. For instance, no additional reimbursement will be made if attempting to bill both 68801 and 68840.*[15]

As per the Centers for Medicare and Medicaid Services guidelines, a few codes can be used when billing the procedure. It is the responsibility of the provider to code the highest level specified. This list isn't exhaustive but some of the relevant ICD-10-CM codes that may be used:

- **H04.20x** (unspecified epiphora)
- **H04.22x** (epiphora because of insufficient drainage)
- **H04.54x** (stenosis of lacrimal canaliculi)
- **H04.55x** (acquired stenosis of NLD)
- **H04.56x** (stenosis of lacrimal punctum)

Codes that ***cannot*** be used and will be denied:

- **H04.21x** (epiphora because of excess lacrimation)

The procedure does have a 10-day global period and ***cannot*** be billed with an evaluation and management (E&M) code on the same day unless a separate identifiable service is documented and provided. A −25 modifier would need to be attached to the E&M code if so.

The CPT code is a unilateral code and a modifier must be used for the site (LT, RT, −50). Only one of these modifiers can be billed on a claim line. A −50 modifier must be used for bilateral services rather than the RT/LT modifiers.

## REFERENCES


1. Ulusoy MO, KJvanç SA, Atakan M, et al. How important is the etiology in the treatment of epiphora? *J Ophthalmol.* 2016;2016:1-6. doi:10.1155/2016/1438376
2. Malvezzi L, Pirola F. The application of the exoscope in lacrimal surgery. In: De Virgilio A, Spriano G, eds. *Exoscope-Assisted Surgery in Otorhinolaryngology.* 1st ed. Elsevier; 2022:97-107. doi:10.1016/b978-0-323-83168-0.00010-0
3. Salmon JF. Lacrimal drainage system. In: Salmon SF, ed. *Kanski's Clinical Ophthalmology: A Systematic Approach.* 9th ed. Elsevier; 2020:99-111.
4. Schaefer JL, Zalzal H, Nguyen J, et al. Endoscopic management of pediatric nasolacrimal obstruction. In: Sindwani R, ed. *Endoscopic Surgery of the Orbit.* 1st ed. Elsevier; 2021:113-117. doi:10.1016/b978-0-323-61329-3.00016-0
5. Hurwitz JJ. The lacrimal drainage system. In: Yanoff M, Duker JS, eds. *Ophthalmology.* 5th ed. Elsevier; 2019:1338-1343. doi:10.1016/b978-0-323-04332-8.00244-4
6. Prokopich CL, Hrynchak P, Flanagan JG, et al. Ocular health assessment. In: Elliot DB, ed. *Clinical Procedures in Primary Eye Care.* 5th ed. 2021:215-225.
7. Soiberman U, Kakizaki H, Selva D, et al. Punctal stenosis: definition, diagnosis, and treatment. *Clin Ophthalmol,*2012; 2012:1011-1018. doi:10.2147/opth.s31904
8. Repka MX, Melia BM, Beck RW, et al. Primary treatment of nasolacrimal duct obstruction with nasolacrimal duct intubation in children less than 4 years old. *J AAPOS.* 2008;12(5):445-450. doi:10.1016/j.jaapos.2008.03.005
9. Remington LA. Ocular adnexa and lacrimal system. In: Remington LA, ed. *Clinical Anatomy and Physiology of the Visual System.* 3rd ed. Elsevier; 2012:159-181. doi:10.1016/b978-1-4377-1926-0.10009-8.
10. Bagheri N, Wajda B, Calvo C, et al. Technique for diagnostic probing and irrigation of the lacrimal system. In: Bagheri N, Wajda D, eds. *The Wills Eye Manual.* 7th ed. Lippincott Williams and Wilkins; 2016:415-416.
11. Jensen PS. Learn how to irrigate the lacrimal system. *Rev Optom.* Published April 4, 2011. Accessed September 28, 2022. https://www.reviewofoptometry.com/article/learn-how-to-irrigate-the-lacrimal-system
12. Provence-Perry M, Smith A, Lighthizer N. How to make your patients stop crying. *Rev Optom.* Published March 15, 2015. Accessed September 28, 2022. https://www.reviewofoptometry.com/article/how-to-make-your-patients-stop-crying
13. Stein HA, Stein RM, Freeman MI, et al. Aseptic technique and minor office surgery. In: Stein HA, Stein RM, Freeman MI, et al, eds. *The Ophthalmic Assistant.* 11th ed. Elsevier; 2023:532-545.
14. Mainville N, Jordan DR. Etiology of tearing: a retrospective analysis of referrals to a tertiary care oculoplastics practice. *Ophthalmic Plast Reconstr Surg.* 2011;27(3):155-157.
15. Centers for Medicare & Medicaid Services. Billing and coding: nasal punctum-nasolacrimal duct dilation and probing with or without irrigation. Updated June 2, 2022. Accessed October 3, 2022. https://www.cms.gov/medicare-coverage-database/view/article.aspx?articleId=57284&ver=6

# 34 Punctal Plug Insertion

**Neal Whittle**

## BACKGROUND

There are times when it is advantageous to mechanically occlude the tear drainage system of the eye. Intentional, permanent punctal occlusion procedures can include surgery, laser cautery, or radiofrequency coagulation.[1] However, the most common method of punctal occlusion is by the use of punctal plugs or intracanalicular plugs. Punctal plugs (and intracanalicular plugs) are small medical implants designed to block the lacrimal drainage system (Figure 34-1). In doing so, the tears produced by the lacrimal system are preserved on the surface of the eye.

The first dumbbell-shaped punctal plug was developed in 1975, and punctal plugs of similar design have been used in clinical practice ever since.[2] Over the years, many other punctal and intracanalicular plugs have been developed with different shapes, sizes, durations, and materials (Figure 34-2). The most common punctal plugs in use today are the collagen intracanalicular plug and the silicone permanent punctal plug.

### Intracanalicular Plugs

Intracanalicular plugs occlude the canaliculus of the lacrimal system (see Figure 34-1f and 34-1c). Because they are placed inside the canaliculus, they cannot be seen after they are inserted.

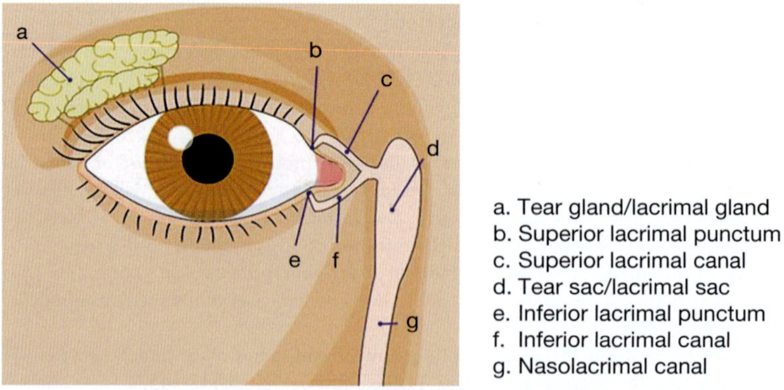


**FIGURE 34-1** Lacrimal system. (Shared by FML and Erin_Silversmith under the Creative Commons Attribution-Share Alike 4.0 International license.)

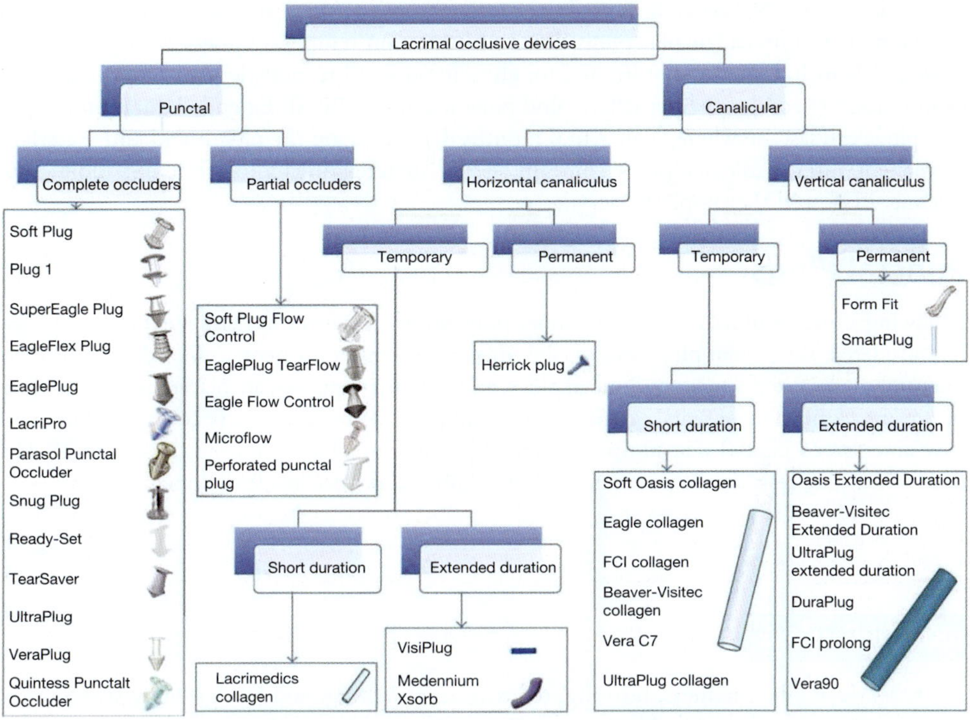


**FIGURE 34-2** Punctal and intracanalicular plugs come in a variety of shapes, functions, materials, and durations. (Figure courtesy of Jehangir et al.[3] under the Creative Commons Attribution License.)

Collagen plugs are temporary intracanalicular plugs that are used diagnostically to determine if lacrimal occlusion would be beneficial (Figure 34-3). Once inserted, collagen plugs will enlarge and gelatinize following hydration by tears, blocking the lacrimal canal. Collagen plugs typically dissolve anywhere from 4 days to 2 weeks.[3]

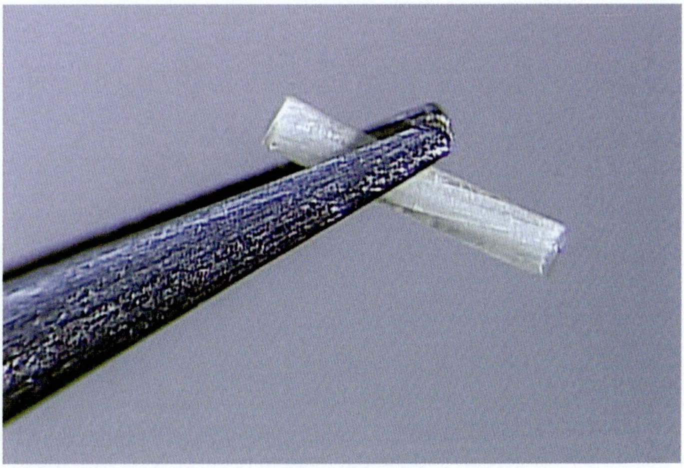

**FIGURE 34-3** Temporary collagen intracanalicular plug.

In addition to the relatively short-lasting collagen plugs, there are also extended duration and permanent intracanalicular plugs. Extended duration temporary plugs come in a variety of materials including, but not limited to, glycolic acid and trimethylene carbonate, epsilon-caprolactone-L-lactide polymer (PCL), and polydioxanone (PDS). Extended duration temporary plugs can last anywhere from 2 to 6 months depending on the plug brand and material.[3] Permanent intracanalicular plugs come in several materials including, but not limited to, silicone, PDS, and thermoplastic acrylic.

## Punctal Plugs

Following a successful trial with a temporary plug, semi-permanent or permanent occlusion can be considered. Permanent plugs are actually considered semi-permanent, as they do not dissolve, but can be removed if necessary. Punctal plugs, as their name suggests, are placed inside the punctum to block outflow of tears. Permanent punctal plugs come in a variety of shapes, but most have an enlarged parasol shaped tip connected by a shaft to a flattened head (Figure 34-4). The head of the plug rests on the punctum with the shaft and parasol inside the canal.

# INDICATIONS

**Key Indications**

- Dry eye relief: redness, burning, reflex tearing, itching, and foreign body sensations that can be relieved by blockage of the punctum or canaliculus
- Increased drug retention time
- Refractive surgery prophylaxis or following refractive surgery to treat postsurgery dryness
- Perforated plugs for punctal stenosis to treat epiphora

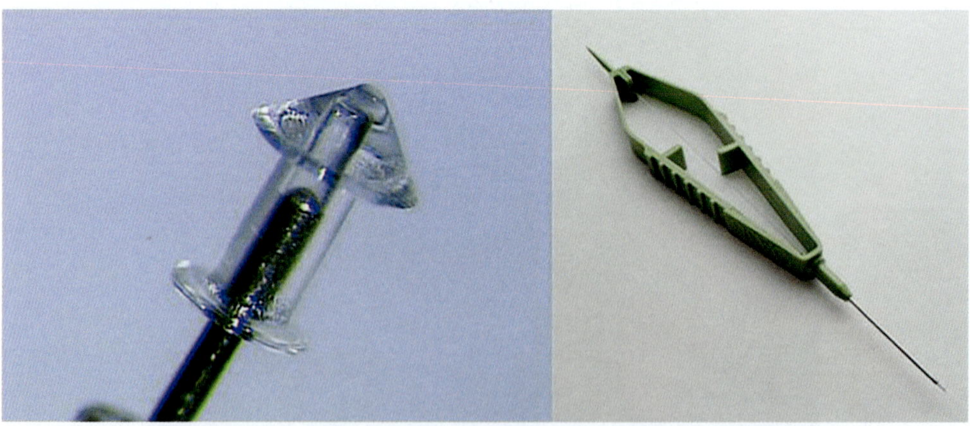

**FIGURE 34-4** (Left) Silicone punctal plug on the end of its included applicator. Note the parasol shape that will be placed into the canaliculus and the flat head that will be level with the punctum opening. (Right) Wide shot of punctal plug applicator. Note the plug on one end and a dilator on the other end.

The most common reason for punctal occlusion and the reason punctal plugs were developed was for the treatment of dry eye.[2] Dry eye has several known causes including, but not limited to, tear evaporation, reduced tear production, inflammation, injury, refractive surgery, and even topical and oral medications. In addition to artificial tears, anti-inflammatory drops, autologous serum, and amniotic membranes, punctal plugs can be an important part of a physician's toolkit to address their patient's dry eye signs and symptoms.

Punctal occlusion might also be used to preserve topical medications on the eye to increase the drug's retention time, such as an intraocular pressure–lowering drop used in the treatment of glaucoma.[4] One of the potential side effects of laser-assisted in situ keratomileusis (LASIK) is dry eye, and punctal plugs can be used prophylactically to minimize the need for continuous lubrication following the procedure.[5] In some cases, punctal plugs can even be used to *increase* tear flow. Patients with epiphora secondary to punctal stenosis can have special perforated punctal plugs inserted. These perforated punctal plugs act like a shunt to allow excess tears to drain from the eye.[6,7]

# CONTRAINDICATIONS

### Key Contraindications

- Inflammation of the eyelid
- Dacryocystitis
- Mucopurulent discharge
- Inflammatory dry eye
- Allergy to materials

Punctal plugs are contraindicated if there is active inflammation or infection present in the lacrimal system or on the ocular surface.[8,9] Any dacryocystitis must be cleared up prior to punctal plug installation to avoid worsening the infection. Likewise, any severe inflammation of the ocular surface or eyelids (e.g., blepharitis) should be treated before punctal plugs are inserted. If punctal plugs are inserted before the inflammation is reduced or resolved, pro-inflammatory cytokines can be retained on the eye, potentially exacerbating the inflammation.[10] If a patient has an allergy or sensitivity to the material of the punctal plug being considered (e.g., silicone, collagen, or any other plug material), a different plug with a different material should be chosen. In particular, collagen plugs can have complications in patients with allergies to bovine collagen, with up to 3% of the population having an allergy or sensitivity to bovine collagen.[11] Allergies to silicone, especially medical grade silicone, are considered to be extremely rare.[12]

# PROCEDURE

Prior to inserting a punctal plug or intracanalicular plug, the patient should sign an informed consent form containing a plain-words description of the procedure, its indications, contraindications, alternative treatments, risks, and potential complications. A note from the

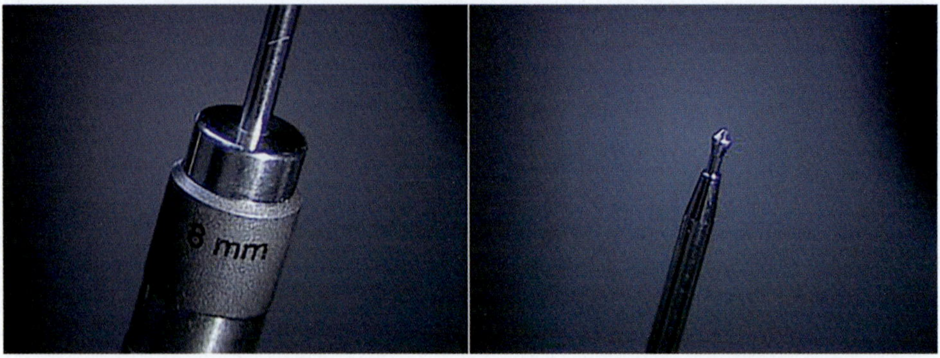


**FIGURE 34-5** Punctum sizer showing the labeled size (left) and the head of the sizer (right).

counseling physician should be included and phrased similar to: "I have counseled this patient as to the nature of the proposed procedure, the attendant risks involved, and the expected results." The patient's and doctor's name should be printed and signed with the date, as well as a witness (typically a staff member).

For both intracanalicular and punctal plug installation, the patient should be instructed to look away from the punctum to avoid scratching the cornea. For example, if occluding the lower punctum, the patient should look up and temporally. The punctum can be anesthetized with either a drop of topical anesthetic or an anesthetic-soaked cotton-tipped applicator (CTA) held to the punctum for 30 seconds.

The appropriate size plug to be used should be determined by using a punctal plug sizing gauge (Figure 34-5). Following installation of anesthetic, insert the head of the sizer into the punctum. There should be slight resistance. If there is no resistance, go up a size. If the tip is too difficult to insert, go down a size. If there is a snug fit with moderate resistance to insertion, that indicates the correct size. The puncta of both eyes should be sized, as the left and right eyes may have different sized puncta.

## COLLAGEN INTRACANALICULAR PLUG PROCEDURE[13]

### Required Instruments

- Collagen plugs
- Sterilized jeweler's forceps
- Slit lamp
- Punctal dilator (optional)
- CTA (optional)
- Topical anesthetic drops (optional)

1. Inspect the punctum to determine size by visual inspection or using a punctal gauge.
2. If necessary, anesthetize with topical anesthetic in the conjunctival sac or an anesthetic-soaked CTA for 30 seconds.
3. If necessary, dilate the punctum with a punctal dilator.

4. Remove the plug from the holder with jewelers' forceps.
5. Insert the plug part-way through the punctal opening while grasping the top half of the plug with the forceps. Release the plug and use the tip of the forceps to push the plug the rest of the way through the punctal opening and into the canaliculus.
6. Repeat the procedure on the upper punctum if desired.
7. Follow up with the patient in 1 to 2 weeks to see if symptoms have improved after plug insertion.

# SILICONE PUNCTAL PLUG PROCEDURE[14]

## Required Instruments

- Silicone plugs
- Punctal size gauge
- Plug inserter and dilator (often included with plug)
- Slit lamp
- CTA
- Topical anesthetic drops

1. Anesthetize with topical anesthetic in the conjunctival sac or an anesthetic-soaked CTA for 30 seconds.
2. Determine plug size with the sizers:
   - Insert head of sizer (see Figure 34-5) into punctum. There should be slight resistance. If there is no resistance, go up a size. If the tip is too difficult to insert, go down a size. If there is a snug fit with moderate resistance to insertion, that indicates the correct size. Both eyes should be sized, as the left and right eyes may have different sized puncta.
3. Dilate:
   - Many companies provide a disposable inserter that comes with a dilator on the other end (see Figure 34-4).
   - Gently dilate the punctum and quickly insert the silicone plug. Insertion must be done within 15 to 30 seconds or the punctum may narrow again, requiring the dilation to be repeated.
4. Insertion:
   - Insert the plug into the punctum until the head of the plug is flush with the punctal opening.
   - The physician's hands should be positioned to squeeze the applicator.
   - When the plug is properly inserted, squeeze and withdraw the inserter to release the plug.
   - Verify that the plug is properly placed. The head of the plug should be resting snugly against the eyelid margin.
   - The tip of the inserter can be used to gently tap the plug down to get it into the proper location if the head of the plug is not flush with the eyelid margin.
5. Repeat the procedure on the upper punctum if desired.
6. Follow up with the patient in 1 to 2 weeks to see if symptoms have improved after permanent plug insertion, to make sure the plug is still retained and to check for any potential adverse events or complications.

# POTENTIAL COMPLICATIONS

## Key Potential Complications

- Intracanalicular plugs
  - Allergy
  - Granuloma formation
  - Scarring
  - Infection
  - Canalicular stenosis
  - Migration
  - Difficult removal
  - Epiphora
- Punctal plugs
  - Extrusion (plug falling out)
  - Granuloma formation
  - Scarring
  - Infection
  - Foreign body sensation
  - Corneal abrasion or ulceration
  - Epiphora
  - Allergy (very rare)

Although punctal plugs and intracanalicular plugs are considered very safe, there are still occasional complications that can occur. Punctal plugs and intracanalicular plugs share several complications, such as granulation tissue (new tissue growth caused by inflammation), pyogenic granuloma formation, epiphora, and infection.[3] Infections can be caused by fungi or bacteria. Dacryocystitis is possible for both plugs. As stated in the Contraindications section, an allergy to the plug material (such as collagen) can cause an allergic reaction that would necessitate plug removal. Chronic irritation caused by the plug can also cause scarring and granuloma formation. Pyogenic granulomas can even push the punctal plug partially out of the punctum. Scar tissue can result in stenosis of the punctum and canaliculus leading to epiphora. It is also possible to damage or even perforate the punctum or canaliculus during installation of the plug. This can cause pain, increased risk of infection, and the possibility that the plug will fall out. In the event of a perforation, placement of the plug should be delayed until the punctum or canaliculus fully heals.

One of the most common potential complications involving punctal plugs is foreign body sensation. Patients will often adjust to this sensation after a few days, similar to a first-time contact lens wearer. Punctal plugs have a unique complication in which they can be partially or fully extruded from the punctum (i.e., they fall out). Extrusion is usually a sign that the punctal plug is the wrong size.[15] If the plug is partially extruded, it can rub on the cornea or conjunctiva, leading to noticeable foreign body sensation, tearing, abrasions, and possibly a corneal ulcer. A partially extruded plug should be removed and the punctum should be rechecked for size.

Intracanalicular plugs can migrate from their original position, possibly resulting in discomfort, infection, and the need for removal with irrigation or surgical removal.

### Removal

If the need arises, permanent punctal plugs are relatively easy to remove. Remove the plug by grasping the shaft of the plug *below* the head with forceps and pull the plug from the punctal opening.

Intracanalicular plugs have an advantage over punctal plugs in that they are typically less irritating to the patient because they sit inside the canaliculus. However, intracanalicular plugs are more difficult to remove if a problem develops. If the intracanalicular plug is a temporary plug, often the doctor and patient will simply wait for the plug to dissolve (~2 weeks for collagen or up to 6 months for extended duration). Alternatively, the plug can be flushed from the canaliculus with dilation and irrigation. Permanent intracanalicular plugs can be much more complicated to remove. In most cases, the plug can be irrigated out, but if the plug gets lodged in the lacrimal canal or lacrimal sac, surgical intervention may be necessary in the form of dacryocystorhinostomy[16] or a canaliculotomy.[17]

### VIDEOS OF PROCEDURES

**Video 34-1**—Punctal sizing—When sizing a punctum, use a punctal gauge. There should be slight resistance when inserting the sizer. If there is no resistance, go up a size. If the tip is too difficult to insert, go down a size. If there is a snug fit with moderate resistance to insertion, that indicates the correct size.

**Video 34-2**—Collagen plug insertion—This video shows the required instruments and the basic process for inserting a temporary collagen plug. Once the size of the plug is determined, remove the plug from the foam holder using jeweler's forceps. Insert the plug using the forceps; using the tip, drive the plug into the canaliculus.

**Video 34-3**—Silicone plug insertion—This video shows the required instruments and the basic process for inserting a silicone punctal plug. Most plugs will come on an inserter with an included dilator. Once the size of the plug is determined, dilate the punctum. Turn the inserter around, an insert the plug until the head of the plug is flush with the punctal opening. Squeeze the sides of the inserter to release the plug.

## EFFICACY

Multiple clinical trials, studies, systematic studies, meta-analyses, and literature reviews have looked at the safety and efficacy of punctal plugs for the treatment of dry eye symptoms. Most studies show a high success rate, with most patients experiencing improvement of their symptoms compared to patients that did not receive punctal plugs.[8,9,18] One large meta-analysis study considered 18 trials (711 participants and 1,249 eyes) from various countries. Each of the trials concluded that punctal plugs were effective for treating dry eye signs and symptoms. However, the meta-analysis concluded that because of the number of types of punctal plugs, the differences in trial methodology, and the risk of bias in each study, they could not come to a solid conclusion as to whether punctal plugs are truly helpful or not.[19]

Regardless, punctal plugs have been shown to be safe and effective in other individual studies; so the reader may rely on them or on their own experiences with punctal plugs to make the best decision for their patients.

Punctal plug extrusion appears to be the most common complication listed across the board in most safety and efficacy studies, with one study showing a retention rate of 49.4% with 85.1 ± 7.3 weeks as the mean survival time.[8] Other reported mild complications included epiphora and irritation. Serious complications such as dacryocystitis and canaliculitis are infrequent.[9]

# CODING/BILLING

## Key Coding/Billing Information

- **CPT code: 68761**—"The closure of the lacrimal punctum, by plug, each."
- Location modifiers:
  - E1—Left upper lid
  - E2—Left lower lid
  - E3—Right upper lid
  - E4—Right lower lid
- 10-day global period

The installation of punctal plugs is considered to be a minor surgical procedure by Medicare, Medicaid, and other private insurance carriers. CPT code 68761 describes "the closure of the lacrimal punctum, by plug, each." Because the code is only describing a single punctum, it will need to be specified which punctum was occluded with the following modifiers: E1—left upper lid; E2—left lower lid; E3—right upper lid; and E4—right lower lid.[20] For example, if only the lower puncta were occluded, modifiers E2 and E4 would be used. Some private insurance carriers will not accept the E1–E4 modifiers, but they will accept RT indicating the right eye and LT indicating the left, with a -50 modifier for bilateral occlusion. In this case, bilateral occlusion would be coded as 68761-50. When billing a procedure code, ensure that the ICD-10 diagnosis codes match the eye that is treated. For example, if it is coded that the patient only has dry eye in one eye, payment for bilateral treatment may be denied. Prophylactic punctal plugs inserted prior to LASIK are considered to be ineligible for reimbursement. However, patients that develop dry eye symptoms following LASIK may be covered.[21]

Because punctal plug insertion is considered a minor surgical procedure, billing for an examination on the same day as the procedure is not allowable, unless there is a separate and identifiable reason for the visit. For example, if a patient being monitored for hydroxychloroquine toxicity also has signs of Sjögren's disease, punctal plugs could be inserted at that visit with the use of a -25 modifier on the visit code. In that example, the patient came in for a hydroxychloroquine eye examination, but was identified as also needing punctal plugs for a separate but identifiable condition. However, if the patient is specifically coming in for dry eye symptoms and is interested in punctal plugs, only the 68761 procedure code will be able to be billed, as that code includes the visit on the day of the procedure as well as any related visits in the global period. CPT 68761 has a 10-day global period.[22]

Most punctal plugs are placed in private offices, but in the rare event that the procedure takes place in an Ambulatory Surgery Center (ASC) or a Hospital-Based Outpatient Department (HOPD), there is the possibility of collecting a facility fee using the Ambulatory Payment Classification (APC) code 5501.

In the event that intracanalicular plugs must be removed, billing for the dilation and irrigation of the lacrimal system using CPT codes 68801 (dilation of lacrimal punctum, with or without irrigation) or 68840 (probing of lacrimal canaliculi, with or without irrigation) is possible. Similar to 68761, 68801 and 68840 are unilateral codes and therefore should have a modifier for the eye irrigated (RT, LT, or –50).[23]

Common ICD-10 codes that support medical necessity for CPT code 68761 (the closure of the lacrimal punctum, by plug, each) include[21]:

- **H04.12** (dry eye syndrome)
- **H16.22** (keratoconjunctivitis sicca)
- **H16.14** (punctate keratitis)
- **H16.20** (keratoconjunctivitis, unspecified)
- **M35.0** (keratoconjunctivitis sicca with Sjögren's syndrome)

## REFERENCES


1. Yaguchi S, Ogawa Y, Kamoi M, et al. Surgical management of lacrimal punctal cauterization in chronic GVHD-related dry eye with recurrent punctal plug extrusion. *Bone Marrow Transplant.* 2012;47(11):1465-1469. doi:10.1038/bmt.2012.50
2. Freeman JM. The punctum plug: evaluation of a new treatment for the dry eye. *Trans Sect Ophthalmol Am Acad Ophthalmol Otolaryngol.* 1975;79(6):OP874-OP879.
3. Jehangir N, Bever G, Mahmood SM, Moshirfar M. Comprehensive review of the literature on existing punctal plugs for the management of dry eye disease. *J Ophthalmol.* 2016;2016:9312340. doi:10.1155/2016/9312340
4. Chen M, Yung Choi S. Preliminary outcomes of temporary collagen punctal plugs for patients with dry eye and glaucoma. *Med Hypothesis Discov Innov Ophthalmol.* 2020;9(1):56-60.
5. Yung YH, Toda I, Sakai C, Yoshida A, Tsubota K. Punctal plugs for treatment of post-LASIK dry eye. *Jpn J Ophthalmol.* 2012;56(3):208-213. doi:10.1007/s10384-012-0125-8
6. Konuk O, Urgancioglu B, Unal M. Long-term success rate of perforated punctal plugs in the management of acquired punctal stenosis. *Ophthalmic Plast Reconstr Surg.* 2008;24(5):399-402. doi:10.1097/IOP.0b013e318185a9ca
7. Lipková B. Perforované zátky v liečbe stenózy slzných bodov [Perforated punctum plugs in treatment lacrimal punctal stenosis]. *Cesk Slov Oftalmol.* 2012;68(4):147-149.
8. Tai MC, Cosar CB, Cohen EJ, Rapuano CJ, Laibson PR. The clinical efficacy of silicone punctal plug therapy. *Cornea.* 2002;21(2):135-139. doi:10.1097/00003226-200203000-00001
9. Marcet MM, Shtein RM, Bradley EA, et al. Safety and efficacy of lacrimal drainage system plugs for dry eye syndrome: a report by the American Academy of Ophthalmology. *Ophthalmology.* 2015;122(8):1681-1687. doi:10.1016/j.ophtha.2015.04.034
10. Yen MT, Pflugfelder SC, Feuer WJ. The effect of punctal occlusion on tear production, tear clearance, and ocular surface sensation in normal subjects. *Am J Ophthalmol.* 2001;131(3):314-323. doi:10.1016/s0002-9394(00)00822-9

11. Mullins RJ, Richards C, Walker T. Allergic reactions to oral, surgical and topical bovine collagen. Anaphylactic risk for surgeons. *Aust N Z J Ophthalmol.* 1996;24(3):257-260. doi:10.1111/j.1442-9071.1996.tb01589.x
12. Prasad A, Reeder MJ. Allergic contact dermatitis to silicone in a continuous positive airway pressure mask. *Contact Dermatitis.* 2021;84(6):460-462. doi:10.1111/cod.13759
13. Oasis. SOFT PLUG Collagen Intracanalicular Plug instructions for use. Published April, 2019. Accessed October 7, 2022. https://www.oasismedical.com/docs/default-source/resources/softplugcollagenplug-ifu.pdf?sfvrsn=163ac1b4_9
14. Oasis. SOFT PLUG Silicone Punctum Plug instructions for use. Published May 2019. Accessed October 7, 2022. https://www.oasismedical.com/docs/default-source/resources/softplugsiliconeplug-ifu.pdf?sfvrsn=3e34c1b4_36
15. Gillogly A, Stout N, Lighthizer N. Plug the drain with lacrimal occlusion. *Rev Optom.* Published June 15, 2016. Accessed October 5, 2022. https://www.reviewofoptometry.com/article/plug-the-drain-with-lacrimal-occlusion
16. White WL, Bartley GB, Hawes MJ, Linberg JV, Leventer DB. Iatrogenic complications related to the use of Herrick Lacrimal Plugs. *Ophthalmology.* 2001;108(10):1835-1837. doi:10.1016/s0161-6420(01)00718-7
17. Hill RH 3rd, Norton SW, Bersani TA. Prevalence of canaliculitis requiring removal of SmartPlugs. *Ophthalmic Plast Reconstr Surg.* 2009;25(6):437-439. doi:10.1097/IOP.0b013e3181b80d63
18. Nava-Castaneda A, Tovilla-Canales JL, Rodriguez L, Tovilla Y Pomar JL, Jones CE. Effects of lacrimal occlusion with collagen and silicone plugs on patients with conjunctivitis associated with dry eye. *Cornea.* 2003;22(1):10-14. doi:10.1097/00003226-200301000-00003
19. Ervin AM, Law A, Pucker AD. Punctal occlusion for dry eye syndrome. *Cochrane Database Syst Rev.* 2017;6(6):CD006775. doi:10.1002/14651858.CD006775.pub3
20. NC Medicaid Division of Health Benefits. Closure of tear duct using plug; CPT Code 68761: billing guidelines. Accessed October 7, 2022. https://medicaid.ncdhhs.gov/blog/2022/01/18/closure-tear-duct-using-plug-cpt-code-68761-billing-guidelines
21. Corcoran Consulting Group. Reimbursement guidelines for punctal or intracanalicular occlusion by plug. Accessed October 7, 2022. https://www.oasismedical.com/docs/default-source/resources/corcoran_plugs-oasis.pdf?sfvrsn=16
22. Corcoran Consulting Group. Medicare reimbursement: punctal occlusion by punctal plug. OASIS. FAQ. Accessed October 7, 2022. https://www.corcoranccg.com/products/faqs/punctal-occlusion-oasis/
23. Centers for Medicare & Medicaid Services. Billing and coding: nasal punctum-nasolacrimal duct dilation and probing with or without irrigation. Accessed October 7, 2022. https://www.cms.gov/medicare-coverage-database/view/article.aspx?articleid=57284&ver=7&

# 35 Thermal Punctoplasty for Involutional Punctal Eversion

**Richard E. Castillo**

Acquired punctal eversion occurs because of the external rotation of the lower medial eyelid margin away from the globe. Although eversion of the punctum may present as a single clinical entity, it is also recognized as one of the earliest signs of ectropion.[1,2] Accompanying signs include epiphora, an increase in the lacrimal lake or lower tear meniscus, and exposure of the palpebral conjunctiva.[1-5] Symptoms reported include redness, irritation, and discharge.[4] This process can eventually lead to ectropion of the lower eyelid with complete keratinization of the palpebral conjunctiva.[3,4]

## INDICATIONS

**Key Indications**

- Involutional or age-related punctal eversion

Evaluation of punctal eversion should focus on etiology. Punctal eversion can result from one or a combination of four primary mechanisms:

1. Involutional[1-4,7]
    a. Horizontal lid laxity
    b. Lamellar disassociation
    c. Disinsertion of the retractors of the lower lid
2. Cicatricial because of shortening or the anterior lamellae[1-4,7]
    a. Trauma including prior surgery
    b. Burns
    c. Autoimmune disease
    d. Chronic inflammation
3. Paralytic [6,8]
    a. Facial nerve palsy—although classically described as a medial or early ectropion, now considered a retraction because of the unopposed action of the retractors of the lower lid.
4. Mechanical causes secondary to a lid mass[4]

The most common cause of punctal eversion is involutional, or age-related, often manifesting as an early sign of involutional ectropion of the lower lid. Involutional ectropion is known to result from horizontal lid laxity, disinsertion, or attenuation of the retractors of the lower lid with combined gravitational pull.[4,7-9]

Cicatricial shortening of the anterior lamellae of the lid is another common etiology behind punctal eversion. Cicatricial changes to the eyelid skin result from causes such as trauma, prior surgery, or chronic inflammatory skin disorders, including autoimmune disease. Chronic rubbing of the eyelid margin in attempts to wipe away tears can result in skin excoriation and cicatricial skin changes in the anterior lamellae leading to punctal eversion. Identifying the underlying etiology of the punctal eversion is critical so that a plan can be developed, which will lead to a successful long-term outcome.[3-5,7,9]

Thermal punctoplasty, performed in the office setting under local anesthesia, is appropriate for mild-to-moderate cases of involutional punctal eversion[2] without significant degrees of ectropion or altered lid biomechanics as evidenced by:

- Disinsertion or dehiscence of the retractors of the lower lid (a white line in the inferior fornix below the level of the tarsus)
- Abnormal snap-back test (inability of the lid to return to its normal position against the globe immediately after being pulled down and away)
- Positive lid distraction test (ability to pull the eyelid >6 mm away from the globe)[3-6]

## CONTRAINDICATIONS[1,3-6,8]

### Key Relative Contraindications

- Lack of patient consent
- Inexperienced practitioner
- Moderate-to-severe ectropion
- Cicatricial ectropion
- Mechanical ectropion because of lid mass

## PREOPERATIVE PREPARATION

- Signed informed consent is obtained and witnessed.
- The preoperative note is documented:
  - Diagnosis is confirmed (e.g., *chronic epiphora secondary to punctal eversion*), including operative site.
  - Allergies and current medications are documented.
  - Proposed procedure: *Thermal punctoplasty inferior puncta (state eye).*
  - Anesthesia given is recorded (e.g., methylcellulose sponge soaked in topical 4% lidocaine held over the palpebral conjunctiva below the involved punctum for 1 minute, combined with *a subconjunctival injection below the level of the tarsus comprised of 0.2 mL of lidocaine 1% or 2% with epinephrine 1:100,000*).

- The operative site is prepared in standard fashion with 5% ophthalmic povidone–iodine (or alternative in the case of iodine allergy).
- A "time-out" is called before starting the procedure whereby patient identity, diagnosis, procedure, and operative site are confirmed by all present.

## Instrument Tray

- Topical anesthetic agent (e.g., 4% lidocaine)
- Ophthalmic sponge spears
- Subconjunctival anesthetic agent (1% or 2% lidocaine with epinephrine 1:100,000)[‡]
- One milliliter sterile syringe
- Half-inch 27- or 30-gauge hypodermic needle
- Five percent ophthalmic povidone–iodine solution
- Bipolar cautery forceps (McPherson-style recommended, Figure 35-1)
    - Angled, insulated shafts with 0.4-mm wide nonstick tips. Flat handle. Overall length: 95 mm
- Bipolar cautery device
- Ophthalmic antibiotic ointment (e.g., erythromycin)

[‡]Consider contraindications to any exogenous agents administered.

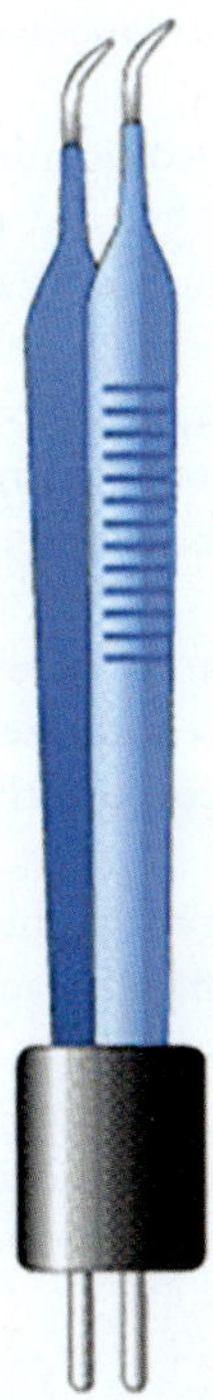

FIGURE 35-1 McPherson-style bipolar forceps.

# PROCEDURE

## Thermal Punctoplasty

Thermal punctoplasty uses a bipolar cautery forceps to cauterize and constrict the palpebral conjunctiva below the border of the involved punctum, functionally shortening the posterior lamellae of the eyelid and causing the punctum to roll backward into the lacrimal lake, it's proper position.[2,4,5] The procedure can be comfortably performed in the office setting with the patient either supine on an examination table or in an examination chair tilted backward to allow the practitioner to be comfortably positioned at the head. Good lighting and proper magnification (loops or operating microscope) allow for adequate visualization. The steps for performing the procedure are as follows:

1. Comfortably position the patient in the supine position.
2. Instill one drop of a topical ophthalmic anesthetic and place an ophthalmic sponge spear soaked in 4% lidocaine over the palpebral conjunctiva directly below the involved punctum for 1 minute.
3. Deliver a subconjunctival injection of approximately 0.2 mL of lidocaine 1% or 2% (with epinephrine 1:100,000, unless contraindicated) into the area directly below the tarsal plate below the involved punctum. Do not overdistend the conjunctiva with anesthetic solution. Close the eye and apply gentle massage over the area to achieve mechanical deturgescence of the infiltrated conjunctiva.
4. Instill one drop of 5% ophthalmic povidone–iodine solution into the inferior conjunctival fornix of the involved eye.
5. Set the bipolar unit to low-power coagulation mode. Verify the bipolar forceps are connected.
6. While everting the lower eyelid and exposing the medial palpebral conjunctiva with the fingers of the nondominant hand, use the bipolar forceps to grasp the conjunctiva immediately below the tarsal plate and place several conjunctival burns in line with the overlying punctal opening. The conjunctiva should at once constrict and turn white in response to the thermal cautery delivered by the bipolar forceps.
   **IMPORTANT NOTE:**
   **Grasp the conjunctiva immediately below the edge of the tarsus and no further down. *DO NOT* grab tissue and cauterize at or near the conjunctival fornix or inadvertently involve the bulbar conjunctiva as a cicatricial symblepharon could result.**
7. Release the eyelid and check the position of the punctum following each application.
8. Procedure is complete when punctum rolls back into normal position. Typically, three to five burns.
9. Hemostasis is rarely necessary. Where indicated, close the eyelid and hold pressure over the area with a 4 × 4 gauze until hemostasis is achieved.
10. Apply an ophthalmic antibiotic ointment to the inferior cul-de-sac.

## POSTOPERATIVE CARE (FOLLOW-UP SCHEDULE)[3,6,8-10]

**Key Postoperative Considerations**

- Topical antibiotic ointment BID for 5 days
- Over-the-counter pain medication as necessary
- Recall 2 to 3 weeks to assess healing

A successful procedure is confirmed on follow-up examination by resolution of the signs and symptoms (e.g., epiphora) and visualization of the punctum in its proper position, apposed to the globe in the lacrimal lake. Instruct the patient to apply an antibiotic ointment to the lateral inferior conjunctival site twice daily for five consecutive days.

## POTENTIAL COMPLICATIONS AND THEIR TREATMENT[3,9,10]

- Failure to achieve proper punctal positioning
- Recurrence of punctal eversion and symptoms
- Infection
  - Prescribing an antibiotic ointment for up to 5 days post-procedure should reduce the risk of infection.
- Cicatricial symblepharon or shortening of the conjunctival fornixes, especially if the cauterization is performed at or near the conjunctival fornix or inadvertently involves the bulbar conjunctiva.
- Pain and discomfort
  - Transient pain secondary to needle trauma and infiltration of tissues with an anesthetic agent
  - Transient pain secondary to procedural trauma
- Transient vision blur
  - Secondary to use of antibiotic ointment

## EFFICACY

Clinical experience has found this procedure to be efficacious.

## CODING/BILLING

- **CPT code: 68705**—Correction of everted punctum, cautery

Common ICD-10 codes that support this procedure include the following:

- **H04.521** (eversion of the right lacrimal punctum)
- **H04.522** (eversion of the left lacrimal punctum)
- **H04.2** (epiphora)

# REFERENCES

1. Lin P, Kitaguchi Y, Mupas-Uy J, et al. Involutional lower eyelid entropion: causative factors and therapeutic management. *Int Ophthalmol.* 2019;39(8):1895-1907.
2. Jones BR. Cautery to cure epiphora from punctal eversion. *Trans Ophthalmol Soc U K.* 1962;82:505-509.
3. O'Donnell B. Age-related medial ectropion of the lower eyelid. *Aust N Z J Ophthalmol.* 1994;22(3):183-186.
4. American Academy of Ophthalmology. *Orbit, Eyelids, and Lacrimal System, Section 7. Basic and Clinical Science Course.* American Academy of Ophthalmology; 2009.
5. Lauer SA. Ectropion and entropion. *Am Acad Ophthalmol Focal Points.* 1994;12(10):1-12.
6. Damasceno RW, Osaki MH, Dantas PE, Belfort R Jr. Involutional ectropion and entropion: clinicopathologic correlation between horizontal eyelid laxity and eyelid extracellular matrix. *Ophthalmic Plast Reconstr Surg.* 2011;27(5):321-326.
7. Barnett BP, Akpek EK, Jun AS. Punctal eversion with silicone plug resulting in ocular surface trauma. *BMJ Case Rep.* 2020;13(5);e232152.
8. Shah-Desai S, Collin R. Role of the lower lid retractors in involutional ectropion repair. *Orbit.* 2001; 20(2): 81-86.
9. AlHarthi AS. Involutional ectropion: etiological factors and therapeutic management. *Int Ophthalmol.* 2023;43(3):1013-1026.
10. Korn EL, Glotzbach RK. Carbon dioxide laser repair of medial ectropion. *Ophthalmic Surg.* 1988;19(9): 653-657.

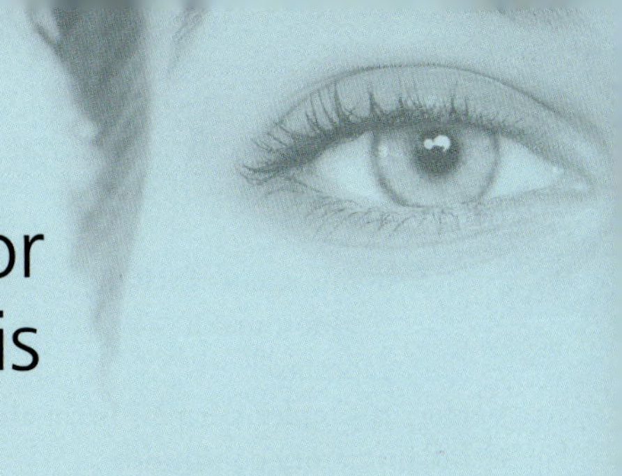

# 36 Three-Snip Punctoplasty for Punctal Stenosis

**Richard E. Castillo**

The three-snip punctoplasty is an office-based surgical procedure that involves the enlargement of the tear ducts' opening, located at the medial canthus of the eyelid, to improve tear drainage. The procedure is performed to correct a blocked or stenotic (narrowed) punctum, and the resulting epiphora, which causes excessive tearing.

Punctal stenosis is a narrowing with partial or complete occlusion of the eyelid's lacrimal punctum (puncta lacrimalia). Studies refer to the condition when the external punctal orifice measures less than 0.3 mm in diameter.[1] Epiphora is typically the presenting complaint.[1-4] Dilation and irrigation of the punctum and nasolacrimal system should be performed to evaluate the patency of the entire ipsilateral nasolacrimal system. Irrigation should also be performed to determine whether stenosis or occlusion distal to the stenotic punctum may contribute to or be primarily responsible for the symptomatology.[3,5,6]

The etiology of punctal stenosis may be multifactorial, ranging from congenital stenosis associated with such conditions as microphthalmos, which may be more appropriately recognized as punctal agenesis, to more common associations, including drug-induced stenosis and inflammatory conditions such as chronic blepharitis.[1,2,6-8] Known etiologies include:

- Chronic blepharitis
- Ectropion
- Drug-induced
  - Topical ophthalmic agents include:
    - Trifluridine
    - Vidarabine
    - Timolol
    - Latanoprost
    - Betaxolol
    - Dipivefrin hydrochloride
    - Echothiophate iodide
    - Pilocarpine

- Systemic agents include:
  - 5-Fluorouracil
  - Docetaxel
- Herpes simplex dermatitis/canaliculitis
- Inflammatory conditions
  - Ocular pemphigoid
  - Stevens–Johnson syndrome

Punctoplasty is employed for the surgical correction of punctal stenosis. Variations of the procedure include the one-snip, two-snip, and three-snip punctoplasty. The three-snip procedure has proven efficacy over the earlier one- or two-snip iterations, with less incidence of re-stenosis because of scarring following the procedure.[3,7-9]

## INDICATIONS

**Key Indications**

- Epiphora secondary to punctal stenosis
- Epiphora with multifactorial etiologies

The three-snip punctoplasty procedure is efficacious in managing epiphora secondary to punctal stenosis.

## CONTRAINDICATIONS

**Key Contraindications**

- Lack of patient consent
- Inexperienced practitioner
- Conditions mimicking punctal stenosis where excessive tearing is not secondary to punctal narrowing or closure
- Active infection

The procedure should not be performed if there is evidence of active infection, uncertainty as to whether or not punctal stenosis is the cause of the epiphora, lack of patient consent, or inexperience in performing the procedure on the part of the practitioner.

# PREOPERATIVE PREPARATION

## Key Preoperative Considerations

- The patient's symptoms should be evaluated and documented through a dye disappearance test such as the Jones I test and slit-lamp examination.
  - Jones I testing involves instilling fluorescein into the lower conjunctival cul-de-sac and then, after 2 to 3 minutes, attempting to retrieve fluorescein from the ipsilateral external naris with a cotton swab. The swab is examined with a cobalt-blue light to check for the presence of fluorescein. If fluorescein is detected on the swab, the nasolacrimal system is patent, and a functional blockage exists at the punctum.
  - Jones II testing involves placing a nasolacrimal cannula into the nasolacrimal sac, bypassing the punctum and canalicular system. Irrigation is then attempted with saline. Failure of the patient to report the taste of saline or fluid down the back of the throat is evidence of an anatomic blockage at the level of the nasolacrimal sac or distal.
- Signed informed consent is obtained and witnessed.
- The preoperative note is documented:
  - Diagnosis is confirmed (e.g., *chronic epiphora secondary to punctal stenosis*), including operative site.
  - Allergies and current medications are documented.
  - Proposed procedure: *Three-snip punctoplasty (state eye)*
  - Anesthesia given is recorded (e.g., methylcellulose sponge soaked in topical 4% lidocaine held over the involved punctum and adjacent palpebral conjunctiva for 1 minute, combined with *a subconjunctival injection adjacent to the punctum comprised of 0.5 mL of lidocaine 1% or 2% with epinephrine 1:100,000*).
- The operative site is prepared in standard fashion with 5% ophthalmic povidone–iodine (or alternative in the case of iodine allergy).
- A "time-out" is called before starting the procedure whereby patient identity, diagnosis, procedure, and operative site are confirmed by all present.

### *Instrument Tray*

- Topical anesthetic agent (e.g., proparacaine, tetracaine, or 4% lidocaine)
- Ophthalmic sponge spears
- Subconjunctival anesthetic agent (1% or 2% lidocaine with epinephrine 1:100,000)*
- One milliliter sterile syringe
- Half-inch 27- or 30-gauge hypodermic needle
- Punctal dilator (have assorted sizes available)
  - A safety pin or hatpin that has been sterilized may offer a starting point for highly stenotic or closed puncta.

- Vannas-style or small iris scissors
- Toothed forceps, 0.12 mm
- Five percent ophthalmic povidone–iodine solution
- Ophthalmic antibiotic ointment (e.g., erythromycin)

*Consider contraindications to any exogenous agents administered.

# PROCEDURE

**Key Procedural Points**

- Can be performed in the office
- Ensure appropriate anesthesia topically and through subconjunctival injection.
- Aggressive punctal dilation is needed to ensure forceps can be inserted.
- Hemostasis is rarely necessary.
- Antibiotic ointment applied postoperatively is indicated to minimize the risk of infection.

## *Three-Snip Punctoplasty*

The three-snip punctoplasty procedure removes a rectangular-shaped segment from the posterior wall (posterior ampullae) of the punctum and vertical canaliculus.[1,3-7,10] The procedure can be comfortably performed in the office setting with the patient either supine on an examination table or in an examination chair tilted backward to allow the practitioner to be comfortably positioned at the head. Good lighting and proper magnification (loupes or operating microscope) allow for adequate visualization. The steps for performing the procedure are as follows:

1. Comfortably position the patient in the supine position.
2. Instill one drop of a topical ophthalmic anesthetic and place an ophthalmic sponge spear soaked in 4% lidocaine over the punctum and adjacent palpebral conjunctiva for 1 minute.
3. Deliver a subconjunctival injection of approximately 0.5 mL of lidocaine 1% or 2% (with epinephrine 1:100,000, unless contraindicated) into the area directly adjacent to the involved punctum and vertical canaliculus (Figure 36-1).
4. Instill one drop of 5% ophthalmic povidone–iodine solution into the inferior conjunctival fornix.
5. Aggressively dilate the punctum with a punctal dilator (Figures 36-2 and 36-3). A sequence of dilators of varying sizes may need to be employed based on the degree of stenosis observed. Occasionally, the point of a small safety pin or hatpin that has been sterilized is helpful to open the punctum wide enough to employ a broader dilator. The punctal opening must be large enough to insert one jaw of the 0.3-mm toothed tissue forceps through the punctal opening and into the vertical portion of the canaliculus.

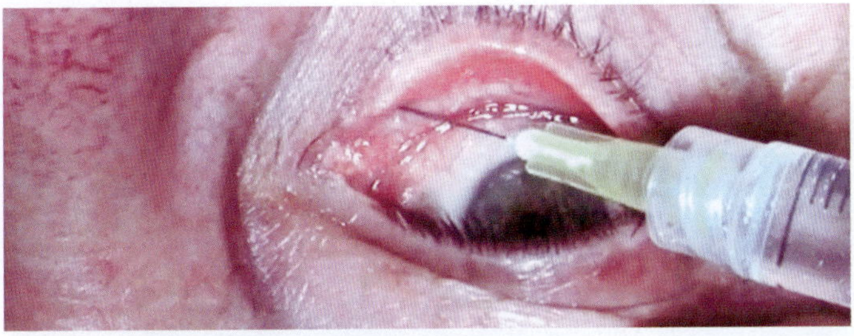

FIGURE 36-1 Local anesthesia is administered via subconjunctival injection of lidocaine 0.5% with epinephrine 1:200,000.

6. Insert one jaw of the 0.12-mm toothed tissue forceps through the dilated punctum into the vertical portion of the canaliculus. The forceps tip should be at the bottom of the vertical canaliculus. Firmly grasp the posterior wall of the punctum between the forceps' jaws. Crimping the tissue at this point by pinching firmly with the forceps may add some degree of "crush" hemostasis to the tissue.
7. With the forceps positioned as detailed above, create a vertical incision with the Vannas scissors on either side of the forceps through the back wall of the vertical canaliculus. These constitute the first two "snips" of the procedure (Figures 36-4 and 36-5). Confirm that the incision(s) extend to the bottom of the vertical canaliculus.
8. Make a horizontal incision with the Vannas (iris) scissors across the bottom of the vertical canaliculus connecting the two prior vertical incisions, effectively removing a rectangular portion of tissue from the posterior wall (Figures 36-6 and 36-7).
9. Hemostasis is rarely necessary. Where indicated, hold pressure over the area with a 4 × 4 gauze and irrigate with sterile saline as needed until hemostasis is achieved. Avoid thermal cautery as this results in more inflammation, which is likely to promote scarring and compromise the procedure's efficacy.
10. Apply an ophthalmic antibiotic ointment to the inferior cul-de-sac.

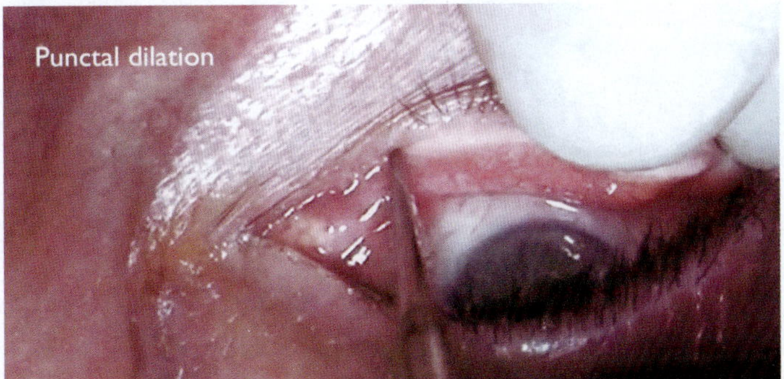


FIGURE 36-2 The punctum is dilated aggressively with a Castroviejo lacrimal dilator.

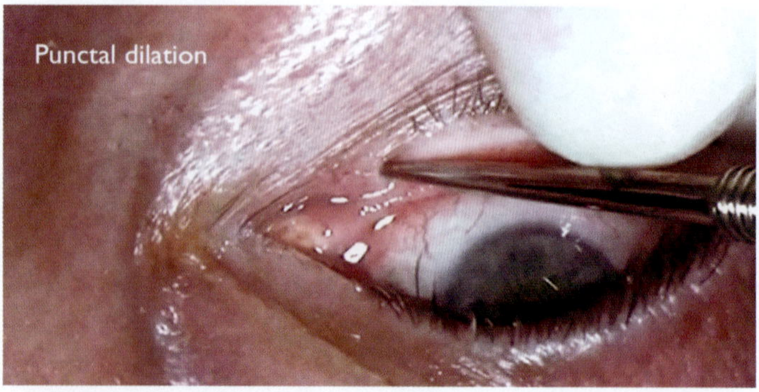


**FIGURE 36-3** The lacrimal dilator is directed medially while the lid margin is stretched laterally, straightening out the canaliculus and facilitating punctal dilation.

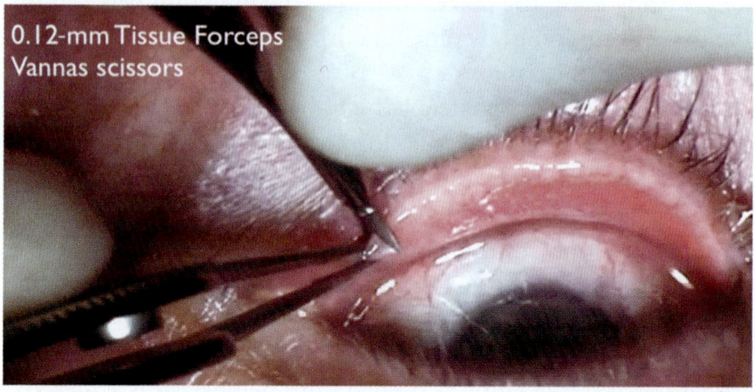


**FIGURE 36-4** The posterior wall of the punctum is grasped with a pair of straight 0.12-mm toothed tissue forceps. A small Vannas-style iris scissor is used to place a vertical incision along the lateral aspect of the forceps.

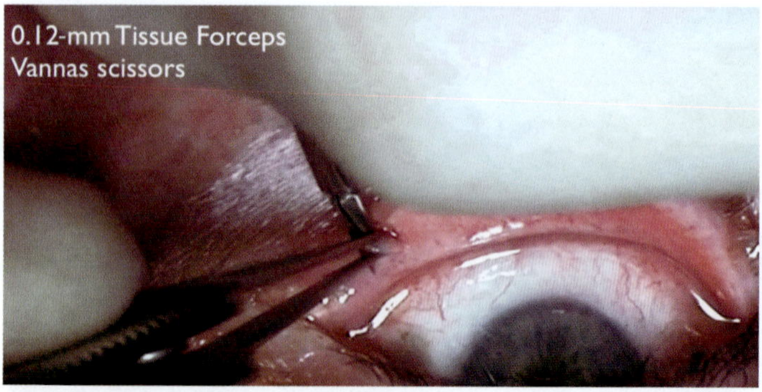


**FIGURE 36-5** The posterior wall of the punctum is grasped with a pair of straight 0.12-mm toothed tissue forceps. A small Vannas-style iris scissor is used to place a vertical incision along the medial aspect of the forceps.

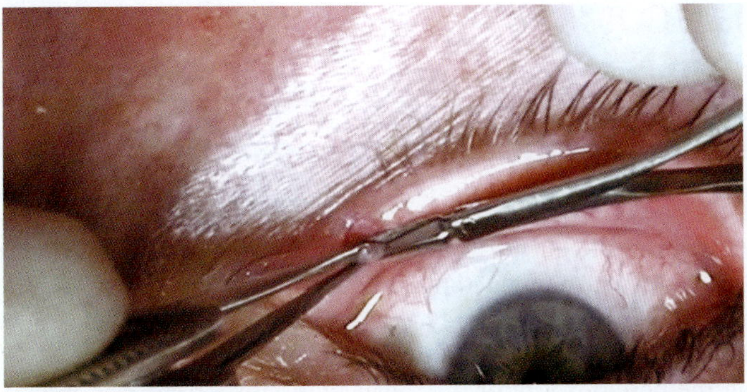

FIGURE 36-6 The third snip incision is placed at the bottom of the flap created, effectively removing a rectangular section of tissue comprising the posterior wall of the punctum.

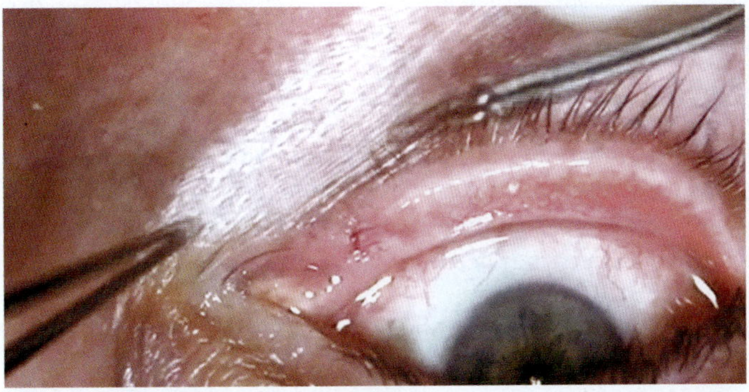

FIGURE 36-7 Completed procedure. Punctum is functionally widened. Hemostasis is rarely necessary.

## POSTOPERATIVE CARE (FOLLOW-UP SCHEDULE)

### Key Postoperative Considerations

- A successful procedure is confirmed on follow-up examination in 1 to 3 months by resolution of the epiphora complaint.
- Instruct the patient to apply an antibiotic ointment to the site twice daily for 5 consecutive days.

# POTENTIAL COMPLICATIONS AND THEIR MANAGEMENT

## Key Potential Complications to Look for

- Recurrence of stenosis secondary to scarring of the tissue[1,3-7,10-14]
  - Observed in greater frequency with prior versions of the three-snip procedure, namely the one-snip and two-snip punctoplasty
  - Recurrence of stenosis may require repeat punctoplasty with the placement of a stent.
- Bleeding and hematoma formation secondary to surgical manipulation[3,4,7,11-13]
  - Crimping the posterior wall of the canaliculus with forceps may minimize the risk of bleeding and hematoma formation.
  - An anesthetic solution containing epinephrine at a dilution of 1:100,000 may decrease the risk of bleeding owing to the vasoconstrictive effect of the epinephrine.
  - Thermal cautery should be avoided as it promotes inflammation and subsequent scarring.
- Infection[1,3-6]
  - Prescribing an antibiotic ointment for up to 5 days post-procedure should reduce the risk of infection.
- Pain and discomfort[1,3-6,11-13]
  - Transient pain secondary to infiltration of tissues with an anesthetic agent
  - Transient pain secondary to surgical trauma
  - Postoperative pain is expected to be transient and short-lived and may be managed with over-the-counter analgesics as needed.
- Transient vision blur[1,3-6]
  - Secondary to use of antibiotic ointment

## VIDEO OF PROCEDURE

**Video 36-1**—Following informed consent, the patient is placed in the supine position. A drop of proparacaine is placed in the operative eye. Next, subconjunctival anesthesia is administered by injecting 0.2 mL of lidocaine 0.5% (with epinephrine 1:200,000 unless contraindicated) into the subconjunctival space directly below the affected punctum. Aggressive dilation of the affected punctum is then carried out using a punctal dilator. One arm of a straight 0.12-mm tissue forceps is then inserted through the dilated punctum down the entire length of the "vertical" portion of the canaliculus, the other arm sandwiching the posterior ampullae (back wall) of the punctum, as shown in the video. A small Vannas (iris) scissor is then used to make two vertical snip incisions along the posterior ampullae of the punctum on either side of the forceps, as shown. The third snip is placed along the bottom, effectively excising a small rectangular bit of tissue (the back wall of the punctum), functionally increasing the diameter of the punctal orifice.

# EFFICACY

According to Kim et al, the most current iteration of the three-snip punctoplasty offers an anatomic success rate (maintenance of patency of the excised canalicular wall without closure or scarring) of between 89% and 96%.[2] Functional success rates, based on patient symptomatology, have been shown to vary between 64% and 93%.[3] Caesar et al conducted a historical review of the various iterations of the snip punctoplasty procedure. After reviewing 102 articles, the authors point to a success rate of 92% using the three-snip procedure.[4]

## CODING AND BILLING

- **CPT code: 68440**—Snip incision of lacrimal punctum (global period 10 days)

Common ICD-10 codes that support snip punctoplasty include the following:

- **H04.2** (epiphora)
- **H04.56** (stenosis of lacrimal punctum)

## REFERENCES


1. Soiberman U, Kakizaki H, Selva D, Leibovitch I. Punctal stenosis: definition, diagnosis, and treatment. *Clin Ophthalmol (Auckland, NZ).* 2012;6:1011-1018.
2. Kim SE, Lee SJ, Lee SY, Yoon JS. Outcomes of 4-snip punctoplasty for severe punctal stenosis: measurement of tear meniscus height by optical coherence tomography. *Am J Ophthalmol.* 2012:153(4):769-773.
3. Chak M, Irvine F. Rectangular 3-snip punctoplasty outcomes: preservation of the lacrimal pump in punctoplasty surgery. *Ophthal Plast Reconstr Surg.* 2009;25(2):134-135.
4. Caesar R, McNab A. A brief history of punctoplasty: the 3-snip revisited. *Eye.* 2005;19:16-18. doi:10.1038/sj.eye.6701415
5. Kashkouli MB, Beigi B, Murthy R, Astbury N. Acquired external punctal stenosis: etiology and associated findings. *Am J Ophthalmol.* 2003;136:1079-1084.
6. Hughes WL, Maris CS. A clip procedure for stenosis and eversion of the lacrimal punctum. *Trans Am Acad Ophthalmol Otolaryngol.* 1967;71(4):653-655.
7. Jones LT. The cure of epiphora due to canalicular disorders, trauma and surgical failures on the lacrimal passages. *Trans Am Acad Ophthalmol Otolaryngol.* 1962;66:506-524.
8. Offutt WN 4th, Cowen DE. Stenotic puncta: microsurgical punctoplasty. *Ophthal Plast Reconstr Surg.* 1993;9(3):201-205.
9. Murdock J, Lee WW, Zatezalo CC, Ballin A. Three-snip punctoplasty outcome rates and follow-up treatments. *Orbit.* 2015;34(3):160-163.
10. Ali MJ, Ayyar A, Naik MN. Outcomes of rectangular 3-snip punctoplasty in acquired punctal stenosis: is there a need to be minimally invasive? *Eye (Lond).* 2015;29:515-518.
11. Shahid H, Sandhu A, Keenan T, et al. Factors affecting outcome of punctoplasty surgery: a review of 205 cases. *Br J Ophthalmol.* 2008;92:1689-1692.
12. Yuen KS, Chan DD, Chan WM, Lam DS. A brief history of punctoplasty: the 3-snip revisited. *Eye (Lond).* 2006;20:402-403.
13. Park SJ, Noh JH, Park KB. et al. A novel surgical technique for punctal stenosis: placement of three interrupted sutures after rectangular three-snip punctoplasty. *BMC Ophthalmol.* 2018;18:70. doi:10.1186/s12886-018-0733-2
14. Kristan RW. Treatment of lacrimal punctal stenosis with a one-snip canaliculotomy and temporary punctal plugs. *Arch Ophthalmol.* 1988;106(7):878-879.

# 37 Dexamethasone Ophthalmic Insert

**Griffin Christenson • Leonid Skorin, Jr**

Cataract formation is the leading cause of vision loss in the United States.[1,2] As the elderly population continues to grow, the number of individuals affected by cataracts is expected to increase proportionally.[1,2] Additionally, among the U.S. Medicare-eligible population, cataract extraction is the most commonly performed surgical procedure.[3] Cataract surgical techniques have come a long way since their likely origin in the ancient world, where procedures such as couching—which involves pushing the crystalline lens into the vitreous and out of the visual axis—were common practice.[4] Likewise, just as surgical treatments have evolved, postoperative care has changed over time as well. Whereas indigenous roots and leaves were once applied to the eye following primitive extracapsular cataract extractions, we now most typically opt for the use of topical eye drop medications.[5] Capsulorhexis, followed by phacoemulsification of the crystalline lens and replacement with an intraocular lens, comprises the current paradigm for modern cataract surgery. Postoperatively, patients are given a combination of ophthalmic antibacterial, steroidal, and nonsteroidal anti-inflammatory topical medications. There are few areas within the perioperative surgical purview that have not changed drastically since phacoemulsification was first described by Kelman in 1967.[6] Although, as Assil et al point out, the delivery mechanism for postoperative therapeutics is one area where inroads to modernization are, just now, being made.[7] An alternative option for decreasing the burden of topical drop regimens is to provide a localized slow release of the active therapeutic ingredient(s) for sustained delivery over time. In addition to being used in postoperative cataract surgical care, the local sustained-release delivery mechanism has broad application potential and is currently being utilized to treat ocular allergies.

## INDICATIONS

### Key Indications

- Treatment of ocular pain following ophthalmic surgery
- Treatment of ocular inflammation following ophthalmic surgery
- Treatment of itching associated with allergic conjunctivitis

Dexamethasone 0.4 mg ophthalmic insert (Dextenza, Ocular Therapeutix) is an intracanalicular insert that elutes a sustained and tapered dose of dexamethasone for 30 days.[8] The 3-mm cylindrical-shaped intracanalicular insert is fluorescent yellow, which helps in visualization after its placement when used with a cobalt blue light source and yellow filter. Dextenza originally received Food and Drug Administration (FDA) approval in November 2018 for treatment of ocular pain following cataract surgery.[8] Subsequently, in 2019, Dextenza received FDA approval for the treatment of ocular inflammation following cataract surgery. Recently, it has been approved for the treatment of itching associated with allergic conjunctivitis.[9]

## CONTRAINDICATIONS

### Key Contraindications

- Active corneal, conjunctival, or canalicular infection
- Glaucoma
- Ocular hypertension
- History of steroid-induced intraocular pressure elevation

As with other steroids, Dextenza is contraindicated in patients with active corneal, conjunctival, or canalicular infections including epithelial herpes, simplex keratitis (dendritic keratitis), vaccinia, and varicella; mycobacterial infections; fungal diseases of the eye; and dacryocystitis.[10] It should be used with caution for patients with glaucoma, ocular hypertension, or a history of steroid-induced intraocular pressure elevation.[10]

## PREOPERATIVE PREPARATION

### Key Preoperative Preparation

- For treatment of ocular pain and inflammation from ophthalmic surgery, the Dextenza insert placement can be done preoperatively or postoperatively in the eye clinic using a slit lamp. For most practical purposes, the Dextenza insert placement is done in the surgical suite immediately after the ophthalmic surgery.
- For itching from allergic conjunctivitis, the Dextenza insert placement is done in the eye clinic using a slit lamp.

When using Dextenza for the treatment of ocular inflammation or ocular pain following ophthalmic surgery, placement of the insert can be done in the office preoperatively or postoperatively. The most practical time to place the Dextenza insert in this situation is actually in the surgical suite immediately after the ophthalmic surgery has been completed. This way the surgical microscope can be utilized and the patient's eye and periocular area are still anesthetized. Placement of Dextenza for the treatment of itching associated with allergic conjunctivitis is performed in the eye clinic utilizing the slit lamp. A topical anesthetic agent may be used prior to insertion of Dextenza, although it is not always necessary.

Usually, the site of insertion is the inferior canaliculus. If the patient has punctal stenosis or ectropion of the lower eyelid, the superior canalicular system can be used instead. Prior to placement of the canalicular insert, the punctum is dilated with a punctal dilator. The Dextenza insert is then removed from the foam housing using blunt (nontoothed) Bishop forceps. Excessive squeezing of the insert may cause deformation and difficulty placing the insert correctly. An assistant can help by holding the foam housing for easier insert removal by the clinician.

## PROCEDURE

After the eye and periocular area is anesthetized and the patient's head positioned appropriately behind the slit lamp, the appropriate eyelid is distracted laterally. Assuming a lower punctum/canaliculus insertion, the patient should be instructed to look up and to their temporal side (away from the site of insertion). Prior to insert placement, the punctal opening and surrounding tissue should be dried with either a cotton-tipped applicator or Weck surgical sponge. The insert can then be placed partially into the punctum vertically. Applying further lateral distraction to the eyelid will allow for straightening of the canalicular system. After the initial placement of the insert into the punctum, progression into the canaliculus can be aided by guiding the insert further down the canaliculus or by tapping it down using the forceps. After the insertion is completed, the patient should be instructed to blink a few times and it should be ensured that the Dextenza insert remains below the punctal opening. As the insert is bathed in tears traveling through the nasolacrimal system, it becomes pharmacologically and morphologically activated. As a result of this activation, the insert begins to widen and decrease in length, which secures it in place within the canaliculi (Figure 37-1). At this time, the insert also begins to elute dexamethasone onto the ocular surface. The Dextenza insert will maintain

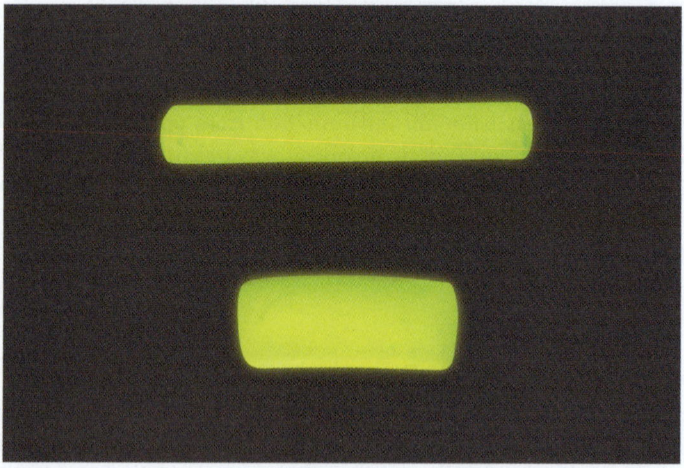

**FIGURE 37-1** After exposure to tears within the canaliculi, the Dextenza insert (top image) widens and decreases in length (bottom image). (Figure courtesy Ocular Therapeutix, Inc.)

its positioning for the next 90 days and will elute dexamethasone in a tapered fashion for the first 30 of those days. The insert dissolves over the 90 days on its own and therefore does not need to be removed.

For patients who are having the insert placed in the surgical suite after cataract surgery, viscoelastic can be injected through the punctum and into the canaliculus to help ease insertion. Any excess viscoelastic on the punctal surface should be removed with a Weck surgical sponge prior to insert placement. The viscoelastic helps the insert glide more freely through the punctum and into the canaliculus. The viscoelastic does not activate the Dextenza insert.

## POSTOPERATIVE CARE/COMANAGEMENT (FOLLOW-UP SCHEDULE)

For clinicians evaluating postoperative cataract surgery patients, who have received the Dextenza intracanalicular insert, much will remain unchanged. Just as for any other postoperative cataract surgery patient, the 1-day, 1-week, and 1-month examinations should include patient history, uncorrected visual acuity, pinhole acuity, and—depending on corneal clarity—refraction. As with postsurgical cataract patients, patients being treated for ocular allergies with the steroid insert, the intraocular pressure should be assessed and a slit-lamp examination should take place at subsequent visits. When performing the slit-lamp examination, the lower lid should be everted to evaluate the inferior punctal region. The Dextenza insert contains fluorescein, which can be seen under cobalt blue light and visualization can be further enhanced with a Wratten #12 yellow filter (Figure 37-2). The insert is easily observable under these settings and can give the

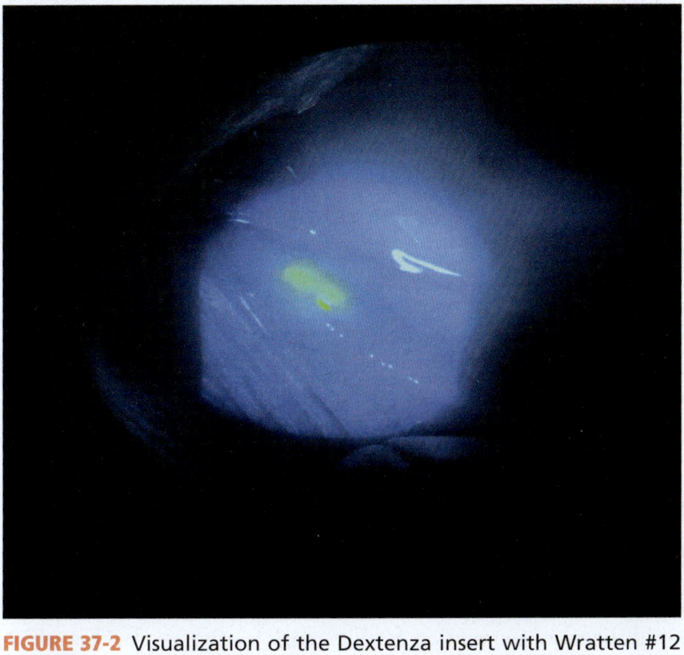

**FIGURE 37-2** Visualization of the Dextenza insert with Wratten #12 yellow filter under cobalt blue light at the 1-day postoperative visit.

doctor confidence that the steroid treatment is being delivered to the patient's ocular surface. Notably absent from the list of duties for the clinician or ophthalmic technician is the need for an exhaustive explanation of the topical therapeutic regimen and taper.

# POTENTIAL COMPLICATIONS AND THEIR TREATMENT

The most common adverse reactions that have been reported in patients receiving Dextenza for the treatment of ocular inflammation and ocular pain following ophthalmic surgery include anterior chamber inflammation such as iritis and iridocyclitis (10%), intraocular pressure increase (6%), visual acuity reduction (2%), cystoid macular edema (1%), corneal edema (1%), eye pain (1%) conjunctival hyperemia (1%), and headache (1%).[10] In nearly all cases, these reactions were manifested within 2 days of surgery and were deemed resultant from the surgery rather than the intracanalicular insert.[7] Despite the limited reports of adverse reactions to the insert itself, it is important to note that hazards related to the effects of corticosteroids on the ocular surface could potentially require the removal of the intracanalicular insert. The Dextenza insert can be removed proximally with manual expression or distally via saline irrigation.[7]

The most common ocular adverse effects reported in patients receiving Dextenza for the treatment of itching for allergic conjunctivitis include intraocular pressure increase (3%–6.5%), lacrimation increase (1%), eye discharge (1%), and visual acuity reduction (1%).[10-12] Intraocular pressure increase can occur as soon as 8 days and as late as 4 weeks after intracanalicular insert placement.[11,12] The intraocular pressure has been found to increase by up to 10 mm Hg within this time frame.[11,12] The most common nonocular adverse reaction was headache (1%).[10]

On rare occasion, the canaliculus may be perforated during dilation or during insert placement. If perforation occurs, do not proceed with insert placement. It would be appropriate to move to the opposite lid punctum/canaliculus on the same side and perform the insertion at this new location.

## VIDEOS OF PROCEDURES

**Video 37-1**—Placement of Dextenza insert immediately after cataract surgery in the surgical suite. Included are two short clips of complicated cases. (Video courtesy of Leonid Skorin Jr and Griffin Christenson.)

**Video 37-2**—Placement of Dextenza insert immediately after cataract surgery in the surgical suite utilizing viscoelastic for ease of insert placement. (Video courtesy of Leonid Skorin Jr and Christian DeJongh.)

# EFFICACY

## Treatment of Ocular Inflammation and Ocular Pain Following Ophthalmic Surgery

Phase III clinical trials report decreased pain, inflammation, and less frequent need for rescue topical steroid therapy intervention for Dextenza relative to placebo vehicles.[13,14] Patients have had "highly favorable" opinions of Dextenza preferring the insert over topical therapy alternatives following surgery.[15] According to the qualitative evaluation of patient satisfaction undertaken by Gira et al, nearly all patients (92%) who received the insert reported that they would recommend the treatment to friends or family, and 84% said they would pay more for the treatment to avoid eye drop therapy.[15]

## Treatment of Itching Associated with Allergic Conjunctivitis

Dextenza has been shown to decrease ocular itching in patients with allergic conjunctivitis for up to 30 days.[11] Dextenza demonstrated lower mean ocular itching scores compared to vehicle group at all points throughout the study in all participants who had a positive history of ocular allergies and positive skin test reaction for perennial and seasonal allergens.[11] If patients require retreatment over the course of their disease, they will need to be re-evaluated by their clinician.[11] Outcomes of repeated doses have not yet been evaluated.[11]

# CODING/BILLING

- **CPT code: 68841**—Insertion of drug delivery implant into tear duct of eye

Common ICD-10 codes that support Dextenza insert include the following:

- **H57.8** (ocular itching)
- **H10.45** (allergic conjunctivitis)
- **H57.11** (ocular pain, right eye)
- **H57.12** (ocular pain, left eye)
- **H25.10** (age-related nuclear cataract)
- **H25.89** (other age-related cataract)

J code for reimbursement of product is billed by the site of care (office, hospital, ambulatory surgical center, etc.): J1096 is billed as 4 units for one Dextenza insert.

# REFERENCES


1. Congdon N, Vingerling JR, Klein BE, et al. Prevalence of cataract and pseudophakia/aphakia among adults in the United States. *Arch Ophthalmol.* 2004;122(4):487-494.
2. Gollogly HE, Hodge DO, St Sauver JL, et al. Increasing incidence of cataract surgery: population-based study. *J Cataract Refract Surg.* 2013;39(9):1383-1389.
3. Schein OD, Cassard SD, Tielsch JM, et al. Cataract surgery among Medicare beneficiaries. *Ophthalmic Epidemiol.* 2012;19(5):257-264.
4. Leffler CT, Klebanov A, Samara WA, et al. The history of cataract surgery: from couching to phacoemulsification. *Ann Transl Med.* 2020;8(22):1551. doi:10.21037/atm-2019-rcs-04
5. Roy PN, Mehra KS, Deshpande PJ. Cataract surgery performed before 800 B.C. *Br J Ophthalmol.* 1975; 59(3):171.
6. Kelman CD. Phaco-emulsification and aspiration. A new technique of cataract removal. A preliminary report. *Am J Ophthalmol.* 1967;64(1):23-35.
7. Assil KK, Greenwood MD, Gibson A, et al. Dropless cataract surgery: modernizing perioperative medical therapy to improve outcomes and patient satisfaction. *Curr Opin Ophthalmol.* 2021; 32(suppl 1):S1-S12.
8. Blizzard C, Desai A, Driscoll A. Pharmacokinetic studies of sustained-release depot of dexamethasone in beagle dogs. *J Ocul Pharmacol Ther.* 2016;32(9):595-600.

9. ClinicalTrials.gov. CLN 0052: a multi-center, randomized, double-masked, vehicle controlled phase 3 study evaluating the efficacy and safety of OTX-DP for the treatment of allergic conjunctivitis using a modified conjunctival allergen challenge model (Ora-CAC). 2020. Accessed October 22, 2022. https://clinicaltrials.gov/ct2/show/NCT04050865
10. Ocular Therapeutix, Inc. Dextenza (dexamethasone ophthalmic insert). Accessed October 25, 2022. https://www.accessdata.fda.gov/drugsatfda_docs/label/2019/208742s001lbl.pdf
11. McLaurin EB, Evans D, Repke CS, et al. Phase 3 randomized study of efficacy and safety of a dexamethasone intracanalicular insert in patients with allergic conjunctivitis. *Am J Ophthalmol.* 2021;229:288-300.
12. Torkildsen G, Abelson MB, Gomes PJ, et al. Vehicle-controlled, phase 2 clinical trial of a sustained-release dexamethasone intracanalicular insert in a chronic allergen challenge model. *J Ocul Pharm Ther.* 2017;33(2):79-90.
13. Walters T, Bafna S, Vold S, et al. Efficacy and safety of sustained release dexamethasone for the treatment of ocular pain and inflammation after cataract surgery: results from two phase 3 studies. *J Clin Exp Ophthalmol.* 2016;7(4):1-11.
14. Tyson SL, Bafna S, Gira JP, et al. Multicenter randomized phase 3 study of a sustained-release intracanalicular dexamethasone insert for treatment of ocular inflammation and pain after cataract surgery. *J Cataract Refract Surg.* 2019;45(2):204-212.
15. Gira JP, Sampson R, Silverstein SM, et al. Evaluating the patient experience after implantation of a 0.4 mg sustained release dexamethasone intracanalicular insert (Dextenza™): results of a qualitative survey. *Patient Prefer Adherence.* 2017;11:487-494.

## SUPPLEMENTAL READING

1. Christenson G, Skorin L. Focus on the cataract patient's experience. *Mod Optom.* 2021;3(7):27-30. https://modernod.com/articles/2021-oct/focus-on-the-cataract-patients-experience?c4src=article:infinite-scroll

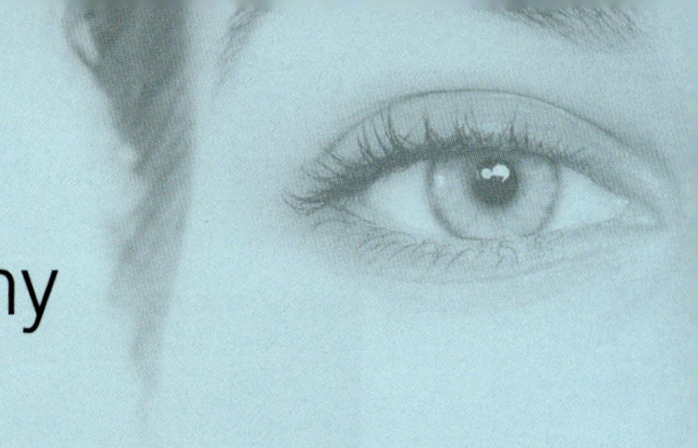

# 38 Canaliculotomy

**Leonid Skorin, Jr • Brianna Johnson**

Canaliculotomy is the gold standard surgical treatment for canaliculitis.[1] Canaliculotomy simply means cutting into the eyelid canaliculus. Canaliculotomy is performed to completely remove concretions from the canaliculus with curettage and open up any blockage or disruption to the canaliculus.[1] Curettage without canaliculotomy has also been supported as an effective way to treat patients affected by canaliculitis.[1] However, this method alone may not reach far enough into the canaliculus to effectively remove all concretions.[1] Canaliculitis can present as acute or chronic, but no matter the chronicity of this infection, prompt surgical therapy is advocated to minimize complications of chronic disease.[1]

## INDICATIONS

### Key Indications

- Canaliculitis
- Lacrimal punctal stenosis

Canaliculitis is a disorder of the excretory lacrimal system characterized by inflammation of the canaliculi, most commonly because of long-term infection, and can have bacterial, viral, or fungal etiology.[2] It is a rare disease that is frequently misdiagnosed.[3,4] Symptoms of this condition are tearing, discharge, red eye, and swelling with tenderness over the medial portion of the upper or lower eyelid (Figure 38-1).[2,4] Signs include erythematous "pouting" of the punctum and erythema of the surrounding area (Figure 38-2).[4,5] Lacrimal sac swelling or distension should be absent.[5] The diagnostic sign of canaliculitis is expression of mucopurulent discharge or concretions (canaliculiths) from the individual's punctum.[2,4] Other signs include recurrent or nonresolving conjunctivitis, which is more severe nasally, periocular skin vesicles when herpes simplex is the underlying cause, and a gritty feeling after contents of the punctum have been expressed.[2,4] Disease etiology is most often *Actinomyces israelii*, a gram-positive rod with fine, branching filaments that produces "sulfur granules" or concretions.[1,4] Other etiologies of primary lacrimal canaliculitis include other bacteria (*Staphylococcus, Streptococcus, Propionibacterium propionicum*), fungal (*Candida albicans, Fusarium, Aspergillus*) or viral (herpes simplex, varicella zoster).[2,4] A retained intracanalicular punctal plug or other lodged foreign body such

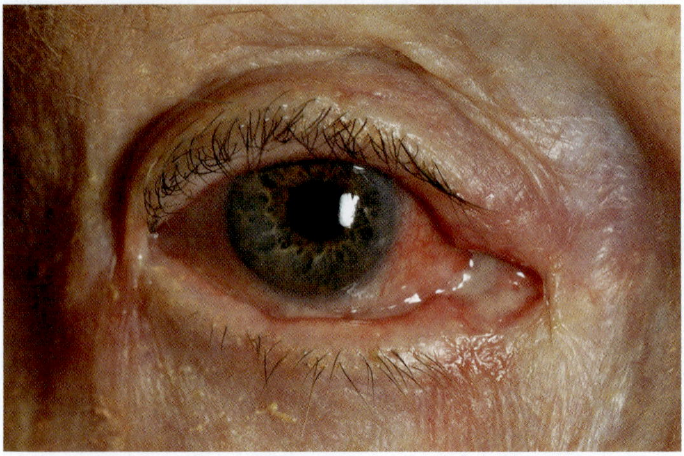

**FIGURE 38-1** Superior canaliculitis.

as a lacrimal stent result in secondary lacrimal canaliculitis and are commonly caused by *Pseudomonas aeruginosa*.[2,4,6]

Lacrimal canaliculitis makes up only 2% to 4% of lacrimal pathologies.[6-8] Although most prevalent as a unilateral condition, bilateral presentation may occur.[9] The lower canaliculus is involved in two-thirds of cases, with multiple canalicular involvement occurring only in a small percentage of cases either at presentation or in subsequent episodes.[9,10] Canaliculitis can affect people of all ages but is more common in the elderly population.[2] There is a 5:1

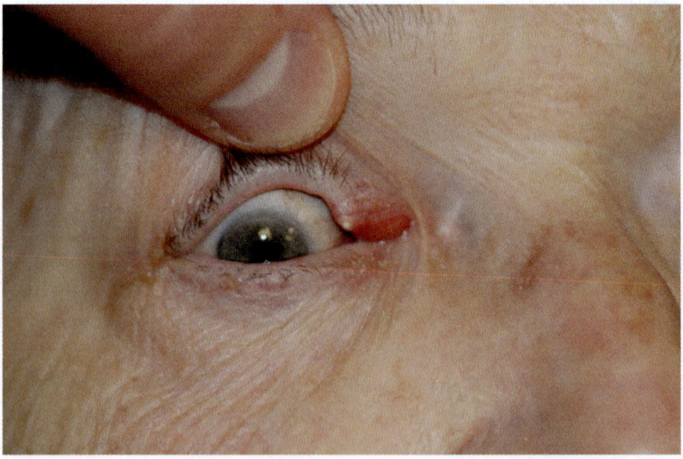

**FIGURE 38-2** Erythema and edema around superior punctum. There is "pouting" of the punctum, and white purulent material can be seen protruding from the punctal orifice. (From Skorin L, Toldo EA. What is the cause of this patient's ocular symptoms? *Consultant*. 2018;58(9):245-248. https://www.consultant360.com/article/consultant360/ophthalmology/what-cause-patients-ocular-symptoms.)

female-to-male ratio.[2,6,11] This may be because of different factors, such as changes in hormones during menopause, which usually affect tear composition and production with an accompanying dry eye.[9] Makeup and other cosmetics also may contribute to blocked canaliculi and promotion of bacterial growth.[9] There is no association with race or ethnicity.[6]

Differential diagnoses include dacryocystitis, chalazion/hordeolum, nasolacrimal duct obstruction, or chronic conjunctivitis/blepharitis.[3,4,7,9] A neoplasm of the lacrimal system may present with unilateral tearing and masquerade as inflammation.[6,12] Carcinoma of the lacrimal canaliculus can include bloody tears, epistaxis, and a mass extending above the medial canthal tendon.[12] These characteristics, along with diagnostic histopathologic findings, differentiate it from canaliculitis and emphasize the importance of submitting excised material for histopathologic analysis.[12] It is important to correctly diagnose canaliculitis before surgical intervention is performed. The rate of clinical misdiagnosis ranges from 45% to 100%,[7] with multiple diagnosis rates of 33% reported in one study.[11] Most cases can be diagnosed clinically; however, dacryocystography and/or ultrasound biomicroscopy should be utilized in uncertain cases.[3]

Lacrimal punctal stenosis can occur because of several reasons. Herpes simplex, varicella zoster, and *Chlamydia trachomatis* are a few infectious etiologies of lacrimal punctal stenosis.[13] Chemotherapeutic agents, topical or systemic, can also cause punctal stenosis.[13] Systemic etiologies (e.g., porphyria cutanea tarda), irradiation, aging changes, and/or tissue atrophy of the fibrous structure of the punctum can cause punctal stenosis as well.[13] In cases of punctal stenosis, punctal dilation is a good first step in the process of opening up the lacrimal system.[13]

## CONTRAINDICATIONS

### Key Contraindications

- Canalicular dilatation
- Abnormal nasolacrimal duct system
- History of punctal plugs

Canalicular dilatation may occur because of long-standing canaliculitis with the chronic stasis of concretions and a prominent, thickened canaliculus.[14] Mean duration of symptoms has been reported to be 10 months.[6] Patients who present with canalicular dilatation require more than just a canaliculotomy, because they will require additional reconstruction of their canaliculus known as a canaliculoplasty.[14] With a canaliculoplasty, excess canalicular tissues are removed and a stent is placed to reconstruct the canaliculus and provide structure to the lacrimal system.[14]

Canaliculotomy and punctoplasty are only suitable surgical treatments for those patients with a relatively normal common canaliculus, lacrimal sac, and nasolacrimal duct.[15] If both upper and lower canaliculi are affected in a patient, visualizing the distal part of the lacrimal duct can be difficult.[15] In these cases where the blockage is suspected to be further down the nasolacrimal duct system, a conjunctivodacryocystorhinostomy should be performed.[15]

A relative contraindication of using canaliculotomy with patients is a history of previous punctal plug use.[16] Some studies discussing canaliculotomy to treat canaliculitis have excluded patients that had a history of punctal plug use because of the difference in the etiology and clinical course of this secondary canaliculitis.[16] Yet in other studies, canaliculotomy that was performed on patients with a previous history of punctal plug use showed a complete resolution of their symptoms.[16] In all such cases, removal of the punctal plug or lacrimal stent is necessary for resolution.[6]

Conservative management of canaliculitis is an option if a patient presents with a contraindication to surgical intervention. Conservative therapy including topical ophthalmic antibiotic drops, oral antibiotics, antibiotic irrigation, or punctal curettage alone is generally not as effective as surgical intervention, which is usually curative.[2,3,17] In one study, as many as 41% of patients who completed conservative therapy alone had recurrences of canaliculitis and needed additional treatment.[3] This may be because of the antibiotics not being able to penetrate through the concretions and debris and not treating soon enough after initial onset of symptoms.[2,3] Prognosis is best if symptoms are treated within the first 30 days of symptom onset.[7,10] The following includes the steps and options for conservative therapy[2]:

- Massage affected area and use warm compresses
- Topical ophthalmic treatment options:
  - Moxifloxacin 0.5% QID then redirected by cultures
  - If cultures are positive for *Actinomyces* sp.: Compounded penicillin or cefazolin four to six times daily (or as directed by patient allergies/sensitivities)
  - If cultures positive for fungus: Natamycin 5% suspension QID
  - Suspected herpetic infection: Trifluridine 1% solution QID
- Oral treatment options:
  - Amoxicillin/clavulanate 500/125 mg BID
  - Cephalexin 250 to 500 mg QID
  - If methicillin-resistant *Staphylococcus aureus* (MRSA) risk factors present: Trimethoprim/sulfamethoxazole 160/800 mg BID or doxycycline 100 mg BID
  - If allergic to penicillin/cephalosporin: Trimethoprim/sulfamethoxazole 160/800 mg BID or clindamycin 150 to 300 mg daily

# PREOPERATIVE PREPARATION

## Necessary Instrumentation

1. Ophthalmic topical anesthetic (e.g., tetracaine 0.5%, proparacaine 0.5%)
2. Lidocaine 1% or 2% with 1:100,000 epinephrine
3. Povidone–iodine 10% swabs for cleaning affected eyelid and surrounding areas
4. Povidone–iodine 5% ophthalmic solution
5. Sterile fenestrated surgical drape
6. Plastic corneal shield
7. Number 11 surgical blade
8. Bowman dilating probe
9. Vannas scissors
10. Two millimeter curette

11. Moxifloxacin 0.5% solution (or comparable antibiotic)
12. Tuberculin syringe (for antibiotic)
13. Lacrimal cannula
14. Three milliliter syringe for anesthetic
15. 30-gauge × ½ inch needle
16. 4 × 4 surgical gauze pads
17. Cotton-tipped applicators
18. 6-0 silk or nylon suture with cutting needle
19. Sterile container for concretions/pyogenic granuloma to send to pathology

## PROCEDURE

1. Before starting surgery, topical anesthetic is applied to the affected eye and an injection of lidocaine 1% or 2% with 1:100,000 epinephrine is administered to the pericanalicular tissues.
2. Povidone–iodine 10% is then utilized to prep the skin area. A drop of 5% ophthalmic povidone–iodine is applied to the eye. A sterile fenestrated surgical drape is placed over the patient's face.
3. Anesthesia is then evaluated to make sure it took effect. A plastic corneal shield is placed on the eye to protect the globe.
4. Four- to five-millimeter incision is made along longitudinal aspect of eyelid canaliculi, sparing the puncta. The contents within the canaliculi are expressed (Figure 38-3).[3,18] These expressed concretions should be sent to pathology.
5. Curettage of inner lining of canaliculi and surrounding areas with 2 mm curette confirms complete removal of concretions and if a pyogenic granuloma is present (Figure 38-4). If a pyogenic granuloma is present, it also should be sent to pathology (Figure 38-5).

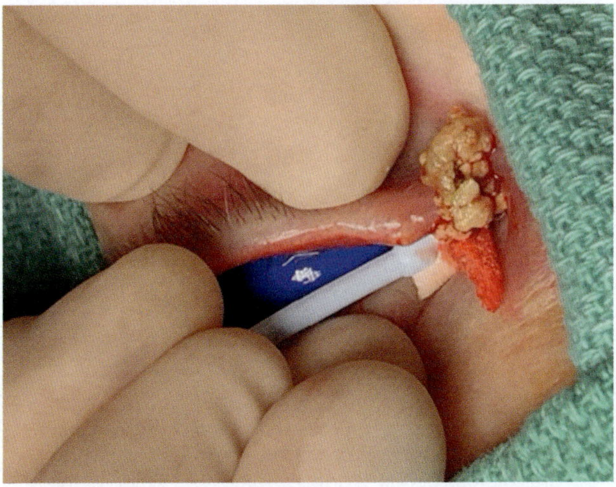

**FIGURE 38-3** Expression of concretions (sulfur granules) during canaliculotomy. (From Skorin L, Toldo EA. What is the cause of this patient's ocular symptoms? *Consultant*. 2018;58(9): 245-248. https://www.consultant360.com/article/consultant360/ophthalmology/what-cause-patients-ocular-symptoms.)

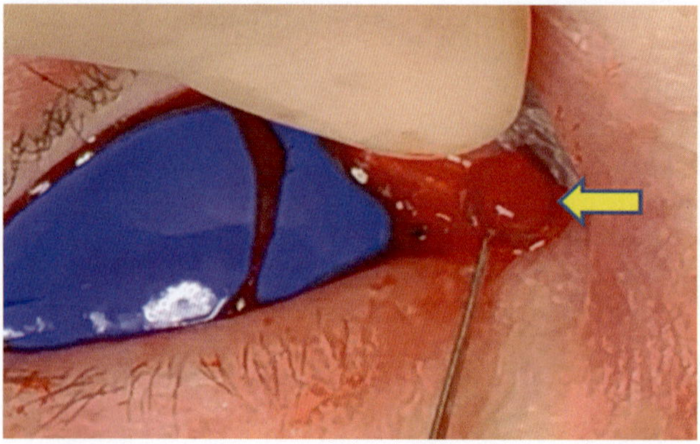

**FIGURE 38-4** Curettage exposing pyogenic granuloma (arrow). (From Skorin L, Toldo EA. What is the cause of this patient's ocular symptoms? *Consultant*. 2018;58(9):245-248. https://www.consultant360.com/article/consultant360/ophthalmology/what-cause-patients-ocular-symptoms.)

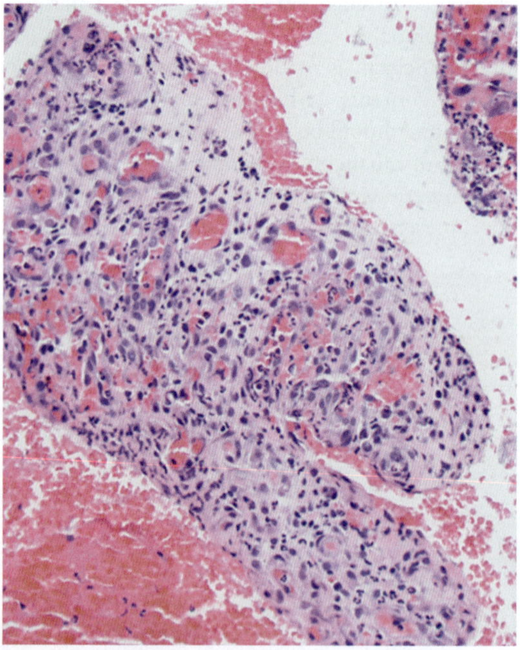

**FIGURE 38-5** Histopathology image showing focal areas of squamous mucosa with underlying vascular congestion and inflammation typical of pyogenic granuloma. (From Skorin L, Toldo EA. What is the cause of this patient's ocular symptoms? *Consultant*. 2018;58(9):245-248. https://www.consultant360.com/article/consultant360/ophthalmology/what-cause-patients-ocular-symptoms.)

6. Bowman dilating probe is passed through the puncta to check for patency.
7. An antibiotic, such as moxifloxacin ophthalmic solution 0.5%, is injected into the canalicular system and into the lacrimal sac using a tuberculin syringe and lacrimal cannula.
8. Digital pressure is applied to ensure hemostasis. The plastic corneal shield is removed and another drop of topical antibiotic is applied to the corneal surface.
9. The horizontal canalicular incision is left open and does not need to be sutured.
10. If a vertical tear develops in the eyelid margin, it should be closed with 6-0 suture to prevent gaping and fistulization.[19]

## POSTOPERATIVE CARE/COMANAGEMENT (FOLLOW-UP SCHEDULE)

### Key Postoperative Considerations

- Topical antibiotic eye drops QID for 2 weeks
- Over-the-counter pain medication as necessary
- Recheck in 1 week.

Topical antibiotic drops are to be applied QID in the affected eye for a duration of 1 week, and the patient should continue any previously prescribed oral antibiotics.[18] Return to clinic for follow-up in 1 week.[18] Carefully place ice packs on the eyelids, and over-the-counter pain medications may be used as necessary.[18] Minimal postoperative pain is experienced, and good cosmetic appearance is achieved once the edema resolves (Figure 38-6).[18]

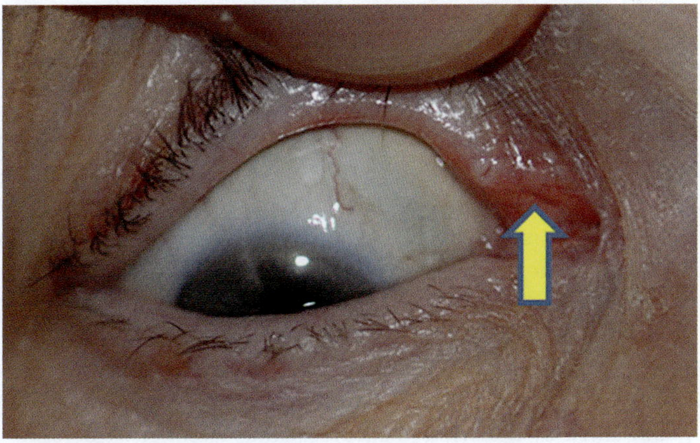

**FIGURE 38-6** One week after canaliculotomy, the longitudinal canalicular incision (arrow) is healing well. (From Skorin L, Toldo EA. What is the cause of this patient's ocular symptoms? *Consultant*. 2018;58(9):245-248. https://www.consultant360.com/article/consultant360/ophthalmology/what-cause-patients-ocular-symptoms.)

Comanaging clinicians should evaluate the pathology and microbiology results to ascertain if the causative organism is sensitive to the prescribed antibiotics.[18,20] If so, the patient should continue the treatment for one more week.[18,20] If not, switch the patient to a treatment therapy based on the results of the culture and continue the regimen for 1 to 2 weeks.[18,20]

# POTENTIAL COMPLICATIONS AND THEIR TREATMENT

## Key Potential Complications

- Canalicular lacrimal narrowing or scarring
- Lacrimal pump dysfunction
- Canalicular fistula formation
- Residual concretions
- Orbital cellulitis
- Abscess formation
- Chronic epiphora

Risks and complications that arise after canaliculotomy increase if both upper and lower canaliculi are involved.[17] Risks of canaliculotomy include canalicular luminal narrowing or scarring, lacrimal pump dysfunction, canalicular fistula formation, misdiagnosis of the disease, inability to treat concretions lodged deeper in the canaliculus, and the need for subsequent surgery, as well as the standard risks associated with any surgical procedure.[6] Some complications that could occur postoperatively with canaliculotomy include needing to reconstruct the canaliculus, intubation, stent placement, canalicular fistula formation, orbital cellulitis, and abscess formation.[6] Epiphora in patients after canaliculotomy was reported in one study, yet long-term follow-up of these patients did not reveal a direct relationship between persistent epiphora and canaliculotomy.[6] Trauma to the canaliculus and the creation of a false passage secondary to aggressive curettage are also possible complications that may arise.[1]

In a study of 40 patients who underwent surgical intervention for their canaliculitis, six experienced postoperative epiphora.[3] Three of those six had canalicular fibrosis, one of them had a partially patent lacrimal system, one developed punctal ectropion, and the final one had punctal stenosis.[3] The authors felt that continued manipulation of the punctum and lacrimal system and increased inflammation were the most likely culprits of canalicular fibrosis.[3] If a patient has a recurrence of canaliculitis after surgical intervention, it is often associated with epiphora and canalicular narrowing.[3]

Anand et al reviewed long-term outcomes after surgical intervention in treating canaliculitis.[11] Out of 15 patients followed and monitored, four of them experienced epiphora postoperatively, but three of these four had preexisting lacrimal pathology.[11] Anand et al's final conclusion was that canaliculotomy is safe and efficacious with no demonstrable risk or epiphora postoperatively.[11]

To treat canalicular stenosis, fibrosis, or stricture, stents or tubes can be put in place to allow for proper drainage of the lacrimal system.[19] Further dilation and irrigation postoperatively may result in scarring of the canaliculus and surrounding tissues.[6] With recalcitrant canaliculitis, more aggressive curettage of the canaliculus with a "cut-down" procedure is often required.[5] Canaliculotomy is a generally well-tolerated procedure with complications occurring rarely.[17] It is important to keep monitoring patients after the surgical intervention was performed and decide whether another surgery is necessary for additional treatment.

## VIDEOS OF PROCEDURES

**Video 38-1**—Canaliculotomy with sparing of the puncta. Expression of "sulfur granules" (concretions). Additional concretions and pyogenic granuloma removed by curettage. The horizontal canalicular incision is left open. (Video courtesy of Leonid Skorin Jr, Sebastian Baker, and Emmalee Toldo.)

**Video 38-2**—Canaliculotomy with sparing of the puncta. Expression of "sulfur granules" (concretions) with cotton-tip applicators. Additional concretions and pyogenic granuloma removed by curettage. Pyogenic granuloma excised with Vannas scissors. The horizontal canalicular incision is left open. (Video courtesy of Leonid Skorin Jr and Scott A. Bauer.)

**Video 38-3**—Pyogenic granuloma blocking punctal opening with concurrent canaliculitis. Excision of pyogenic granuloma with expression of "sulfur granules" (concretions) using cotton-tip applicators. Patency of canaliculi confirmed with punctal dilator. No need for canaliculotomy. For further details of this case please, see Supplemental Reading #3. (Video courtesy of Leonid Skorin Jr and Dessie Westall.)

# EFFICACY

Repeat injections of intracanalicular antibiotic is an alternative to surgery in the management of chronic suppurative canaliculitis, but surgical treatment by canaliculotomy and canalicular curettage remains the mainstay of treatment.[21] In one study, patients who underwent canaliculotomy had a lower recurrence rate (16%) than those with conservative treatment (33%), but this difference was not statistically significant ($p = 0.348$).[21] Canaliculotomy with canalicular curettage is associated with a high resolution rate and is one of the more effective surgical interventions with curative results.[14] Alam et al found complete resolution of canaliculitis to be 97.5% after canaliculotomy in their patients.[3] Alam et al observed that long-term efficacy of canaliculotomy was as high as 85% in their patients and that this was comparable to other studies that they reviewed.[3]

# CODING/BILLING AND MODIFIERS

- **CPT code: 68525**—Biopsy of lacrimal sac
- **CPT code: 68840**—Probing of lacrimal canaliculi
- **CPT code: 68815**—Canalicular curettage
- **Modifier 57**—Major surgical procedure performed same day or the day before

Common ICD-10 codes that support this procedure include the following:

- **H04.33** (acute canaliculitis of lacrimal passage)
- **H04.42** (chronic canaliculitis of lacrimal passage)
- **H04.56** (stenosis of lacrimal punctum)
- **H04.54** (stenosis of lacrimal canaliculi)

## REFERENCES


1. Ebroon DA, Hornblass A. Canaliculitis and acquired canalicular stenosis. In: Mauriello JA, ed. *Unfavorable Results of Eyelid and Lacrimal Surgery.* Butterworth Heinemann; 2000:427-437.
2. Jones HN, Mick AB. Canaliculitis. In: Onofrey BE, Skorin L, Holdeman NR, eds. *Ocular Therapeutics Handbook: A Clinical Manual.* 4th ed. Wolters Kluwer; 2020:311-312.
3. Alam MS, Poonam NS, Mukherjee B. Outcomes of canaliculotomy in recalcitrant canaliculitis. *Saudi J Ophthalmol.* 2019;33(1):46-51.
4. Bagheri N, Wajda BN, Calvo CM, et al. Canaliculitis. In: Bagheri N, Wajda BN, eds. *The Wills Eye Manual.* 7th ed. Wolters Kluwer; 2017:138-139.
5. Hirshbein MJ, Stasior GO. Lacrimal system. In: Chen WP ed. *Oculoplastic Surgery: The Essentials.* Thieme; 2001:263-288.
6. Freedman JR, Markert MS, Cohen AJ. Primary and secondary lacrimal canaliculitis: a review of literature. *Surv Ophthalmol.* 2011;56(4):336-347.
7. Singh M, Gautam N, Agarwal A, et al. Primary lacrimal canaliculitis—a clinical entity often misdiagnosed. *J Curr Ophthalmol.* 2018;30:87-90.
8. Xiang S, Lin B, Pan Q, et al. Clinical features and surgical outcomes of primary canaliculitis with concretions. *Medicine (Baltimore).* 2017;96(9):e6188.
9. Kaliki S, Ali MJ, Honavar SG, et al. Primary canaliculitis: clinical features, microbiological profile, and management outcome. *Ophthalmic Plast Reconstr Surg.* 2012;28(5):355-360.
10. Zaldivar RA, Bradley EA. Primary canaliculitis. *Ophthalmic Plast Reconstr Surg.* 2009;25(6):481-484.
11. Anand S, Hollingworth K, Kumar V, et al. Canaliculitis: the incidence of long-term epiphora following canaliculotomy. *Orbit.* 2004;23(1):19-26.
12. Charles NC, Lisman RD, Mittal KR. Carcinoma of the lacrimal canaliculus masquerading as canaliculitis. *Arch Ophthalmol.* 2006;124(3):414-416.
13. Kristan RW. Treatment of lacrimal punctal stenosis with a one-snip canaliculotomy and temporary punctal plugs. *Arch Ophthalmol.* 1988;106(7):878-879.
14. Su Y, Zhang L, Li L, et al. Surgical procedure of canaliculoplasty in the treatment of primary canaliculitis associated with canalicular dilatation. *BMC Ophthalmol.* 2020;20(1):1-7.
15. Zhuang A, Sun J, Shi WD. Treatment of upper and lower lacrimal punctal occlusion using retrograde canaliculotomy and punctoplasty. *Int J Ophthalmol.* 2019;12(9):1498-1502.
16. Perumal B, Meyer DR. Vertical canaliculotomy with retrograde expression of concretions for the treatment of canaliculitis. *Ophthalmic Plast Reconstr Surg.* 2015;31(2):119-121.
17. Khu J, Mancini R. Punctum-sparing canaliculotomy for the treatment of canaliculitis. *Ophthalmic Plast Reconstr Surg.* 2012;28(1):63-65.
18. Skorin L, Toldo E, Baker S. Snip and squeeze: canaliculitis. *Rev Optom.* 2018;155(6):101.
19. Dailey RA, Chavez MR. Surgery of the lacrimal system. In: Yen MT, ed. *Surgery of the Eyelids, Lacrimal System, and Orbit.* 2nd ed. Oxford Univ. Press; 2012:189-202.
20. Skorin L Jr, Toldo EA. What is the cause of this patient's ocular symptoms? *Consultant.* 2018;58(9):245-248.
21. Lin SC, Kao SC, Tsai CC, et al. Clinical characteristics and factors associated the outcome of lacrimal canaliculitis. *Acta Ophthalmol.* 2011;89(8):759-763.


## SUPPLEMENTAL READINGS


1. Skorin L, Toldo E, Baker S. Snip and squeeze: canaliculitis. *Rev Optom.* Published June 15, 2018. https://www.reviewofoptometry.com/article/snip-and-squeeze-canaliculitis
2. Skorin L Jr, Toldo EA. What is the cause of this patient's ocular symptoms? *Consultant.* Published September 2018. https://www.consultant360.com/article/consultant360/ophthalmology/what-cause-patients-ocular-symptoms
3. Skorin L, Westall DD. A new eyelid growth. *Osteopath Fam Physician.* 2019;11(5):32-35. https://www.ofpjournal.com/index.php/ofp/article/view/640/546

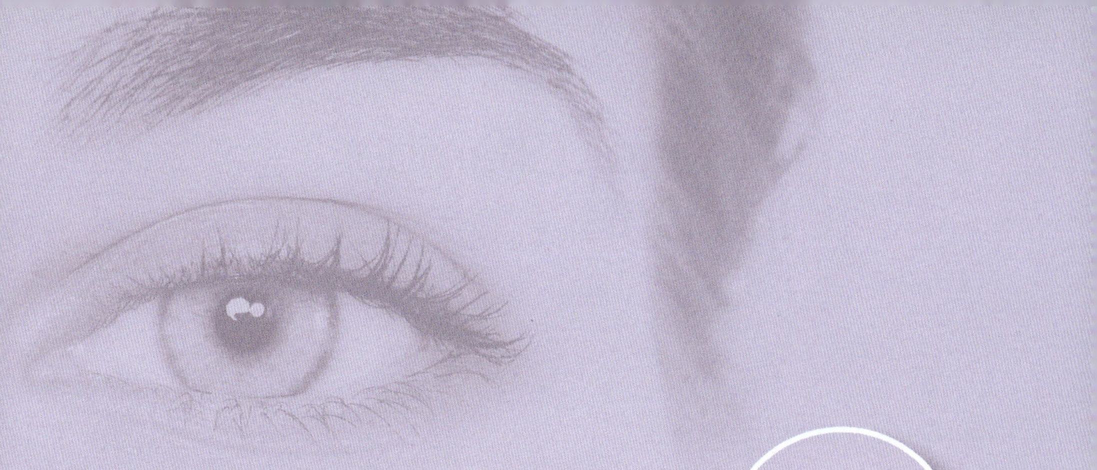

# SECTION 7

# Intraocular Procedures

# 39 Anterior Chamber Implants

I. Paul Singh • Nate Lighthizer

There has been a paradigm shift in the management of glaucoma over the last decade. With the introduction of the iStent (microinvasive glaucoma surgery [MIGS]) back in 2012, along with the renewed interest in first-line selective laser trabeculoplasty (SLT), and now drug delivery in the form of intracameral bimatoprost (Durysta, Allergan), clinicians are appreciating the importance of earlier intervention and the impact of compliance on long-term glaucoma control. In our practices, compliance with topical glaucoma medications has been the most significant barrier to preventing glaucoma progression. A 2015 study of over 1,200 patients newly diagnosed with glaucoma who were started on one topical medication therapy found only 20% of patients had good treatment adherence at 1 year.[1] Historically, we have preferred brand name medications over generic medications because of the consistency of inactive ingredients and bottle manufacturing. Unfortunately, aside from patient costs, it takes significant time and staff resources for patients to initiate and continue brand name medications. In an unpublished in-office study, we were able to save 4 minutes of technician time per patient per visit after reducing one topical medication post-SLT and/or MIGS surgery. This time saving resulted from a combination of less call backs, less faxes being sent to the pharmacy, and less verification of medications at the patient's office visits. Studies have found that up to 60% of our patients with glaucoma have a concomitant dry eye, which has also been related to the number of topical glaucoma medications.[2-4] Because of the symptoms of dry eye and ocular surface disease (OSD) such as tearing, burning, pain, and fluctuating vision, patients often blame their glaucoma drops and often reduce or even stop taking their glaucoma drops. Baudouin demonstrated a 30% reduction in compliance when patients with glaucoma also had dry eye.[5]

Addressing compliance is crucial because poor compliance can lead to fluctuating intraocular pressure (IOP). Studies such as the Advanced Glaucoma Intervention Study (AGIS) have demonstrated that patients with advanced open-angle glaucoma (OAG) who fluctuated more than 4 mm Hg throughout the course of the study had a higher risk of progression than those who had less fluctuation.[6] Another study from 2019 demonstrated increased short-term IOP fluctuation as a risk factor for glaucoma progression on visual field (VF).[7]

We now also have reliable data supporting the positive impact of reducing the drop burden on patient's quality of life and progression of disease post-SLT and MIGS procedures. The Laser in Glaucoma and Ocular Hypertension Trial (LiGHT) trial, which compared first-line SLT to topical latanoprost, demonstrated less risk for progressing to incisional glaucoma surgery in the SLT group versus latanoprost group despite similar IOP reductions.[8] After a 6-year follow-up, the SLT arm had a better Glaucoma Symptoms Score than the drops arm (83.6 [SD 18.1] vs. 81.3 [SD 17.3], respectively).[8] Up to 69.8% of eyes in the SLT arm remained at or below target IOP without the need for medical or surgical treatment.[8] More eyes in the drops arm exhibited disease progression (26.8% vs. 19.6%, respectively, $p = 0.006$).[8] Trabeculectomy was required in 32 eyes in the drops arm compared to 13 eyes in the SLT arm ($p < 0.001$), and there were more cataract surgeries in the drops arm (95 compared to 57 eyes, $p = 0.03$).[8] There were no serious laser-related adverse events.[8]

The 5-year data of the Horizon trial, which compared cataract surgery alone to cataract surgery with the Hydrus microstent, also revealed less medication burden in the Hydrus group and a 60% less chance of mild-to-moderate patients progressing to needing incisional glaucoma surgery (such as trabeculectomy or tube surgery) than the cataract surgery alone group.[9] In addition, the Hydrus microstent lowered the rate of VF loss by 47% versus cataract surgery alone.[9] In a study we helped publish in 2021, based on the iStent inject phase 3 pivotal trials, a higher percentage of patients who received the iStent inject showed meaningful improvements in quality-of-life (QOL) scores, including Ocular Surface Disease Index (OSDI) and Visual Function Questionnaire (VFQ-25), when compared with patients who received cataract surgery alone. Patients who were medication-free had the greatest improvement in QOL scores.[10]

Now that we have established the importance of reducing the topical drop burden, where do anterior chamber (AC) implants, in the form of sustained-release glaucoma medications, fit into the glaucoma treatment paradigm? Since June 2020, we have had access to the Durysta intracameral implant, which has allowed us to decrease the drop burden in a variety of patients in multiple situations. Durysta is a 1-mm preservative-free implant infused with 10 μg of bimatoprost, which actively releases medication 24 hours per day for approximately 4 months. It is a preloaded device with an ergonomic injector system (Figure 39-1), like the dexamethasone intravitreal steroid implant (Ozurdex).

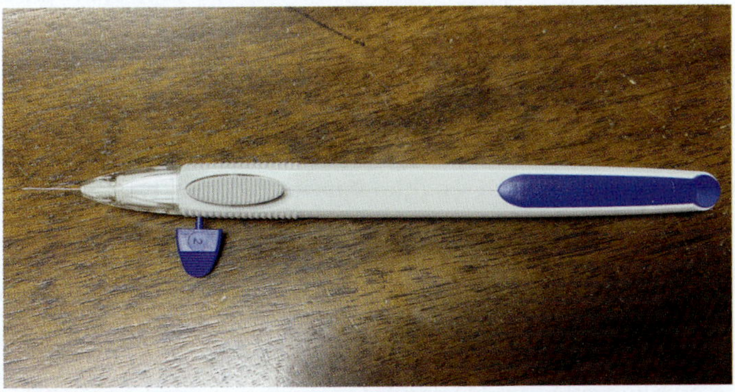

**FIGURE 39-1** Bimatoprost implant (Durysta) injector apparatus showing the 28-gauge needle at the end, the blue safety pin, and the white actuator button in the middle of the device.

# INDICATIONS

## Key Indications

- OAG
- Ocular hypertension (OHT)
- Secondary OAG

The indication is very broad. It is indicated for the reduction of IOP in patients with OAG or OHT. It is an option regardless of starting IOP or disease severity (mild, moderate, or severe). It is also approved for secondary OAG, including pigmentary, pseudoexfoliation, angle recession, and steroid-induced glaucoma.

# CONTRAINDICATIONS

## Key Contraindications

- Narrow angles or those whose angles may have sloping of the iris that could potentially cause the implant to sit more anterior to the trabecular membrane.
- Patients with active or suspected ocular or periocular infections
- Corneal endothelial cell dystrophy (e.g., Fuchs' dystrophy)
- Prior corneal transplantation or endothelial cell transplants (e.g., Descemet's stripping automated endothelial keratoplasty [DSAEK])
- Absent or ruptured posterior lens capsule, because of the risk of implant migration into the posterior segment
- Hypersensitivity to bimatoprost or to any other components of the product

The biodegradation rate of the implant varies between patient to patient, and thus in some patients, the vehicle (shell) can remain in the angle even a year later. In the two independent multicentered phase 3 trials, three implants were injected 4 months apart.[11,12] In a small percentage of patients, the second and even third implant ended up stacking on top of the previous implant causing the implants to make contact with the corneal endothelium. At 2 years, after three implants had been placed, 5.4% of patients were found to have endothelial cell loss more than 30%, whereas in the phase 1/2 trials, where patients received only one implant and were followed over 2 years, 0.9% of patients were found to have endothelial cell loss.[13] Until phase 4 studies are completed to determine the optimal timing between implantation, the U.S. Food and Drug Administration (FDA) decided to approve Durysta for a single administration only. It is important to note that no patient in the phase 1 to 3 studies developed complications because of endothelial cell loss. It was a numerical adverse event, and no patients developed clinically significant edema or loss of vision.

## PREOPERATIVE PREPARATION

### Key Preoperative Considerations

- Gonioscopy performed to confirm an open angle
- Confirming presence of indications and absence of contraindications
- Confirming patient noncompliance, reduction of quality of life, or lifestyle burdens created by eye drops
- Patient education regarding:
  - The nature of the procedure
  - The temporary nature of the implant
  - Single administration
- Consent form reviewed and signed
- Topical anesthetic eye drops (e.g., proparacaine 0.5%), topical antibiotic eye drops, and 5% povidone–iodine (Betadine) eye drops instilled into eye. One to two drops of each
- Sterile surgical gloves are set out and ready to be used.

Although the implant is actively releasing bimatoprost for 4 months, it is important to recognize the duration of IOP lowering after implantation has been seen for up to 2 years in up to 25% of patients and 1 year in 36% of patients with a single implant.[13] There seems to be a potential remodeling of the target tissues, including the ciliary body and trabecular meshwork (TM). Studies have demonstrated an increased expression of metalloproteinase (MMP) and a decreased expression of tissue inhibitor of metalloproteinase (TIMP) with both topical and intracameral bimatoprost.[14] The magnitude has been found to be significantly higher with intracameral administration.[14] This overexpression of MMP and significant inhibition of TIMP could be why we are seeing the prolonged duration of effect. In our own clinical experience, 70% of patients at 9 months and over 45% at 1 year do not need rescue therapy.

So how do we pick the right patient? First, the patient should have an open angle on gonioscopy. The patient should have a Shaffer grade 3 or greater opening. The contour of the iris is also a critical factor to take into account. If there is a significant sloping of the iris or a significant ridge as its approaches the angle, avoid implanting Durysta, as the implant may sit on the "ridge" and make contact with the corneal endothelium. We have learned the key to identifying a patient is not to wait for the "ideal" patient. Any patient with compliance issues could be a candidate. It's important to pay attention to clues of poor compliance, whether because of cost, side effects, forgetfulness, physical limitations, or OSD, these patients are in our offices every day. Patients are routinely telling us they are not compliant, but we are often busy and not able to pick up on their complaints. Involving the technicians can help to identify these patients. For instance, a patient may ask for "samples" every time they come in, indicating cost is an issue, may complain of fluctuating vision, indicating OSD, or may not even be able to recall the color of the top of the eye drop bottle, indicating likely forgetfulness. Regardless of the IOP or stability of the optic nerve head (ONH) and VF, if the patient indicates a high likelihood of poor compliance, has an open angle, and healthy corneal endothelium, they could be a candidate for Durysta.

Although the patient on topical prostaglandin (PGA) monotherapy is a great candidate, we have found patients on multiple drops can benefit from Durysta. This is true for not only being able to get off the topical PGA, but also in patients on multiple drops and poor compliance, getting off more than just the PGA. We have also found patients post-SLT tend to be open to the idea of a procedure and are motivated to avoid topical drops. If the IOP has risen post-SLT, or is not at target after treatment, Durysta can be a good option. We have also found it useful post-MIGS, when the IOP is not at target whether after a combination cataract surgery/MIGS or standalone MIGS, Durysta can help achieve that drop-free outcome for some time. We have noticed patients who received Durysta and refused an MIGS procedure in the past, ended up opting for an MIGS procedure once the Durysta effect wore off. Durysta seemed to serve as a bridge, helping them feel comfortable with the idea of a procedure. Those patients who may need a subconjunctival surgery like a trabeculectomy or XEN Gel Stent and have significant ocular surface inflammation can benefit from Durysta. This may permit the patient to discontinue the topical PGA in hopes of decreasing surface inflammation and thus less risk of postoperative bleb failure. In patients who have a more severe stage of glaucoma and are awaiting a subconjunctival surgery, we will also reduce the aqueous suppressants and start oral acetazolamide.

So how do we discuss this AC implant with our patients? Once you have identified a compliance-related issue, use the idea of "compliance" as the rationale to discuss the implant. You are offering a solution to their problem. When describing the procedure, express confidence. Avoid words such as "needle" or "injection." We will often say,

> Mrs. Smith, that eye drop you are taking at night seems to be causing some redness (insert any other compliance issue for that patient). We can help you. There is a product available that has the equivalent of 1 drop of the medication you are already taking in a small dissolvable pellet. Right here (behind the slit-lamp), where you get your pressures checked, I can press a button and gently place the pellet in your eye. The pellet releases the medication 24 hour a day for 4 months. The effect of the medication can last even longer. In some patients it can last even up to 2 years. We will follow you like we do now and when the eye pressure increases again, we can restart medications or consider alternative options. I think this would help you with the issues you are having and would be nice to give you a break from that drop.

Some clinicians are concerned with the single administration approval and feel it is a barrier for adoption. To us, it's all about the risk–benefit ratio. We tell patients there is no cure for glaucoma and no treatment that lasts forever. At any given time, we recommend treatments to help protect them from losing vision while also trying to maintain a high quality of life. Because the safety and patient experience is so positive with Durysta, the expectation of duration of effect is not as high as a surgical option, such as a conventional outflow MIGS procedure for example. When we offer SLT, which we tell patients work about 80% of the time, the effect is like a topical drop, and the effect can last anywhere from a few months to a few years. It is a similar discussion with Durysta. A benefit of Durysta over SLT is the responder rate seems to be a bit higher, well over 90% of patients have significant efficacy.[12] Once they understand the risks and benefits, patients do not seem to be turned off with the idea of Durysta being a temporary solution. Patients tell us the insertion procedure is easier than getting their eye pressures checked. To this day, we have not had a patient upset with us or regret having Durysta implanted even after the effect wore off. They routinely thank us for the time they had off the drop.

## PROCEDURE

Durysta implantation can be performed in the office at the slit lamp or in a minor procedure room. It can also be done at the ambulatory surgical center (ASC) or hospital outpatient department (HOPD). There is a facility fee associated with the procedure, which does make it realistic to perform at the ASC and HOPD. In the beginning, as an investigator in the phase 2 and 3 trials, I (IPS) performed the procedure in a minor procedure room using an operating microscope. Because of commercialization, I have transitioned all my cases to the slit lamp.

Regardless of where you perform the procedure, it is important to follow three important criteria.

1. Use good magnification, whether loops, a slit lamp, or a microscope.
2. Provide good patient head stabilization, that is, having a technician hold the patient's head still if performed at the slit lamp.
3. Follow good aseptic sterile technique, using 5% povidone–iodine (Betadine) prep, sterile gloves, and the option of peri-procedure topical antibiotics.

The basic steps to guide you on the slit-lamp implantation technique are as follows:

- Prior to your first case, spend time in a dry lab holding the device in each hand and using a model eye to practice the steps.
- After your first few cases, consider not using a speculum. The speculum can often get in the way of your hand and induce a squeeze reflex from the patient.
- Anesthetize the nonprocedure eye as well. This will prevent the patient from blinking either eye.
- Have the patient and the slit lamp in proper position before you take the device from your assistant.
- Once you have control of the device, remove the safety tabs of the device (Figure 39-2).
- Rest your hand on the cheek of the patient to stabilize the device (Figure 39-3).
- Have the patient focus on one part of the slit lamp. This will provide natural countertraction. This can allow you to avoid using a second instrument (cotton tip swab or 0.12 forceps) to keep the eye in primary position. Initially, you still may want to use a second instrument to stabilize the eye. You can apply a little countertraction using a soft cotton

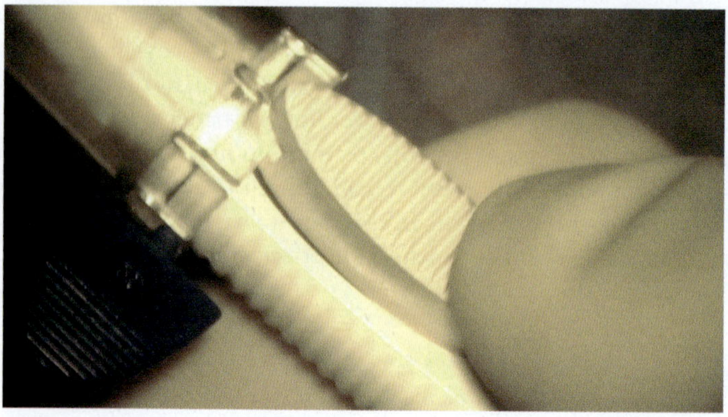

FIGURE 39-2 Magnified view of the blue safety pin (bottom left), and the white actuator button, which when pressed will release the implant. Notice the thumb pressing the back half of the button.

tip swab positioned 180° away from where you enter with the device needle. The second instrument can help to generate enough counterforce for a straightforward entry into the AC (Figure 39-4).

- The insertion is performed by entering the AC via the loader's 28-gauge needle (Figure 39-5) through the clear cornea, engaging just anterior to the limbal vessels (Figure 39-6).
- The goal is to enter the AC parallel to the iris and maintain the needle over the iris for the entire procedure.

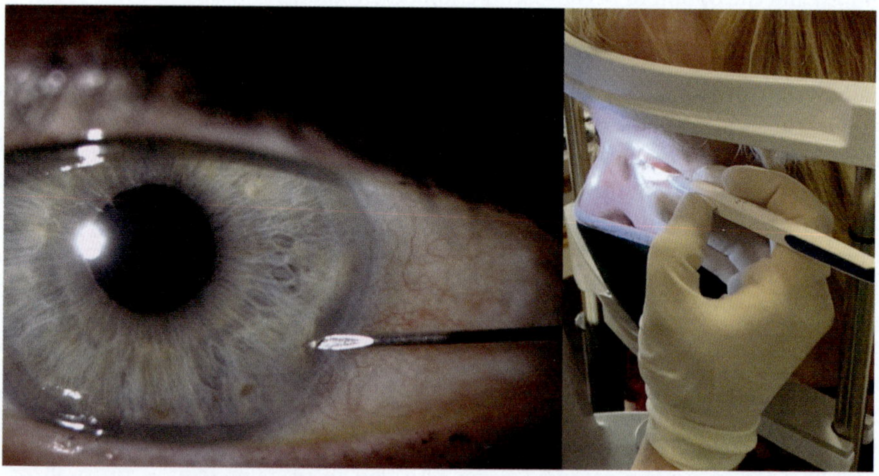

FIGURE 39-3 Proper hand placement showing stabilization of the hand and fingers on the patient's face (right side of the photo). Proper approach and entry of the needle through the cornea. Notice the needle is entering through the cornea at approximately the 4 to 5 o'clock position in this left eye.

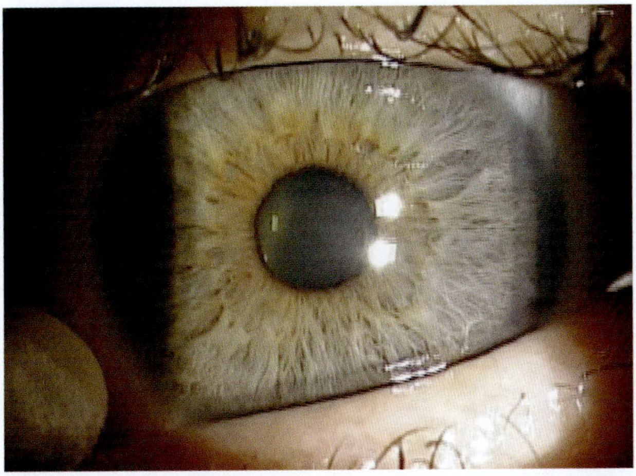

FIGURE 39-4 A secondary device, in this case a cotton-tipped applicator, is being used to apply a little countertraction opposite the needle as the procedure is about to be performed.

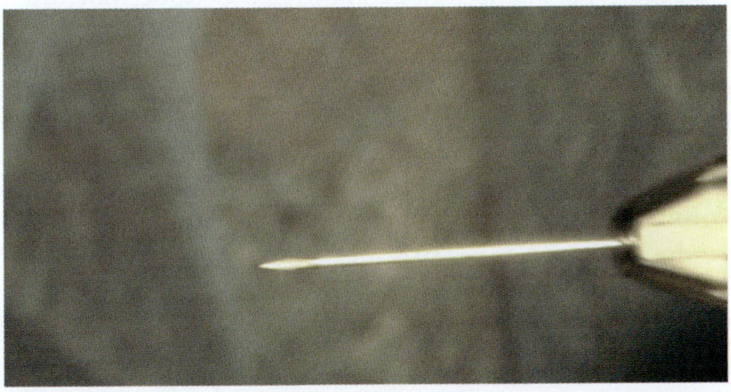

FIGURE 39-5 Magnified view of the 28-gauge needle at the end of the device. Of note, the implant is not visible in this photo.

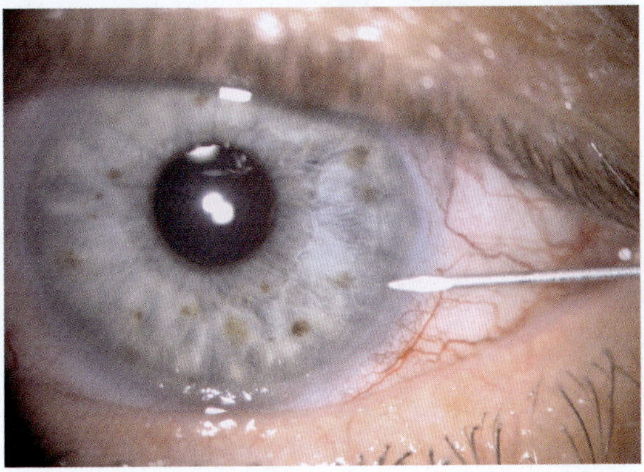

FIGURE 39-6 Proper placement and orientation of the needle as the procedure begins. Notice the placement at approximately the 4 o'clock position, with the needle located just anterior to the limbal blood vessels.

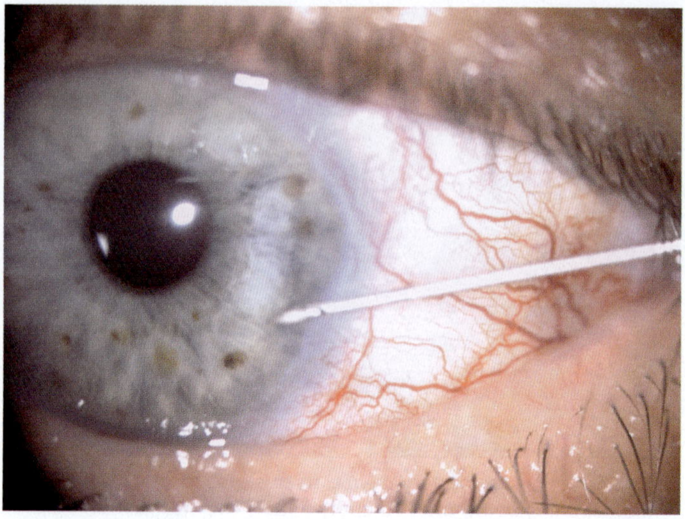

**FIGURE 39-7** Needle making its way through the cornea. A clear corneal injection is being performed in this photo. Notice how the eye has moved slightly nasal compared to Figure 39-6, this is because of the traction forces of moving the needle through the cornea. A countertraction device such as a cotton-tipped applicator or a forceps was not used in this procedure, and again is optional.

- One should enter at the clock hour that is most convenient to your hand position and the anatomy of the orbit and eye. We tend to enter around 7 or 8 o'clock for the right eye and 4 or 5 o'clock for the left eye (Figures 39-7 and 39-8).

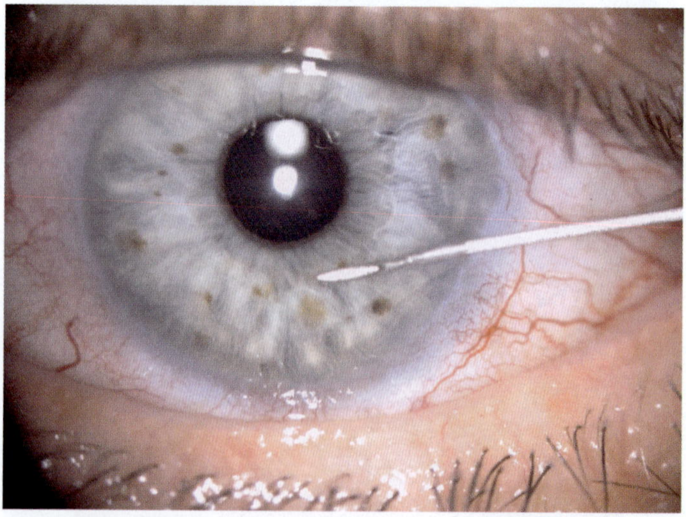

**FIGURE 39-8** The needle is now in the anterior chamber (AC) at the proper position for insertion of the pellet, approximately two bevel lengths into the AC. Notice how the needle is properly placed in front of the iris.

- If you are ambidextrous, for the right eye, use your left hand to hold the device to allow you to enter temporally near the 7 or 8 o'clock position, whereas for the left eye, you will want to use your right hand to enter near the 4 to 5 o'clock position. Entering at these clock hour positions will allow you to enter directly perpendicular to the cornea and maximize the area over the iris.
- After entering and ensuring you are two needle bevel lengths into the AC, press the posterior aspect of the actuator button (Figure 39-2), which is located on the device, to release the implant. Once the implant is released (Figures 39-9 and 39-10), come straight back out of the eye (Figure 39-11). It is important to remove the needle straight back out of the track to avoid tangential forces on the wound, which could cause aqueous to escape and the implant to migrate back to the wound. Also, make sure your thumb is already on the actuator button so you can press it without having to take your eyes away from the slit-lamp oculars. One pearl: press the oval button with conviction, for if you are too slow, the implant may get stuck to the needle.
- Check the wound using a surgical spear sponge or cotton tip swab to check for a wound leak (Figure 39-12). We do place a drop of antibiotic after the procedure, but do not give a prescription for eye drops to use at home.
- With gravity, the implant sinks to the inferior angle where it resides and slowly biodegrades into two inert substances, glycolic and lactic acid (Figure 39-13). Again, gonioscopy is crucial before considering Durysta.

We have found the slit-lamp technique flows well with our clinic schedules and provides a very low stress and overall positive experience for the patient. In fact, many patients have commented the procedure was more comfortable than an "eye pressure check." Again, we do not use a speculum or second instrument anymore because we enter the eye between 7 and 8 o'clock for the right eye and 4 and 5 o'clock for the left eye. This way, we do not need the patient's eyes

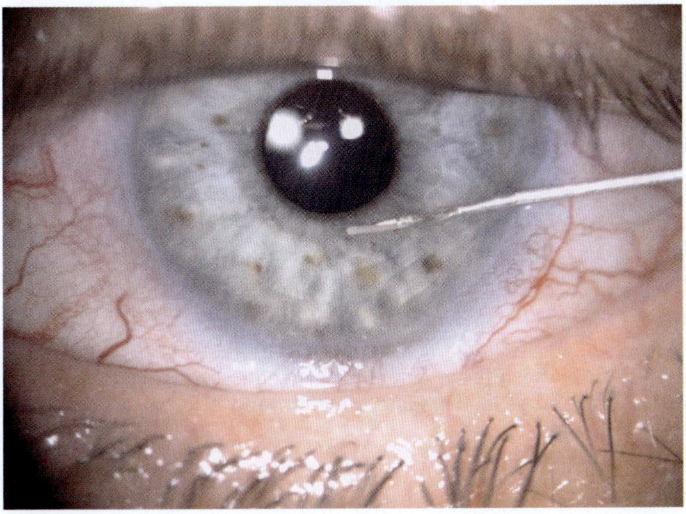

**FIGURE 39-9** The actuator button is being depressed, and the implant is starting to be released from the device.

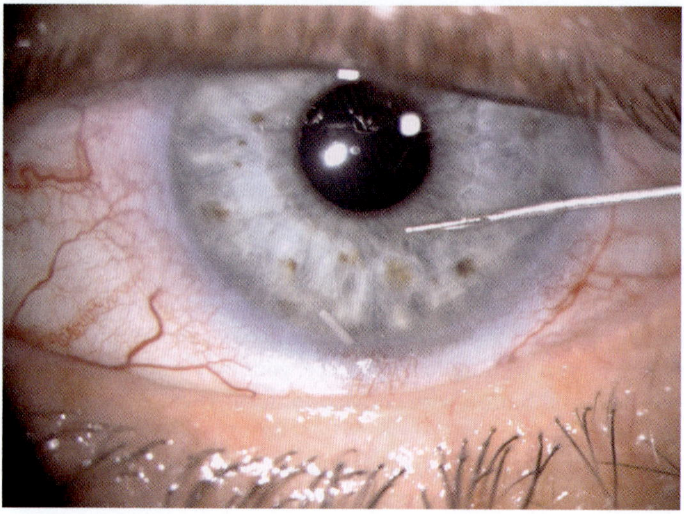

FIGURE 39-10 The actuator button has been fully depressed, and the implant has been released and immediately falls toward the inferior angle.

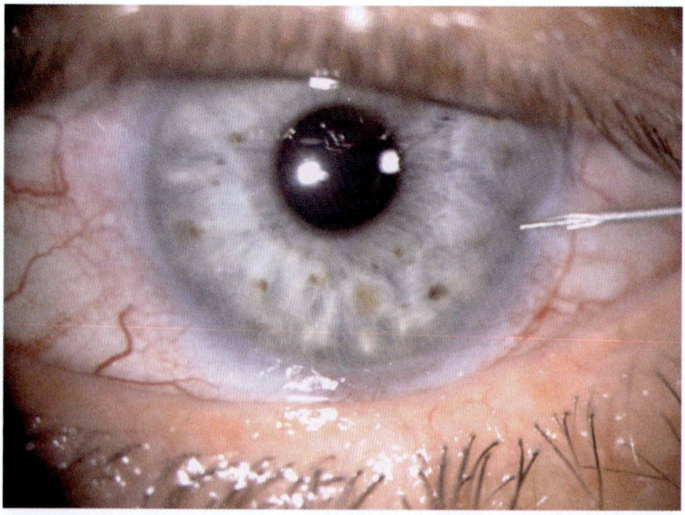

FIGURE 39-11 The implant is no longer visible as it has fallen completely into the inferior angle. The needle is removed from the anterior chamber in the same direction and orientation as it was inserted.

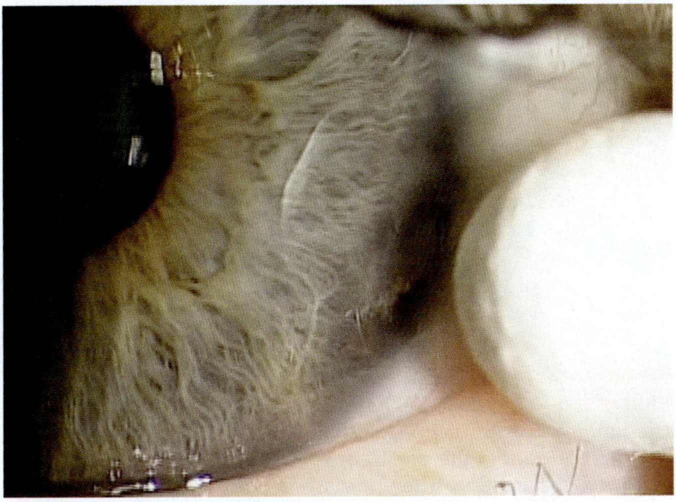

**FIGURE 39-12** A cotton-tipped applicator is being used to gently tamponade the wound to ensure wound closure and a negative Seidel sign.

wide open. We can have them keep their eye open naturally and have them stare at a part of the slit lamp to provide eye stability and countertraction without using a second instrument. We do anesthetize both eyes, even if only performing the procedure in one eye, which helps to prevent the patient from squeezing the nonprocedure eye. We use the cheek bones to rest our wrist and last three fingers, which helps to stabilize our hand. By avoiding a speculum or second

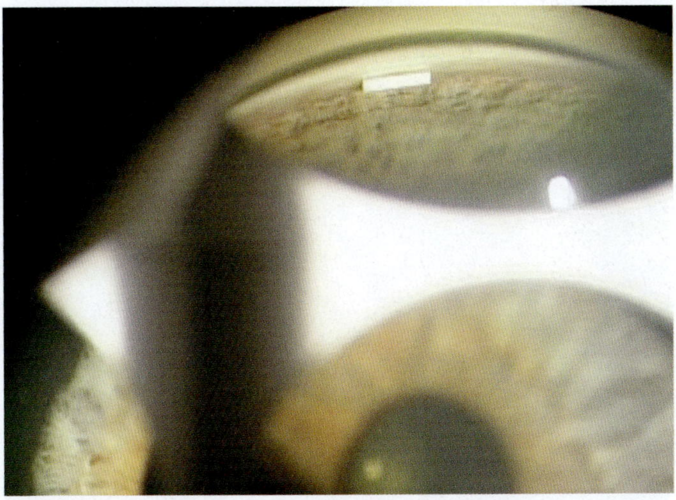

**FIGURE 39-13** Gonioscopic view of the inferior angle showing perfect position of the bimatoprost pellet (Durysta) a few minutes after the procedure was completed.

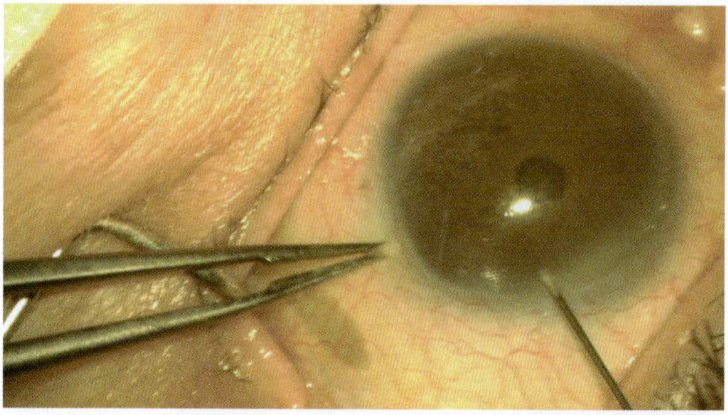

**FIGURE 39-14** Durysta being inserted into the anterior chamber with the patient in the supine position. Notice a lid speculum is being used to better hold the eyelids open, and forceps are being used to apply countertraction. The approach is more temporal in this procedure with the needle entering at around the 2 o'clock position in this left eye.

instrument, patients do not tend to view the insertion as a surgery or even minor procedure, rather they think of it as part of the routine eye examination. We verbally count down from 10 to 0 to give them a goal, which helps them continue to keep their eyes open.

If performing the procedure in the supine position, whether in office, ASC, or HOPD, the above steps should be followed with a few possible adjustments below.

- We do recommend a speculum, which does not seem to get in the way of your hand and device (Figure 39-14).
- We sit and enter the eye more temporal than when at the slit lamp (9 or 10 o'clock right eye, 2 or 3 o'clock left eye), aiming over the iris toward the inferior angle (Figures 39-14 and 39-15).

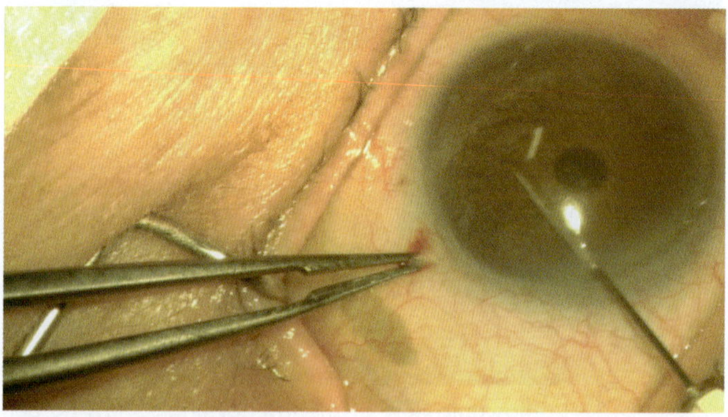

**FIGURE 39-15** The bimatoprost implant has been successfully ejected from the applicator in the same patient as Figure 39.14. The implant will rest on the iris until the patient sits up, at which time it will fall into the inferior angle.

- Tell the patient to focus on the microscope lights.
- We tend to use a second instrument to stabilize the eye.
- If at the ASC or HOPD, I tend to schedule the procedures at the end of the surgical day, whereas in the office via the slit-lamp technique, I schedule patients throughout the day. For the office implantations, I do not implant the same day as the consult, rather I order the procedure and have my staff send for insurance verification and set up another time for the implantation.

The majority of clinicians implant Durysta in one eye, then have the patient come back for the other eye a week or 10 days later. In my clinic, if a patient needs the implant in both eyes, I insert Durysta in both eyes at the same visit. This helps with scheduling and number of patient visits. It is important to note that although you will receive full reimbursement for the cost of goods for both implants, you will receive 50% of the physician reimbursement for the second eye if you implant in both eyes on the same day. I have found the patient perception of the procedure to be even more positive by implanting both eyes on the same day, which makes it again, more like an eye pressure check, rather than a "procedure," in their minds. We have trained a few technicians to prep the patients with 5% povidone–iodine and topical anesthetic and antibiotic drops. Therefore, when we get in to the room, the consent has been signed and the slit lamp, product, and our sterile surgical gloves are on the table. There is very little disruption to the flow of the clinic. We don't have a special Durysta day. We basically incorporate these visits into our normal clinic days. Patients go home with instructions to call us if any pain, increased redness or decreased vision develops, or any other new symptoms occur. We have not yet seen an infection, and no cases of infection were identified in the trials.[11,12]

## POSTOPERATIVE CARE/COMANAGEMENT (FOLLOW-UP SCHEDULE)

### Key Postoperative Considerations

- Topical ophthalmic antibiotic eye drop instilled in office immediately after the procedure
- Patient education regarding:
  - Keep head elevated for the first day
  - Do not rub your eyes for the first 48 to 72 hours
- Return to clinic (RTC) in 4 to 6 weeks for an IOP check and gonioscopy to check positioning of the implant

We do not prescribe topical antibiotic drops after the procedure. Good aseptic conditions during the implantation are crucial to preventing infection. We do tell patients to keep their head elevated for the first day to allow the implant to settle in the inferior angle. We remind them not to rub their eye for at least 2 days to prevent infection. We have patients return to the clinic in 4 to 6 weeks for a follow-up IOP check and gonioscopy to check positioning of the implant. Assuming the IOP is at target, we will have them return based on their disease severity. For a patient with mild OAG, assuming the IOP is at target at the 4 to 6 weeks visit, we have them come back in 6 months. For a patient with moderate-to-severe OAG, we have them return in 3 to 4 months. Based on the phase 3 trials, the IOPs did not return to baseline rapidly and there was often a slow rise in the IOP.[11,12] Therefore, you should be able to identify patients as their IOPs are rising and then decide if they need to restart drops or consider an alternative treatment. We have often kept patients off drops even if the IOP is a couple mm Hg higher at the follow-up visit, especially if they are still in the target range. We would rather have a patient 1 or 2 mm Hg higher but without compliance issues than a patient noncompliant with drops that could potentially lead to fluctuating IOPs. It will take some time and experience to decide when you reinitiate topical therapy or recommend another intervention.

## POTENTIAL COMPLICATIONS AND THEIR TREATMENT

Although the procedure and product are safe, there are potential complications that can arise during and after the implantation. One must be aware of these complications and be comfortable managing them.

### Troubleshooting Scenarios

- Touching the iris with the needle—If you enter too far anteriorly, you increase the chances of pointing toward the iris. If this happens, back up and change the angle of your needle more parallel to the iris. If need be, come out and re-engage more back toward the limbus.
- Touching the phakic lens—If the anterior capsule is not ruptured, there are changes to the postoperative regimen. Watch for cataract formation. If there is a rupture to the anterior capsule, watch for an AC reaction, address a potential inflammatory reaction, and consider natural lens removal. Initially, we recommend implanting Durysta in pseudophakic eyes, then after a few cases, include phakic eyes. Currently, 70% of the implanted eyes in our practice are phakic eyes. Phase 3 trials confirmed no cataract formation post-Durysta implantation in phakic eyes.[11,12]
- The implant sticks to the needle tip—The implant tends to stick to the end of the 28-gauge needle tip. If this should occur, first wait for a few seconds to see if it will disengage. If it does not, gently press the implant against the anterior iris to engage it and slightly rotate the applicator to disconnect the implant from the needle tip. If this does not work, you can come back out as planned, the implant will usually separate from the needle as the needle comes in contact with the inner aspect of the wound.
  - See Video 39-2 of the "Double Press" technique to avoid the implant from getting stuck on the needle tip. Once the needle is two bevel lengths in the AC, press the button halfway until you see the implant coming out of the needle. Hold your position and wait for a second to allow aqueous to come in contact with the implant. This will prevent an air bubble from causing the implant to stick to the needle. After waiting a second, further depress the button all the way with conviction, to release the implant.

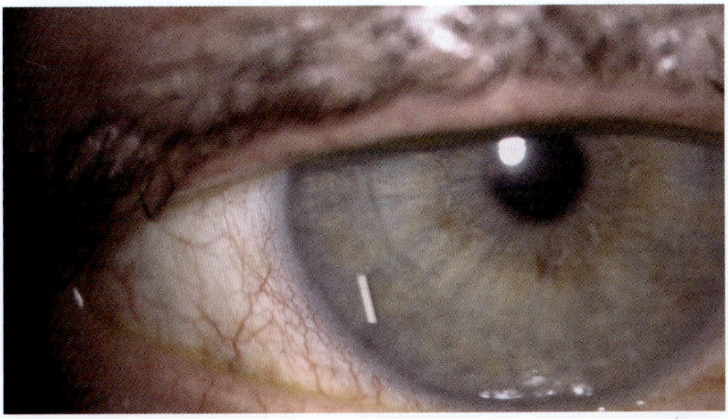

FIGURE 39-16 The implant stuck to the inside of the wound. A cotton-tipped applicator could be used to tap over the area to see if that dislodges the implant. If that doesn't work, an anterior chamber probe can be used to dislodge the implant.

- If the implant adheres to the inside of the wound (Figure 39-16), you can tap the cornea externally with a cotton tip swab or a forceps and the implant should separate and eventually sink to the inferior angle. If needed, one can use an "AC probe" supplied by Allergan to enter the needle track and push the implant away from the wound (Figure 39-17).
- The implant separates from the needle, but an air bubble causes it to rise toward the superior angle (Figure 39-18)—The air bubble will eventually evaporate and the implant will sink to the inferior angle (Figures 39-19 and 39-20). There is no additional intervention needed.

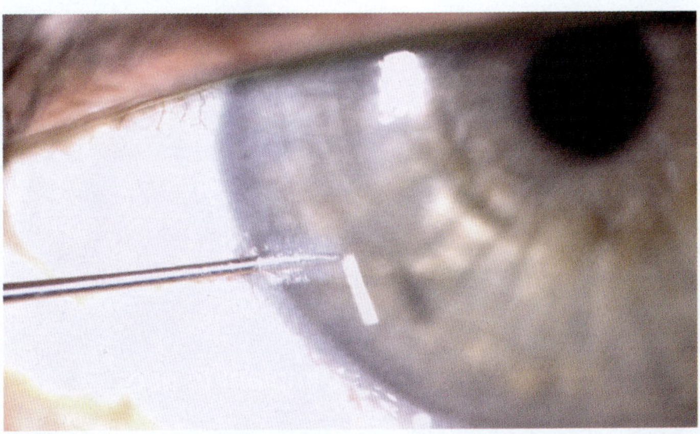

FIGURE 39-17 An anterior chamber probe being used to dislodge the stuck bimatoprost implant.

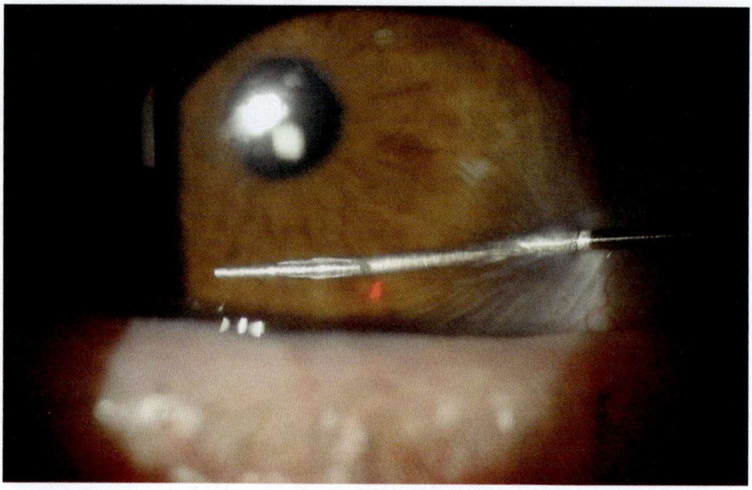

**FIGURE 39-18** In this procedure, an air bubble caused the implant to immediately rise after it was ejected from the applicator. Notice the implant immediately to the left of the pupil in the dark portion of the photo. The implant is oriented perfectly vertical in this photo.

- The implant sinks behind the iris—There is no need to remove the implant or go chasing after it. There is no harm if the implant resides behind the iris. In fact, in the phase 3 trials, a few of the implants initially resting behind the iris were found to migrate, with the flow of aqueous, anteriorly into the inferior angle.

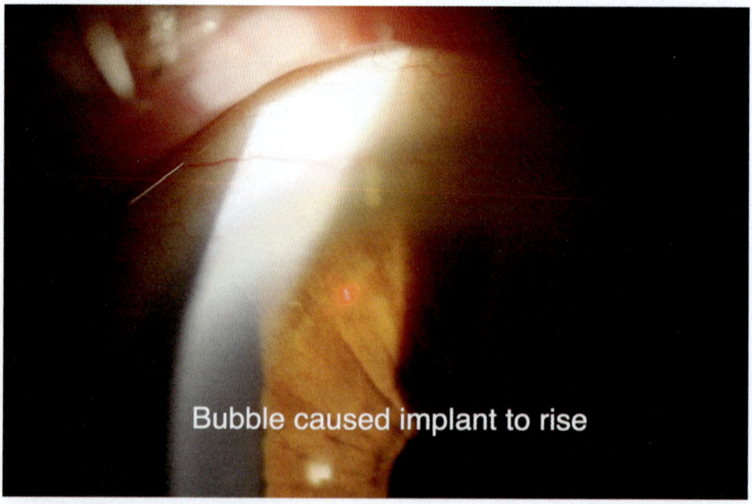


**FIGURE 39-19** The air bubble continued to cause the implant to rise all the way up into the superior angle.

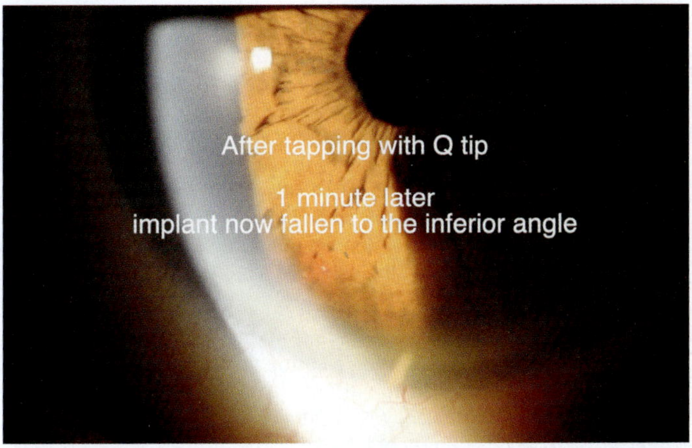


**FIGURE 39-20** After tapping the area with a cotton-tipped applicator and waiting for a minute or two, the bimatoprost implant fell into the inferior angle.

## Complications

- Postoperative inflammation: Rarely, a patient may have an AC reaction to the vehicle, even more rare, to the active ingredient. Topical nonsteroidal anti-inflammatory drug (NSAID) for a week or even a short course of a topical steroid can reduce the inflammation and remain quiescent more long term.
- Corneal edema: Although there were no reported cases of corneal edema in the trials, corneal edema has occurred in clinical practice. Most often this is because of implants being placed in eyes with risky angles or in patients with compromised corneas. If peripheral edema occurs, one can observe if it is localized, because the implant will biodegrade. If there are any signs of progression, one can remove the implant.

## VIDEOS OF PROCEDURES

**Video 39-1**—This video demonstrates the sterile technique for Durysta insertion at the slit lamp. First, prior to the clinician coming into the room, the technician preps the patient. The technician first places a drop of anesthetic drops into both eyes (so the patient does not blink the nonprocedure eye), then 5% povidone–iodine solution in the procedure eye followed by a flush of balanced salt irrigating solution. Using a sterile 4 × 4 gauze, the technician wipes the external lids to remove any potential povidone–iodine and debris and then places a drop of antibiotic on the eye. The patient is then brought to the slit lamp and positioned by the clinician. Using sterile gloves, the product is removed from the packaging and the protective shipping portion is also removed. The patient is told to fixate on a spot of the slit lamp and their head is stabilized by the technician. The clinician stabilizes their hand on the cheek of the patient, holding the Durysta loader with the thumb on the actuator button. The needle of the loader enters the eye just anterior to the limbal vessels through the clear cornea and maintaining the needle parallel to the iris. Once two bevel lengths of the needle is in the anterior chamber (AC), the back portion of the button is pressed with conviction to release the implant into the AC. The needle is retracted in the same direction as it was inserted. (Video courtesy of I. Paul Singh.)

**Video 39-2**—This video demonstrates the "Double Press" technique, without the need for a speculum. The patient has already been prepped, anesthetized, and positioned at the slit lamp. Using the cheek of the patient to stabilize the hand, enter the eye through the clear cornea (anterior to the limbal vessels) at approximately the 4 o'clock position (8 o'clock for the right eye). There is some slight torquing of the eye, which is why it is important for verbal reminders to look at a fixation spot on the slit lamp. Once you are two bevel lengths into the AC with the needle, depress the white actuator button halfway until one sees the implant outside of the needle. Hold for a split second to allow aqueous to bathe the implant and prevent an air bubble from keeping the implant stuck to the needle tip. After the split second hold, further depress the button to fully release the implant into the AC. Remove the needle and then watch the implant sink to the inferior angle. (Video courtesy of I. Paul Singh.)

**Video 39-3**—This video demonstrates how the implant may rise up to the superior angle when released into the AC. If this happens, one can use a cotton tip applicator to apply pressure externally at the limbus to help the air bubble release from the implant. Alternatively, one can wait for the air bubble to naturally separate and the implant will eventually fall to the inferior angle without need for any further intervention. (Video courtesy of I. Paul Singh.)

**Video 39-4**—This video demonstrates a Durysta implantation procedure using a supine approach. The patient has been prepped and has a speculum between the eyelids. The clinician is sitting temporal to the patient. After inspecting the Durysta delivery device, hold the eye with a second instrument (optional) and engage the eye superior temporally with the needle. Enter parallel to the iris and stay over the iris. Once two bevel lengths of the needle is in the AC, press the white actuator button to release the implant. Then remove the needle in the same direction as you entered. You can see the implant in the inferior angle immediately after the procedure. (Video courtesy of I. Paul Singh.)

**Video 39-5**—This video demonstrates a slit-lamp insertion of Durysta. The needle of the loader enters the eye at the 4 o'clock position in this left eye, keeping the needle over the iris the entire time. Once two bevel lengths of the needle is in the AC, the actuator button is pressed to release the implant in the AC. The implant can be seen sinking immediately to the inferior angle. (Video courtesy of I. Paul Singh.)

**Video 39-6**—This video demonstrates the use of the AC probe supplied by Allergan to "dislodge" the implant from the cornea. If the implant should get stuck to the corneal endothelium, one can tap the cornea externally using a second instrument or a cotton tip applicator to help facilitate separation. One can also use the AC probe to "push" the implant away from the endothelium and allow it to sink to the inferior angle. (Video courtesy of I. Paul Singh.)

**Video 39-7**—This video demonstrates a slit-lamp insertion of Durysta. The needle of the loader enters the eye at the 4 o'clock position in this left eye, keeping the needle over the iris the entire time. Notice a little countertraction is applied using a soft cotton tip swab positioned 180° away from where the needle entered the cornea. Once two bevel lengths of the needle is in the AC, the actuator button is pressed to release the implant in the AC. The implant can be seen sinking immediately to the inferior angle. A cotton-tipped applicator is used to gently tap on the wound to ensure a sealed entry site with a negative Seidel sign. Lastly, a quick gonioscopy view shows the Durysta implant settled nicely into the inferior angle. (Video courtesy of Nate Lighthizer.)

## EFFICACY

The ARTEMIS 1 and ARTEMIS 2 phase 3 clinical trials were two multicenter, randomized, parallel-group, controlled studies comparing the 10-μg bimatoprost implant to twice-daily timolol 0.5% topical drops. Parallel groups of patients diagnosed with OAG or OHT (with a baseline IOP of 22–32 mm Hg at hour 0 after washout) were followed for a period of

20 months, including an 8-month extended follow-up. Durysta lowered mean IOP by up to 33% from baseline over the 12-week primary efficacy period. This works out to be about 5 to 8 mm Hg of reduction from the mean baseline IOP of 24.5 mm Hg.[15]

The trials involved 1,122 subjects that were randomized to treatment with the implant versus topical timolol eye drops. Patients that were randomized to the bimatoprost implant had the drug administered in the study eye on day 1, week 16, and week 32. Patients randomized to topical timolol were treated with twice-daily dosing. By week 12, patients randomized to the bimatoprost implant achieved an IOP reduction from 24.6 to 17.7 mm Hg, representing approximately a 30% reduction from baseline. The bimatoprost implant met predefined criteria for noninferiority compared to timolol.

To evaluate the ideal dose and duration of effect, the phase I/II dose-ranging study enrolled 63 participants who were randomized to 6, 10, 15, or 20 μg bimatoprost implant administration in their study eye and topical bimatoprost once daily in their fellow (control) eye and followed for 24 months.[13] Eyes were permitted to receive a single repeat implant administration or rescue topical IOP-lowering medication during the study period. By 24 months, IOP was reduced from baseline by 7.5, 7.3, 7.3, and 8.9 mm Hg in the 6, 10, 15, and 20 μg bimatoprost implant groups, respectively. A single administration of the bimatoprost implant was found to control IOP in 40% of patients for up to 12 months and in 28% of patients for up to 24 months. In eyes treated with topical bimatoprost, mean IOP reduction from baseline was 8.2 mm Hg at 24 months.

A 24-month, open-label, multicenter, long-term safety and efficacy extension of the phase 3 trial enrolled patients with OAG or OHT after their completion of a bimatoprost implant phase 3 clinical trial.[16] Enrollment was optional. This analysis included patients who had received 10 or 15-μg bimatoprost implant in the study eye on day 1 and weeks 16 and 32 in a 20-month, randomized, phase 3 ARTEMIS trial. Rescue with topical drops was allowed if the study eye did not meet/maintain IOP expectations (investigator decision). The analysis evaluated IOP and the number of patients who received no additional (rescue) IOP-lowering treatment in the study eye for 2 or more years after the last implant administration during the ARTEMIS trial. Among 181 implant-treated patients who completed ARTEMIS and enrolled in the study extension, 48 had not been rescued at the study extension screening, and 32 did not require rescue for 2 or more years after their last implant administration. For these 32 patients (16 treated with 10-μg implant, 16 with 15-μg implant), mean (±SD) time without rescue after the last implant administration was 2.6 ± 0.5 years (range, 2.0–4.0), and mean (±SD) IOP was 23.4 ± 1.9 mm Hg at initial (ARTEMIS study) baseline and 18.1 ± 3.1 mm Hg at the last recorded visit (still without rescue). Seven patients remained untreated for 3 or more years (range, 3.1–4.0); their mean (±SD) IOP was 22.8 ± 1.5 mm Hg at baseline and 18.0 ± 4.1 mm Hg at the last recorded visit (still without rescue). This data reconfirmed the phase I/II data that Durysta can have a sustained IOP lowering and require no IOP-lowering treatment for 2 or more years after their last administration.

## CODING/BILLING

There are two codes needed when billing for Durysta: a procedure code (Current Procedural Terminology [CPT] code) and a drug code (Healthcare Common Procedure Coding System [HCPCS] code), commonly referred to as a J-code. The CPT code for Durysta, 66030, is an established Category I code for injecting medication into the AC. If you administer Durysta into both eyes on the same date of service, the standard multiple procedure rules apply. The CPT code for Durysta carries a 10-day global period.

The J-code is for the drug. A product-specific J-code has been established and is valid for dates of service on or after October 1, 2020, for all sites of service. This product-specific code is a Level II HCPCS code and is J7351, "Injection, bimatoprost, intracameral implant, 1 μg." It's important to note that the billing description for Durysta is 1 μg, yet it is a 10-μg implant, so you need to bill J7351 as 10 units. When offices are checking a patient's benefits, they will need to check for both the CPT code and the J-code. Also include J7351 along with the CPT code on the CMS-1500 form.

Common ICD-10 diagnostic codes that support the use of Durysta implants into the AC include:

**Open-angle glaucoma**

- **H40.10X** (unspecified OAG)
- **H40.111** (primary OAG, right eye)
- **H40.112** (primary OAG, left eye)
- **H40.113** (primary OAG, bilateral)
- **H40.119** (primary OAG, unspecified eye)
- **H40.131** (pigmentary glaucoma, right eye)
- **H40.132** (pigmentary glaucoma, left eye)
- **H40.133** (pigmentary glaucoma, bilateral)
- **H40.139** (pigmentary glaucoma, unspecified eye)
- **H40.141** (capsular glaucoma with pseudoexfoliation of lens, right eye)
- **H40.142** (capsular glaucoma with pseudoexfoliation of lens, left eye)
- **H40.143** (capsular glaucoma with pseudoexfoliation of lens, bilateral)
- **H40.149** (capsular glaucoma with pseudoexfoliation of lens, unspecified eye)

**Ocular hypertension**

- **H40.051** (OHT, right eye)
- **H40.052** (OHT, left eye)
- **H40.053** (OHT, bilateral)
- **H40.059** (OHT, unspecified eye)

## FUTURE TECHNOLOGIES

Several other sustained-release devices are in development, including a travoprost intracameral implant (OTX-TIC; Ocular Therapeutix) similar in technology to the Durysta implant, a latanoprost microdose device (MicroProst; Eyenovia), and a travoprost-latanoprost punctal plug (Evolute; Mati Therapeutics). Recently, a single-piece, hydrophobic acrylic intraocular lens (IOL) and bimatoprost drug-eluting pads securely attached to the haptics of the IOL implanted directly into the capsular bag during routine cataract surgery have been studied (Spyglass Pharma). Six-month data were presented at the 2023 Glaucoma 360 New Horizons meeting.

There are other glaucoma drug delivery devices in phase 2 or 3 FDA trials that can be subdivided into nonsurgical external modalities and surgically implanted devices. The external modalities include latanoprost microdose delivery with Optejet (Microprost, Eyenovia) and latanoprost or travoprost delivery via a punctal plug (L-evolute and T-evolute, Mati Therapeutics). Surgically implanted devices in trials include two travoprost delivery vehicles, ENV515 (Envisia Therapeutics) and iDose (Glaukos).[17-19]

However, the next drug delivery product likely to be approved in the United States is the iDose TR intracameral travoprost-releasing implant from Glaukos. I (IPS) was a principal investigator for both the phase 2 and phase 3 clinical trials for iDose TR. The device is a 1.8-mm × 0.5-mm biocompatible titanium implant that releases a proprietary formulation of travoprost inside the AC.[20,21] Like Durysta, eluting a PGA inside the eye bypasses the corneal surface permeability issues, allowing for a consistent 24-hour delivery of the active drug over time without the significant side effects of topical PGAs on the surface and extraocular tissues. The implant has three parts: a scleral anchor that passes through the TM and sits within the scleral wall; the body of the device, which serves as the drug reservoir; and the elution membrane, which allows for the consistent release of travoprost over time.

We implanted the iDose in our sterile in-office surgical suite, but most surgeons performed the procedure at an ambulatory surgery center or hospital. This standalone implantation procedure was efficient and intuitive—the process will seem familiar to surgeons who have implanted an iStent Inject. We created a 2.2-mm incision and filled the AC with a cohesive viscoelastic. We then rotated the head and scope nasally, and with a gonioprism and viscoelastic on the cornea, we viewed the nasal angle in the same way as our MIGS procedures. We then introduced the ergonomic iDose loader and aimed it at the TM. We then applied direct perpendicular pressure to anchor the implant into the scleral wall and released the prongs. We confirmed its stability by using the loader to nudge the device from side to side and made sure the device was not pointing down toward the iris. We used manual irrigation and aspiration to remove viscoelastic and hydrated the wounds with balanced salt solution.

The phase 2 trial enrolled 154 patients with OAG or OHT. Patients in the study were randomly assigned to receive a fast-elution implant, a slow-elution implant, or sham surgery followed by twice-daily topical timolol maleate 0.5%. Post-procedure IOP was measured over 12 months. At 3 months, mean IOP reductions for both iDose groups and the control group were similar, ranging from 8.5 mm Hg (a 33% decrease from baseline) in the fast implant group, 8 mm Hg (32% decrease) in the slow implant group, and 7.6 mm Hg (30% decrease) in the timolol group. IOP was controlled without additional medications in 82% of the two iDose groups and 74% in the control group. At 12 months, IOP in both iDose groups remained around 32% below baseline. IOP in sham (patients treated with topical medications) was similar at around 30%.

Safety outcomes were favorable, as there were no serious adverse events. Through 12 weeks, there was no increased conjunctival hyperemia in either treatment arm, and travoprost was not detected in any study patient's blood serum. In addition, the mean number of glaucoma medications ranged from 0.54 to 0.56 at 12 months in the fast- and slow-elution iDose TR groups, respectively, compared to 0.72 mean medications in the timolol group.[10]

The recently reported phase 2b results are based on an analysis conducted at 36 months for all 154 subjects randomized into the trial. Subjects in the iDose TR arms received a single intracameral implant, whereas the subjects randomized to the timolol active comparator received twice-daily eye drops over the 36-month evaluation period, which equates to approximately 2,190 eye drops per eye, per protocol. In the fast- and slow-release iDose TR arms, 70% and 68% of subjects, respectively, were well controlled, with the same or fewer IOP-lowering topical medications at 36 months versus screening, compared to 46% of subjects in the timolol control arm. In this responder group, average IOP reductions from baseline observed at 36 months were 8.3 and 8.5 mm Hg in the fast- and slow-release iDose TR arms, respectively, versus 8.2 mm Hg in the timolol control arm. Overall, iDose TR subjects performed similarly to timolol subjects at 36 months in terms of mean IOP reductions with fewer topical medications versus timolol. The 36-month phase 2b data also continued to demonstrate a favorable safety profile for iDose TR, with no clinically significant corneal endothelial cell loss, no serious corneal adverse events, and no adverse events of periorbital fat atrophy or conjunctival hyperemia reported to date in either elution arm.[13]

The TR phase 3 trial compared iDose TR devices at both fast- and slow elution rates to twice-daily topical timolol. The phase 3 trials randomized a total of 1,150 subjects across 89 clinical sites, most of which are in the United States.[14] The phase 3 trial results are expected to support Glaukos's new drug application (NDA) submission (submitted February 2023), with Prescription Drug User Fee Act (PDUFA) date of December 22, 2023.

## REFERENCES


1. Newman-Casey PA, Blachley T, Lee PP, et al. Patterns of glaucoma medication adherence over four years of follow-up. *Ophthalmology.* 2015;122(10):2010-2021.
2. Fechtner RD, Godfrey DG, Budenz D, et al. Prevalence of ocular surface complaints in patients with glaucoma using topical intraocular pressure-lowering medications. *Cornea.* 2010;29(6):618-621.
3. Erb C, Gast U, Schremmer D, et al. German register for glaucoma patients with dry eye. I. Basic outcome with respect to dry eye. *Graefes Arch Clin Exp Ophthalmol.* 2008;246(11):1593-1601.
4. Leung EW, Medieros FA, Weinreb RN, et al. Prevalence of ocular surface disease in glaucoma patients. *J Glaucoma.* 2008(5);17:350-355.
5. Baudouin C. Detrimental effect of preservatives in eyedrops: implications for the treatment of glaucoma. *Acta Ophthalmol.* 2008;86(7):716-726.
6. Ederer F, Gaasterland DE, Sullivan EK; AGIS Investigators. The Advanced Glaucoma Intervention Study (AGIS): 1. Study design and methods and baseline characteristics of study patients. *Control Clin Trials.* 1994;15(4):299-325. doi:10.1016/0197-2456(94)90046-9
7. Matlach J, Bender S, König J, et al. Investigation of intraocular pressure fluctuation as a risk factor of glaucoma progression. *Clin Ophthalmol.* 2018;13:9-16. doi:10.2147/OPTH.S186526
8. Gazzard G, Konstantakopoulou E, Garway-Heath D, et al; LiGHT Trial Study Group. LiGHT trial: 6-year results of primary selective laser trabeculoplasty versus eye drops for the treatment of glaucoma and ocular hypertension. *Ophthalmology.* 2023;130(2):139-151. doi: 10.1016/j.ophtha.2022.09.009
9. Ahmed IIK, De Francesco T, Rhee D, et al; HORIZON Investigators. Long term outcomes from the HORIZON randomized trial for a Schlemm's canal microstent in combination cataract and glaucoma surgery. *Ophthalmology.* 2022;129(7):742-751. doi:10.1016/j.ophtha.2022.02.021
10. Samuelson TW, Singh IP, Williamson BK, et al. Quality of life in primary open-angle glaucoma and cataract: an analysis of VFQ-25 and OSDI from the iStent inject® pivotal trial. *Am J Ophthalmol.* 2021;229:220-229. doi:10.1016/j.ajo.2021.03.007
11. Medeiros FA, Walters TR, Kolko M, et al; ARTEMIS 1 Study Group. Phase 3, randomized, 20-month study of bimatoprost implant in open-angle glaucoma and ocular hypertension (ARTEMIS 1). *Ophthalmology* 2020;127:1627-1641.

12. Bacharach J, Tatham A, Ferguson G, et al; ARTEMIS 2 Study Group. Phase 3, randomised, 20-month study of the efficacy and safety of bimatoprost implant in patients with open-angle glaucoma and ocular hypertension (ARTEMIS 2). *Drugs* 2021;81:2017-2033.
13. Craven ER, Walters T, Christie WC, et al. 24-month phase I/II clinical trial of bimatoprost sustained-release implant (bimatoprost SR) in glaucoma patients. *Drugs*. 2020;80:167-179.
14. Yamada H, Yoneda M, Gosho M, et al.. Bimatoprost, latanoprost, and tafluprost induce differential expression of matrix metalloproteinases and tissue inhibitor of metalloproteinases. *BMC Ophthalmol.* 2016;16:26
15. ClinicalTrials.gov. Safety and efficacy of bimatoprost sustained-release in patients with open-angle glaucoma or ocular hypertension. https://classic.clinicaltrials.gov/ct2/show/NCT02250651
16. Medeiros FA, Nagar S, Bejanian M, et al. Extended duration of IOP lowering with bimatoprost implant in a phase 3 open-label extension study. *Invest Ophthalmol Vis Sci.* 2021;62(8):2778.
17. Schweitzer J, Ibach M. Sustained-release drug delivery: the future of glaucoma treatment? *Glaucoma Today.* Accessed June 12, 2020. https://glaucomatoday.com/articles/2016-nov-dec/sustained-release-drug-delivery-the-future-of-glaucoma-treatment
18. Goldberg DF, Williams R. A phase 2 study evaluating safety and efficacy of the latanoprost punctal plug delivery system (L-PPDS) in subjects with ocular hypertension (OH) or open-angle glaucoma (OAG). *IOVS ARVO Journals*. https://iovs.arvojournals.org/article.aspx?articleid=2358808 (accessed 22 November 2019).
19. Helzner J. Microdose latanoprost delivery set for broad patient base. Glaucoma Physician. Accessed June 12, 2020. https://www.glaucomaphysician.net/issues/2019/june-2019/microdose-latanoprost-delivery-set-for-broad-patie.
20. Ibach M. Interim results of a prospective phase II study of travoprost intraocular implants. Paper presented at: The American Academy of Optometry Annual Meeting; November 9, 2018; San Antonio, TX.
21. ClinicalTrials.gov. Prospective, randomized phase II study comparing two elution rates of Glaukos travoprost intraocular implants to timolol maleate ophthalmic solution, USP, 0.5%. Updated April 30, 2021. Accessed April 20, 2022. https://clinicaltrials.gov/ct2/show/NCT02754596

# 40 Anterior Chamber Paracentesis

Michael D. Greenwood • Nicholas C. Risbrudt • Seth J. Stofferahn

The anterior chamber of the eye has gained more attention from eye care clinicians in recent years as the field continues to learn more about ocular anatomic structure and physiology. Anterior chamber paracentesis (ACP) is performed by passing a needle or surgical blade through the clear cornea to the space posterior to the corneal endothelium and anterior to the iris (Figure 40-1). In the past, ACP was utilized as a surgical procedure to remove aqueous humor (AH) from the anterior chamber of the eye (in a controlled fashion), thus decreasing the intraocular eye pressure (IOP) in acute angle-closure glaucoma (AACG).[1] ACP may also be indicated for any ocular pathology that poses an immediate threat to vision in which IOP lowering or AH sampling is indicated.

ACP is no longer only used in acute emergency situations to lower IOP. Perhaps in more relevant terms, ACP should be considered in eye care today as the insertion or removal of content from the anterior chamber of the eye via a needle. ACP is now more commonly being used for many different clinical indications other than IOP lowering. Technologies continue to emerge for treatment in which ACP is becoming more commonly performed routinely in clinic and no longer only in emergency situations.

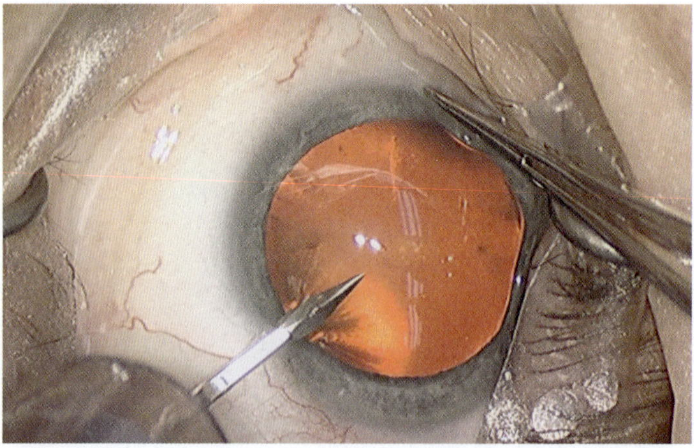

**FIGURE 40-1** The globe is stabilized with a forceps and then a 1.0-mm blade is used to enter the anterior chamber near the limbus and parallel to the iris. Once the widest part of the blade has entered the anterior chamber, the blade is withdrawn.

# INDICATIONS

**Key Indications**

- Acute IOP lowering
- Drug delivery
- AH sampling/anterior chamber tap
- Anterior chamber gas placement for Descemet membrane endothelial keratoplasty (DMEK)

## Acute Intraocular Eye Pressure Lowering

Historically, the most common indication for ACP was to quickly lower IOP in AACG. However, with increases in access to health care, advancement in surgical devices, diagnostics, lasers, and ophthalmic medications, ACP for AACG is not performed as often as it was in the past. AH is secreted from the anterior most portion of ciliary body called the ciliary processes.[2] It then flows through the pupil and drains via two different pathways—the conventional outflow and uveoscleral outflow pathways.[3] In AACG, the drainage angles of both pathways become obstructed by the anterior position of the iris and thus causes acutely elevated IOP. Treatment is promptly needed as patients suffering from AACG will experience symptoms of ocular pain, epiphora, decreased vision, headache, nausea, and abdominal discomfort.[4] High IOP in AACG also puts the patient at risk for permanent vision loss. ACP allows for rapid reduction in IOP and further therapy to take place.

Patients can also suffer AACG in neovascular glaucoma (NVG). NVG occurs when new blood vessels and fibrovascular tissue grow into the anterior chamber, which can occlude the drainage angle causing extremely high IOP. In the majority of AACG cases, more conservative treatment may be able to effectively lower IOP to make the patient more comfortable before needing ACP. Ophthalmic and systemic medications, laser peripheral iridotomy, clear lens exchange, cataract surgery, and glaucoma filtering surgeries are more effective long-term treatments for AACG.

ACP has perhaps gained more attention once again after anti-vascular endothelial growth factor (anti-VEGF) medications came to the market to treat wet macular degeneration and various other vascular retinal pathologies. IOP may be acutely elevated after an anti-VEGF injection has been performed. Although this IOP spike is usually short lived, clinicians may perform ACP to lower IOP prophylactically before or after anti-VEGF treatment to prevent patients from suffering an acute IOP spike. One study indicated that there was a need to perform an ACP in 33% ($n = 87$) out of 230 intravitreal anti-VEGF injections after the patients developed an IOP spike.[5] This study also advocated for the benefits of ACP.[5]

It is not uncommon for patients with glaucoma who undergo cataract, cataract plus minimally invasive glaucoma surgeries (MIGS), or stand-alone MIGS to have an IOP spike 1 day postoperatively. There are different ways for lowering IOP 1 day after surgery. A provider may prescribe topical IOP-lowering drops, use oral IOP-lowering medications, or perform a surgical wound burp. A wound burp is performed by using a rounded blunt sterile device (cotton-tipped applicator or punctum dilator) to gently apply pressure right next to the clear corneal incision or paracentesis. Pressure is applied until AH is released from the incision. The provider will then check the patient's IOP and repeat as needed until IOP reaches the desired target pressure. Sodium fluorescein (NaFl) may be used to help with visualization of the AH exiting the incision site. A NaFl strip is then used to "paint" the incision from which the wound burp was performed to ensure the incision has resealed and no Seidel sign is detected.

## Drug Delivery

The hydrophilic nature of the tears and hydrophobic nature of the corneal epithelium pose a challenge to all topical drugs trying to penetrate the cornea. The cornea itself is a very complex cellular tissue and acts as a strong defense barrier. Tight junctions (zonula occludens) efficiently barricade the epithelial cells, creating an effective seal to keep out foreign objects and substances. Although topical instillation of drugs is very popular in eye care, topically applied drugs are rapidly eliminated from the precorneal area.[6] Systemic medications also have difficulty penetrating the blood–aqueous and blood–retinal barrier. ACP can be used to bypass the eyes' natural defense barriers. ACP is used in drug delivery to transport medications to target tissues in the anterior chamber. ACP can be used to treat a multitude of ocular pathologies. In cases of bacterial or fungal endophthalmitis, antibiotics or antifungal medications can be injected directly into the anterior chamber to fight the infection.

Extended-release intracameral glaucoma medications can also effectively lower IOP in patients with primary open-angle glaucoma (POAG). Topical IOP-lowering medications continue to be the mainstay in POAG treatment. However, patient compliance with these drops continues to be a burden. Consistent use of glaucoma medications is generally considered to be poor, with studies reporting that fewer than 25% of patients use their eye drops consistently for 12 months.[7] Also, it is well known that once a second topical IOP-lowering medication is added, patient compliance is reduced even further. Presence of ocular surface disease secondary to the use of topical IOP-lowering medications is also heavily supported in literature. Glaucoma is associated with significant ocular surface disease, and severity of corneal staining appears to be directly correlated with the frequency of topical glaucoma therapy administration.[8]

Extended-release intracameral medications are a large focus of many ongoing Food and Drug Administration (FDA) clinical trials for the treatment of multiple disease states.

## Aqueous Humor Sampling/Anterior Chamber Tap

There are a few reasons why an eye care clinician may decide to sample the AH. In cases of any intraocular infection, it is important to know the causative organism to accurately treat the infection. Intraocular identification of antibodies to certain microorganisms or DNA of viruses, bacteria, fungi, or parasites by means of the polymerase chain reaction (PCR) or laboratory culture assists in early and specific diagnosis.[9,10] Once AH has been removed from the anterior chamber, it can be sent off to the lab for identification via culture or PCR. When the causative etiology has been determined, the patient can receive therapy with medications to specifically target the infectious organism. Because identifying organisms via culture or PCR can take days or even weeks, the patient should receive treatment based on the presumed diagnosis until the organism can be properly identified. AH sampling can also determine whether an anterior uveitis is infectious or noninfectious so that appropriate treatment can be prescribed.

AH sampling can also be used to determine pharmacokinetics and bioavailability of drugs in the eye. One study used AH sampling to compare the pharmacokinetics of levofloxacin 1.5% versus moxifloxacin hydrochloride 0.5% ophthalmic solutions after multiple doses prior to cataract surgery.[11] Another study used AH sampling to measure the levels of VEGF in patients with diabetic macular edema, central retinal vein occlusion, branched retinal vein occlusion, and neovascular age-related macular degeneration.[12]

### Anterior Chamber Gas Bubble For Descemet Membrane Endothelial Keratoplasty

In Fuchs' corneal dystrophy, the endothelium of the cornea gradually deteriorates. Early in the disease process, patients are generally asymptomatic. However, late in the disease process, the patient will experience blurry vision secondary to corneal edema. A DMEK is performed to replace the patient's endothelium with a new donor layer of endothelial cells. During the surgery, once the corneal specialist has removed the patient's unhealthy endothelium and has the new donor endothelial layer in position, a gas bubble is put into the anterior chamber to stabilize the donor graft. Postoperatively, if the donor graft is not properly attached, the patient will be experiencing blurry vision and light sensitivity secondary to corneal edema. The corneal specialist will then inject gas into the anterior chamber to provide support for the donor graft again. Because the function of the endothelium is to pump fluid from the corneal stroma into the anterior chamber, the corneal edema will quickly resolve once the donor endothelium graft adheres sufficiently, resulting in vision restoration. To prevent an IOP spike from the presence of the anterior chamber gas bubble, all patients undergoing DMEK surgery are prophylactically treated with a laser peripheral iridotomy to prevent the eye from going into pupillary block.

## CONTRAINDICATIONS

**Key Contraindications**

- Patient is allergic to topical anesthetics (relative contraindication).
- Patient is unable to cooperate for the procedure (relative contraindication).

There are no absolute contraindications to performing ACP for any of the indications listed above. In most patients undergoing ACP, their vision is at risk without further treatment. The majority of these patients have already undergone more conservative measures for treatment prior to performing ACP. Relative considerations include patients that are allergic to topical anesthetics or patients unable to cooperate doing the procedure.

# PREOPERATIVE PREPARATION

## Key Preoperative Considerations

- Appropriate signed informed consent
- Decision if procedure to be done in clinic or in operating room
- Proper positioning of patient behind slit lamp or reclined clinic chair

First, proper informed consent is received from the patient. ACP can be performed either in an operating room setting or in the clinic. Patient positioning is determined by the clinician either having the patient lay supine or remain sitting up. ACP may also be performed behind the slit lamp or with the patient lying back in the exam chair. Supplies needed are the physician's preferred gauge needle and plunger, topical anesthetic drops, povidone–iodine 5% ophthalmic solution with gauze sponges or povidone–iodine swab sticks, an eyelid speculum, and sterile gloves (Figure 40-2). In the case of an uncooperative patient due to ocular discomfort, headache, or nausea, some clinicians may choose to perform ACP under local anesthesia.

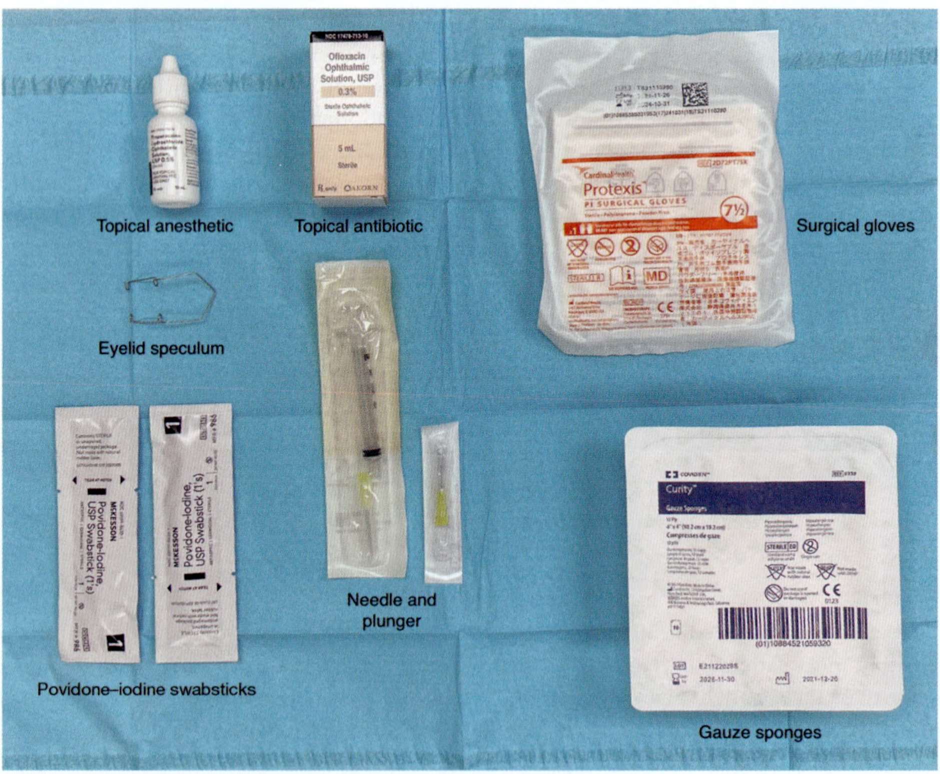


**FIGURE 40-2** Supplies and instruments necessary for anterior chamber paracentesis.

## PROCEDURE

Prior to the incision, the patient is given one or more drops of topical anesthetic. The eye is then prepped with a drop of broad-spectrum topical antibiotic. The patient's eyelids are also cleaned with povidone–iodine 5% ophthalmic solution. Once the patient's eye has been properly cleaned, a sterile eyelid speculum is placed to prevent the patient from blinking. The patient is now prepared for the incision. The needle should be attached to a syringe prior to starting the procedure. The needle bevel should face upward. This needle is then used to make an incision in the peripheral cornea 3 mm from the limbus, thus avoiding the corneal limbal stem cells or limbal vasculature. If operating on the patient's right eye, the incision is typically made at 9 o'clock. If operating on the patient's left eye, the incision is typically made at 3 o'clock. The angle of the needle during incision is to remain parallel to the iris to avoid making contact with corneal endothelium, iris, or the crystalline lens. Once the needle is fully inserted into the anterior chamber, AH can be removed in a steady and controlled manner by slowly pulling on the syringe plunger. This procedure will lower the IOP. AH is aspirated in small increments until the target IOP is achieved. In the case of AH sampling, once AH has been aspirated, it is sent to the laboratory for further testing. The procedure remains the same as mentioned previously when injecting contents into the anterior chamber whether that may be intracameral medications or a second gas bubble after DMEK surgery. The ideal gas bubble size should fill approximately 80% of the anterior chamber and will fully dissolve within 3 to 5 days. After the procedure, the patient is given another drop of a broad-spectrum topical antibiotic before leaving the clinic.

## POSTOPERATIVE CARE/COMANAGEMENT SCHEDULE

### Key Postoperative Considerations

- For AACG, seen every day until target IOP achieved
- After anti-VEGF injection, normal follow-up with a retina specialist
- After postoperative wound release, follow-up in 1 week
- For infectious cases, seen every day until improvement, then weekly
- For extended-release procedure, seen in 1 to 2 weeks
- After gas bubble for DMEK, follow-up in 1 week

The postoperative care schedule is relative to the indication in which ACP is being performed. For AACG, the patient may be followed every day or every other day to repeat ACP until further surgery to control IOP can be performed. ACP for AACG does acutely lower IOP; however, the IOP lowering is short lived. Further treatment must be initiated to control IOP for the long term. Because IOP spikes after anti-VEGF injections are very short lived, patients receiving ACP after anti-VEGF injections will resume their normal follow-up schedule with their retinal specialist. A patient receiving a wound burp at their 1-day postoperative appointment will continue their normal follow-up schedule and be seen a week later. For infectious cases in which medications are being injected into the anterior chamber, these patients should be seen every day or every other day until improvement is seen. Once improvement is seen, the patient can follow up weekly until the infection has been eradicated. For intracameral extended-release bimatoprost injections for the treatment of POAG, the patient is typically seen 1 to 2 weeks after the injection for an IOP check to establish efficacy of the treatment. For a repeat bubble after DMEK, the patient is seen 1 week after the procedure to determine if the DMEK is properly adhering and corneal edema is resolving. If needed, a third bubble can be placed.

## POTENTIAL COMPLICATIONS

### Key Potential Complications

- Intraocular hemorrhages and hyphema
- Decompression retinopathy
- Endophthalmitis

When performing ACP, AH should be removed in small increments to prevent complications. Rapid IOP lowering can lead to intraocular hemorrhages or more frequently decompression retinopathy and hyphema.[13] In majority of cases, the abovementioned complications resolve without further treatment, but occasionally a vitrectomy may be needed to clear an unresolving hemorrhage.[14] Although extremely rare, anytime an incision is made through the cornea, endophthalmitis is a possible complication.

## VIDEOS OF PROCEDURES

**Video 40-1**—After the patient has been correctly positioned in the slit lamp, the patient is directed to look down so the clinician can securely lift the upper lid out of the field of view. The patient is then directed to look up and toward their nose to obtain a clear view of the clear corneal incision. A wound burp is then performed using a round blunt sterile instrument (punctum dilator or cotton-tipped applicator) by pushing gently near the limbus adjacent to the clear corneal incision until aqueous is released from the eye. Multiple burps may be needed until the target intraocular eye pressure (IOP) is achieved.

**Video 40-2**—The globe is stabilized with a forceps and then a 1.0-mm blade is used to enter the anterior chamber near the limbus and parallel to the iris. Once the widest part of the blade has entered the anterior chamber, the blade is withdrawn.

## EFFICACY

The efficacy of the ACP is relative to the indication in which ACP is performed, but in general, it has good success. ACP for AACG is not a permanent or long-term treatment, but it may be needed to make a patient more comfortable in acute situations prior to initiating further treatment or surgery. The cause for AACG needs to be addressed and treated to prevent future acute angle-closure attacks and permanent vision loss. ACP will acutely lower IOP, but if left without further treatment, the IOP will spike again, usually within a couple of days. ACP is repeatable. A patient may need multiple ACPs to control IOP until further surgery therapy can be initiated. As stated earlier, more effective long-term treatments for AACG include laser peripheral iridotomy, clear lens exchange/cataract surgery, and/or filtering glaucoma surgeries.

## BILLING AND CODING MODIFIERS

ACP can be billed using Current Procedural Terminology (CPT) code 65800—Paracentesis of the anterior chamber of the eye (separate procedure), with diagnostic aspiration removal of aqueous. Global period for CPT code 65800 is 0 day. This code applies both for acute IOP lowering and AH sampling.

ACP for medications injected into the anterior chamber of the eye can be billed using CPT code 66030—Injection, anterior chamber of eye (separate procedure); medication. Global period for CPT code 66030 is 10 days.

Although CPT code 65800 also describes the procedure of a wound burp performed for an IOP spike 1-day after cataract, cataract plus MIGS, or stand-alone MIGS, it is generally considered nonbillable as it falls under the global period under the primary surgery. The same rule applies for anterior chamber gas placement for DMEK.

## REFERENCES


1. Cioboata M, Anghelie A, Chiotan C, et al. Benefits of anterior chamber paracentesis in the management of glaucomatous emergencies. *J Med Life*. 2014;7(2):5-6.
2. Goel M, Picciani RG, Lee RK, Bhattacharya SK. Aqueous humor dynamics: a review. *Open Ophthalmol J*. 2010;4:52-59. doi:10.2174/1874364101004010052
3. van Zyl T, Yan W, McAdams A, et al. Cell atlas of aqueous humor outflow pathways in eyes of humans and four model species provides insight into glaucoma pathogenesis. *Proc Natl Acad Sci U S A*. 2020;117(19):10339-10349. doi:10.1073/pnas.2001250117
4. Galloway G, Wertheim M, Broadway D. Acute glaucoma with abdominal pain. *J R Soc Med*. 2002;95(11):555-556. doi:10.1177/014107680209501111
5. Lorenz K, Zwiener I, Mirshahi A. Subconjunctival reflux and need for paracentesis after intravitreal injection of 0.1 ml bevacizumab: comparison between 27-gauge and 30-gauge needle. *Graefes Arch Clin Exp Ophthalmol*. 2010;248:1573-1577.
6. Sasaki H, Yamamura K, Mukai T, et al. Enhancement of ocular drug penetration. *Crit Rev Ther Drug Carrier Syst*. 1999;16(1):85-146.
7. Schwartz GF. Compliance and persistency in glaucoma follow-up treatment. *Curr Opin Ophthalmol*. 2008;16(2):114-121. doi:10.1097/01.icu.0000156139.05323.26
8. Mathews PM, Ramul, PY, Friedman DS, et al. Evaluation of ocular surface disease in patients with glaucoma. *Ophthalmology*. 2013;120(11):2241-2248. doi:10.1016/j.ophtha.2013.03.045
9. de Boer JH, Verhagen C, Bruinenberg M, et al. Serologic and polymerase chain reaction analysis of intraocular fluids in the diagnosis of infectious uveitis. *Am J Ophthalmol*. 1996;121(6):650-658. doi:10.1016/s0002-9394(14)70631-2
10. Boer de JH, Luyendijk L, Rothova A, Kijlstra A. Analysis of ocular fluids for local antibody production in uveitis. *Br J Ophthalmol*. 1995;79:610-616.
11. Bucci F Jr, Teuma Nguimfack I, Fluet AT. Pharmacokinetics and aqueous humor penetration of levofloxacin 1.5% and moxifloxacin 0.5% in patients undergoing cataract surgery. *Clin Ophthalmol*. 2016;10:783-789. doi:10.2147/OPTH.S91286
12. Campochiaro PA, Choy DF, Do DV, et al. Monitoring ocular drug therapy by analysis of aqueous samples. *Ophthalmology*. 2009;116(11):2158-2164. doi:10.1016/j.ophtha.2009.04.038
13. Dumitrache M, Anisescu M, Ciocalteu A. *Non-traumatic eye emergency*. Carol Davila University Publishing House; 2009. Acute Glaucoma, Mocanu C. 267/295.
14. Reddy S, Doshi S, Pathengay A, Panchal B. Ocular decompression retinopathy following intracameral bevacizumab injection in a case of proliferative diabetic retinopathy with neovascular glaucoma. *Ind J Ophthalmol*. 2020;69(6):1206-1209. doi:10.4103/ijo.IJO_1401_19

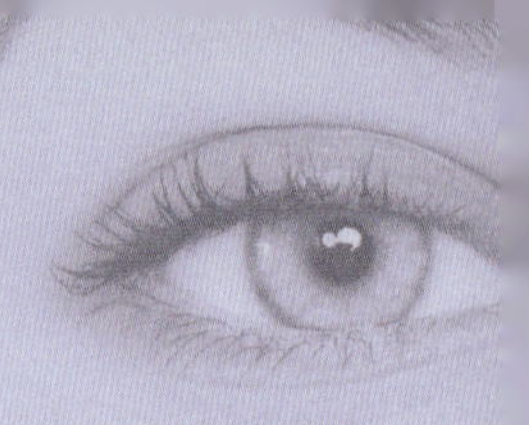

# 41 Intravitreal Injection of Anti-Vascular Endothelial Growth Factor Agents

**Vlad M. Matei • Carolyn Majcher**

The introduction of anti-vascular endothelial growth factor (anti-VEGF) agents into eye care in the 2000s revolutionized the management of exudative age-related macular degeneration (AMD), macular edema secondary to diabetic retinopathy (DR), and retinal vein occlusions (RVOs).[1] More recently, anti-VEGF therapy has been applied to moderately severe and severe nonproliferative diabetic retinopathy (NPDR) to prevent vision-threatening complications, whereas previously anti-VEGF therapy in DR was primarily used for diabetic macular edema (DME) and proliferative diabetic retinopathy (PDR). The current method of anti-VEGF administration, via repeated intravitreal injections, places a significant burden on patients.[2] Sustained-release devices, extending the duration of action of anti-VEGF medications, and drugs targeting other molecular targets, are currently under development and may overcome some of these burdens.

While reading this chapter, keep in mind that details of intravitreal injection protocols vary widely among various practitioners, in part because of limited evidence to support superior efficacy and safety of one particular technique over others.

## INDICATIONS

### Key Indications

- Neovascular (wet) age-related macular degeneration (nAMD)
- Macular edema following RVO
- Diabetic macular edema: Although anti-VEGF therapy may be used on-label for any degree of DME, it is often instituted for eyes with center-involved DME and decreased visual acuity.
- Diabetic retinopathy: More specifically, anti-VEGF therapy may be used in eyes with active PDR to induce regression of neovascularization. It may also be used in eyes with moderate-to-severe NPDR to improve the stage of retinopathy and prevent the onset of vision-threatening complications such as center-involved DME and PDR. Anti-VEGF is also often used prior to vitrectomy in eyes with severe PDR to reduce intraoperative bleeding that may occur when preretinal fibrovascular tissue is dissected from the retina.
- Myopic choroidal neovascularization (mCNV)

The following is a list of anti-VEGF agents commercially available in the United States, along with their U.S. Food and Drug Administration (FDA)-approved indications:

- Lucentis (ranibizumab) 0.5 mg (0.05 mL): nAMD, mCNV, RVO[3]
- Lucentis (ranibizumab) 0.3 mg (0.05 mL): DR, DME[3]
- Eylea (aflibercept) 2 mg (0.05 mL): nAMD, RVO, DME, DR[4]
- Eylea HD (aflibercept) 8 mg (0.07 mL of 114.3 mg/mL solution): nAMD, DME, DR[5]
- Beovu (brolucizumab) 6 mg (0.05 mL of 120 mg/mL solution): nAMD, DME[6]
- Vabysmo (faricimab-svoa) 6 mg (0.05 mL of 120 mg/mL solution): nAMD, DME[7]
- Byooviz (ranibizumab-nuna) 0.5 mg (0.05 mL): nAMD, RVO, mCNV[8]

Although lacking FDA-approved ocular indications, bevacizumab is often used off-label intravitreally to treat these same diseases because of its lower cost and similar efficacy to FDA-approved agents.

Other off-label indications for which anti-VEGF therapy is frequently employed in a clinical setting include other conditions that may cause macular edema because of increased vascular permeability or retinal ischemia as well as other conditions that cause retinal, choroidal, iris, or angle neovascularization[1,9]:

Ischemic or exudative retinopathies:

- Radiation retinopathy
- Proliferative sickle cell retinopathy
- Ocular ischemic syndrome
- Retinopathy of prematurity
- Coats disease
- Familial exudative vitreoretinopathy
- Pseudophakic cystoid macular edema (CME)
- Uveitic CME
- Retinal arterial macroaneurysm
- Vasoproliferative tumor
- Eales' disease

Causes of choroidal neovascularization[1,9]:

- Presumed ocular histoplasmosis syndrome
- Pachychoroid spectrum diseases, such as central serous chorioretinopathy and polypoidal choroidal vasculopathy
- Posterior uveitis (punctate inner choroidopathy multifocal choroiditis, toxoplasmosis)
- Angioid streaks
- Trauma
- Choroidal tumors (choroidal osteoma)
- Idiopathic choroidal neovascularization
- Peripapillary choroidal neovascularization
- Idiopathic macular telangiectasia
- Macular dystrophies such as Best disease and adult-onset foveomacular vitelliform dystrophy

# CONTRAINDICATIONS

## Key Contraindications

- Active ocular or periocular infections such as conjunctivitis, meibomianitis, or blepharitis[3-8,10]
- Active intraocular inflammation[3-8,10]
- Known hypersensitivity to the active medication or other inactive vehicle components[3-8]
- Pregnancy[3-8]: The use of intravitreal anti-VEGF in patients who are pregnant is usually avoided, although controversy exists because of lack of sufficient evidence supporting safety or risk.[11] The physician should weigh the potential patient benefits against the risks for fetal harm for each case, discuss them with the patient, and list them on the informed consent document.[11] Particular caution should be exercised in women with a history of miscarriage.[12] Nonpregnant women of childbearing age planning to begin anti-VEGF therapy should be advised to use contraception prior to the initial dose and continue contraceptive use until at least 3 months after the final dose.[7]

**Relative Contraindications**

- End-stage glaucoma or preprocedure elevated intraocular pressure (IOP)[13-17]
- Vitreoretinal traction[18,19]
- Recent stroke, myocardial infarction, gastrointestinal bleeding, or history of multiple past strokes[1,20]
- Breastfeeding[3-8,21]: Evidence has demonstrated that anti-VEGF medications are found in breast milk, but limited evidence exists to support safety or risk with regards to the newborn child. As with pregnancy, the risks to the child must be weighed against the benefit to the mother. Limited research suggests that medication concentration levels in breast milk may be lower with ranibizumab compared to bevacizumab and aflibercept. Factors to consider include the necessity of anti-VEGF treatment, the postnatal age of the newborn, and whether breastfeeding can be avoided during therapy.

# INFORMED CONSENT CONSIDERATIONS

## Key Informed Consent Adverse Events Listed

- Conjunctival hemorrhage: Conjunctival hemorrhage is the most common side effect, occurring in approximately 7%, caused by the intravitreal injection procedure itself.[3-8] Conjunctival hemorrhage is benign but can appear alarming to patients, so it is important to counsel patients about this common occurrence ahead of time.
- Elevated IOP
- Endophthalmitis

- Retinal detachment
- Arterial thromboembolic events (ATEs, nonfatal stroke, nonfatal myocardial infarction, or vascular death): A causal effect from intravitreal anti-VEGF injections has not been demonstrated, and at this time this remains merely an association to include in the informed consent.
- Intraocular inflammation
- Transient blurring of vision
- Hypersensitivity reaction
- Corneal abrasion
- Floaters
- Cataract
- Vitreous hemorrhage

Informed consent should include a description of the procedure in plain, nontechnical words in the patient's preferred language. For example: "An intravitreal injection is a procedure to place a medication directly into the space in the back of the eye called the vitreous cavity, which is filled with a jelly-like fluid called the vitreous gel. The medication to be used is an anti-vascular endothelial growth factor (anti-VEGF) that helps reduce fluid leakage in the central portion of the vision (macular edema), and decreases damaging new blood vessel growth."[22]

Potential alternative treatments, such as eye drops, monitoring, or invasive surgery, should be listed if applicable. Risks and complications inherent to the intravitreal injection procedure itself include, but are not limited to, conjunctival hemorrhage, increased IOP, ocular surface irritation or corneal abrasion, eye pain or discomfort, floaters, temporary blurring of vision, endophthalmitis, retinal detachment, vitreous hemorrhage, cataract, permanent vision loss, and loss of the eye.[3-8,22]

A note from the counseling clinician should be included and phrased similar to: "I have counseled this patient as to the nature of the proposed procedure, the attendant risks involved, and the expected results." The patients', doctors', and witness' names should be printed, signed, and dated.

Females or males of reproductive age and potential should be screened for pregnancy or breastfeeding (see Contraindications).[3-8]

If bevacizumab is to be used, patients should be informed that its use for ocular conditions is off-label.

## PREOPERATIVE CARE

### Key Preoperative Considerations

- Macular optical coherence tomography (OCT) and vitreoretinal examination
- Allergies
- Physical setting: In-office versus operating room

- Same-day versus alternate-day bilateral injections
- Sterile supplies
- Medication preparation: Varies depending upon the anti-VEGF agent to be used
- Size of needle used for injection
- Lid inspection for blepharitis
- Absence of other active ocular infection or inflammation
- Crystalline lens status
- Location of injection on the eye

On the same day, prior to the procedure, the following tests should be performed: (1) visual acuities with correction including pinhole as appropriate, (2) slit-lamp examination of the anterior segment, (3) dilated fundus examination, and (4) IOP. Note that some practitioners do not dilate the procedural eye if the patient is following up after injections on prior visit and if the patient denies any vision changes since the previous visit. If IOP is found to be significantly elevated (generally >30 mm Hg), an attempt to lower the IOP medically prior to injection should be made, either medically or with an anterior chamber paracentesis. Lens status (phakic, pseudophakic, or aphakic) should be assessed and noted because this informs how far posterior to the limbus the injection is given.[10] Injection should be withheld if any signs of active infection or inflammation such as uveitis, conjunctivitis, vitritis, or keratitis are present.[2-8,10] If blepharitis is found, this should be managed appropriately, and the procedure postponed, if possible, pending treatment of the blepharitis. Examine the conjunctiva and sclera for a suitable injection location: avoid injecting in areas that contain scleral or glaucoma implants or trabeculectomy blebs.[2,10] The typical location of injection is inferotemporal, but the injection may be administered in any quadrant.[23] Macular OCT and vitreoretinal examination should be recent or same day.

Although historically intravitreal injections were performed in the operating room, more recent guidelines allow for performing this procedure in the clinic, without a sterile suite required.[24] The patient chair should allow the patient to comfortably recline, and good lighting is essential.[25]

It is important to have a sterile 0.5-inch 30-gauge needle ready to perform anterior chamber paracentesis in case of optic disc hypoperfusion because of elevated IOP following injection.[2,25,26]

The eye undergoing injections should be clearly marked and confirmed against the record and with the patient. A "time out" should be performed to confirm the correct patient identity (with at least two patient identifiers), the correct medication and dose (and use prior to the expiration date), and the correct eye laterality.

The physician performing the injection and staff involved in the patient/medication preparation should wear surgical masks during the procedure. A "no-talking" policy is an alternative to wearing a mask, and optimally the patient and everyone present in the room should keep their mouths closed at all times during the injection procedure. Gloves are optional.

In a recent survey, about half of American retinal specialists indicated that they perform same-day bilateral injections if indicated, and certainly this practice pattern reduces the already significant burden on patients and caregivers inherent to anti-VEGF therapy.[23] If bilateral injections are to be performed, each eye should be treated as a separate procedure and prepped accordingly.[2,10] Separate instrumentation and medication from different compounding lots (different lot numbers) should be used for each eye.[2,10] The patient should be counseled about the possibly increased risk of endophthalmitis in the setting of same-day bilateral injections.

Medication preparation depends upon the anti-VEGF agent being used and how it is supplied. In all cases, medication preparation should be performed using aseptic techniques on a sterile field by a gloved individual wearing a surgical face mask. The medication should be visually inspected for particulates, cloudiness, and discoloration.[4] Most anti-VEGF agents come supplied in a prefilled syringe. A 30- to 33-gauge needle of 0.5 inch or shorter length is most commonly used for anti-VEGF intravitreal injection.[10]

Medication preparation utilizing a prefilled syringe:

- Twist off the syringe cap and replace it with a sterile needle that will be used to penetrate the eye.[10,27]
- Inspect for air bubbles with the needle pointing upward. If bubbles are present, tap the syringe, encouraging the bubbles to rise to the top.[27]
- Expel any bubbles and excess drug by slowly depressing the plunger to align the cylindrical base of the plunger dome edge with the line corresponding to the exact dosage desired.[27]

Medication preparation utilizing a medicine vial:

- Remove the plastic protective cap from the vial, taking care to not touch the underlying surface of the vial.[4]
- Use an alcohol wipe to clean the rubber top of the medication vial.[4]
- Attach a 19-gauge or 18-gauge filter needle to a 1-mL syringe and insert the needle into the center of the rubber vial top with the needle pointing down and the vial upright until the needle touches the bottom edge of the vial.[2,4]
- Withdraw the medication by pulling back on the plunger. Extract slightly more than the desired dosage. The vial may need to be tilted slightly if all contents of the vial are to be withdrawn.[4]
- Exchange the filter needle for a 30-gauge, 0.5-inch needle.[2]
- Inspect for air bubbles with the needle pointing upward. If bubbles are present, tap the syringe encouraging the bubbles to rise to the top.[4,27]
- Expel any bubbles and excess drug by slowly depressing the plunger to align the cylindrical base of the plunger dome edge with the line corresponding to the exact dosage desired.[4,27]

## PROCEDURE

### Key Procedural Points

- **Handwashing, glove, and mask:** The individual performing the injection and any assistants should thoroughly wash their hands before the procedure. Gloves are optional. The individual performing the procedure should ideally wear a mask. The patient should not be wearing a mask, or, if a mask is necessary for the patient, the top edge of the mask should be taped firmly against the cheek to avoid aerosolized bacteria directed toward the injection site.

- **Time out**: Time should be taken to verify patient identity, check that the eye to be injected is correctly marked, and that an informed consent has been signed. Also ensure that the prepared medication name, concentration, and dosage are correct, and that the medication has not expired.
- **Anesthesia**: Various methods of anesthesia have been described, including topical drops such as proparacaine 0.5% or tetracaine 0.5%, anesthetic-soaked cotton tip applicator or pledget, lidocaine gels, and subconjunctival injection.[25,28] A common method of topical anesthesia is proparacaine 0.5% instilled two to three times with an interval of 4 to 5 minutes between each application, followed by holding one or two cotton tip applicators soaked in either 4% lidocaine solution or proparacaine 0.5% for 1 minute on the injection site. If lidocaine gel is used, it should be instilled after povidone–iodine asepsis, because gel anesthetic may reduce the efficacy of povidone–iodine.[2,29,30]
- **Lid retraction**: A sterile metal lid retractor is ideal for eyelid retraction and is the most common method of lid retraction employed, but so long as the sterility of the injection site is maintained during and after lid retraction, the use of a speculum is optional (Figure 41-1).[23,25]

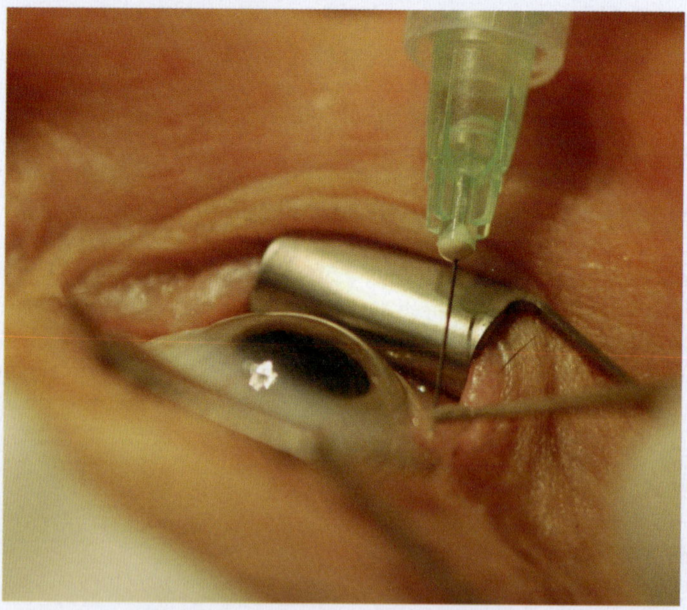

**FIGURE 41-1** Intravitreal anti-VEGF injection. Note solid blade speculum to reflect the eyelashes away from the ocular surface. VEGF, vascular endothelial growth factor. (Image courtesy of Leonid Skorin Jr, DO, MS.)

- **Conjunctival asepsis**: Povidone–iodine 5% should be liberally instilled onto the conjunctival surface (including the fornices), eyelid margins, and eyelashes.[2,10,31,32] It is important to ensure that povidone–iodine is applied directly to the intended injection site as well. If additional anesthesia needs to be subsequently instilled, it is important to reapply povidone–iodine to the conjunctiva of the intended injection site.[2,29,30] The povidone–iodine should be allowed to soak on the conjunctiva for at least 30 seconds. Additionally, a povidone–iodine swab stick may be used to swipe the inferior and superior conjunctival fornices. To minimize the risk of corneal toxicity, it is important to avoid using a concentration greater than 5% of povidone–iodine (Figure 41-2). More recently, the use of either lower concentrations of povidone–iodine or dilute aqueous chlorhexidine in place of povidone–iodine 5% has been demonstrated in some studies to provide similarly effective antisepsis.
- **Measure and mark the point of needle entry**: Using sterile ophthalmic calipers or the tip of a sterile 1 mL tuberculin syringe, measure either 3 to 3.5 mm (pseudophakic or aphakic eyes) or 3.5 to 4 mm (phakic eyes) posterior to the limbus in the inferior temporal quadrants, although the injection can be administered in any quadrant (Figure 41-3).[10] Apply gentle pressure to the posterior caliper tip to create a small

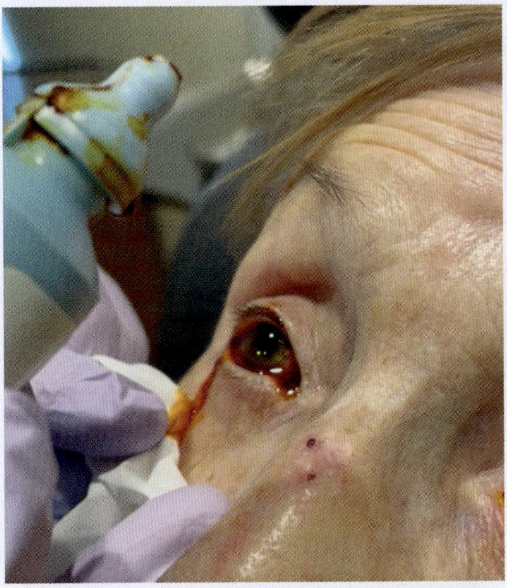

**FIGURE 41-2** Intravitreal anti-VEGF injection. Five percent povidone–iodine is liberally instilled onto the conjunctival surface and into conjunctival sac. VEGF, vascular endothelial growth factor. (Image courtesy of Vlad Matei, MD.)

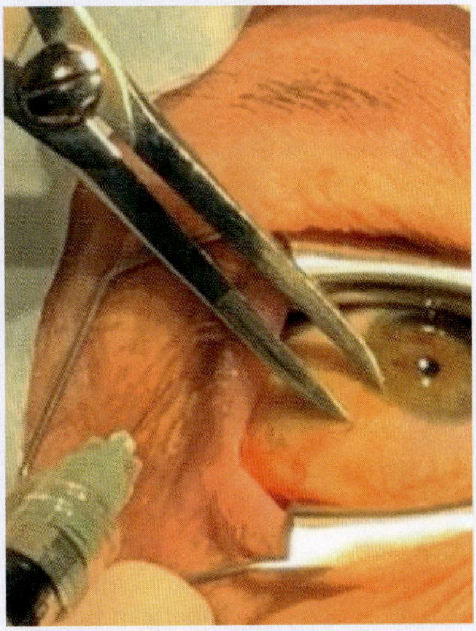

**FIGURE 41-3** Intravitreal anti-VEGF injection. Ophthalmic calipers are used to measure the appropriate distance posterior to the limbus and mark the point of needle entry. VEGF, vascular endothelial growth factor. (Image courtesy of Leonid Skorin Jr, DO, MS.)

scleral indentation at the intended site of needle entry. An additional drop of povidone–iodine 5% can then be instilled on the injection site and allowed to pool into the indentation, making the targeted point of entry easy to identify (Figure 41-4).[10]

- **Needle insertion and medication injection**: For better visualization and access, ask the patient to look away (usually superior nasal) from the injection site. The needle should be inserted perpendicularly to the globe to avoid touching the lens or retina (Figure 41-5).[31] The needle should be advanced at least 4 mm into the vitreous cavity, but advancing the needle all the way to its hub is not necessary. The plunger should be slowly and steadily depressed until all medication is injected into the vitreous. The needle is then removed along the same perpendicular path. Optionally, a sterile cotton tip applicator is placed and gentle pressure is held for a few seconds on the injection site to prevent and/or minimize external vitreous reflux, but reflux of vitreous fluid is common and benign (Figure 41-6).[10,31] Immediately place the used needle still attached to the empty syringe in a sharp disposal container and remove the lid speculum (Figure 41-7).

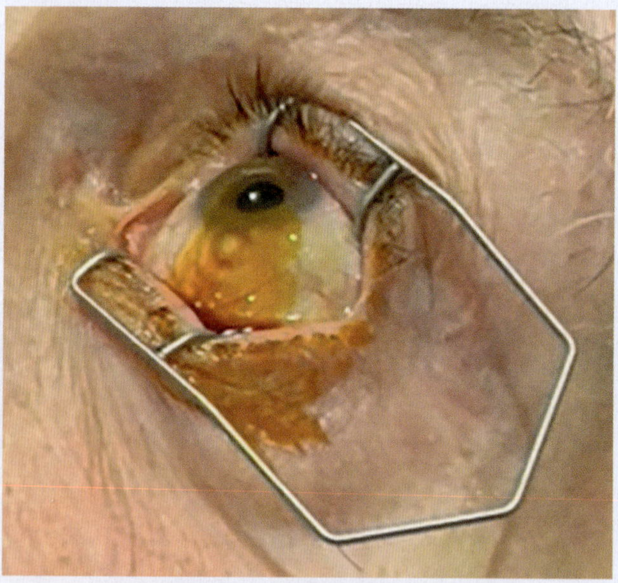

**FIGURE 41-4** Intravitreal anti-VEGF injection. The instrument or caliper can be used to create a small conjunctival indent at the intended site of needle entry. An additional drop of povidone–iodine 5% can then be instilled on the injection site and allowed to pool into the indention, making the intended point of entry easy to identify. VEGF, vascular endothelial growth factor. (Image courtesy of Vlad Matei, MD.)

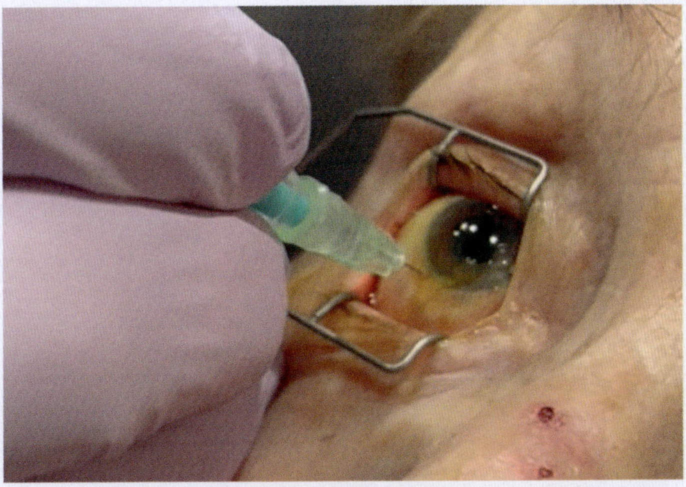

FIGURE 41-5 Intravitreal anti-VEGF injection. The patient is asked to look away from the injection site and the needle is inserted perpendicularly to the globe. VEGF, vascular endothelial growth factor. (Image courtesy of Vlad Matei, MD.)

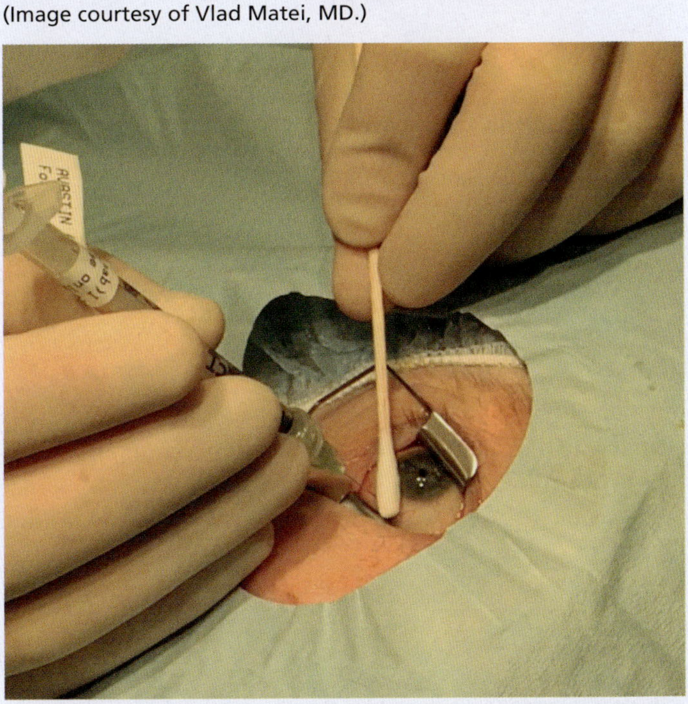

FIGURE 41-6 Intravitreal anti-VEGF injection. After needle removal, a sterile cotton tip applicator is held on the injection site to prevent and/or minimize external vitreous reflux. VEGF, vascular endothelial growth factor. (Image courtesy of Leonid Skorin Jr, DO, MS.)

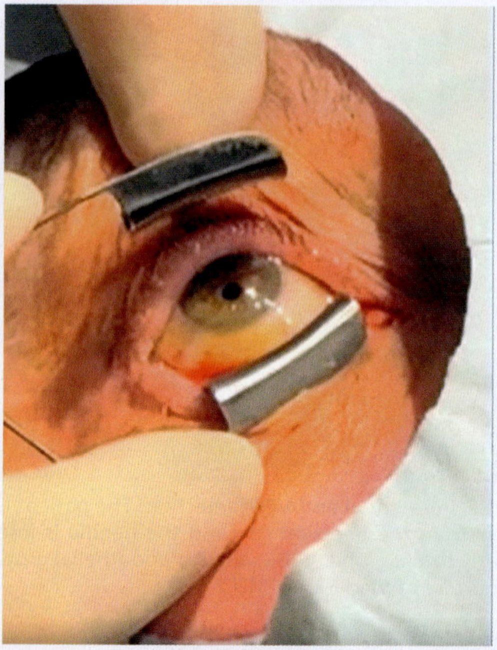

**FIGURE 41-7** Intravitreal anti-VEGF injection. The lid speculum is removed post injection. VEGF, vascular endothelial growth factor. (Image courtesy of Leonid Skorin Jr, DO, MS.)

# POSTOPERATIVE CARE/FOLLOW-UP SCHEDULE

## Key Postoperative Considerations

- Confirmation of central retinal artery (CRA) perfusion
- Thorough irrigation of povidone–iodine from the ocular surface with sterile balanced salt solution or artificial tears
- Patient education regarding symptoms and signs of endophthalmitis and retinal detachment
- Liberal preservative-free artificial tear use by the patient as needed
- Documentation

Immediately after injection, confirm retinal perfusion by determining whether the patient can count fingers in the procedural eye. Alternatively, one may perform ophthalmoscopic examination of the optic nerve to confirm perfusion of the optic disc. If the patient is unable to count fingers or the CRA appears hypoperfused (there should at least be pulsations of the

CRA), then this is because of a high IOP, which should be immediately lowered. Measurement of the IOP is not necessary so long as the CRA is perfused. In cases of advanced glaucoma, IOP may be checked and prophylactic anterior chamber paracentesis performed at the clinician's discretion even if the CRA is perfused. Remove the lid speculum. The eye should be irrigated thoroughly with sterile balanced salt solution or artificial tears to ensure that no povidone–iodine remains on the ocular surface, which could cause corneal epithelial disruption.

A notation similar to "The patient tolerated the procedure well without any complications and left in no apparent distress" should be added to the chart. Documentation in the patient's medical record must reflect the drug name, concentration, dosage, expiration date, lot number, and the eye that was injected. Documentation should include that excess medication remaining in the syringe or vial beyond the required dose that was discarded.

Consider recommending preservative artificial tear use at least four times a day in the postoperative eye to help with discomfort following povidone–iodine application.

Provide the patient with verbal and written instructions to return/notify the doctors' office immediately if signs or symptoms of endophthalmitis or retinal detachment occur. These may include pain, flashes, mucopurulent discharge, photophobia, decreased vision, and curtain or veil-like visual obstruction. New-onset floaters are expected immediately postprocedure because of introduction of medication into the vitreous cavity; however, patients should be warned to return if floaters worsen after they leave the office.

A postprocedural follow-up is typically unnecessary and patients can often be seen back in 4 to 6 weeks for consideration of repeat injection. Patients should be instructed to return if any signs or symptoms of retinal detachment or endophthalmitis arise as described earlier.

## POTENTIAL COMPLICATIONS AND THEIR TREATMENT

### Key Potential Complications

- **Conjunctival hemorrhage:** Conjunctival hemorrhage is an expected, common (~7%), and benign complication of any intravitreal injection procedure.[3-8] Punctate subconjunctival hemorrhage can be seen at the site of needle insertion in almost all eyes, and a diffuse conjunctival hematoma may rarely occur (Figure 41-8).[10]
- **Corneal abrasion:** Corneal compromise and abrasions may occur because of povidone–iodine epithelial compromise or, less likely, insertion/removal of the lid speculum. Use of bandage contact lens or pressure patching is generally discouraged and may promote infection. We recommend conservative management of corneal abrasions including topical antibiotic, liberal preservative artificial tear use, and pain management as needed (Figure 41-9).
- **IOP elevation:** IOP elevation of some degree commonly occurs because additional volume is being added into an enclosed cavity, and the risk of IOP elevation is expected to increase with greater volumes of medication injected.[2,3-8] Elevations in IOP typically are transient and often resolve within 60 minutes of the injection.[3-8] Patients

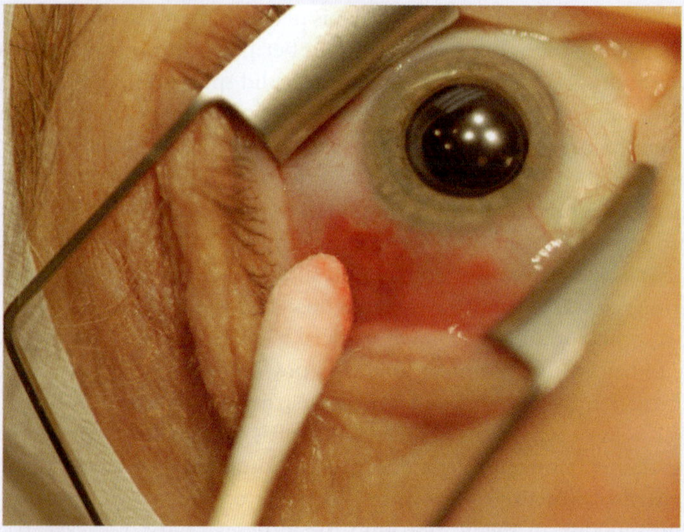

FIGURE 41-8 Subconjunctival hemorrhage after intravitreal anti-VEGF injection. VEGF, vascular endothelial growth factor. (Image courtesy of Leonid Skorin Jr, DO, MS.)

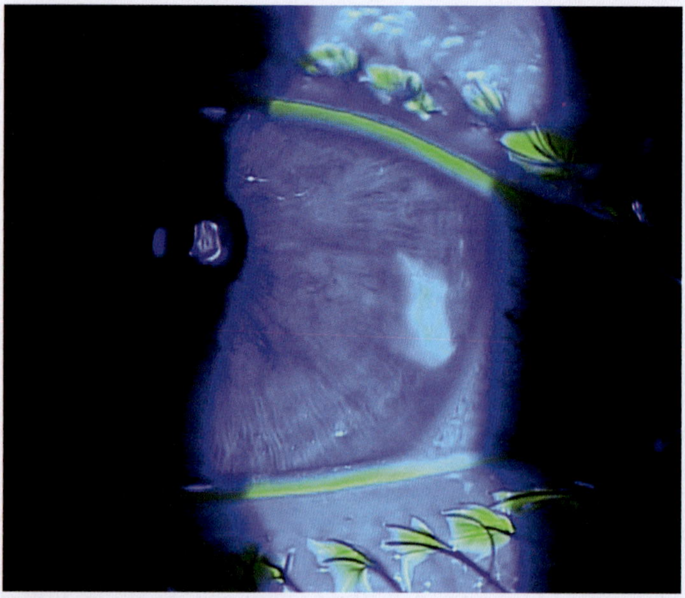

FIGURE 41-9 Corneal abrasion. (Image courtesy of Komal Patel, OD.)

with a history of glaucoma appear to be at greater risk for postprocedure IOP elevation.[2,10] Paracentesis should be considered for eyes found to have significant postprocedural IOP elevation (≥40 mm Hg), especially if they have a history of advanced glaucoma. Aggressive digital ocular massage should be avoided as this could result in meibomian gland expression, which could contaminate the ocular surface.[2] Some studies have reported development of glaucoma, ganglion cell layer loss, and retinal nerve fiber layer decrease in eyes treated with long-term anti-VEGF therapy.[13-17,26]

- **Cataract or traumatic lens damage:** Cataract was reported in approximately 7% of patients in phase 3 studies using aflibercept and brolucizumab but can occur with injection of any anti-VEGF agent [4,6,10]
- **Intraocular inflammation:** The incidence of acute-onset sterile intraocular inflammation or inflammatory pseudo-endophthalmitis ranges from 0.02% to 0.37%.[10,33] It frequently occurs within 1 day of injection, and prognosis for recovery is often good even without treatment.[10,33] Common signs of pseudo-endophthalmitis include vitreous cells and anterior chamber reaction (Figure 41-10). Hypopyon may be present but is uncommon.[10,33] Typical symptoms include blurred vision, floaters, pain, and photophobia.[10,33] Cases of occlusive retinal vasculitis have been associated with intravitreal brolucizumab injection and may result in unrecoverable vision loss.[34] The estimated incidence of this complication is up to approximately 3.3%.[35]
  - Inflammatory occlusive retinal vasculitis following intravitreal brolucizumab—Intraocular inflammation with evidence of retinal vasculitis occurred in approximately 3.3% of brolucizumab-treated eyes in post hoc analysis of the phase 3 HAWK and HARRIER trials.[6,34,35] Cases of retinal vasculitis were usually preceded

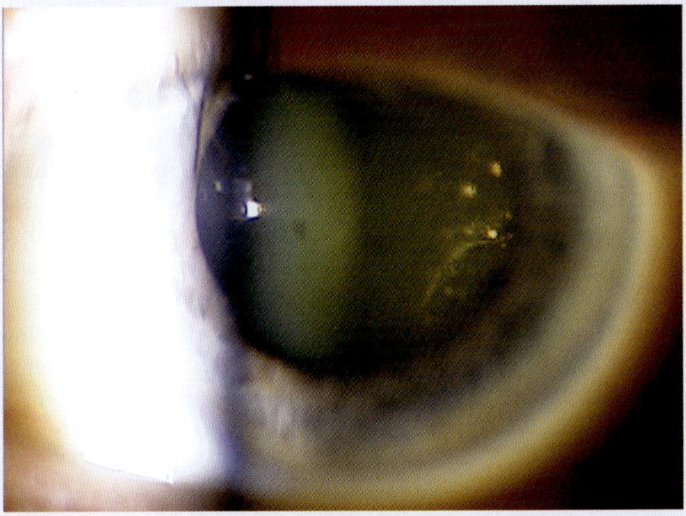

**FIGURE 41-10** Vitreous cells and anterior chamber reaction. (Image courtesy of Laura Chan, OD.)

by intraocular inflammation of delayed onset, with presentation at a mean of 25 days after the most recent injection.[35] In an analysis of 26 eyes with retinal vasculitis, 46% had a greater than 3-line decrease in visual acuity at final follow-up and 46% had final acuity of 20/200 or worse.[35]

- **Endophthalmitis:** Infectious endophthalmitis may be procedure-related or caused by nonsterile medication compounding/manufacturing methods. The pooled infectious endophthalmitis rate from 20 large retrospective case series of anti-VEGF injections reported by Merani and Hunyor was found to be 0.028%.[36] The use of povidone–iodine and lid retraction are critical procedural steps that reduce the risk of subsequent infectious endophthalmitis.[32] Routine use of prophylactic topical antibiotics is discouraged.[10,37] Endophthalmitis should be suspected in individuals complaining of decreasing vision and pain postprocedure that present with severe anterior chamber reaction and hypopyon, vitreous cells and haze, and severe conjunctival hyperemia.[38] Additionally, periorbital eyelid and corneal edema may be seen.[38] Sachdeva et al. reported a mean time to presentation of endophthalmitis of 4.3 days following injection with a range of 1 to 15 days.[37] A vitreous tap should be performed if endophthalmitis is suspected for Gram stain, culture, and sensitivities.[38] Positive culture results are yielded in up to 75% of cases, with coagulase-negative *Staphylococcus* being the most commonly identified organism.[37] Additionally, intravitreal broad-spectrum antibiotics such as vancomycin 1 mg per 0.1 mL and ceftazidime 2.25 mg per 0.1 mL such be injected empirically.[10,38] Urgent vitrectomy may also be considered.[10] If therapy is effective, some clinical improvement should be seen within 48 hours.[38] Following intravitreal antibiotics, oral and/or intravitreal steroids can be added on a case-by-case basis. Although infectious endophthalmitis can be visually devastating, Chaudhary et al. found that 90% of patients regained visual acuity within 1 line of baseline when treated with vitreous tap and intravitreal antibiotics, whereas 46% regained visual acuity within one line of baseline when treated with vitreous tap, intravitreal antibiotic injection and subsequent pars plana vitrectomy.[39]
- **Retinal detachment or break:** Retinal tear and retinal detachment occur at a rate of approximately 0.06% and 0.1% per anti-VEGF injection, respectively (Figure 41.11).[10,40] Prophylactic barrier laser photocoagulation should be considered to prevent rhegmatogenous retinal detachment when retinal tears are discovered. Retinal detachments may require pneumatic retinopexy, pars plana vitrectomy, and/or scleral buckle depending upon the location and extent of the detachment.
- **Vitreous hemorrhage:** The incidence of vitreous hemorrhage following intravitreal injection is low (~0.23% per injection) and if encountered, B-scan ultrasonography should be performed to rule out a concurrent retinal detachment.[40] Most vitreous hemorrhages can be managed conservatively and observed for spontaneous clearing (Figure 41-12).
- **ATEs:** There is likely a low but potential risk of ATEs, defined as nonfatal stroke, nonfatal myocardial infarction, or vascular death (including deaths of unknown cause), with intravitreal anti-VEGF therapy especially in patients being treated for DME.[7]

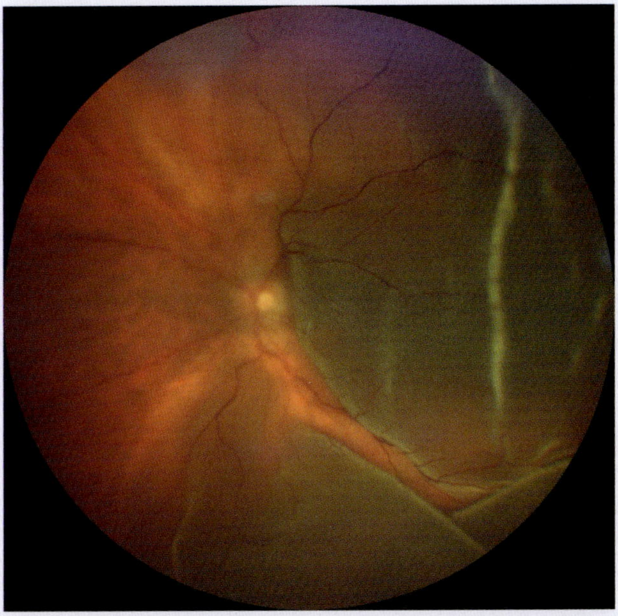

**FIGURE 41-11** Rhegmatogenous retinal detachment. (Image courtesy of Laura Chan, OD.)

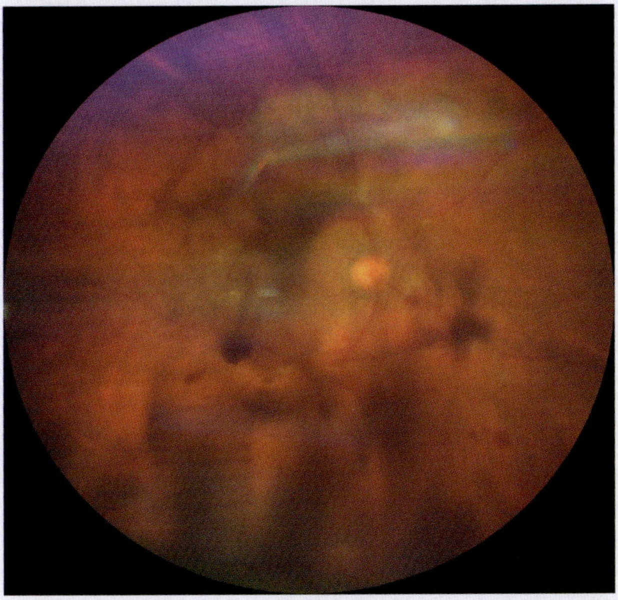

**FIGURE 41-12** Vitreous hemorrhage. (Image courtesy of Carolyn Majcher, OD.)

The estimated rate of ATE within the first year of treatment in patients with neovascular AMD is approximately 1% to 2% of patients, although definite data demonstrating a causal link to an increased risk of stroke, major cardiovascular events, arteriothrombotic events, or mortality with anti-VEGF therapy in patients with neovascular AMD is lacking.[3-7,20] Rates of ATEs occurring in patients treated with anti-VEGF therapy included in DME trials appear to be higher than patients included in neovascular AMD studies, because these individuals likely have an inherently greater risk because of the presence of systemic vasculopathic conditions.[3-7,20,41] Serious systemic adverse events have been reported to occur more frequently with bevacizumab compared with ranibizumab.[42] The reported incidence of ATEs in DME studies of aflibercept during the first 52 weeks was 3.3% in the combined group of patients treated with aflibercept compared with 2.8% in the control group.[41] Similarly, the reported incidence of ATEs in DME studies of faricimab during the first year was 2% in patients treated with faricimab and 2% in patients treated with aflibercept.[7] It would seem prudent to carefully weigh the risk-to-benefit profile and make attempts to lower the risk of ATEs in patients with a history of recent stroke, multiple strokes, or recent myocardial infarction.[20]

- **Vitreous reflux:** If vitreous reflux occurs using a 30-gauge or smaller needle, it is usually minimal and can be observed without intervention. It can be reduced by applying pressure to the injection site with a sterile cotton tip applicator immediately after the needle is withdrawn from the eye, but this is unnecessary in most cases.[2]
- **Retinal pigment epithelium (RPE) rip or tear:** The rate of RPE tear in eyes with neovascular AMD was 3% in the HAWK and HARRIER trials and 2% in the VIEW 1 and VIEW 2 trials.[4,6] It is thought that eyes with large pigmented epithelial detachments, causing mechanical RPE strain, may be at greater risk.[43]
- **RPE atrophy:** Eyes being treated with long-term anti-VEGF therapy for neovascular AMD may be at greater risk for RPE atrophy, but the evidence for this is not robust, and anti-VEGF therapy should not be withheld solely because of this concern.[44]
- **Anti-VEGF "crunch" syndrome:** In eyes with PDR and extensive preretinal neovascularization, rapid regression may cause contraction of neovascular membranes that produces or exacerbates a tractional retinal detachment.[1,19]
- **Hypersensitivity reaction**

Patients are typically reevaluated at 4- to 6-week intervals initially but may be evaluated sooner if postprocedural complications arise or symptoms of endophthalmitis or retinal detachment are noted.[1] Patients with extensive vitreoretinal traction or those with extensive areas of preretinal neovascularization at risk of anti-VEGF "crunch" syndrome should be evaluated sooner, as early as 1-week postprocedure.[1,19] There is often a need for repeated or serial intravitreal anti-VEGF therapy; however, injections should be separated by at least 4 weeks or more depending upon the duration of action of the particular anti-VEGF agent being used.

## VIDEOS OF PROCEDURES

**Video 41-1**—Intravitreal anti-vascular endothelial growth factor (anti-VEGF) injection. After topical and/or subconjunctival anesthesia, several drops of povidone–iodine 5% are applied to the ocular surface, enough so that the antiseptic extends onto the eyelashes. The patient is then asked to sit quietly without talking or touching the procedural eye for at least 60 seconds, to allow the antiseptic to take effect. A sterile eyelid speculum is inserted. The patient is instructed to look up and the intended point of needle entry is marked 3 to 4 mm posterior to the limbus in the inferotemporal quadrant. Note that the marking in this video is achieved using a 1-mL Slip-Tip syringe, the tip of which has a diameter of approximately 4 mm. An additional drop of povidone–iodine 5% is instilled onto the injection site, which has the additional benefit of making the scleral mark easier to identify. The needle is then inserted perpendicular to the globe and advanced at least 4 mm into the vitreous cavity. The plunger is slowly and steadily depressed until all medication is injected, and then the needle is removed along the same perpendicular path. (Video courtesy of Dr. Vlad Matei.)

**Video 41-2**—Intravitreal anti-VEGF injection. After topical and/or subconjunctival anesthesia, several drops of povidone–iodine 5% are applied to the ocular surface, enough so that the antiseptic extends onto the eyelashes. The patient is then asked to sit quietly without talking or touching the procedural eye for at least 60 seconds, to allow the antiseptic to take effect. A sterile eyelid speculum is inserted. The patient is instructed to look up, and the intended point of needle entry is marked 3 to 4 mm posterior to the limbus in the inferotemporal quadrant. Note that the marking in this video is achieved using a 1-mL Slip-Tip syringe, the tip of which has a diameter of approximately 4 mm. An additional drop of povidone–iodine 5% is instilled onto the injection site, which has the additional benefit of making the scleral mark easier to identify. The needle is then inserted perpendicular to the globe and advanced at least 4 mm into the vitreous cavity. The plunger is slowly and steadily depressed until all medication is injected, and then the needle is removed along the same perpendicular path. (Video courtesy of Dr. Vlad Matei.)

**Video 41-3**—Intravitreal anti-VEGF injection. (Video courtesy of Leonid Skorin Jr and Taylor Lauermann.)

**Video 41-4**—Intravitreal anti-VEGF injection. (Video courtesy of Leonid Skorin Jr and Andrew Mackner.)

# EFFICACY

## Neovascular Age-Related Macular Degeneration

- **Vabysmo**—TENAYA and LUCERNE were two parallel phase 3 randomized trials that compared Vabysmo 6 mg up to every 16 weeks (following four monthly doses) to Eylea 2 mg every 8 weeks (following three monthly doses).[45] The adjusted mean change in best-corrected visual acuity (BCVA) from baseline at 48 weeks in TENAYA was 5.8 letters in the Vabysmo group and 5.1 letters in the Eylea group. In LUCERNE, the adjusted mean change in BCVA from baseline was 6.6 in both treatment arms (noninferior).[45]
- **Eylea**—VIEW1 and VIEW2 were two parallel randomized controlled clinical trials that compared Eylea 2 mg administered every 8 weeks following three initial monthly doses to Lucentis 0.5 mg administered every 4 weeks.[4,46] Clinical equivalency was demonstrated at 52 weeks. The proportion of patients who maintained vision, defined as losing fewer than 15 Early Treatment Diabetic Retinopathy Study (ETDRS) severity scale letters of

BCVA at week 52 compared to baseline, in the Eylea 2 mg every 8 weeks group was 94% in VIEW1 and 95% in VIEW2.[4,46] The proportion of patients maintaining vision in the Lucentis 0.5 mg every 4 weeks group was identical (94% in VIEW1 and 95% in VIEW2) at 52 weeks. The mean change in BCVA from baseline at week 52 was +7.9 letters in the Eylea 2 mg every 8 weeks group and +8.1 letters in the Lucentis 0.5 mg every 4 weeks group. In both groups, 31% of patients gained at least 15 letters at week 52.[4,46]

- **Eylea HD 8 mg**—PULSAR was a phase 3 randomized controlled clinical trial that included 1,009 patients with treatment naïve nAMD and compared the following treatment options: (1) Eylea HD 8 mg every 12 weeks following three initial monthly injections, (2) Eylea HD 8 mg every 16 weeks following three initial monthly injections, or (3) Eylea 2 mg every 8 weeks following three initial monthly injections.[47] If disease progression was noted during the first year of the study, the dosing interval for Eylea HD 8 mg groups could be shortened to 8 weeks.[47] At 48 weeks, 79% of patients among the Eylea HD 8 mg every 12-week group maintained 12-week dosing and 77% of patients in the Eylea HD 8 mg every 16-week group maintained 16-week dosing.[48] Clinically equivalent vision gains were achieved in Eylea HD 8 mg groups compared to Eylea 2 mg group. The mean gain in acuity at 48 weeks was +7.6 letters in the Eylea 2 mg group, +6.7 letters in the Eylea HD 8 mg every 12-week group, and +6.2 letters in the Eylea HD 8 mg every 16-week group.[49] No new safety signals with Eylea HD were identified.[50]

  During the second year of the study, Eylea HD 8 mg patients could extend the dosing interval up to 24-weeks if stability criteria were met. At 2 years, 70% of patients among the Eylea HD 8 mg every 16-week group maintained 16-week or longer dosing intervals. Additionally, 47% met the criteria for 20-week or longer dosing intervals.[51]
- **Lucentis**—MARINA was a large randomized controlled trial that compared the efficacy of Lucentis 0.5 mg every 4 weeks to sham injection in eyes with patients with minimally classic or occult choroidal neovascularization.[3] The proportion of patients who maintained vision, defined as losing fewer than 15 ETDRS letters of BCVA at 12 months was 91% in the Lucentis-treated group and 60% in the sham group. At 4 months, 89% in the Lucentis-treated group and 56% in the sham group maintained vision. The mean change in BCVA from baseline at month 24 was +5.5 letters in the Lucentis group and −15 letters in the sham group. At 24 months, 30% of patients gained at least 15 letters in the Lucentis group compared to 4% of those receiving sham.[3,52]
  - HARBOR was a randomized, double-masked, active treatment–controlled study that compared different dosing schedules of Lucentis 0.5 mg, (1) Lucentis every 4 weeks (monthly) or (2) pro re nata (PRN) treatment following three monthly doses.[52] A mean of 13.3 injections were given in the PRN treatment group over the course of the 2-year study. The mean change in BCVA from baseline at 2 years was +9.1 letters in the monthly treatment group compared to +7.9 letters in the PRN treatment group. At 2 years, 34.5% of patients gained at least 15 letters in the monthly Lucentis group compared to 33.1% of those receiving Lucentis PRN.[52]
- **Beovu**—HAWK and HARRIER were two parallel randomized active-controlled clinical trials that compared Beovu 6 mg administered every 8 or 12 weeks (following three monthly doses) to Eylea 2 mg administered every 8 weeks (following three monthly doses). At 96 weeks in HAWK, the mean change in BCVA from baseline was +5.9 letters in the

Beovu group and +5.3 letters in the Eylea group. In HARRIER, mean acuity gains were 6.1 and 6.6 letters in the Beovu and the Eylea groups, respectively. The proportion of patients gaining at least 15 letters by week 96 in HAWK was 34.2% in the Beovu group and 27% in the Eylea group. In the sister trial HARRIER, 29.1% gained at least 15 letters by week 96 in the Beovu group and 31.5% in the Eylea group.[6]

## Diabetic Macular Edema

- **Vabysmo—**YOSEMITE and RHINE were two parallel randomized active-controlled clinical trials that compared (1) Eylea administered every 8 weeks (following five monthly doses), (2) Vabysmo administered every 8 weeks (following six monthly doses), and (3) Vabysmo initially administered monthly for 4 months followed by a variable injection interval depending upon disease activity.[7,53] In both YOSEMITE and RHINE, the mean change from baseline in both Vabysmo groups compared to patients treated with Eylea. In YOSEMITE, the mean change in BCVA from baseline at week 56 was +10.7 letters in the Vabysmo administered at a fixed interval every 8 weeks, +11.6 letters in the Vabysmo with variable administration group, and +10.9 letters in the Eylea group. In RHINE, the mean change in BCVA from baseline at week 56 was +11.8 letters in the Vabysmo administered at a fixed interval every 8 weeks, +10.8 letters in the Vabysmo with variable administration group, and +10.3 letters in the Eylea group.[7,53]
- **Eylea 2 mg—**VISTA and VIVID were two parallel phase 3 randomized controlled clinical trials that included 872 eyes with center-involved DME and compared the following treatment options: (1) Eylea 2 mg every 8 weeks following five initial monthly injections, (2) Eylea 2 mg monthly, or (3) macular laser photocoagulation.[54] From week 24 through week 100, eyes in the Eylea groups were eligible to receive rescue laser photocoagulation and eyes in the macular photocoagulation groups were eligible to receive rescue Eylea every 8 weeks. At week 100 in VISTA and VIVID, the mean change in BCVA from baseline was +11.5 and +11.4 letters in the monthly Eylea group, +11.1 and + 9.4 letters in the Eylea every 8 weeks group, and +0.9 and +0.7 letters in the macular photocoagulation group. At week 100 in VISTA and VIVID, the proportion of eyes gaining at least 15 ETDRS letters or more was 38.8% and 38.2% in the monthly Eylea group, 33.1% and 31.1% in the Eylea every 8 weeks group, and 13% and 12.1% in the macular photocoagulation group.[54]
- **Eylea HD 8 mg—**PHOTON was a phase 3 randomized controlled clinical trial that included 658 patients with center involved DME and compared the following treatment options: (1) Eylea HD 8 mg every 12 weeks following three initial monthly injections, (2) Eylea HD 8 mg every 16 weeks following three initial monthly injections, or (3) Eylea 2 mg every 8 weeks following five initial monthly injections.[47] If disease progression was noted during the first year of the study, the dosing interval for Eylea HD 8 mg groups could be shortened to 8 weeks.[47] At 48 weeks, 91% of patients among the Eylea HD 8 mg every 12-week group maintained 12-week dosing and 89% of patients in the Eylea HD 8 mg every 16-week group maintained 16-week dosing.[55] Clinically equivalent vision gains were achieved in Eylea HD 8 mg groups compared to Eylea 2 mg group. The mean gain in acuity at 48 weeks was +9.2 letters in the Eylea 2 mg group, +8.8 letters in the Eylea HD 8 mg every 12-week group, and +7.9 letters in the Eylea HD 8 mg every 16-week group.[56] No new safety signals with Eylea HD were identified.[57]

During the second year of the study, Eylea HD 8 mg patients could extend the dosing interval up to 24-weeks if stability criteria were met. At 2 years, 84% of patients among the Eylea HD 8 mg every 16-week group maintained 16-week or longer dosing intervals. Additionally, 44% met the criteria for 20-week or longer dosing intervals.[58]

- **Lucentis**—RISE and RIDE were parallel phase 3 randomized controlled clinical trials including 377 and 382 patients, respectively, with DME and BCVA of 20/40 to 20/320.[59] Patients were randomized to either monthly Lucentis or sham injections. At 24 months in RISE and RIDE, the proportion of eyes gaining at least 15 ETDRS letters or more was 44.8% and 33.6% in the 0.3 mg Lucentis group compared to 18.1% and 12.3% in the sham group.[59]
- **Beovu**—KESTREL and KITE were two parallel randomized active-controlled clinical trials that compared Beovu 6 mg administered every 8 or 12 weeks depending upon disease activity (following five monthly doses) to Eylea 2 mg administered every 8 weeks (following five monthly doses).[6] At week 52, the mean change in BCVA from baseline was +9.2 letters in the Beovu group and +10.5 letters in the Eylea group in KESTREL. In KITE, the mean letter gain was +10.6 in the Beovu group and +9.4 in the Eylea group.[6]

## Effect of Anti-VEGF on Diabetic Retinopathy in Eyes with Diabetic Macular Edema

- **Eylea**—Although VISTA and VIVID were designed to evaluate the efficacy of Eylea in eyes with DME, secondary analysis showed that significantly more eyes in the Eylea groups had an improvement in DR stage compared to the macular photocoagulation group. A two-step or greater improvement in the Diabetic Retinopathy Severity Score (DRSS) at 100 weeks was noted in 37% and 29.3% of the monthly Eylea group, 37.1% and 32.6% in the Eylea every 8 weeks group, and 15.6% and 8.2% in VISTA and VIVID, respectively.[54]
- **Lucentis**—Similarly, RIDE and RISE were designed to evaluate the efficacy of Lucentis in eyes with DME; however, secondary analysis showed that monthly Lucentis significantly reduced the rate of DR progression while increasing the chances of DR regression. The proportion of eyes achieving a two-step or greater improvement in the ETDRS severity scale was 37.2% in the monthly 0.3 mg Lucentis group compared to 5.4% in the sham group. Furthermore, the proportion with mild NPDR increased from 16% to 44% at 24 months in the monthly 0.3 mg Lucentis group.[60]

## Effect of Anti-VEGF on Diabetic Retinopathy in Eyes without Diabetic Macular Edema

- Eylea—PANORAMA was a randomized clinical trial that evaluated the efficacy of Eylea to improve retinopathy in 402 eyes with moderately severe to severe NPDR (DRSS levels 47–53), no DME, and acuity of 20/40 or better at baseline.[61] Eyes were randomized to one of three groups: (1) Eylea 2 mg every 16 weeks following three initial monthly injections and one 8-week interval, (2) Eylea 2 mg every 8 weeks following five initial monthly injections with PRN dosing starting at week 56, or (3) sham injections. At 52 weeks, 65.2% in the Eylea every 16 weeks, 79.9% in the Eylea every 8 weeks, and only 15% in the sham groups showed a two-step or more improvement in the DRSS. Significantly less eyes developed vision-threatening complications (proliferation or anterior segment neovascularization) or center-involved DME at week 100 (16.3% in the Eylea every 16 weeks group, 18.7% in the Eylea every 8 weeks followed by PRN dosing group, and 50.4% in the sham group).[61]

The Diabetic Retinopathy Clinical Research Network (DRCR.net) Protocol W was set out to evaluate the potential benefits of periodic anti-VEGF therapy in preventing vision-threatening complications.[62] The study included 399 eyes with moderate-to-severe NPDR without center-involved DME and randomized them to either immediate periodic anti-VEGF injections (three monthly Eylea 2 mg injections, one at an 8-week interval, followed by injections every 4 months) or observation until center-involved DME with vision loss or high-risk PDR developed. The 2-year results showed that Eylea significantly reduced the rate of development of vision-threatening complications such as center-involved DME with vision loss or PDR (incidence of 16.3% of eyes in the Eylea group compared to 43.5% in the sham group at 2 years). However, there was no significant acuity benefit at 2 years, and the mean change in BCVA from baseline was −0.9 letters in the Eylea group compared to −2.0 letters in the sham group.[62]

## Macular Edema Following Retinal Vein Occlusion

- **Eylea**
  - **Branch retinal vein occlusion (BRVO)**—VIBRANT study was a randomized controlled trial that randomized 183 patients with macular edema secondary to BRVO to either 2 mg Eylea injections every 8 weeks following six monthly doses or grid laser photocoagulation at baseline.[63] The Eylea group was able to receive rescue grid laser at week 36 if needed and the grid laser photocoagulation group was eligible to receive Eylea after 6 months. The proportion of eyes gaining at least 15 EDTRS letters at week 52 was 52.7% in the Eylea group and 26.7% in the grid laser group. The mean change in BCVA from baseline at week 52 was +17.1 letters in the Eylea group and +12.2 letters in the grid laser group.[63]
  - **Central retinal vein occlusion (CRVO)**—COPERNICUS was a randomized controlled trial that randomized 188 patients with macular edema secondary to CRVO to monthly injections of either Eylea 2 mg or sham for 6 months, followed by PRN Eylea injections (monthly evaluation during weeks 25 through 52, and quarterly evaluation during weeks 52–100) for all groups up to 1 year depending upon disease activity.[64] The proportion of patients gaining at least 15 letters at 6 months (prior to the sham eyes being eligible for Eylea treatment) was 56% in the monthly Eylea group and 12% in the sham group. At 2 years, 49% in the group initially treated with monthly Eylea and 23% in the initial sham group gained at least 15 letters compared to baseline, suggesting that early treatment results in better long-term visual outcomes.[64]
- **Lucentis**
  - **BRVO:** BRAVO was a large randomized, double-masked study including 397 patients with center-involved macular edema secondary to BRVO that compared monthly injections of either 0.5 mg Lucentis or sham for 6 months, followed by PRN Lucentis

injections for all groups up to 1 year depending upon disease activity.[3,65] After 3 months, all eyes could receive rescue grid laser photocoagulation if no improvement from baseline was seen. By 6 months, 54% of eyes in the sham group received rescue grid laser photocoagulation. The proportion of patients gaining at least 15 letters at 6 months (prior to the sham eyes being eligible for Lucentis treatment) was 61% in the monthly Lucentis group and 29% in the sham group. At 1 year, 71% in the group initially treated with monthly Lucentis and 50% in the initial sham group gained at least 15 letters from baseline, suggesting that early Lucentis treatment provides the best visual prognosis.[3,65]

HORIZON was an open-label 1-year extension study of BRAVO, during which all eyes received 0.5 mg Lucentis no sooner than every 3 months depending upon disease activity.[66] A similar number of injections, approximately 2, was performed in both the initial 0.5 mg Lucentis and sham groups. The mean change in BCVA at the end of the 1-year follow-up period was −0.7 letters in the initial 0.5 mg Lucentis group and 0.9 letters in the initially sham group.[66]

- **CRVO**—CRUISE was a large prospective randomized, controlled trial including 392 patients with foveal involved macular edema secondary to CRVO that compared monthly injections of either 0.5 mg Lucentis or sham for 6 months, followed by PRN Lucentis injections for all groups up to 1 year depending upon disease activity.[67] At 6 months, 48% of patients gained at least 15 letters in the 0.5 mg Lucentis group compared to 17% of those receiving sham. At 12 months, the mean change in BCVA from baseline was +13.9 letters in the 0.5 mg Lucentis group and +7.3% in the group initially randomized to sham.[3,67] HORIZON was an open-label 1-year extension study of BRAVO, during which all eyes received 0.5 mg Lucentis no sooner than every 3 months depending upon disease activity. The mean change in BCVA at the end of the 1-year follow-up period demonstrated a loss of initial acuity gains and was −4.1 letters in the initial 0.5 mg Lucentis group and −4.2 letters in the initially sham group.[66]

## Myopic Choroidal Neovascularization

- **Lucentis**—RADIANCE was a phase 3 active-controlled clinical trial that included 277 eyes with active choroidal neovascularization secondary to pathologic myopia and Snellen acuity of 20/32 to 20/320. Patients were randomized to (1) two monthly injections of Lucentis 0.5 mg followed by PRN treatment determined by the visual acuity stabilization criterion, (2) an initial injection of Lucentis 0.5 mg followed by PRN treatment determined by the disease activity criterion, or (3) verteporfin photodynamic therapy (PDT) with an option for rescue Lucentis 0.5 mg starting at month 3. Both Lucentis groups were superior to PDT with regards to gain in acuity. The mean change in BCVA at 1 year was +13.8 letters in the Lucentis followed by PRN acuity-guided treatment, +14.4 letters in the Lucentis followed by PRN disease-guided treatment, and +9.3 letters in the PDT group. The median number of injections given in the Lucentis followed by PRN acuity-guided treatment group was 4, whereas a median of two injections over the course of the year was given in the other two treatment groups.[68]

## CODING/BILLING

For an intravitreal anti-VEGF injection, Current Procedural Terminology (CPT) code 67028 is used: "Vitreous Procedures on the Posterior Segment of the Eye" and appended with a modifier depending on the eye injected (RT, LT) or 50 for bilateral injections. In addition, the appropriate HCPCS J-code depending upon the medication used should also be billed and the total dosage administered should be noted within the claim "Remarks"[69-71]:

- **J7999**—Bevacizumab compounded 1.25 mg, additionally add a description such as "1.25 mg of Avastin for ophthalmological use" in the narrative field[69,70]
- **J2778**—Lucentis (ranibizumab) 0.1 mg per unit (typical unilateral dose is 3 or 5 units)
- **Q5124**—Byooviz (ranibizumab-nuna) 0.1 mg per unit (typical unilateral dose is 5 units)
- **J0178**—Eylea (aflibercept) 1 mg per unit (typical unilateral dose is 2 units)
- **J2777**—Vabysmo (faricimab-svoa) 0.1 mg per unit (typical unilateral dose is 60 units)
- **J0179**—Beovu (brolucizumab) 1 mg per unit (typical unilateral dose is 6 units)

The medically necessary ICD-10 code should be linked to the 67028 code and the J-code (see eTable 41-1 for commonly used billable ICD-10 codes).[70] CPT code 67028 has a 0-day postoperative global period.[69-71]

## REFERENCES


1. Karmel M. Off-label anti-VEGF therapy: targeting new conditions [Internet]. 2012. Accessed December 7, 2022. https://www.aao.org/eyenet/article/off-label-anti-vegf-therapy-targeting-new-conditio
2. Myers LA (Provencher), Almeida D, Abràmoff MD. Intravitreal injection technique: A primer for ophthalmology residents and fellows [Internet]. 2015. Accessed December 7, 2022. http://www.EyeRounds.org/tutorials/intravitreal-injection/
3. LUCENTIS (ranibizumab). Package insert. Genentech, Inc; 2018.
4. Eylea (aflibercept). Package insert. Regeneron Pharmaceuticals, Inc; 2021.
5. Eylea (aflibercept) HD. Package insert. Regeneron Pharmaceuticals, Inc; 2023.
6. Beovu (brolucizumab). Package insert. Novartis; 2020.
7. VABYSMO. Package insert. Genentech, Inc; 2022.
8. Byooviz. Package insert. Biogen Inc., Ltd; 2021.
9. Gunther JB, Altaweel MM. Bevacizumab (Avastin) for the treatment of ocular disease. *Surv Ophthalmol.* 2009;54(3):372-400.
10. Wilson ME, Scott AW. How to give intravitreal injections [Internet]. 2013. Accessed December 7, 2022. https://www.aao.org/eyenet/article/how-to-give-intravitreal-injections
11. Polizzi S, Mahajan VB. Intravitreal anti-VEGF injections in pregnancy: case series and review of literature. *J Ocul Pharmacol Ther.* 2015;31(10):605-610.
12. Kianersi F, Ghanbari H, Naderi Beni Z, Naderi Beni A. Intravitreal vascular endothelial growth factor (VEGF) inhibitor injection in patient during pregnancy. *J Drug Assess.* 2021;10(1):7-9.
13. SooHoo JR, Seibold LK, Kahook MY. The link between intravitreal antivascular endothelial growth factor injections and glaucoma. *Curr Opin Ophthalmol.* 2014;25(2):127-133.
14. Pershing S, Bakri SJ, Moshfeghi DM. Ocular hypertension and intraocular pressure asymmetry after intravitreal injection of anti-vascular endothelial growth factor agents. *Ophthalmic Surg Lasers Imaging Retina.* 2013;44:460-464.
15. Beck M, Munk MR, Ebneter A, et al. Retinal ganglion cell layer change in patients treated with anti-vascular endothelial growth factor for neovascular age-related macular degeneration. *Am J Ophthalmol.* 2016;167:10-17.
16. Saleh R, Karpe A, Zinkernagel MS, et al. Inner retinal layer change in glaucoma patients receiving anti-VEGF for neovascular age related macular degeneration. *Graefes Arch Clin Exp Ophthalmol.* 2017;255(4):817-824.

17. Kopić A, Biuk D, Barać J, et al. Retinal nerve fiber layer thickness in glaucoma patients treated with multiple intravitreal anti-VEGF (bevacizumab) injections. *Acta Clin Croat.* 2017;56:406-414.
18. Chang CK, Cheng CK, Peng CH. The incidence and risk factors for the development of vitreomacular interface abnormality in diabetic macular edema treated with intravitreal injection of anti-VEGF. *Eye (Lond).* 2017;31(5):762-770.
19. Tan Y, Fukutomi A, Sun MT, et al. Anti-VEGF crunch syndrome in proliferative diabetic retinopathy: a review. *Surv Ophthalmol.* 2021;66(6):926-932.
20. Zarbin MA. Anti-VEGF agents and the risk of arteriothrombotic events. *Asia Pac J Ophthalmol (Phila).* 2018;7(1):63-67.
21. Dalal PJ, Patel AL, Carle M, et al. Review of ophthalmic and breastfeeding medicine evidence: real and theoretical risks of intravitreal anti-vascular endothelial growth factor administration in lactating women. *Retina.* 2020;40(11):2065-2069.
22. The Foundation American Society of Retina Specialists. Retina health series: intravitreal injections [Internet]. 2017. Accessed December 7, 2022. https://www.asrs.org/patients/retinal-diseases/33/intravitreal-injection
23. Chaturvedi R, Wannamaker KW, Riviere PJ, et al. Real-world trends in intravitreal injection practices among American retina specialists. *Ophthalmol Retina.* 2019;3(8):656-662.
24. Yorston D. Intravitreal injection technique. *Community Eye Health.* 2014;27(87):47.
25. Avery RL, Bakri SJ, Blumenkranz MS, et al. Intravitreal injection technique and monitoring: updated guidelines of an expert panel. *Retina.* 2014;34(suppl 12):S1-S18.
26. Saxena S, Lai TY, Koizumi H, et al; International Pharmacokinetic Collaboration. Anterior chamber paracentesis during intravitreal injections in observational trials: effectiveness and safety and effects. *Int J Retina Vitreous.* 2019;5:8.
27. Bayer AG Leverkusen, Germany. Preparation and handling of the EYLEA (aflibercept) prefilled syringe [Internet]. 2020. Accessed December 7, 2022. https://ophthalmology.bayer.com/sites/g/files/vrxlpx4811/files/2020-08/EYLEA%20PFS%20Instructions%20for%20Use%20A4%20PDF.pdf
28. Blaha GR, Tilton EP, Barouch FC, et al. Randomized trial of anesthetic methods for intravitreal injections. *Retina.* 2011;31(3):535-539.
29. Boden JH, Myers ML, Lee T, et al. Effect of lidocaine gel on povidone-iodine antisepsis and microbial survival. *J Cataract Refract Surg.* 2008;34(10):1773-1775.
30. Doshi RR, Leng T, Fung AE. Povidone-iodine before lidocaine gel anesthesia achieves surface antisepsis. *Ophthalmic Surg Lasers Imaging.* 2011;42(4):346-349.
31. https://www.reviewofophthalmology.com/article/updated-guidelines-for-intravitreal-injection
32. Friedman DA, Mason JO 3rd, Emond T, McGwin G Jr. Povidone-iodine contact time and lid speculum use during intravitreal injection. *Retina.* 2013;33(5):975-981.
33. Cox JT, Eliott D, Sobrin L. Inflammatory complications of intravitreal anti-VEGF injections. *J Clin Med.* 2021;10(5):981.
34. Witkin AJ, Hahn P, Murray TG, et al. Occlusive retinal vasculitis following intravitreal brolucizumab. *J Vitreoretin Dis.* 2020;4(4):269-279.
35. Monés J, Srivastava SK, Jaffe GJ, et al. Risk of inflammation, retinal vasculitis, and retinal occlusion-related events with brolucizumab: post hoc review of HAWK and HARRIER. *Ophthalmology.* 2021;128(7):1050-1059.
36. Merani R, Hunyor AP. Endophthalmitis following intravitreal anti-vascular endothelial growth factor (VEGF) injection: a comprehensive review. *Int J Retina Vitreous.* 2015;1:9.
37. Sachdeva MM, Moshiri A, Leder HA, et al. Endophthalmitis following intravitreal injection of anti-VEGF agents: long-term outcomes and the identification of unusual micro-organisms. *J Ophthalmic Inflamm Infect.* 2016;6(1):2.
38. Bagheri N, Wajda B, Calvo C, et al. *The Wills Eye Manual: Office and Emergency Room Diagnosis and Treatment of Eye Disease.* 7th ed. Lippincott Williams & Wilkins; 2017.
39. Chaudhary KM, Romero JM, Ezon I, et al. Pars plana vitrectomy in the management of patients diagnosed with endophthalmitis following intravitreal anti-vascular endothelial growth factor injection. *Retina.* 2013;33(7):1407-1416.
40. Day S, Acquah K, Mruthyunjaya P, et al. Ocular complications after anti-vascular endothelial growth factor therapy in Medicare patients with age-related macular degeneration. *Am J Ophthalmol.* 2011;152(2):266-272.
41. DR: anatomy outcomes [Internet]. Regeneron Pharmaceuticals, Inc. 2021. Accessed December 7, 2022. https://hcp.eylea.us/about/diabetic-retinopathy-anatomy-outcomes/
42. Nguyen CL, Oh LJ, Wong E, Wei J, Chilov M. Anti-vascular endothelial growth factor for neovascular age-related macular degeneration: a meta-analysis of randomized controlled trials. *BMC Ophthalmol.* 2018;18(1):130.

43. Sarraf D, Joseph A, Rahimy E. Retinal pigment epithelial tears in the era of intravitreal pharmacotherapy: risk factors, pathogenesis, prognosis and treatment (an American Ophthalmological Society thesis). *Trans Am Ophthalmol Soc.* 2014;112:142-159.
44. Munk MR, Ceklic L, Ebneter A, et al. Macular atrophy in patients with long-term anti-VEGF treatment for neovascular age-related macular degeneration. *Acta Ophthalmol.* 2016;94:e757-e764.
45. Heier JS, Khanani AM, Quezada Ruiz C, et al; TENAYA and LUCERNE Investigators. Efficacy, durability, and safety of intravitreal faricimab up to every 16 weeks for neovascular age-related macular degeneration (TENAYA and LUCERNE): two randomised, double-masked, phase 3, non-inferiority trials. *Lancet.* 2022;399(10326):729-740.
46. Heier JS, Brown DM, Chong V, et al; VIEW 1 and VIEW 2 Study Groups. Intravitreal aflibercept (VEGF trap-eye) in wet age-related macular degeneration. *Ophthalmology.* 2012;119(12):2537-2548.
47. Regeneron Pharmaceuticals. Afibercept 8 mg meets primary endpoints in two global pivotal trials for DME and wAMD with a vast majority of patients maintained on 12- and 16- week dosing intervals [Internet]. 2022. Accessed September 12, 2023. https://investor.regeneron.com/news-releases/news-release-details/aflibercept-8-mg-meets-primary-endpoints-two-global-pivotal
48. Regeneron Pharmaceuticals. Wet AMD: extended dosing [Internet]. 2023. Accessed September 12, 2023. https://eyleahcp.us/s/eyleahd/wet-amd-extended-dosing
49. Regeneron Pharmaceuticals. Wet AMD: vision outcomes [Internet]. 2023. Accessed September 12, 2023. https://eyleahcp.us/s/eyleahd/wet-amd-vision-outcomes
50. Regeneron Pharmaceuticals. Wet AMD: safety [Internet]. 2023. Accessed September 12, 2023. https://eyleahcp.us/s/eyleahd/wet-amd-safety-data
51. Regeneron Pharmaceuticals. Two-year PULSAR trial results for aflibercept 8 mg demonstrate durable vision gains at extended dosing intervals in wet age-related macular degeneration [Internet]. 2023. Accessed September 12, 2023. https://investor.regeneron.com/news-releases/news-release-details/two-year-pulsar-trial-results-aflibercept-8-mg-demonstrate
52. Ho AC, Busbee BG, Regillo CD, et al; HARBOR Study Group. Twenty-four-month efficacy and safety of 0.5 mg or 2.0 mg ranibizumab in patients with subfoveal neovascular age-related macular degeneration. *Ophthalmology.* 2014;121(11):2181-2192.
53. Wykoff CC, Abreu F, Adamis AP, et al; YOSEMITE and RHINE Investigators. Efficacy, durability, and safety of intravitreal faricimab with extended dosing up to every 16 weeks in patients with diabetic macular oedema (YOSEMITE and RHINE): two randomised, double-masked, phase 3 trials. *Lancet.* 2022;399(10326):741-755.
54. Brown DM, Schmidt-Erfurth U, Do DV, et al. Intravitreal aflibercept for diabetic macular edema: 100-week results from the VISTA and VIVID studies. *Ophthalmology.* 2015;122(10):2044-2052.
55. Regeneron Pharmaceuticals. DME: extended dosing [Internet]. 2023. Accessed September 12, 2023. https://eyleahcp.us/s/eyleahd/dme-extended-dosing
56. Regeneron Pharmaceuticals. DME: vision outcomes [Internet]. 2023. Accessed September 12, 2023. https://eyleahcp.us/s/eyleahd/dme-vision-outcomes
57. Regeneron Pharmaceuticals. DME: safety [Internet]. 2023. Accessed September 12, 2023. https://eyleahcp.us/s/eyleahd/dme-safety-data
58. Regeneron Pharmaceuticals. Aflibercept 8 mg two-year results from pivotal PHOTON trial in diabetic macular edema presented at ASRS [Internet]. 2023. Accessed September 12, 2023.https://investor.regeneron.com/news-releases/news-release-details/aflibercept-8-mg-two-year-results-pivotal-photon-trial-diabetic
59. Nguyen QD, Brown DM, Marcus DM, et al; RISE and RIDE Research Group. Ranibizumab for diabetic macular edema: results from 2 phase III randomized trials: RISE and RIDE. *Ophthalmology.* 2012;119(4):789-801.
60. Ip MS, Domalpally A, Hopkins JJ, et al. Long-term effects of ranibizumab on diabetic retinopathy severity and progression. *Arch Ophthalmol.* 2012;130(9):1145-1152.
61. Brown DM, Wykoff CC, Boyer D, et al. Evaluation of intravitreal aflibercept for the treatment of severe nonproliferative diabetic retinopathy: results from the PANORAMA randomized clinical trial. *JAMA Ophthalmol.* 2021;139(9):946-955.
62. Maturi RK, Glassman AR, Josic K, et al; DRCR Retina Network. Effect of intravitreous anti-vascular endothelial growth factor vs sham treatment for prevention of vision-threatening complications of diabetic retinopathy: the Protocol W randomized clinical trial. *JAMA Ophthalmol.* 2021;139(7):701-712.
63. Clark WL, Boyer DS, Heier JS, et al. Intravitreal aflibercept for macular edema following branch retinal vein occlusion: 52-week results of the VIBRANT study. *Ophthalmology.* 2016;123(2):330-336.

64. Heier JS, Clark WL, Boyer DS, et al. Intravitreal aflibercept injection for macular edema due to central retinal vein occlusion: two-year results from the COPERNICUS study. *Ophthalmology.* 2014;121(7):1414-1420.e1.
65. Campochiaro PA, Heier JS, Feiner L, et al; BRAVO Investigators. Ranibizumab for macular edema following branch retinal vein occlusion: six-month primary end point results of a phase III study. *Ophthalmology.* 2010; 117(6):1102-1112.e1.
66. Heier JS, Campochiaro PA, Yau L, et al. Ranibizumab for macular edema due to retinal vein occlusions: long-term follow-up in the HORIZON trial. *Ophthalmology.* 2012;119(4):802-809.
67. Brown DM, Campochiaro PA, Singh RP; CRUISE Investigators. Ranibizumab for macular edema following central retinal vein occlusion: six-month primary end point results of a phase III study. *Ophthalmology.* 2010; 117(6):1124-1133.e1.
68. Wolf S, Balciuniene VJ, Laganovska G, et al; RADIANCE Study Group. RADIANCE: a randomized controlled study of ranibizumab in patients with choroidal neovascularization secondary to pathologic myopia. *Ophthalmology.* 2014;121(3):682-692.e2.
69. Centers for Medicare & Medicaid Services. Billing and coding: information regarding uses, including off-label uses, of anti-vascular endothelial growth factor for the treatment of ophthalmological diseases [Internet]. 2023. Accessed January 30, 2023. https://www.cms.gov/medicare-coverage-database/view/article.aspx?articleId=53121
70. Novitas Solutions. Avastin for ophthalmological use, J7999 [Internet]. 2023. Accessed January 30, 2023. https://www.novitas-solutions.com/webcenter/portal/MedicareJL/pagebyid?contentId=00240103
71. American Academy of Ophthalmology. Coding for injectable drugs [Internet]. 2023. Accessed January 30, 2023. https://www.aao.org/practice-management/coding/injectable-drugs

# 42 Intravitreal Steroid Injections

Vlad M. Matei • Jessica Haynes

## BACKGROUND

Intravitreal steroid injections are an important therapeutic option for noninfectious intermediate, posterior, and panuveitis, as well as for macular edema (ME) of various etiologies, including uveitis, diabetes, retinal vein occlusions, and other ischemic retinopathies.[1,2] Both off-label and on-label steroid preparations have demonstrated efficacy. Although fundamentally the injection procedure is similar to that of intravitreal anti-vascular endothelial growth factor (anti-VEGF) injections, for some medications the procedure varies slightly. This chapter surveys the uses, techniques, and complications of intravitreal steroid use.

## INDICATIONS

### Key Indications

- Diabetic macular edema (DME)
- ME secondary to retinal vein occlusions
- Uveitic ME
- Idiopathic cystoid macular edema (CME)
- Noninfectious intermediate, posterior, and panuveitis

Triamcinolone acetonide (TA) suspension—Intravitreal injections of both off-label and on-label preparations of TA have been employed. Kenalog-10 (10 mg/mL) and Kenalog-40 (40 mg/mL) (both Bristol-Myers-Squibb, Princeton, NJ) are commercially available TA preparations that are off-label for intravitreal use; the latter has been used more commonly as an injection of 4 mg, which is more effective than the lower dose.[3] Preservative-free triamcinolone 40 mg/mL (Triesence, Alcon Laboratories Inc., Fort Worth, TX) is approved for treatment of sympathetic ophthalmia, temporal arteritis, uveitis, and ocular inflammatory conditions unresponsive to topical corticosteroids. Triesence is approved at a dose of 4 mg per 0.1 mL for all the above listed in-office indications. Some practitioners prefer to inject only 0.05 mL (2 mg) of Triesence to minimize the intraocular pressure (IOP) increase following intravitreal injection. The use of Triesence for non-uveitic ME is off-label.

Dexamethasone intravitreal implant 0.7 mg (Ozurdex, Allergan Inc., Irvine, CA)—This sustained-release intravitreal dexamethasone implant (IDI) is approved for the treatment of ME following branch retinal vein occlusion (BRVO) or central retinal vein occlusion (CRVO), noninfectious posterior uveitis, and DME in those who are pseudophakic or phakic and planning for cataract surgery.

Fluocinolone acetonide intravitreal implant 0.19 mg (ILUVIEN, Alimera Sciences Inc., Alpharetta, GA)—This sustained-release fluocinolone acetonide intravitreal implant (FAI9) is U.S. Food and Drug Administration (FDA)-approved for the treatment of DME.

Fluocinolone acetonide intravitreal implant 0.18 mg (YUTIQ, Eyepoint Pharmaceuticals Inc., Watertown, MA)—This sustained-release fluocinolone acetonide intravitreal implant (FAI8) is approved for the treatment of patients with chronic noninfectious posterior uveitis. It is very similar to FAI9, with the primary difference between the two being their on-label uses.

Fluocinolone acetonide intravitreal implant 0.59 mg (Retisert, Bausch + Lomb, Bridgewater, NJ)—Unlike FAI9 and FAI8, which are injected transconjunctivally into the eye as an in-office procedure, the fluocinolone acetonide intravitreal implant 0.59 mg (FAI5) is implanted surgically in the operating room.

## CONTRAINDICATIONS

### Key Contraindications

- Advanced glaucoma (>0.8 cup-to-disc ratio)
- Active ocular or periocular infection
- Aphakia or anterior chamber intraocular lens (ACIOL) (IDI, FAI9, and FAI8)
- Hypersensitivity to the medications used

**Relative Contraindications**

- Mild-to-moderate glaucoma
- Ocular hypertension
- Phakic status
- Pseudophakia with lack of an intact posterior lens capsule (IDI, FAI9, and FAI8)

Ocular corticosteroid use may result in increased IOP. This makes advanced glaucoma a contraindication for intravitreal corticosteroid use and mild-to-moderate glaucoma or ocular hypertension—which may be more amenable to medical control—relative contraindications.

Corticosteroids are immunosuppressants and may potentially worsen an active ocular or periocular infection. This is especially important in the setting of uveitis, where every effort must be made to rule out an infectious etiology prior to the use of steroids.

The IDI[4] and, less commonly, the fluocinolone acetonide implants[5] can migrate to the anterior chamber when there is no lens capsule to serve as a barrier to this migration. This is a much greater concern in aphakic patients or patients with an ACIOL, rather than in pseudophakic patients with a posterior-chamber IOL following an uncomplicated planned posterior capsulotomy.

All ocular corticosteroids increase the incidence of cataract formation—a consideration that should be taken into account when using steroids in phakic patients.

# PROCEDURE

For preoperative preparation of intravitreal injections, please see Chapter 41 on intravitreal anti-VEGF injections, as this procedure will apply similarly to intravitreal steroid injections. Following informed consent and a procedural time-out, either topical or subconjunctival anesthesia should be used and allowed to take effect. The most important component of the preparation is sterilization of the ocular surface and eyelashes via the topical application of povidone–iodine 5%.[6] The use of sterile gloves, a sterile drape, and a sterile eyelid speculum are no longer required, although many practitioners prefer to use a speculum. Short needles, with a maximum length of 13 mm, are typically used. Although 30-gauge needles are often used for delivery of anti-VEGF medications, these are less appropriate when injecting TA, as the diameter of these needles is too small to allow smooth passage of the TA particles through the needle; instead, most practitioners use short 27-gauge needles when injecting TA intravitreally.[7]

After sterilization of the ocular surface and eyelashes, the eyelid should be retracted (with or without a speculum), followed by injection of the medication into the vitreous, as described in Chapter 41. As for anti-VEGF injections, the distance of the scleral entry site posteriorly from the corneal limbus should be approximately 3 mm in aphakic or pseudophakic patients and 3.5 to 4.0 mm in phakic patients. Although the injections may be performed in any meridian, most practitioners prefer an inferior meridian for intravitreal steroid injections, because an inferior injection may reduce the degree of floaters experienced by the patient following a TA suspension injection, and for the IDI, it may reduce the risk of the IDI settling on the postequatorial retina or migrating into the anterior chamber. Many practitioners prefer the inferotemporal quadrant over the inferonasal quadrant because of the improved exposure and easier access in the former. For similar reasons, placing the patient with the head in an upright or nearly upright position prior to injection is advisable.

Each medication has additional procedural details, as follows:

## Triamcinolone Suspensions[4]

After shaking the vial of a TA suspension to help to homogeneously distribute the particles in the suspension, withdraw the contents of the vial into a sterile 1-mL syringe using a 27-gauge (or larger) needle. Place a new sterile 27-gauge needle on the syringe and rest the syringe with the needle pointed upward for a few minutes to allow the TA crystals to settle to the bottom of the suspension in the syringe. Eject excess supernatant from the syringe by advancing the plunger until 0.1 mL remain in the syringe. Some practitioners prefer to inject only 0.05 mL to minimize the increase in IOP following the injection. Each vial should only be used once and for the treatment of only one eye.[8]

## Dexamethasone Intravitreal Implant 0.7 mg (Ozurdex)

This IDI comes in a prepackaged applicator. Prior to injection, remove injector from the foil pouch and inspect it for any damage. Take the applicator in one hand and remove the cap with the other hand, maintaining aseptic technique and not allowing the cap to touch the needle. Pull off the safety tab on the side of the applicator; do not bend or twist the safety tab. Approach the eye with the needle parallel to the limbus, entering into the sclera at an oblique angle with the bevel of the needle pointed upward. Many practitioners prefer to displace the conjunctiva with a sterile cotton tip applicator prior to injecting. Advance forward into the sclera at that oblique angle for at least 1 mm, then redirect the needle into the center of the eye and continue advancing the needle until the needle hub is flush with the sclera or there is full needle penetration into the vitreous cavity. This makes a shelved wound. Some practitioners prefer to advance the needle to its entire extent without redirecting it toward the center of the vitreous cavity. Do not advance the needle past the point where the sleeve of the applicator touches the conjunctiva. Finally, press the actuator button on the injector slowly until you hear a click and the button is pressed all the way down. Make sure that the actuator button is fully engaged and flush with the applicator surface before removing the needle. When removing the needle, follow the same path as for its insertion.[9] Making a shelved wound and displacing the conjunctiva is helpful for minimizing leakage of the wound postoperatively, which is a greater concern following the IDI injection compared to following other intravitreal injections because of the larger 22-gauge needle of the IDI.

## Fluocinolone Acetonide Intravitreal Implant 0.19 mg (ILUVIEN)

The FAI9 comes in a prepackaged applicator. The applicator is packaged in a tray inside of a box. The interior, but not the exterior, of the tray is sterile. The tray should be inspected to ensure that it is not damaged. If there are signs of compromise, the unit should be discarded.

The implant should be visually inspected through the viewing window of the applicator to ensure that it is properly positioned inside (Figure 42-1). Then remove the applicator from the tray. The applicator tip must be kept above a horizontal plane prior to injection to ensure that the implant remains in proper position in the applicator, as it otherwise may slide out of position prior to injection (Figure 42-2).[10]

Gently press the white applicator button down and slide it forward to the black curved line (Figures 42-3 to 42-5). At this first stop position, the white button should click upward into the up position (Figure 42-6). If it does not, do not use the unit. Remove the protective cap of the applicator and inspect the needle to ensure that the tip of the needle is not bent and that the implant has not protruded into the beveled opening of the needle tip (Figure 42-7). The unit is now ready for injection. Carefully displace the conjunctiva so the conjunctiva and scleral injection sites do not align postinjection and insert the needle through the conjunctiva and sclera at the desired injection site, 4 mm posterior to the limbus (Figure 42-8). Because the 25-gauge needle of the injector is delicate and may bend easily, it is very important to inject the needle directly perpendicular to the sclera, unlike for the IDI (Figure 42-9). With the white button remaining in the up position, place finger over the bottom three lines of the white button (Figure 42-10) and slide the button forward until it reaches the end of its track. Remove finger from the white button. Do not move the button backward after the implant has been injected. Then remove the needle from the eye.[10]

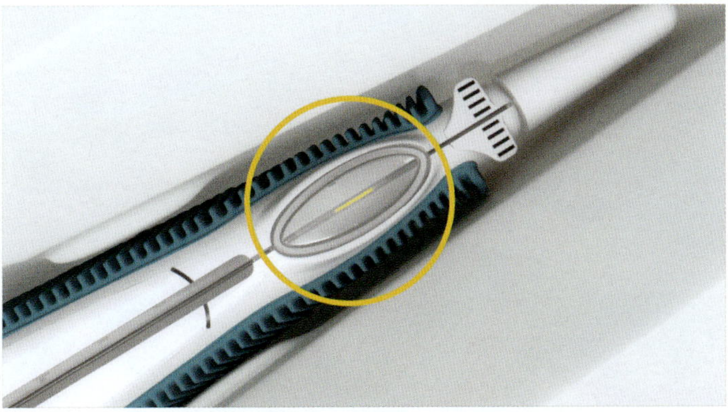

FIGURE 42-1 Visually check through the viewing window of the preloaded applicator to ensure that there is a drug implant inside.

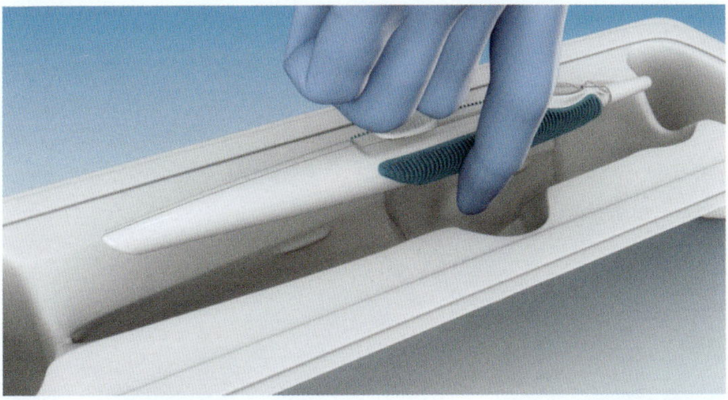

FIGURE 42-2 Remove the applicator from the tray with sterile gloved hands touching only the sterile interior tray surface and applicator. The protective cap on the needle should not be removed until the patient is ready to be injected.

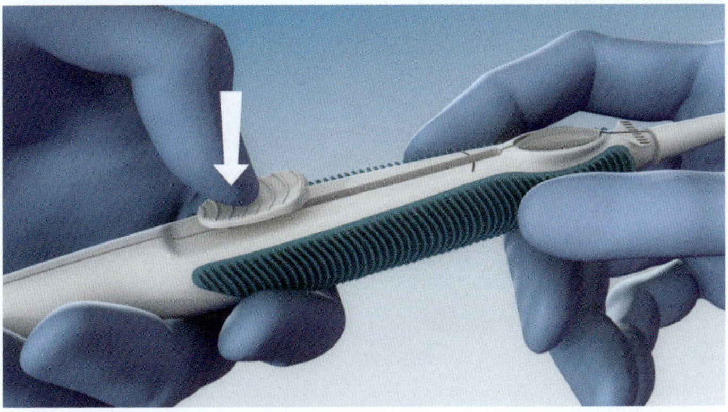

FIGURE 42-3 Incline the device with the tip pointing upward. Using the thumb, press the button down. Prior to the injection, the applicator tip must be kept above the horizontal plane.

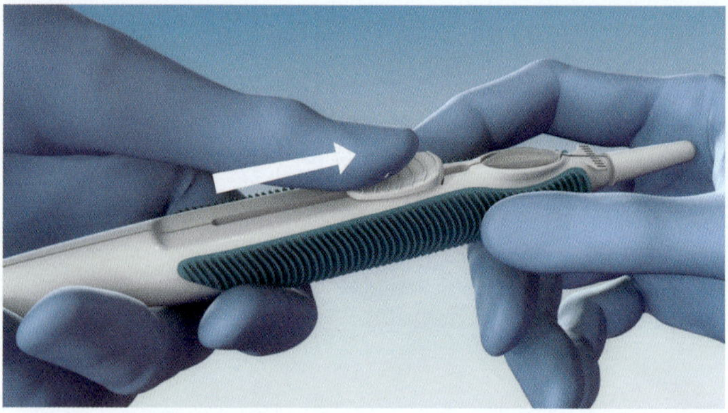

**FIGURE 42-4** With deliberate downward pressure, slide the button forward in one continuous motion until it stops at the curved black line.

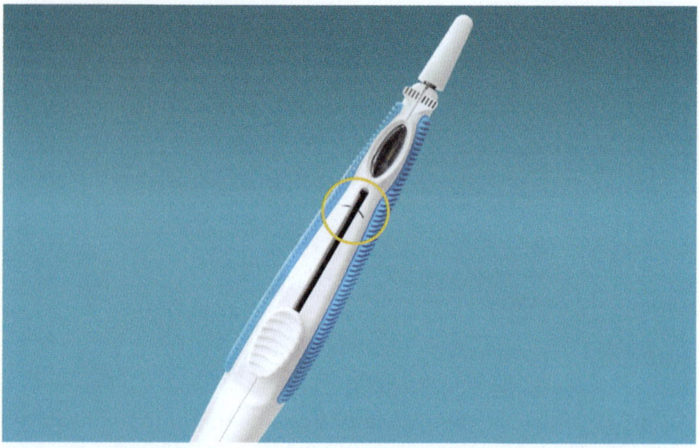

**FIGURE 42-5** Yellow circle shows the black line where the button will come to a stop.

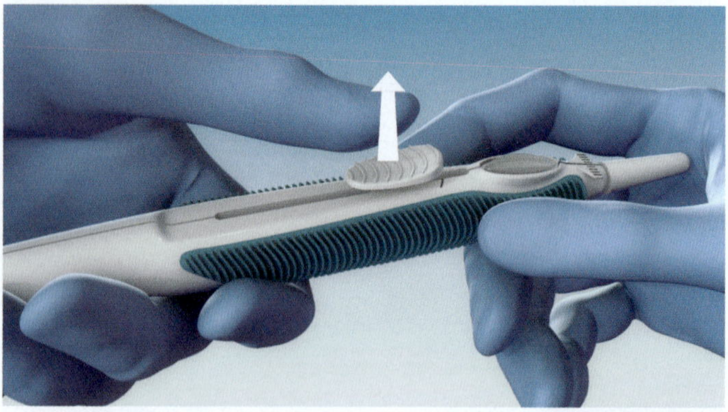

**FIGURE 42-6** Release the button and it will rise into the UP position. The ILUVIEN applicator is now primed for the injection. If the button does not rise, do not proceed with the injection.

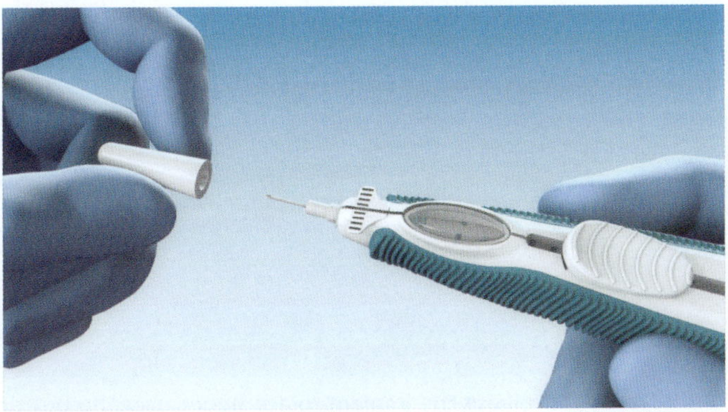

FIGURE 42-7 Maintain the injector tip above the horizontal plane. Carefully remove the protective cap from the needle and inspect the needle tip to ensure the implant has not protruded into the beveled opening at the needle tip.

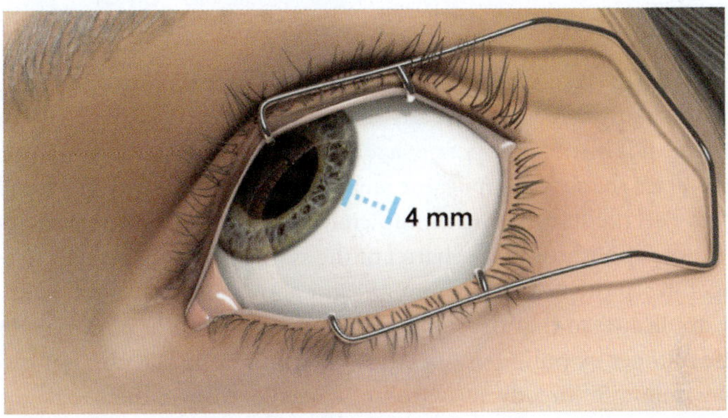


FIGURE 42-8 Optimal placement of the implant is inferior to the optic disc and posterior to the equator of the eye. Measure 4 mm inferotemporal from the limbus with calipers.

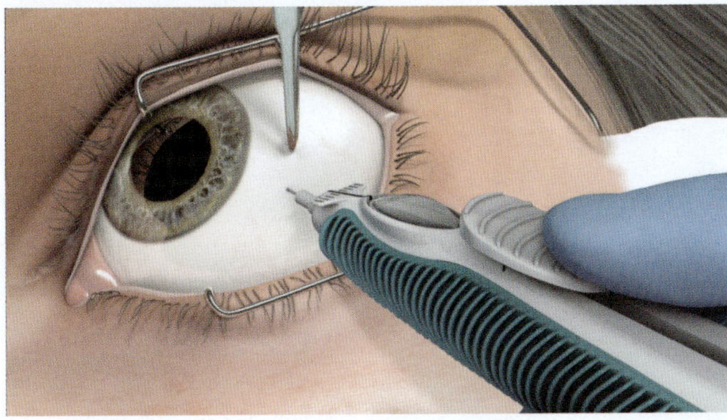

FIGURE 42-9 To release the implant, place finger over the bottom three lines, then slide forward until the button stops at the end of the track.

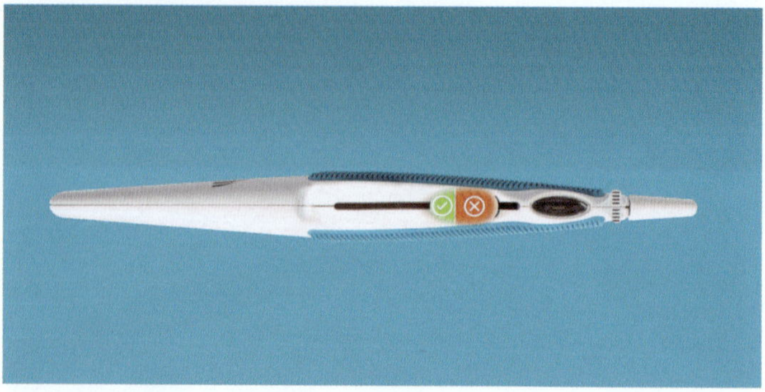

**FIGURE 42-10** To release the implant, place finger over the bottom three lines (as illustrated in green), then slide forward until the button stops at the end of the track.

## Fluocinolone Acetonide Intravitreal Implant 0.18 mg (YUTIQ)

As for the FAI9, the FAI8 is packaged inside its own applicator (Figure 42-11). Begin by opening the YUTIQ carton, taking care not to use any sharp objects to open the carton. Inside the carton, the YUTIQ applicator is in a double pouch: a sealed external nonsterile pouch and a sealed internal sterile pouch. Place the sealed applicator on a tray. Remove the external pouch by opening it and slipping it off. Peel the sterile pouch completely open, exposing the entire applicator.[11] With one hand pick up the applicator by the barrel of the syringe. Do not hold or handle the applicator by the plunger. Keep the needle of the applicator above the horizontal plane throughout the handling of the applicator so that the implant does not slide out of position. Remove the black stopper from the plunger by pulling it directly away from the applicator. Remove the cap covering the needle by pulling it directly away from the needle. Inspect the needle to ensure that it is not bent. There is a metal piece shaped like a trombone inserted into the needle (Figure 42-12). Remove it by pulling it straight off the needle. (You may choose to use sterile forceps for this.)

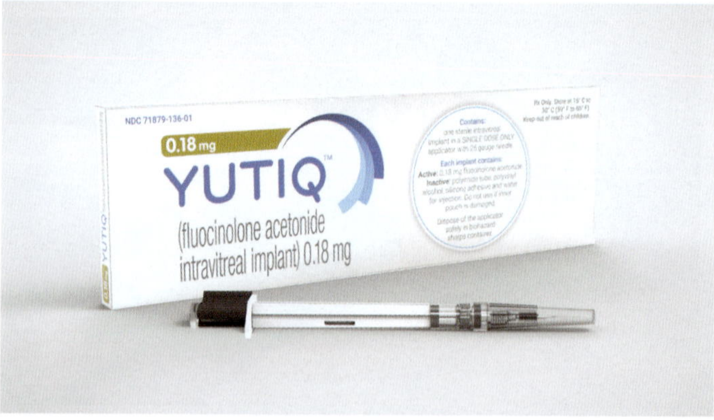


**FIGURE 42-11** YUTIQ applicator.

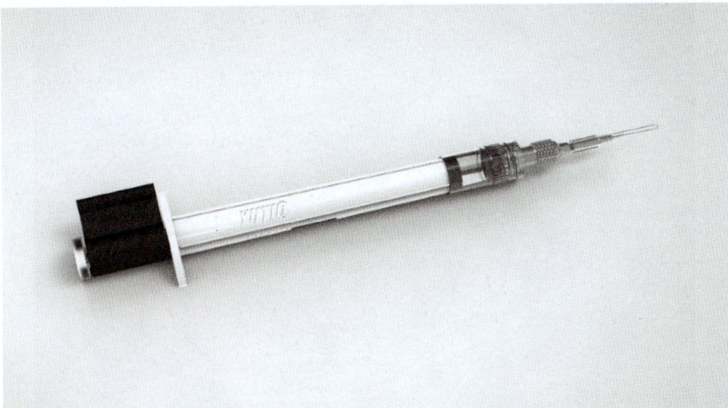

**FIGURE 42-12** YUTIQ applicator with cap removed showing metal trombone.

Carefully displace the conjunctiva so the conjunctival and scleral entry sites do not align postinjection. Insert the needle through the conjunctiva and sclera at the desired injection site, 4 mm posterior to the corneal limbus. Insert the needle up to the positive stop of the applicator. As with the FAI9, it is important to insert the needle directly perpendicular to the sclera. Then press the plunger fully to insert the implant. Withdraw the needle from the eye.[11]

### Fluocinolone Acetonide Intravitreal Implant 0.59 mg (Retisert)

In a sterile operating room, once the eye has been prepped and draped in a customary fashion for ophthalmic procedures, a sterile eyelid speculum is placed, and a localized conjunctival peritomy is made in the quadrant desired for injection. Hemostasis of the episcleral vessels with cautery may be necessary. Then, a microvitreoretinal (MVR) blade is used to make a 3.5-mm circumferential sclerotomy, making sure to penetrate all the way through the choroid into the vitreous cavity with the blade. Clear any prolapsed vitreous at the site of the wound with a vitrector. The FAI5 is comprised of a plate with an 8-0 polypropylene suture at one end. Insert the opposite end into the sclerotomy, with the longest side of the plate perpendicular to the sclera, until the plate is entirely within the vitreous cavity. Then, pass each end of the attached polypropylene suture partial-thickness through the sclera to close the sclerotomy. Pass additional, separate sutures as needed to ensure that the sclerotomy is well-sealed. Finally, close the conjunctiva with polyglactin or plain-gut suture.

## POSTOPERATIVE CARE/COMANAGEMENT (FOLLOW-UP SCHEDULE)

Immediately after the injection of a TA suspension, confirm that the optic disc appears perfused with binocular indirect ophthalmoscopy (BIO). The patient should also be confirmed to have at least count-fingers vision. If neither of these conditions are present within 5 minutes,

**FIGURE 42-13** Ozurdex implant well positioned within the vitreal cavity. (Image courtesy of Leonid Skorin Jr, DO, MS.)

an anterior chamber paracentesis should be performed to reduce the IOP and allow adequate optic disc perfusion. The chance of needing to perform an anterior chamber paracentesis is greater following injection of 0.1 mL compared to following an injection of 0.05 mL. Once optic disc perfusion is restored, the patient may leave the clinic and further IOP monitoring is not necessary. Immediately following the injection of a steroid implant, an increase in IOP is much less likely than following an injection of a TA suspension. However, following injection, an IDI should be visualized in the vitreous cavity with BIO, ensuring that it is not on the macula and that no damage to fundus structures has occurred during the injection process (Figure 42-13).

Patients should be counseled to return to clinic if they experience pain, redness, photophobia, or a significant decrease in vision. Package inserts and prescribing information for FDA-approved medications Triesence, IDI, FAI8, and FAI9 all suggest performing biomicroscopy within 2 to 7 days following the procedure.[8-11] In-office follow-up is often performed in 4 to 6 weeks, including measurement of IOP, a comprehensive dilated fundus examination, and additional retinal imaging such as optical coherence tomography (OCT) to evaluate the efficacy of the medications and monitor for adverse events.

## POTENTIAL COMPLICATIONS AND THEIR TREATMENT

### Key Potential Complications

- Superficial punctate keratitis
- Subconjunctival hemorrhage
- Cataract formation

- Increased IOP and/or glaucoma
- Corneal abrasion
- Infectious endophthalmitis
- Inflammation (pseudo-endophthalmitis or sterile endophthalmitis)
- Vitreous hemorrhage
- Retinal detachment

**Superficial punctate keratitis (SPK)** is a common complication of intravitreal injection and is primarily related to use of needed topical anesthetics and/or povidone–iodine prior to the injection. Symptoms include pain, light sensitivity, epiphora, and blurry vision. Unlike endophthalmitis, symptoms of SPK usually begin immediately following the injection. Treatment is typically palliative with the use of lubricating eye drops. Care should be taken to manage ocular surface disease in those requiring frequent injections, as these patients are more likely to have ocular surface discomfort following injections.

**Subconjunctival hemorrhages** are a common, benign occurrence following intravitreal injection. Patient reassurance is the main aspect of management, as these hemorrhages will clear spontaneously, usually within 2 weeks. Use of topical ocular lubricants may be needed for comfort.

**Cataract** formation is perhaps the most common long-term adverse effect in phakic patients receiving intravitreal steroid medications. Once again, cataract progression is more common with repeated injections and in those who receive longer-acting agents. For example, in phakic patients who receive ILUVIEN, up to 80% ultimately require cataract surgery.[10]

**Increased IOP** can occur immediately following any type of intravitreal injection. Greatly elevated IOP can cause nonperfusion of the central retinal artery and care should be taken to ensure prompt reperfusion of the eye, as described above. Long-term, up to one-third of patients may develop an elevated IOP following intravitreal injections, as early as 1 to 2 weeks and usually within 2 months. The risk increases with the need for repeat injections or longer-acting agents. For example, in those receiving ILUVIEN, up to 38% required IOP-lowering medication and up to 5% required surgical intervention.[10] Most cases can be managed with topical medical therapy alone.

**Corneal abrasion** can occur, either from corneal contact with the eyelid speculum or from the patient's accidental trauma to the eye following the injection. Abrasions can be treated with topical antibiotic prophylaxis, lubricating drops, cycloplegia, and a bandage contact lens, as needed.

**Infectious endophthalmitis** is a rare, but very serious, complication of intravitreal injections. The incidence of endophthalmitis in the setting of intravitreal steroid injections has been reported to be higher than that for intravitreal anti-VEGF (0.13% for intravitreal steroid injection vs. 0.019% for intravitreal anti-VEGF).[12] Thus, careful observation and patient education are necessary to evaluate for signs or symptoms of endophthalmitis, which may occur as early as 24 to 48 hours following injection. Symptoms may include floaters, decreased vision, ocular redness, light sensitivity, and pain. Signs may include chemosis, conjunctival injection, anterior chamber cells with or without hypopyon, corneal edema with or without corneal infiltration, and vitritis.

Because of the devastating effects of infectious endophthalmitis, even a low degree of suspicion should warrant consideration of a vitreal tap-and-inject procedure, whereby broad-spectrum intravitreal antibiotics (most commonly vancomycin and ceftazidime) are delivered into the vitreal cavity. In those with light perception vision or worse, the Endophthalmitis Vitrectomy Study suggests prompt pars plana vitrectomy (PPV) should instead be performed, but this study only included patients with endophthalmitis following cataract surgery, and this conclusion may not be generalizable to endophthalmitis following intravitreal injections.[13] The decision of whether and when to add PPV to the treatment of endophthalmitis following intravitreal injections remains controversial, but, in general, PPV should be strongly considered if virulent organisms, such as streptococci or gram-negative organisms, are suspected, or if the patient is not improving within 48 hours following a tap-and-inject procedure.[14,15] The benefit of adjunct systemic antibiotics such as moxifloxacin also remains controversial. The prognosis is guarded and depends on the organism involved in the infection.

**Inflammation (pseudo-endophthalmitis)** is also a concern following intravitreal steroid injections. It is more common than infectious endophthalmitis and has also been suggested to be more common following intravitreal injection of steroids such as TA than anti-VEGF agents, with incidence ranging between 0.1% and 7.3% for TA[16] versus 0.05% and 4.4%[17] for anti-VEGF agents. The incidence varies based on the agent used for both categories of drugs. Signs and symptoms may be similar to infectious endophthalmitis but tend to be much less severe, and patients characteristically have minimal to no pain or light sensitivity.[18] Unlike infectious endophthalmitis, the course is typically much more benign, with a much better prognosis. Sterile endophthalmitis can be managed with topical steroids and cycloplegic agents. Great care should always be taken to properly rule out infectious endophthalmitis and monitor carefully for signs of worsening that could suggest infection. The threshold for performing a tap-and-inject procedure in questionable cases should be very low.[19]

**Vitreous hemorrhage** can usually be observed, as it will resolve spontaneously in most cases. However, all patients with a new onset of vitreous hemorrhage should be carefully evaluated with a scleral-depressed peripheral fundus examination to rule out any retinal tear or detachment, as well as to rule out any neovascular complications of disease which could be causing the hemorrhage. Vitrectomy may be required in instances of nonclearing vitreous hemorrhage.

**Retinal detachment** requires prompt intervention with surgical repair.

## VIDEOS OF PROCEDURES

**Video 42-1**—ILUVIEN mechanism of action.

**Video 42-2**—YUTIQ injection guide demonstrating how to prepare the patient and the applicator, safely perform the YUTIQ injection, and evaluate the patient following the procedure.

# EFFICACY

## General Efficacy of Medications

Because of landmark trials[3] and because of the long-term adverse effects of cataract and elevated IOP, anti-VEGF agents remain the mainstay of non-uveitic ME treatment. However, intravitreal steroids remain a vital component of therapy for non-uveitic ME.[20,21] Most practitioners use intravitreal steroids when ME proves resistant to one or more anti-VEGF injections, or as planned, staged combination therapy in severe cases of ME. In most cases, the effect of IDI lasts about 3 months and requires the reinjection of another IDI implant following that period. Because of key differences such as pH value, dissolution rate, and particle size of formulations of TA, the effect of TA may be less predictable than that of IDI, and the effect of TA suspensions is short-lived than that of IDI, particularly in postvitrectomy eyes. Nonetheless, off-label use of compounds such as Kenalog-40 is common because of its accessibility and cost.[22]

Although non-uveitic ME often responds well to anti-VEGF medications, uveitic ME is much less responsive to this class of medications, and intravitreal steroids remain the mainstay of the treatment of uveitic ME not responsive to topical therapy and/or to systemic immunosuppressives alone.[23]

For both uveitis and non-uveitic ME, the fluocinolone acetonide implants provide a much longer-acting effect of up to 3 years.[24,25] However, patients often need additional IDI and/or anti-VEGF injections during this time for breakthrough ME. A direct comparison of the efficacy of all of the steroid implants to one another is not currently available. Finally, the FAI5 is used much less commonly than the other steroid medications because of its higher risk of cataract and IOP-related complications, its need for surgical implantation, and in light of the high degree of efficacy of FAI8.

## Alternatives for Macular Edema (Diabetic Macular Edema, Central Retinal Vein Occlusion, and Branch Retinal Vein Occlusion)

All formulations of intravitreal steroid injections carry risk of cataract formation and glaucoma, making their side-effect profiles higher than the use of intravitreal anti-VEGF agents. This remains a key factor in why intravitreal anti-VEGF medications continue to be preferred first-line agents for most providers over intravitreal steroid injections for the treatment of DME and ME secondary to retinal vein occlusion. Consideration for intravitreal steroids may be given in patients who have suboptimal response to anti-VEGF.[21,26,27] In addition, when considering long-acting agents such as FAI9, potential benefits include the need for fewer injections and a more stable macular thickness.[28] These benefits must always be weighed against the increased risk of glaucoma and cataract formation.

Focal or grid photocoagulation also remains an alternative for the treatment of DME and ME from BRVO, but its use has diminished because of the risk of macular scarring and its reduced efficacy when compared to intravitreal medications.

## Efficacy and Alternatives for Noninfectious Uveitis

Intravitreal steroid injections are a treatment option for noninfectious intermediate, posterior, and panuveitis to reduce inflammation and prevent complications from inflammation. Long-acting agents such as FAI8 can also aid in the prevention of episodic uveitis flare-ups.[25] Most cases of bilateral uveitis are treated with systemic steroid-sparing therapy, instead of bilateral steroid injections, because of its similar or superior long-term visual outcomes, more even control of disease, and avoidance of the risks of bilateral intravitreal therapy.[29] Other alternative and adjunct treatment options include topical, periocular, and oral steroids; topical and oral nonsteroidal anti-inflammatory drugs, cycloplegic agents, systemic steroids, and suprachoroidal injection of TA injectable suspension 40 mg/mL (Xipere, Bausch + Lomb Bridgewater, NJ) approved for ME associated with uveitis.

# CODING/BILLING AND MODIFIERS

Intravitreal injection of medication uses Current Procedural Terminology (CPT) code 67028 with an eye modifier (-RT or -LT). Bilateral injections use −50 modifier. Appropriate medication codes are then used for reimbursement for medications. Use JW code to indicate medication wastage.

**Kenalog-40**

- **Healthcare Common Procedure Coding System (HCPCS) code J3301**
- Multiple National Drug Code (NDC) codes per manufacturer

**Triesence**

- **HCPCS code J3300**, injection, TA, preservative-free, 1 mg
- **NDC code 0065-0523-01**, one glass vial of 1 mL Triesence 40 mg/mL

**Ozurdex**

- **HCPCS code J7312**, injection dexamethasone, intravitreal implant 0.1 mg
- **NDC code 00023-3348-07**, Ozurdex (dexamethasone intravitreal implant) 0.7 mg
- **Potential ICD-10 codes:** E10.311, E10.3211, E10.3212, E10.3213, E10.3311, E10.3312, E10.3313, E10.3411, E10.3412, E10.3413, E10.3511, E10.3512, E10.3513, E11.311, E11.3211, E11.3212, E11.3213, E11.3311, E11.3312, E11.3313, E11.3411, E11.3412, E11.3413, E11.3511, E11.3512, E11.3513, H34.8110, H34.8120, H34.8130, H34.8310, H34.8320, H34.8330, H30.001, H30.002, H30.003, H30.011, H30.012, H30.013, H30.021, H30.022, H30.023, H30.031, H30.032, H30.033, H30.041, H30.042, H30.043

**ILUVIEN**

- **HCPCS code J7313**, injection fluocinolone acetonide intravitreal implant, 0.01 mg
- **NDC code 68611-190-02**, ILUVIEN (fluocinolone acetonide intravitreal implant) 0.19 mg

- **Potential ICD-10 codes:** E08.311, E08.321, E08.331, E08.341, E08.351, E09.311, E09.321, E09.331, E09.341, E09.351, E10.311, E10.321, E10.331, E10.341, E10.351, E11.311, E11.321, E11.331, E11.341, E11.351, E13.311, E13.321, E13.331, E13.341, E13.351

## YUTIQ

- **HCPCS code J7314**, injection fluocinolone acetonide intravitreal implant (YUTIQ), 0.01 mg
- **NDC code 71879-136-01**, YUTIQ (fluocinolone acetonide intravitreal implant) 0.18 mg
- **Potential ICD-10 codes:** H30.21, H30.22, H30.23, H30.20, H44.111, H44.112, H44.113, H44.119, H35.021, H35.022, H35.023, H35.029, H35.061, H35.062, H35.063, H35.069, H30.91, H30.92, H30.93, H30.90, H30.891, H30.892, H30.893, H30.899, H30.811, H30.812, H30.813, H30.819, H20.821, H20.822, H20.823, H20.829, H30.041, H30.042, H30.043, H30.049, H30.101, H30.102, H30.103, H30.109, H30.111, H30.112, H30.113, H30.119, H30.121, H30.122, H30.123, H30.129, H30.131, H30.132, H30.133, H30.139, H30.001, H30.002, H30.003, H30.009, H30.011, H30.012, H30.013, H30.019, H30.021, H30.022, H30.023, H30.029, H30.031, H30.032, H30.033, H30.039

# REFERENCES


1. Gao L, Zhao X, Jiao L, Tang L. Intravitreal corticosteroids for diabetic macular edema: a network meta-analysis of randomized controlled trials. *Eye Vis (Lond)*. 2021;8(1):35.
2. Abdulla D, Ali Y, Menezo V, Taylor SRJ. The use of sustained release intravitreal steroid implants in non-infectious uveitis affecting the posterior segment of the eye. *Ophthalmol Ther*. 2022;11(2):479-487.
3. Diabetic Retinopathy Clinical Research Network. A randomized trial comparing intravitreal triamcinolone acetonide and focal/grid photocoagulation for diabetic macular edema. *Ophthalmology*. 2008;115(9):1447-1449.
4. Celik N, Khoramnia R, Auffarth GU, et al. Complications of dexamethasone implants: risk factors, prevention, and clinical management. *Int J Ophthalmol*. 2020;13(10):1612-1620.
5. Li AS, Nguyen HV, Do DV. Migration of a fluocinolone acetonide intravitreal implant into the anterior chamber. *JAMA Ophthalmol*. 2020;138(10):e201388.
6. Avery RL, Bakri SJ, Blumenkranz MS, et al. Intravitreal injection technique and monitoring: updated guidelines of an expert panel. *Retina*. 2014;34:S1-S18.
7. Anijeet DR, Hanson RJ, Bhagey J, Bates RA. National survey of the technique of intravitreal triamcinolone injection in the United Kingdom. *Eye*. 2007;21(4):480-486.
8. Triesence. Package insert. Alcon Laboratories; 2014.
9. Ozurdex. Package insert. Allergan; 2018.
10. ILUVIEN. Prescribing information. Alimera Sciences; 2016.
11. YUTIQ. Prescribing information. EyePoint Pharmaceuticals, Inc; 2018.
12. VanderBeek BL, Bonaffini SG, Ma L. The association between intravitreal steroids and post-injection endophthalmitis rates. *Ophthalmology*. 2015;122(11):2311-2315.e1.
13. Results of the Endophthalmitis Vitrectomy Study. A randomized trial of immediate vitrectomy and of intravenous antibiotics for the treatment of postoperative bacterial endophthalmitis. Endophthalmitis Vitrectomy Study Group. *Arch Ophthalmol*. 1995;113(12):1479-1496.
14. Feng HL, Robbins CB, Fekrat S. A nine-year analysis of practice patterns, microbiologic yield, and clinical outcomes in cases of presumed infectious endophthalmitis. *Ophthalmol Retina*. 2020;4:555-559.
15. Soundararajan S, Robbins CB, Feng HL, Fekrat S. Management patterns and outcomes for intravitreal injection–related endophthalmitis. *J Vitreoretin Dis*. 2022;6(3):188-193.

16. Mahjoub A, Ben Abdesslem N, Ben Abderrazek A, et al. Sterile endophthalmitis after intravitreal triamcinolone acetonide injection: a case report series. *Ann Med Surg.* 2022;76:103537.
17. Anderson WJ, da Cruz NFS, Lima LH, et al. Mechanisms of sterile inflammation after intravitreal injection of antiangiogenic drugs: a narrative review. *Int J Retina Vitreous.* 2021;7(1):37.
18. Schwartz SG, Flynn HW, Emerson GG, et al. Distinguishing between infectious endophthalmitis and noninfectious inflammation following intravitreal anti-VEGF injection. *J Vitreoretin Dis.* 2019;3(1):42-44.
19. Şuţă M, Karancsi O, Muşat O, et al. Triamcinolone acetonide induces sterile endophthalmitis in patients with intermediate uveitis: a case report series. *Exp Ther Med.* 2020;20(3):2524-2528.
20. Boyer DS, Yoon YH, Belfort R, et al. Three-year, randomized, sham-controlled trial of dexamethasone intravitreal implant in patients with diabetic macular edema. *Ophthalmology.* 2014;121(10):1904-1914.
21. Maturi RK, Glassman AR, Liu D, et al. Effect of adding dexamethasone to continued ranibizumab treatment in patients with persistent diabetic macular edema: a DRCR network phase 2 randomized clinical trial. *JAMA Ophthalmol.* 2018;136(1):29-38.
22. Chen H, Sun S, Li J, et al. Different intravitreal properties of three triamcinolone formulations and their possible impact on retina practice. *Invest Ophthalmol Vis Sci.* 2013;54(3):2178-2185.
23. Thorne JE, Sugar EA, Holbrook JT, et al. Periocular triamcinolone vs. intravitreal triamcinolone vs. intravitreal dexamethasone implant for the treatment of uveitic macular edema: the PeriOcular vs. INTravitreal corticosteroids for uveitic macular edema (POINT) trial. *Ophthalmology.* 2019;126(2):283-295.
24. Singer MA, Sheth V, Mansour SE, et al. Three-year safety and efficacy of the 0.19-mg fluocinolone acetonide intravitreal implant for diabetic macular edema: the PALADIN study. *Ophthalmology.* 2022;129(6):605-613.
25. Jaffe GJ, Pavesio CE; Study Investigators. Effect of a fluocinolone acetonide insert on recurrence rates in noninfectious intermediate, posterior, or panuveitis: three-year results. *Ophthalmology.* 2020;127:1395-1404.
26. Zhioua I, Semoun O, Lalloum F, Souied EH. Intravitreal dexamethasone implant in patients with ranibizumab persistent diabetic macular edema. *Retina.* 2015;35(7):1429-1435.
27. Lazic R, Lukic M, Boras I, et al. Treatment of anti-vascular endothelial growth factor-resistant diabetic macular edema with dexamethasone intravitreal implant. *Retina.* 2014;34(4):719-724.
28. Eaton A, Koh SS, Jimenez J, Riemann CD. The USER study: a chart review of patients receiving a 0.2 μg/day fluocinolone acetonide implant for diabetic macular edema. *Ophthalmol Ther.* 2019;8(1):51-62.
29. Tomkins-Netzer O, Lightman SL, Burke AE, et al. Seven-year outcomes of uveitic macular edema: the multicenter uveitis steroid treatment trial and follow-up study results. *Ophthalmology.* 2021;128(5):719-728.

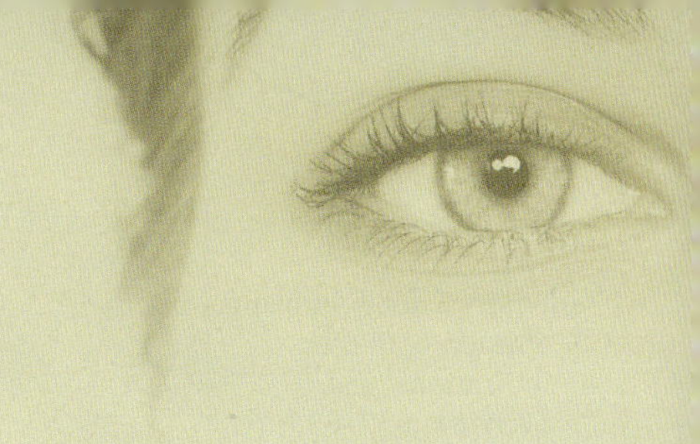

# INDEX

Note: Page numbers in italic and bold refer to figures and tables, respectively.

## A

## B



## C